Principle-Based Stepped Care and Brief Psychotherapy for Integrated Care Settings

Alexandros Maragakis
William T. O'Donohue
Editors

Principle-Based Stepped Care and Brief Psychotherapy for Integrated Care Settings

Springer

Editors
Alexandros Maragakis
Eastern Michigan University
Ypsilanti, MI
USA

William T. O'Donohue
Department of Clinical Psychology
University of Nevada
Reno, NV
USA

ISBN 978-3-030-09967-1 ISBN 978-3-319-70539-2 (eBook)
https://doi.org/10.1007/978-3-319-70539-2

Softcover re-print of the Hardcover 1st edition 2018

Printed on acid-free paper

This Springer imprint is published by the registered company Springer International Publishing AG part of Springer Nature
The registered company address is: Gewerbestrasse 11, 6330 Cham, Switzerland

Preface

The healthcare system in the United States has changed dramatically in the last few decades and will continue to change rapidly. This is due to the fact that there are many intractable underlying problems that contribute to the healthcare crisis that will necessitate continued modifications to find better resolution. However, another factor to the complexity of the situation is that there are many different point of views (and different vested interests) on how to define, prioritize, and respond to the subproblems. For mental health providers, one of the biggest changes has come in the form of integrating behavioral health—thought to be an important cost driver—within the primary care medical setting and providing the necessary brief, team-based interventions that integrate care requires. These integrated care delivery systems require mental health providers to shift from traditional methods of delivering longer-term therapeutic interventions and aim to eliminate all symptoms and make a shift to focus on brief interventions that aim to alleviate a wider range of problems (e.g., treatment adherence, chronic pain) sufficiently to restore functioning. For behavioral health practitioners, there is a developing literature on how to set up a functional and effective integrated care system. However, there is a lack of scholarship and research on the "what to do clinically" when implementing these brief interventions in integrated care system that are essential to its success. This book has been created as a "bridge" to provide integrated care providers with specific information on how to effectively implement multiple clinical tasks (e.g., screening and assessment, stepped-care interventions, when to refer, the role of the medical team) for delivering care for a wide array of mental and behavioral health problems. The chapters in this book have been written by experts in the field and provide readers with explicit tools and methods for conducting interventions that are consistent with an integrated care model. It is important to note that many of these methods still require further empirical testing and that many of the methods provided in this book are either derived from principles of empirically supported treatments or are truncated versions of manualized treatments that have been supported by randomly controlled trials in specialized care. We hope that this book will help close the gap between traditional interventions found in specialty care and brief effective interventions required in specialty care and aid providers within integrated care settings to deliver high-quality care. We would like to thank the authors for their willingness to collaborate on the project by writing excellent chapters. We would also like to thank our editor Janice Stern for her patience, good cheer, and expertise in this project. Without her this book would not have been completed.

Ypsilanti, MI, USA
Reno, NV, USA

Alexandros Maragakis
William T. O'Donohue

Contents

Contributors

Angeleque Akin-Little Akin-Little and Little Behavioral Psychology Consultants, Malone, NY, USA

Mana K. Ali, Ph.D. Department of Physical Medicine and Rehabilitation, Johns Hopkins University, Baltimore, MD, USA

Eamonn Arble, Ph.D. Psychology, Eastern Michigan University, Ypsilanti, MI, USA

David Austern, Psy.D. Veterans Affairs Maryland Healthcare System (VAMHCS), Baltimore, MD, USA

The Steven A. Cohen Military Family Clinic at NYU Langone Medical Center, New York, NY, USA

David E. Bauman, Psy.D. Family Medicine, Central Washington Family Medicine Residency, Yakima, WA, USA

Bridget R. Beachy, Psy.D. Behavioral Health, Community Health of Central Washington, Yakima, WA, USA

Daniel S. Bromberg Special Psychological Services, L.L.C., Bloomfield, NJ, USA

Tom Buqo, B.A. Department of Psychology, Hofstra University, Hempstead, NY, USA

Michelle Byrd Eastern Michigan University, Ypsilanti, MI, USA

Gwendolyn C. Carlson Department of Psychology, University of Nevada, Reno, Reno, NV, USA

Jeffrey A. Cigrang, Ph.D., A.B.P.P. Wright State University, Dayton, OH, USA

James V. Cordova, Ph.D. Department of Psychology, Clark University, Worcester, MA, USA

Michael A. Cucciare, Ph.D. Center for Mental Healthcare and Outcomes Research, Central Arkansas Veterans Affairs Healthcare System, Little Rock, AR, USA

Department of Psychiatry, University of Arkansas for Medical Sciences, Little Rock, AR, USA

VA South Central Mental Illness Research, Education, and Clinical Center, Central Arkansas Veterans Healthcare System, Little Rock, AR, USA

Caroline Cummings Department of Psychology, University of Nevada, Reno, NV, USA

Claudia Drossel Eastern Michigan University, Ypsilanti, MI, USA

Melanie P. Duckworth, Ph.D. Department of Psychology, University of Nevada, Reno, Reno, NV, USA

Eddie C. Erazo Department of Psychology, University of Nevada, Reno, Reno, CA, USA

Ashley L. Evans, B.S. Wright State University, Dayton, OH, USA

Michelle A. Fernando Department of Psychology, Eastern Michigan University, Ypsilanti, MI, USA

Megha Garg Department of Psychology, Eastern Michigan University, Ypsilanti, MI, USA

J. Arthur Gillaspy Jr., Ph.D. Psychology and Counseling, University of Central Arkansas, Conway, AR, USA

Stephen R. Gillaspy The University of Oklahoma Health Sciences Center, Oklahoma City, OK, USA

Peter A. Girolami Department of Behavior Psychology, Kennedy Krieger Institute, Johns Hopkins University School of Medicine, Baltimore, MD, USA

Melissa L. González Pediatric Development and Therapy Center, Our Lady of the Lake Physicians Group, Baton Rouge, Louisiana, USA

Margaret T. Gopaul Department of Psychology, Walden University, Malone, NY, USA

Tatiana D. Gray, Ph.D. Department of Psychology, Clark University, Worcester, MA, USA

Marianthi N. Hatzigeorgiou University of Michigan, Ann Arbor, MI, USA

Brittany M. Hayden, Ph.D. Outpatient Behavioral Health Department, Sarah A. Reed Children's Center, Erie, PA, USA

Ann F. Haynos Department of Psychiatry, University of Minnesota Medical Center, Minneapolis, MN, USA

Holly Hazlett-Stevens Department of Psychology, University of Nevada, Reno, Reno, CA, USA

Melissa Castle Heatly, Ph.D. Pediatric Behavioral Health and Wellness, University of Rochester Medical Center, Rochester, NY, USA

Amy Hufsteader, B.S. Behavioral Medicine, Winthrop P. Rockefeller Cancer Institute, University of Arkansas for Medical Sciences, Little Rock, AR, USA

Tony Iezzi Behavioural Medicine Service, London Health Sciences Center, London, ON, Canada

Karen Kersting, Ph.D. Department of Family and Community Medicine, Medical College of Wisconsin, Milwaukee, WI, USA

Ellen I. Koch Department of Psychology, Eastern Michigan University, Ypsilanti, MI, USA

Laura Krasean, Ph.D. Rainbow Rehabilitation Centers, Livonia, MI, USA

Kate Happel Krautbauer Eastern Michigan University, Ypsilanti, MI, USA

Stu Law, M.A. Department of Psychology, University of Nevada, Reno, NV, USA

E.B. Lee Utah State University, Logan, UT, USA

Phyllis Lee, Ph.D. University of Connecticut Health Center, Farmington, CT, USA

Sarah M. Lindeman, M.S. Department of Psychology and Counseling, University of Central Arkansas, Conway, AR, USA

Steven G. Little Department of Psychology, Walden University, Malone, NY, USA

Mark Malady, M.S., B.C.B.A. Bx Plus, Reno, NV, USA

Alexandros Maragakis, Ph.D. Eastern Michigan University, Ypsilanti, MI, USA

Heather Martens University of Central Arkansas, Conway, AR, USA

Melody Mickens, Ph.D. Hunter Holmes McGuire Veterans Affairs Medical Center, Richmond, VA, USA

Cindy W. Mikeal, Ph.D. Psychology, CHI St. Vincent, Little Rock, AR, USA

Thomas D. Mulderink Pediatric Feeding Disorders Program, St. Vincent, Evansville, IN, USA

Rory Newlands Department of Clinical Psychology, University of Nevada, Reno, NV, USA

William T. O'Donohue, Ph.D. Department of Clinical Psychology, University of Nevada, Reno, NV, USA

Stacy A. Ogbeide, Psy.D. Departments of Family and Community Medicine and Psychiatry, UT Health San Antonio, San Antonio, TX, USA

C.W. Ong Utah State University, Logan, UT, USA

Lauren Ostarello Department of Psychology, Eastern Michigan University, Ypsilanti, MI, USA

Anthony Papa, Ph.D. Department of Psychology, University of Nevada, Reno, Reno, NV, USA

Brittany R. Patterson, Ph.D. Department of Psychiatry, University of Maryland School of Medicine, Center for School Mental Health, Baltimore, MD, USA

Carol B. Peterson Department of Psychiatry, University of Minnesota Medical Center, Minneapolis, MN, USA

The Emily Program, Minneapolis, MN, USA

Stefanie Poehacker, M.S. Department of Psychology, Eastern Michigan University, Ypsilanti, MI, USA

Sheila A. Rauch, Ph.D., A.B.P.P. Emory University School of Medicine and Atlanta VA Medical Center, Atlanta, GA, USA

John M. Ray, Ph.D. Center for Mental Healthcare and Outcomes Research, Central Arkansas Veterans Affairs Healthcare System, North Little Rock, AR, USA

Department of Psychiatry, University of Arkansas for Medical Sciences, Little Rock, AR, USA

VA South Central Mental Illness Research, Education, and Clinical Center, Central Arkansas Veterans Healthcare System, North Little Rock, AR, USA

Bradford C. Richards, Ph.D., A.B.P.P. Cognitive Behavioral Institute of Albuquerque, Albuquerque, NM, USA

Sarah L. Russell Department of Social Work, St. Catherine University and the University of St. Thomas, St. Paul, MN, USA

Brandon T. Sanford Department of Psychology, University of Nevada, Reno, Reno, NV, USA

M. Todd Sewell, Ph.D. Cognitive Behavioral Institute of Albuquerque, Albuquerque, NM, USA

Allen C. Sherman, Ph.D. Behavioral Medicine, Winthrop P. Rockefeller Cancer Institute, University of Arkansas for Medical Sciences, Little Rock, AR, USA

Stephanie Simonton-Atchley, Ph.D. Behavioral Medicine, Winthrop P. Rockefeller Cancer Institute, University of Arkansas for Medical Sciences, Little Rock, AR, USA

M.P. Twohig Utah State University, Logan, UT, USA

Rachel VanPutten Department of Psychology, Eastern Michigan University, Ypsilanti, MI, USA

Catalina Vechiu, M.A. Department of Clinical Psychology, University of Nevada, Reno, NV, USA

Michael Vriesman Eastern Michigan University, Ypsilanti, MI, USA

Thomas J. Waltz Department of Psychology, Eastern Michigan University, Ypsilanti, MI, USA

Casiana Warfield Eastern Michigan University, Ypsilanti, MI, USA

Nicholas D. Wignall, Ph.D. Cognitive Behavioral Institute of Albuquerque, Albuquerque, NM, USA

Larry Williams, Ph.D., B.C.B.A.-D. Department of Psychology, University of Nevada, Reno, NV, USA

Morgan Wright Department of Psychology, Eastern Michigan University, Ypsilanti, MI, USA

Martha Zimmermann, B.A. Department of Psychology, University of Nevada, Reno, Reno, NV, USA

1 Introduction: Integrated Care—The Promise and the Challenges

William T. O'Donohue

In the last few decades, integrated care has received a wide amount of favorable comment and even fairly widespread adoption. Histories of our field will likely note that this dramatic shift has been nearly unprecedented in the first century of applied psychology: perhaps only the role of the Veteran Affairs after WWII has behavioral health demonstrated such a significant shift in both the way services are delivered and in the way behavioral health professionals are trained. However, it is also fair to say that the changes brought forth by the rise of integrated care are perhaps even larger as integrated care represents a new paradigm: consultation and brief screening and interventions with a high volume of patients in a primary care setting are simply a new paradigm for the delivery of behavioral health services. To be sure, the traditional behavioral health delivery paradigm is generally fine: in fact, integrated care with its case finding in the primary care setting requires a robust specialty care delivery system to refer more complex or long-term patients. However, there are many unresolved questions about the new integrated care paradigm.

It is important to contrast the two service delivery models in order to gain a clearer understanding of the integrated care paradigm (see Hunter, Goodie, Orrdt, & Dobmeyer, 2016; O'Donohue, Cummings, Cucciarre, Runyan, & Cummings, 2005; Robinson & Reiter, 2015). The traditional specialty care service delivery model is the one that has been around for decades and thus is the more familiar one. In this model the patient is usually seen in a setting that is independent from where they receive their medical care. Referrals come from a variety of sources including self-referral, and the presenting problem is often described solely or at least mainly in behavioral/psychological terms, particularly in DSM diagnoses such as major depression, panic disorder, delusional disorder, and so on. The individual becomes the client of the mental health professional. The focus is not on a population but rather on the individual client. Assessment and diagnosis are the first task of professional contact, and this can take from one to several 60-minute sessions. Next, treatment is delivered usually again in 60-minute sessions that can last from a few to several dozen weekly sessions—or even in some therapy models for years. The goal in this paradigm is often complete elimination of symptoms. Again, there are some nuances missed in this description, but in broad strokes it is a faithful description of the traditional specialty care model of delivering mental health services.

The integrated care model, properly construed, is distinct along each of the dimensions described above. The patient is seen in the

W.T. O'Donohue, Ph.D.
Department of Clinical Psychology,
University of Nevada, Reno, NV, USA
e-mail: williamodonohue@yahoo.com

A. Maragakis, W.T. O'Donohue (eds.), *Principle-Based Stepped Care and Brief Psychotherapy for Integrated Care Settings*, https://doi.org/10.1007/978-3-319-70539-2_1

medical clinic—usually a primary care clinic such as a family practice, internal medicine, or pediatrician office—the healthcare services are "colocated." The patient is usually referred to this colocated behavioral health provider by the primary care provider. This is often done through a "warm handoff" where the primary care provider (PCP) briefly introduces the patient and the referral question to the behavioral care provider (BCP). The emphasis is on population health not just the individual's health—with the population often defined as the cohort the medical clinic serves which can be in the range of 1500 to 2000 patients/PCP (O'Donohue et al., 2005). Thus, epidemiology is used to target high-frequency problems that result in medical presentations such as smoking, obesity, depression, and anxiety. The individual does not usually become the patient of the behavioral health provider but remains the patient of the PCP or the primary care team. The referral often comes with a very specific referral question, e.g., "Is the patient depressed?" The model of service delivery is often consultation—in the above example—the BCP task then is to correctly and efficiently answer this question so the PCP can be in a better position to understand the patient and formulate a more accurate or comprehensive diagnosis and treatment plan. In an important sense, the primary client of the BCP is the PCP, not the patient. Assessment is much briefer—usually done in a half hour or less—as it is best if the information loop between PCP and BCP is closed before the patient leaves that day. The number of episodes of service is fewer—ideally ranging from 1 to 4. This allows more total patients to be seen—it is a "low-touch, high-volume" delivery model. The time period for each contact is also less—usually from 15 to 30 min—mirroring the pace of the primary care clinic. The focus is often on restoring functional status—e.g., helping the patient get back to work or to parent—rather than total symptom resolution. Behavioral health services are more diverse, dealing not only with traditional DSM diagnostic categories but also with behavioral health issues like diet, exercise, treatment compliance, pain, sleep, stress, and the like. Stepped care (see O'Donohue & Draper, 2011; and Chap. 2 this volume) is often used, and a variety of service modalities are used including watchful waiting, eHealth, the provision of psychosocial information, bibliotherapy, group therapy, and individual therapy. If the problem is more intense, requiring more than 1–4 20-minute sessions—again much like primary care medicine—the BCP manages a referral to an appropriate specialty care provider.

Thus, the contrasts between these two behavioral health service delivery models are sharp—or at least can be. Part of the current problem in the field is that the phrase "integrated care" has achieved the status of an honorific—and it is used to describe a wide variety of treatment models often inchoate models. Sometimes this phrase is simply used to describe specialty care that perhaps only has better information flow between it and medical care. Perhaps notes are routinely sent to the PCP. Sometimes it is simply used to describe "colocated care" in which traditional mental healthcare (e.g., 60-minute sessions for DSM diagnoses) is provided in a medical clinic. Sometimes it is used to describe when only one behavioral health problem is targeted in the primary care setting, for example, depression is screened for and treated if found, but no other behavioral health problem is addressed. The variety in these dimensions of service delivery is important because choice points on each dimension have implications on the extent to which the goals of integrated care are achieved. This raises the question of why attempt to integrate care at all?

It is well known that healthcare in the United States has been and currently is in a crisis. The crisis itself has various dimensions. Costs are considered too high; in 1960 healthcare was approximately 5% of GDP; currently it is about 18% and thought to be as high as 25% by 2050 (Wendell, Seratt, & O'Donohue, 2017). Most consider that such spending is excessive and inefficient—nearly 1 in every 5 dollars going to healthcare squeezes other legitimate spending such as dollars for education, infrastructure, and housing and food for the poor. Quality is also considered to be low—the Institute of Medicine's influential Crossing the Quality Chasm (2001) suggests that thousands of Americans die each year due to medical errors. The reason the report used the word "chasm" instead of gap was to illustrate the wide difference between healthcare that is ideal and healthcare that we have. There is a myriad of other quality problems: diagnoses are missed, evidence-based treatments are not delivered, and treatment at times is delivered due to financial self-interest not due to the patient's best interest. Also importantly patient and provider satisfaction is low.

This has given rise to the well-known "Triple Aims" of healthcare reform: improving the patient experience of care (including quality and satisfaction), improving the health of populations, and reducing the per capita cost of healthcare.

Integrated care is generally thought of as helping to achieve these triple aims by:

1. Increasing patient satisfaction because more services are delivered in a single setting where both physical and behavioral services are coordinated. (In integrated setting there are often other services that are integrated such as dental, physical therapy, dietician, and so on.) There is some evidence that this can happen (see Chaffee, Laygo, & O'Donohue, 2013).
2. Improving the quality of care by better capturing the patient's actual problem through not missing diagnoses (such as depression or substance abuse), by being able to make more accurate diagnoses (by having input of a variety of professionals with diverse core competencies), by providing more evidence-based treatment by having a BCP trained in these, and by increasing patient "uptake" of needed behavioral health services (e.g., a stop smoking program) by allowing a coordinated team approach which both can reinforce messaging and provide convenient onsite treatment. There is not a lot of current evidence that this is occurring.
3. An important part of improving the health of populations is engaging in healthier lifestyle behaviors and improving treatment compliance, and a focus on wellness and prevention often has a large behavioral component which can be addressed when behavioral health services are integrated in medical services.
4. Costs can be lowered—sometimes called "medical cost offset" (see Cummings, O'Donohue, & Ferguson, 2002)—due to the following: (a) proper and more efficient diagnosis can lead to lower costs by more appropriate efficient care; (b) improving lifestyle and treatment compliance can lower future medical costs by creating healthier individuals; (c) substituting lower-cost but needed behavioral health services for higher-cost and unneeded medical services can lower cost (e.g., more efficiently diagnosing the problem as depression rather than doing a series of medical tests to evaluate physiological pathways); and (d) targeting the behavioral health needs of high-cost medical utilizers can produce substantial savings.

However, two situations are apparent:

1. There is a paucity of data regarding the extent to which integrated care delivery systems actually produce these outcomes. Some version of integrated care is often adopted because it is supposed to produce these desirable effects. However, there have been few randomized controlled trials of integrated care compared to traditional care. There are even too few pre-post studies of the adoption of an integrated paradigm.
2. In addition, there have been too few reports of quality improvement projects (O'Donohue & Maragakis, 2016) involving integrated care showing the extent to which a particular integrated care delivery system achieves these aims and what innovations were necessary to improve these outcomes.

Developing a better healthcare system is a very complex matter, and this complexity is one reason why progress is slow. There are important *workforce issues* that need to be resolved (see O'Donohue & Maragakis, 2014)—how workers ought to be trained and the number of people needed to fill all the diverse roles that the delivery system needs—this has stymied the development of quality integrated care as there has been a severe shortage of workers trained in this skill set. Another important workforce issue is how many BCPs are needed relative to PCPS? Too often there have been too few BCPs as organizations put only a cautious toe in the water—which, in turn, can hamper achieving the aims of integrated care. There are *financial issues*: Who will pay for the integrated care service delivery system with its increases in behavioral health costs? This is a particular concern when physical health and mental health have fractionated payment systems—the behavioral health managed care company is tasked with reducing costs not increasing these—and any cost reductions from integrated care are then experienced by the medical insurer or managed care company not the behavioral health entity. In addition, there are often roadblocks to integrated care in the financial system—from pre-authorizations, which can interfere with warm handoffs and same-day services, to separate copays, to prohibitions against billing for same-day services for behavioral and medical services, and to diagnostic coding that is not appropriate for the actual work done by BCPs. There are also *workflow issues*: Where does the BCP work—in the medical exam room or a separate office? Who is responsible for ensuring that the behavioral health screen is completed? How is the behavioral health note integrated into the electronic record? Who rooms the BCP's patients and so on? There are *clinical pathway issues*: How much should integrated care focus on prevention and wellness vs. treatment of currently existing problems? How much ought it to focus on behavioral medicine issues like pain, treatment compliance, diet, and exercise vs. a focus on traditional mental health issues such as depression and anxiety? How much should behavioral health services be oriented toward other general healthcare goals like healthcare literacy and shared decision-making? Finally, there is a group of issues relating to the *management of integrated care*: Who is in charge of integrated care? What are reasonable expectations for a BCP's performance? What can be done if these are not achieved? What should a BCP's productivity be like? What qualifications should be sought in hiring a BCP? How ought a BCP be incented? How is burnout ought to be prevented? What sort of professional development activities ought to be available? All these are again choice points and decisions can again affect the extent to which the aims of integrated care are achieved.

It is reasonable to construe that the core of integrated care is clinical—there is screening for a wide range of behavioral health problems and subsequent clinical assessment to rule in or rule out these problems, and then there is a clinical response to these. These clinical processes are at the core of integrated care because to a large extent the quality of these clinical processes will determine the extent to which the overall aims of integrated care are achieved. Moreover, there is a consensus that these clinical responses ought to be "evidence based." Evidence based generally has come to mean that the clinical response has been evaluated by at least a few randomized controlled clinical trials and found to be superior to no-treatment or an attention-placebo condition (see Chambless & Hollon, 1998). Thus a further issue becomes actual adoption of these clinical protocols (as opposed to an approach that does not have such evidence) and faithful implementation of these protocols. In screening and assessment, this often means that the assessment measures are appropriate and have acceptable psychometrics, such as sensitivity, specificity, interrater reliability, treatment utility, and so on (see Haynes, Smith, & Hunsley, 2011). Unfortunately, currently, it is fair to say that these integrated care protocols do not exist. There are few studies on the effectiveness of protocols that are consistent with the paradigm—1–4 sessions of 20 min—aimed at restoring functioning and for the many problems encountered in primary care such as:

- Treatment nonadherence (for a variety of treatments)
- Stress
- Pain
- Depression
- Anxiety
- Sleep

- Relationship problems
- Obesity
- Child management
- Smoking
- Social isolation

Integrated care—like primary care medicine—needs to take all comers and be ready to at least deal with (if only to find an acceptable referral source) every behavioral health problem. This should not be unexpected as in an important sense integrated care becomes primary care psychology. And like primary care medicine, it is meant to be the gateway into the entire healthcare system where the gatekeeper is able to assess, triage, and possibly treat (with first-order treatments) everything from head to toe. Thus, this results in a large research agenda regarding psychometrically adequate screens, assessments, consultations, and interventions that are appropriate for the ecology of primary care. These brief protocols need to be developed and evaluated for dozens of problems. The worry of course is threefold:

1. That there will be a dosage problem—that the brief intervention model of integrated care with 3 or 4 sessions of 20 min simply will not be sufficient to produce sufficient change.
2. That there will be complex comorbidities found in many patients in integrated care that will interact with each other and also need to be researched—e.g., what if the diabetic patient is noncompliant but also depressed and obese and how ought quality integrated care treatment look like for these complex (but far too common) patients?
3. Can a BCP be trained in this large number of protocols so that they can faithfully implement each?

This is a mammoth research undertaking—and it would involve a lot of resources as well as a lot of talent to successfully navigate. Unfortunately, perhaps because of its enormity, it is largely being ignored. To be sure part of the problem is that granting agencies—often divided up by organ system—have not been willing to fund research into the development and evaluation of such comprehensive systems. However unfortunately to date this leaves the field with the fact that integrated care delivery systems are being developed in a context where these issues about the evidence based of their clinical interventions are largely being ignored. The question is complex: Are there iatrogenic effects of integrated care? What problems are being effectively treated, and which are not? What problems are screens missing? What problems have unacceptable relapse rates with integrated care treatment? What ought to be the priorities for treatment in integrate care? What is to be done if there is a need for a specialty care referral but no such specialist exists in the area or that accepts the patient's insurance (or noninsurance)? Instead, over the years, one can see that a number of the controversies and mistakes of specialty care are not being incorporated into integrated care. For example:

1. *There is a willingness to deliver clinical services in ways that are not evidence based.* This may be inevitable given the paucity of data described above, but one can also see BCPs incorporate problematic therapies into integrated care such as dance therapy, power therapies, psychodynamic approaches, Rogerian approaches, Gestalt approaches, and so on. For example, Robinson, Gould, and Strosahl (2011) recently published a problematic book in which acceptance and commitment therapy is advanced as the cure-all for every problem that is encountered in integrated care. One can see the emergence of therapeutic allegiance instead of a data orientation that has long existed in specialty care. It seems now that all the controversies surrounding treatment effectiveness research (dodo effect, cure-alls) will now enter into integrated care.
2. *There is a willingness to be unconcerned about both treatment fidelity and fidelity to an integrated care delivery model.* Too often placing anybody doing anything in a medical system is sufficient for someone to consider it as integrated care. There is too little concern about fidelity to a distinct treatment model and how that treatment delivery system needs

to be designed to actually produce desired outcomes.

3. *There is a willingness to ignore quality improvement and data generation.* Integrated care is itself a quality improvement initiative—it seeks to improve quality along the lines of the Triple Aims, and it would appear to be consistent with a quality improvement orientation—it would be operated only within the context of a constant quality improvement system which would consistently provide data on patient satisfaction, financial outcomes, clinical outcomes, provider satisfaction, and so on. However, this is more of the exception rather than the rule.
4. *There is a willingness to ignore psychometrics.* Although at times BCPs are using standard measures like the Beck Depression Index which has some reasonable psychometric data, at times, screening devices and other assessment measures are being used (including brief clinical interviews) that need more psychometric study.
5. *There is a willingness to ignore cultural considerations.* Although "cultural competences" has been emphasized and perhaps overemphasized in specialty care (see Frisby & O'Donohue, in press), there has been much less emphasis on this in integrated care. The reason for this is perplexing especially as integrated care is often implemented in settings such as community health centers that serve a large number of minority patients. Of course this can add complexity to the research agenda above as not only do researchers need to find an effective brief intervention for, say, depression, but they also then need to find if any cultural tailoring is needed for the vast number of cultures that will be served by integrated care.
6. *There is a willingness to ignore training needs and workforce development issues.* Too often the individuals hired to work in an integrated care setting have little to no training in integrated care. Training programs have developed, but the output of these does not meet the demand—O'Donohue and Maragakis (2014) suggested in a workforce analysis that the shortfall may be on the order of 50,000 or so. Clearly, innovations in training for integrated care need to be a priority.
7. *There is a willingness to ignore financial outcomes.* There are too few data showing medical cost offset. One can conduct integrated care in a way that increases cost rather than decreases overall costs, e.g., by providing ineffective clinical services, by not billing appropriately for these, by poor BCP productivity, and by not targeting high-cost medical utilizers. More data are desperately needed on financial outcomes of integrated care.
8. *Overall there is a lack of a thoroughgoing commitment to innovation.* Integrated care is itself an innovation but an innovation that needs and is dependent upon other innovations. The field needs comprehensive, sensitive, and specific screen that can cover a wide range of problems in one easy-to-score screen. It needs adaptations for other primary care environments such pediatrics and gynecology. It needs improved EHRs that have decision tools and resources for BCPs and a format that is behavioral health-friendly. It needs benchmarks for BCP productivity. It needs a variety of clinical support tools such as stepped care treatments for a wide variety of clinical problems including comorbidities.

This book was initiated and developed to help with some of these problems. It is based on this reasonable assumption: that the best interventions in integrated care ought to be based on principles that have been shown to be effective in specialty care. That is, cognitive behavioral interventions such as behavioral activation and cognitive disputation of irrational beliefs are found to be effective in specialty care for depression than an adoption of these principles to a briefer format and are ought to be current best practices for integrated care. In addition, an examination is ought to be conducted to see what evidence-based treatments might exist at the different levels of stepped care, e.g., bibliotherapy, eHealth, group therapy, and individual interventions. Of course, there is a question of dose—usually (but not always) these would involve a lower dose. This might be acceptable for two reasons: (1) the goal is often different (symptom reduction to restore functioning instead of a complete cure); (2) if the integrated care intervention is not effective, a referral for more prolonged and intense specialty care treatment can be made.

Thus authors were asked to follow the following format for their chapters:

- A Brief Description of the Problem
- Screens
- Follow-Up Assessments if Screen Is Positive
- Evidence-Based Stepped Care and Brief Interventions
- Generally stepped care is thought to have the following steps (see O'Donohue & Draper, 2011):
  - Watchful waiting
  - Psychoeducation
  - eHealth
  - Bibliotherapy
  - Group intervention
  - Individual therapy
  - Medication
  - Inpatient Tx
  - However it is possible that there are no evidence-based interventions at one or more of these steps.
- When to Refer
- The Role of the PCP/Team
- What Does Not Work
- Quality Improvement

This is certainly only a beginning—it is not a substitute for quality outcome research but a reasonable place to begin. The research agenda is huge and hopefully will be less neglected in the near future. The screens, assessments, and treatments described in these chapters are generally based on sound psychological principles of change and usually have a good database in specialty care for the efficacy or effectiveness. It is recommended that further research be conducted on the effectiveness in integrated care and that these be implemented only in the context of a quality improvement system (the last topic in the chapter) so that they can be assessed for safety, satisfaction, and clinical impact and improvements can be made.

References

Chaffee, B., Laygo, R., & O'Donohue, W. (2013). The Hawaii integrated care project, (unpublished manuscript).

Chambless, D. L., & Hollon, S. D. (1998). Defining empirically supported therapies. *Journal of Consulting and Clinical Psychology.*, *66*(1), 7–18.

Committee on Quality Health Care in America, Institute of Medicine. (2001). *Crossing the quality chasm : A new health system for the 21st century*. Washington, D.C.: National Academy Press.

Cummings, N., O'Donohue, W., & Ferguson, K. (2002). *The impact of medical cost offset*. Reno, NV: Context Press.

Frisby, C., & O'Donohue, W. (in press). *Handbook of cultural competence*. New York: Springer.

Haynes, S., Smith, G., & Hunsley, J. (2011). *Scientific foundations of clinical assessment*. New York: Routledge.

Hunter, C., Goodie, J., Orrdt, M., & Dobmeyer, A. (2016). *Integrated behavioral health in primary care*. Washington, D.C.: American Psychological Association.

O'Donohue, W., Cummings, N. A., Cucciarre, M., Runyan, T., & Cummings, J. (2005). *Integrated care: A guide to effective intervention*. New York: Humanity Books.

O'Donohue, W., & Draper, C. (2011). *Stepped care and e-health: Practical applications to behavioral disorders*. New York: Springer.

O'Donohue, W., & Maragakis, A. (2014). Healthcare reform means training reform. *Journal of Online Doctoral Education*, *1*, 73–88.

O'Donohue, W., & Maragakis, A. (2016). *Quality improvement in behavioral health*. New York: Springer.

Robinson, P., Gould, D., & Strosahl, K. (2011). *Real behavior change in primary care*. New York: New Harbinger.

Robinson, P., & Reiter, J. (2015). *Behavioral consultation and primary care: A guide to integrating services*. New York: Springer.

Wendell, J., Seratt, T., & O'Donohue, W. (2017). *Understanding healthcare economics* (2nd ed.). New York: Productivity Press.

2 The Transformation of the Healthcare System: Integrated Primary Care and the Role of Stepped Care Interventions for Behavioral Health Providers

Alexandros Maragakis
and Marianthi N. Hatzigeorgiou

Recent Healthcare Reform

Most countries spend a significant portion of their gross domestic product (GDP) on healthcare expenses. As of 2013, the OECD average healthcare expense per GDP was 8.9%, and in the United States (US), one of the most fragmented examples of healthcare, over 16.4% of the nation's GDP was spent on healthcare expenses (OECD, 2015). Furthermore, healthcare costs are steadily increasing at an annual rate of 3%, well above the inflation rate (Moses et al., 2013). Though US healthcare expenditures surpass that of any other developed country, data indicates that American healthcare fails to achieve proportionately higher outcomes and quality, typically trailing behind many middle-income countries (Berwick, Nolan, & Whittington, 2008; Moses et al., 2013). The mismatch between spending and quality, in conjunction with the ever-increasing costs of healthcare, has spurred the need for reform and has become a major political and social discussion point.

A. Maragakis (✉)
Eastern Michigan University, Ypsilanti, MI, USA
e-mail: amaragak@emich.edu

M.N. Hatzigeorgiou
University of Michigan, Ann Arbor, MI, USA

Given that reform is complex and multifaceted, a full literature review on how to improve healthcare is beyond the scope of this chapter. However, there have been key themes to healthcare reform that are highly relevant for the future practice and utility of behavioral health providers in the overall healthcare system. A primary goal of healthcare reform has been the focus on improving the quality of care while simultaneously lowering overall healthcare costs (Rittenhouse & Shortell, 2009). In an attempt to achieve higher-quality care at lower costs, the framework of the "Triple Aim," which focuses on improving quality of care, population health outcomes, and reducing costs (Berwick et al., 2008), has been the center of many discussions and driven reform attempts. While the authors highlight many of the inefficiencies in current healthcare practices (e.g., payments linked to volume rather than outcomes), and offer multiple recommendations, a key piece to ensuring the Triple Aim's goals would require the incorporation of an entity called an "integrator." The responsibilities of the integrator would include engaging individuals and their families in care plans to increase transparency and compliance, facilitate patient-centered informed decisions around care, and engage in population health management. Through the delivery of these integrated services, healthcare practices and models would shift from

A. Maragakis, W.T. O'Donohue (eds.), *Principle-Based Stepped Care and Brief Psychotherapy for Integrated Care Settings*, https://doi.org/10.1007/978-3-319-70539-2_2

the delivery of costly, reactive care to models that encourage patient engagement in affordable, proactive, and preventative care. In theory, achievement of the Triple Aim, the intersection of all three goals, would reduce overall healthcare spending while simultaneously providing higher-quality care. Various attempts have been made to successfully introduce integrators in healthcare settings; in an effort to effectively achieve the goals of the integrator, reform and redesign of primary care settings is an identified key strategy to serve as this introduction platform. Allowing behavioral health providers (BHPs) to serve as integrators in primary care settings, in which services include the provision of preventive services and brief targeted behavioral health services, is one possibility that may strengthen the healthcare system while encouraging successful achievement of the Triple Aim.

The reengineering and transformation of primary care settings has been part of an attempt to improve how the United States provides care, with the goal of providing higher-quality, consistent, affordable care at reduced costs (Reid et al., 2009). This redesign has been led by the advent of patient-centered medical home (PCMH). Promoted as a new way to consider primary care delivery, these clinical settings integrate multiple providers and healthcare workers, creating teams that work together on a patient to drive patient-centric practices, outcomes, and goals. Though multiple physicians may be part of these PCMH teams, the PCMH also strives to connect a patient with community resources, enabling patient-driven results and compliance, without the necessity of multiple visits (Stange et al., 2010). Unlike many current primary care settings, PCMHs are driven by results, not services provided, and payment/reimbursement is adjusted based on the results. Additionally, PCMHs have been found to reduce avoidable emergency department utilization among patients with chronic illnesses (David, Gunnarsson, Saynisch, Chawla, & Nigam, 2015). Results and care plans are to be discussed thoroughly with patients and families, keeping each individual's case unique and adjusting care plans based on comorbidities and specific diagnoses (Rittenhouse & Shortell, 2009). The continuous adjustments in patient care plans are part of the transition toward better managed care in the primary care setting that paves way for better control of chronic issues and illnesses (David et al., 2015), including behavioral health issues. In the context of behavioral issues and psychological disorders, this individualization and comprehensiveness, particularly in the connection to community resources and patient follow-through using healthcare providers, would be pinnacle to creating an effective delivery system. The role of behavioral issues and psychological disorders and their adverse impact of health have been nationally recognized, as these conditions add to overall patient and population healthcare spending. It is well known that individuals with psychological disorders are more likely to make a visit to a physician than those without one and that many chronic illnesses (e.g., diabetes, obesity) have behavioral factors that compound the severity of the disease and are key components to treatment (Blount et al., 2007). Given the challenges and opportunities associated with improving behavioral health delivery, integrating BHPs into primary care settings, a process called integrated care (IC), has become a key professional objective for the field of psychology (Rozensky, 2012) and other behavioral health fields in an effort to properly address behavioral health issues.

Transforming the Primary Care Setting Through Integrated Care

It is estimated that 60–70% of adult visits to primary care physicians are complicated by behavioral health issues (Cummings, O'Donohue, & Cummings, 2011). These behavioral health issues create challenges in primary care settings (e.g., improper use of medical expertise, repeated visits to primary care providers or emergency rooms), as patients fail to receive the proper care needed to alleviate underlying behavioral health problems. Additionally, physicians are not properly trained to detect or treat these problems (Blount et al., 2007), leading to the delivery of suboptimal treatments for behavioral health issues. Though patients with behavioral health issues often do not receive proper care, primary care appointments usually take 30–60 min when behavioral health concerns are present, two to three times the length normally allotted for a typical primary care visit (Cummings, 2003). Deviation from typical appointment times reduces physician efficiency and physician job satisfaction (Meadows, Valleley, Haack, Thorson, & Evans, 2011). IC approaches that integrate behavioral health specialists as part of the primary care team are growing in popularity and practice as they are also found to increase physician efficiency and properly address and care for behavioral health issues (Christian & Curtis, 2012).

Patients who receive IC interventions have higher satisfaction ratings with regard to the quality of care they are receiving. Additionally, physicians report higher job satisfaction, and hospitals and clinics report savings due to medical cost offset from providing behavioral health treatments on-site (Christian & Curtis, 2012; Oser & O'Donohue, 2009). IC also reduces the stigma patients experience from receiving mental health treatment in traditional settings by making intervention a seamless part of primary care treatment (Christian & Curtis, 2012), thereby limiting the steps and locations needed to receive care.

For IC to be successful, it is imperative that empirically supported assessments and treatments are used. Failure to use empirically supported behavioral health treatments will result in increased medical utilization and further leads to a dramatic increase in healthcare spending, with little-to-no positive effect on outcome (Cummings et al., 2011). The most famous example of this is the Fort Bragg study. Behavioral health services were offered free of charge to whomever wished to receive them, and there was no system to ensure that the behavior health services consisted of evidence-based care. This resulted in a tenfold increase in healthcare costs and did not produce any significant results in regard to the quality of care for patients (Bickman, 1996). Therefore, it is important to be cognizant that simply providing access to behavioral health services as the solution to fragmented care is not enough; rather, these behavioral health services must be evidence-based and occur within well-coordinated systems.

Another important factor for the success of IC is the shift away from the traditional psychotherapy model. BHPs in the primary care setting do not have the luxury of the traditional 50-minute weekly sessions, nor do they have the schedule flexibility required to hold longer patient appointments needed to administer hours' worth of assessments. Rather, BHPs are allotted few (usually two to three) 15–20-minute sessions to identify and treat behavioral health issues (Cummings, 2011). The goal of redesigned primary care models is to allow BHPs to practice primary care psychology similar to and consistent with primary care medicine. This is described as a "high-volume, low-touch" approach, where patients requiring more intensive behavioral health interventions are triaged to behavioral health specialty care in a similar manner to medical primary care patients who require specialty care (Strosahl, 2005). Therefore, a goal of successful IC is for BHPs to be as efficient and effective as possible, given the constraints of the primary care setting.

Furthermore, before appropriate behavioral health treatment can be administered, effective and efficient assessments and screening devices must be used (Byrd & Alschuler, 2009). There have been several successful measures that have been developed for primary care use. These measures are relatively short (i.e., fit on one page) and do not require expertise in psychology or much additional time or resources when scoring (e.g., if the total value is above a certain number, then further investigation is warranted (Curtis & Christian, 2012)). These short, easy-to-use measures are extremely useful for the primary care provider (PCP), as they are able to quickly detect the potential presence of behavioral health issues without requiring additional time on the part of either the patient or the physician. In the primary care setting, this quick detection allows the PCP to either refer to a psychologist or, if in an integrated care setting, hand off to the BHP. This rapid response to behavioral health issues from the integration of a BHP would result in an overall decrease in the long-term cost of care, a process that has been coined as "medical cost offset."

When effectively utilized within the IC setting, BHPs can serve as the integrator of healthcare delivery systems, helping providers and systems achieve the Triple Aim. If IC models are to use PCMH strategies, and connect patients to community resources in addition to further medical and behavioral interventions, overall population health should improve given the strengthening of community networks and delivery models. BHPs in this role are able to consider more than DSM criteria when handling patient cases, allowing for a more comprehensive care episode, and focus on improving patient function, rather than reducing symptoms (Robinson & Strosahl, 2009).

There have been several discussions in the literature regarding how to successfully create IC settings that best facilitate improved care and the general role of a BHP (Christian & Curtis, 2012; O'Donohue & Maragakis, 2015; Robinson & Reiter, 2016). However, these discussions have typically lacked in providing details on what specific strategies BHPs could utilize during treatment in order to successfully accomplish the "high-volume, low-touch" mandate of the IC setting. In order to fill this gap in the literature, we propose that the utilization of stepped care interventions for specific behavioral health concerns provides a structured format for BHPs to be successful in the fast-paced primary care setting.

The Application of Stepped Care

In order for IC to be most effective and efficient, BHPs would benefit from delivering care in a stepped fashion, an approach that is consistent with medical treatment delivery in primary care settings (Von Korff, Glasgow, & Sharpe, 2002; Zeiss & Karlin, 2008); transitioning patients to more complex and costly interventions only after simpler, reasonable interventions has demonstrated inadequacy in improving patient conditions (O'Donohue & Draper, 2011; Von Korff et al., 2002). Stepped care posits that providers offer care that (1) causes the least disruption in the patient's life; (2) is the least extensive; (3) is the least intensive; (4) is the least expensive, in order to produce overall results (O'Donohue & Draper, 2011); and (5) is the most efficient in terms of team-based integrated care. These attributes contribute to increased patient choice regarding medical treatment and an opportunity for increased coordination between interdisciplinary team members.

For example, Snipes, Maragakis, and O'Donohue (2015) provide an example of a stepped care model when considering the diagnosis of depression:

1. *Watchful waiting* (used for patients that test positive but at very low levels, perhaps subclinical reactive depression such as a breakup of a romance; this includes following up with patient and asking them to monitor symptoms)
2. *Psychoeducational interventions* (brochures provided on behavioral activation, seeking social support, and exercise used to combat mild depression)
3. *eHealth* (the patient is referred to excellent evidence-based eHealth sites such as the Australian Beacon sites)
4. *Bibliotherapy* (the patient is referred to excellent evidence-based self-help books such as Burns' *Feeling Good*)
5. *Group psychotherapy* (the patient is referred to an ongoing cognitive behavioral mood management group where 10 or so patients can be simultaneously treated)
6. *Individual psychotherapy* for more severe depression
7. *Medication intervention* for more severe depression and due to patient preference
8. *Inpatient treatment* for the severest depression, perhaps associated with substantial suicidality

Under the auspice of stepped care is a common language by which all team members can be involved in triage, coordination, and treatment. Most PCPs are trained to provide intervention in a stepped manner, and application of this model in behavioral health intervention can enhance care provided at this level. Incorporating BHPs at the primary care setting level also helps to increase the number of patients that are assessed and appropriately cared for, aiming to further reduce disease burden and subsequent visits.

Empirical Evidence for the Use of Stepped Care

Multiple studies have demonstrated the effectiveness of stepped care methodology in reducing or delaying behavioral health issues (Andrews, Cuijpers, Craske, McEvoy, & Titov, 2010; Rucci et al., 2012; Seekles, van Straten, Beekman, van Marwijk, & Cuijpers, 2009; van't Veer-Tazelaar et al., 2010). In addition to driving down associated costs by delivering care directly at primary care settings and avoiding the need for inpatient admission, integrated stepped care also initiates a greater understanding and acceptance around behavioral health issues and is thought to facilitate earlier conversations between patients and providers surrounding diagnosis and treatment (Rucci et al., 2012). Patients enrolled in stepped care were found to withdraw enrollment from treatment group at higher rates than patients treated via treatment-as-usual (TAU) methods (Rucci et al., 2012) but also had significantly better outcomes.

Stepped care also offers the patient the greatest amount of choice in the intervention they receive. This choice creates a "buy-in" between the patient and provider, enabling patients to feel more in control of treatment and lead to the inclination for higher compliance (O'Donohue & Draper, 2011) (Richards, 2012). For example, patients who are uncomfortable using online treatment platforms may instead elect to engage in bibliotherapy. In the case of high-severity patients, patients are given access to consultation regarding the potential benefits of antidepressants versus individual psychotherapy (or a combination thereof) via interaction with the multidisciplinary care team. From a provider lens, this encourages multiple practitioners to be engaged in patient care plans and treatment options, leading to care that is individualized using standardized platforms. Regarding behavioral health issues, increased individualization can help to address deterrents and mitigate issues in receiving IC as enhanced patient choice renders integrated stepped care "consumer-centric."

As part of the Triple Aim initiative, health of the specified population (i.e., catchment area) should be managed and improved in any successful healthcare setting. Population health management is the application of interventions to defined groups of patients in an effort to improve the health of the individuals within the group at the lowest cost (HealthCatalyst, 2015). Through identification of patient severity, stepped care delivers the least invasive and least costly intervention to patients overall. In addition, those patients identified as high severity or high utilizers can be targeted to receive the highest level of professional care (or use of the most team resources), reducing the misallocation of resources to patients that do not require intensive care. Though additional care workers are needed to effectively implement stepped care models, overall cost-effectiveness should be demonstrated when considering downstream charges generated from untreated and exacerbated behavioral health issues.

Outside of the traditional diagnoses of care, collaborative stepped care has been shown to increase population impact for various behavioral health concerns. For example, the treatment of posttraumatic stress disorder has benefited from stepped care (Zatzick et al., 2013). Shifting disease burden from trauma centers to primary care settings enables providers and BHPs to appropriately begin interventions with patients early on and allow patients the opportunity to manage disease prior to the necessity for trauma center admission.

Through implementation of stepped care, and effective population management as a result thereof, medical cost offset is more likely to be achieved than in traditional integrated care. Integrated care has been shown to reduce costs by approximately 20% overall, across a range of implementation approaches (Chiles, Lambert, & Hatch, 1999). However, in some cases, integrated care fails to deliver medical cost offset (California Mental Health Service Authority, 2015) due to a number of systemic challenges. Team-based stepped care can address these problems by allocating collaborative resources in the most effective manner. Specifically, team-based stepped care aims to neither over- nor undertreat.

Conclusion

As political and administrative discussions continue to focus on the growing costs of care, and the drive to further push the United States as the innovative provider of healthcare systems and delivery, it would be of benefit to pursue stepped care pathways as primary care settings are reformatted and redesigned. Doing so will help to triage and treat patients who struggle to receive adequate care and often succumb to debilitating side effects before reactive treatment is used to try and manage more serious symptoms. The use of stepped care provides a clear framework for BHPs operating within IC systems, and if utilized, this stepped care framework may provide consistency among providers as efforts are initiated to reform and redesign primary care methodologies.

References

Andrews, G., Cuijpers, P., Craske, M., McEvoy, P., & Titov, N. (2010). Computer therapy for the anxiety and depressive disorders is effective, acceptable and practical health care: A meta-analysis. *PLoS One*, *5*(10), e13196.

Berwick, D., Nolan, T., & Whittington, J. (2008). The triple aim: Care, health, and cost. *Health Affairs*, *27*(3), 759–769.

Bickman, L. (1996). A continuum of care: More is not always better. *American Psychologist*, *51*, 689–701.

Blount, A., Schoenbaum, M., Kathol, R., Rolman, B., Thomas, M., O'Donohue, W., & Peek, C. (2007). The economics of behavioral health services in medical settings: A summary of the evidence. *Professional Psychology: Research and Practice*, *38*(3), 290–297.

Byrd, M. R., & Alschuler, K. N. (2009). Behavioral screening in adult primary care. In L. C. James & W. T. O'Donohue (Eds.), *The primary care toolkit: Practical resources for the integrated behavioral care provider* (pp. 121–130). New York: Springer.

California Mental Health Service Authority. (2015). Why pursue integrated behavioral health care? Retrieved from http://ibhp.org/index.php?section=pages&cid=104

Chiles, J. A., Lambert, M. J., & Hatch, A. L. (1999). The impact of psychological interventions on medical cost offset: A meta-analytic review. *Clinical Psychology: Science and Practice*, *6*, 204–220.

Christian, E., & Curtis, R. (2012). Introduction to integrated care. In R. Curtis & E. Christian (Eds.), *Integrated care: Applying theory to practice* (pp. 3–20). New York: Routledge.

Cummings, N. A. (2003). Advantages and limitations of disease management—A practical guide. In N. A. Cummings, W. T. O'Donahue, & K. E. Ferguson (Eds.), *Behavioral health as primary care: Beyond efficacy to effectiveness* (pp. 31–44). Reno: Context Press.

Cummings, N. A. (2011). Our 50-minute hour in the nanosecond era. The need for a third "E" in behavioral healthcare efficiency. In N. A. Cummings & W. T. O'Donohue (Eds.), *Understanding the behavioral healthcare crisis: The promise of integrated care and diagnostic reform* (pp. 19–32). New York: Routledge.

Cummings, N. A., O'Donohue, W. T., & Cummings, J. L. (2011). The financial dimension of integrated behavioral/primary care. In N. A. Cummings & W. T. O'Donohue (Eds.), *Understanding the behavioral healthcare crisis: The promise of integrated care and diagnostic reform* (pp. 33–54). New York: Routledge.

Curtis, R., & Christian, E. (2012). A screening and assessment primer. In R. Curits & E. Christian (Eds.), *Integrated care: Applying theory to practice* (pp. 35–58). New York: Routledge.

David, G., Gunnarsson, C., Saynisch, P., Chawla, R., & Nigam, S. (2015). Do patient-centered medical homes reduce emergency department visits. *Health Services Research*, *50*(2), 418–439.

HealthCatalyst. (2013). Burton DA. Population health management—Conceptual outline. Salt Lake City. 2013. Retrieved from https://www.healthcatalyst.com/wpcontent/uploads/2013/07/WhitePaper_PopulationHealthManagement.pdf

Meadows, T., Valleley, R., Haack, M., Thorson, R., & Evans, J. (2011). Physician "costs" in providing behavioral health in primary care. *Clinical Pediatrics*, *50*(5), 447–455.

Moses, H., III, Matheson, D., Dorsey, E., George, B., Sadoff, D., & Yoshimura, S. (2013). The anatomy of health care in the United States. *JAMA*, *310*(18), 1947–1963.

O'Donohue, W. T., & Draper, C. (2011). The case for evidence-based stepped care as part of a reformed delivery system. In W. T. O'Donohue & C. Draper (Eds.), *Stepped care and e-health: Practical applications to behavioral disorders* (pp. 1–16). New York: Springer.

O'Donohue, W., & Maragakis, A. (2015). *Integrated primary and behavioral care: Role in medical homes and chronic disease management*. Cham: Springer International.

OECD. (2015). *Health at a glance 2015: OECD indicators*. Paris: OECD Publishing.

Oser, M., & O'Donohue, W. T. (2009). How to determine the need: A readiness assessment system. In L. C. James & W. T. O'Donohue (Eds.), *The primary care toolkit: Practical resources for the integrated behavioral care Provider* (pp. 3–13). New York: Springer.

Reid, R., Fishman, P., Yu, O., Ross, T., Tufano, J., Soman, M., & Larson, E. (2009). Patient-centered medical home demonstration: A prospective, quasi-experimental, before and after evaluation. *The American Journal of Managed Care, 15*, e71–e87.

Richards, D. (2012). Stepped care: A method to deliver increased access to psychological therapies. *Canadian Journal of Psychiatry, 57*(4), 210–215.

Rittenhouse, D., & Shortell, S. (2009). The patient-centered medical home: Will it stand the test of health reform? *JAMA, 301*, 2038–2040.

Robinson, P., & Reiter, J. (2016). *Behavioral consultation and primary care: A guide to integrating services* (2nd ed.). Cham: Springer International Publishing.

Robinson, P. J., & Strosahl, K. D. (2009). Behavioral health consultation and primary care: Lessons learned. *Journal of Clinical Psychology in Medical Settings, 16*, 58–71.

Rozensky, R. (2012). Health care reform: Preparing the psychology workforce. *Journal of Clinical Psychology in Medical Settings, 19*, 5–11.

Rucci, P., Piazza, A., Menchetti, M., Berardi, D., Fioritti, A., Mimmi, S., & Fantini, M. (2012, 2012). Integration between primary care and mental health services in Italy: Determinants of referral and stepped care. *International Journal of Family Medicine*, 507464.

Seekles, W., van Straten, A., Beekman, A., van Marwijk, H., & Cuijpers, P. (2009). Stepped care for depression and anxiety: From primary care to specialized mental health care: A randomised controlled trial testing the effectiveness of a stepped care program among primary care patients with mood or anxiety disorders. *BMC Health Services Research, 9*, 90.

Snipes, C., Maragakis, A., & O'Donohue, W. (2015). Team based stepped care in integrated delivery settings. *Family Medicine and Community Health, 3*(1), 39–46(8).

Stange, K., Nutting, P., Miller, W., Jaen, C., Crabtree, B., Flocke, S., & Gill, J. (2010). Defining and measuring the patient-centered medical home. *Journal of General Internal Medicine, 25*(6), 601–612.

Strosahl, K. (2005). Training behavioral health and primary care providers for integrated care: A core competencies approach. In W. O'Donohue, M. Byrd, N. Cummings, & D. Henderson (Eds.), *Behavioral integrative care: Treatments that work in the primary care setting* (pp. 15–52). New York: Brunner-Routledge.

van't Veer-Tazelaar, P., Smit, F., van Hout, H., van Oppen, P., van der Horst, H., Beekman, A., & van Marwijk, H. (2010). Cost-effectiveness of a stepped care intervention to prevent depression and anxiety in late life: Randomised trial. *The British Journal of Psychiatry, 196*, 319–325.

Von Korff, M., Glasgow, R. E., & Sharpe, M. (2002). ABC of psychological medicine: Organising care for chronic illness. *BMJ: British Medical Journal, 325*(7355), 92.

Zatzick, D., Jurkovich, G., Rivara, F., Russo, J., Wagner, A., Wang, J., … O'Connor, S. K. (2013). A randomized stepped care intervention trial targeting posttraumatic stress disorder for surgically hospitalized injury survivors. *Annals of Surgery, 257*(3), 390–399.

Zeiss, A. M., & Karlin, B. E. (2008). Integrating Mental Health and Primary Care Services in the Department of Veterans Affairs Health Care System. *Journal of Clinical Psychology in Medical Settings, 15*, 73–78.

Advanced Cancer

3

Allen C. Sherman, Amy Hufsteader, and Stephanie Simonton-Atchley

Individuals with advanced cancer are confronted by a range of difficult challenges. As treatment options narrow in response to metastatic or progressive disease, many patients encounter jarring changes in multiple spheres of daily life, including emotional, physical, social, and spiritual domains. In this chapter, we focus on the experience of advanced cancer patients receiving outpatient palliative care. Palliative care involves efforts to manage symptoms and maximize quality of life. Although historically the term has evoked images of patients in their final days, these services are designed to assist patients at any stage of disease, from those with highly curable malignancies to those with acutely terminal illness. Here we consider the needs of ambulatory patients with late-stage disease, for whom the goals are generally life extension or symptom management rather than cure. Some of these individuals experience an interval of stable disease, and others have moved toward end-of-life care. We review some of the common problems that emerge, discuss screening measures to help identify those at elevated risk for psychosocial difficulties, and examine brief interventions that might be useful as initial components in stepped care.

Mental health clinicians have a salient role to play in the multidisciplinary care of these patients. The importance of psychosocial concerns has long been recognized in oncology, and these have been the focus of a rather vast and vibrant body of research. The actual integration of psychosocial services into routine care, however, has been more slow and uneven. In recent years, these efforts have received greater impetus by the development by several professional groups of standards for psychosocial care of cancer patients (e.g., American College of Surgeons, Commission on Cancer, 2012; Institute of Medicine, 2008; National Comprehensive Care Network, 2008; American Society of Clinical Oncology/Oncology Nursing Society, Neuss et al., 2013). We anticipate that health psychologists and other mental health specialists will have a growing presence in oncology settings in the years to come.

Brief Description of the Problem

The difficulties that cancer patients experience are shaped in part by the basic clinical characteristics of their illness, including disease stage (e.g., early vs. advanced), type of malignancy (e.g., colon vs. multiple myeloma), and phase in the trajectory of care (e.g., initial diagnosis

A.C. Sherman, Ph.D. (✉) • A. Hufsteader, B.S.
S. Simonton-Atchley, Ph.D.
Behavioral Medicine, Winthrop P. Rockefeller Cancer Institute, University of Arkansas for Medical Sciences, Little Rock, AR, USA
e-mail: ShermanAllenC@uams.edu; ahufstedler1@CUB.UCA.edu; simontonatchleystep@uams.edu

A. Maragakis, W.T. O'Donohue (eds.), *Principle-Based Stepped Care and Brief Psychotherapy for Integrated Care Settings*, https://doi.org/10.1007/978-3-319-70539-2_3

vs. long-term survivorship or terminal illness). Patients with intractable disease face disquieting questions about shifting the focus of treatment from curative efforts to life prolongation or comfort care. They must adapt to disruptions in quality of life and increased functional limitations, as well as a foreshortened future. Although most patients cope well with these daunting demands, problems with reactive distress (e.g., anxiety or depressive symptoms, grief, uncertainty) are not uncommon (e.g., Delgado-Guay, Parsons, Li, Palmer, & Bruera, 2009). In addition, there is an elevated prevalence of psychiatric morbidity. For example, a meta-analysis (Mitchell et al., 2011) encompassing over 4000 palliative care patients who had been assessed with diagnostic interviews suggested that 29% met the criteria for a mood or anxiety disorder. (More specifically, 16.5% were diagnosed with major depressive disorder, 9.6% were diagnosed with minor depression, 15.4% were classified with adjustment disorders, and 9.8% struggled with anxiety disorders.) Not surprisingly, rates of subsyndromal distress and diagnosable mental health disorders are notably higher than those in the general population. Despite their prevalence, these problems are notoriously overlooked and undertreated across the spectrum of cancer care (e.g., Fallowfield, Ratcliffe, Jenkins, & Saul, 2001). Insufficient treatment is especially troubling because of the potential adverse impact of psychiatric difficulties on other aspects of care. For example, depression has been associated with greater nutritional deficits, poorer adherence, and increased hospitalizations among various types of medical patients (DiMatteo, Lepper, & Croghan, 2000; Kitagawa, Yasui-Furukori, Tsushima, Kaneko, & Fukuda, 2011).

Aside from emotional distress, problems may emerge in a number of other areas as well. Existential concerns take on greater immediacy in response to advanced or progressive disease, as patients are confronted with a limited future. Difficult decisions may need to be made about end-of-life care (e.g., goals of treatment, life-sustaining interventions, communication of preferences, etc.). At the same time, unsettling questions may arise regarding the broader meaning, purpose, or legacy of one's life. Spiritual issues may assume greater salience as well; many patients find solace and meaning in their spiritual orientations, but some wrestle with painful doubts or alienation (Sherman et al., 2015).

As a result of diminished functional capacity, patients may struggle with the loss of routine roles, increased dependency on others, or an altered sense of identity. Many worry that they have become a burden to their families. Some patients experience unwelcome changes in body image or sexual functioning (Mercadante, Vitrano, & Catania, 2010). Sleep disruption is a common concern (Parker et al., 2008). Financial pressures can be oppressive as well (e.g., loss of income, onerous medical expenses, lack of insurance coverage).

The burden of physical symptoms becomes more pronounced with advanced disease. By the time they have transitioned to palliative care, most patients have weathered taxing treatment regimens and demanding toxicities. Fatigue is among the most common problems generated by the illness and its treatments (Seow et al., 2011). Other frequent sequelae include pain, nausea, anemia, infectious complications, constipation, and dyspnea. Palliative treatments (e.g., radiotherapy, chemotherapy), intended to diminish tumor burden and improve quality of life, are generally delivered at lower doses that are more readily tolerated, but these too may carry their own toxicities.

The physical and psychosocial difficulties that the patient experiences have a considerable impact on family life as well (Sherman & Simonton, 2001). Levels of emotional distress reported by the partner are often comparable to and sometimes higher than those of the patient (Hodges, Humphris, & Macfarlane, 2005). Shifts in the health-care system have meant that family members now assume extensive responsibility for assisting with day-to-day care. Thus, in addition to coping with grief and uncertainty, families must accommodate new tasks and altered roles. Caregivers tend to experience greater burdens when the patient's functioning is more compromised or requires greater disruption in the caregiver's routines, when they feel less confident in their ability to provide appropriate care, when they receive less support from others, and when they have greater concomitant responsibility for caring for other family members (Wadhwa et al., 2013).

Effective Ways to Screen

Systematic screening is intended to help identify patients at heightened risk or those in need of psychosocial services. In recent years, routine screening of cancer patients has been advocated internationally by a growing number of professional standards and practice guidelines (e.g., National Comprehensive Care Network, 2008; American College of Physicians, Qaseem et al., 2008; Butow et al., 2015; Cancer Care Ontario, Dudgeon et al., 2012). Despite widespread endorsement, this approach is not without its critics (Coyne, 2013; Garssen & de Kok, 2008), and there are questions about the extent to which screening translates into improved psychosocial outcomes for patients (specifically those who have not already been receiving mental health care). Clearly, screening processes need to include a mechanism to share results with patients and medical providers, and to provide appropriate follow-up for clinical evaluation and intervention. (There is little point in screening problems if no resources are available to treat them.) Several cancer centers have used electronic kiosks or tablets to facilitate the collection, tracking, and sharing of screening results. Importantly, uptake of services may be greater when patients receive personal contact rather than only automatically generated recommendations (Carlson et al., 2012). Moreover, patients may have pressing unmet needs in areas that fall outside the narrow confines of the particular screening instrument being used (e.g., family difficulties or existential uncertainties rather than emotional distress). In our view, screening should not be the only pathway to psychosocial services.

A large number of standardized instruments are available to assist with the screening process, as an initial component of stepped care. They vary in focus, with some intended to evaluate a single concern (e.g., distress or depression) and others designed to capture a broader range of common psychosocial and physical problems (e.g., mood, dyspnea, pain, nausea, etc.). Selection of an appropriate measure is not a one-size-fits-all proposition, and should be tailored to the needs and goals of the particular practice setting.

Brief, self-report measures of distress have been compared to diagnostic interviews to help evaluate their psychometric performance. In general, brief instruments tend to perform adequately in screening patients, as a first step in provision of services (i.e., they appropriately rule out those without distress, without mislabeling as healthy those individuals who are in fact distressed). However, they tend to perform poorly in case identification (i.e., they are not so good at ruling in individuals who are distressed, and often mislabel as distressed those who are managing well) (Mitchell, 2007; Mitchell et al., 2012; Ryan, Gallagher, Wright, & Cassidy, 2012). Simply stated, patients who screen positive on distress measures generally require a more comprehensive clinical assessment to determine their status and needs.

"Ultrashort" measures seek to screen distress using only a few items, in an effort to maximize acceptability and minimize patient burden. The most widely used of these instruments in oncology is the distress thermometer (DT; Ryan et al., 2012), which simply asks respondents to indicate how distressed they have felt in the past week by marking a "thermometer" or visual analogue scale that ranges from 0 ("no distress") to 10 ("extreme distress"). Usually the DT is accompanied by a 36-item problem checklist (which may render its brevity a bit less "ultra"). Another example involves use of one or two items from the Patient Health Questionnaire (Kroenke, Spitzer, & Williams, 2003), concerning depressed mood and anhedonia.

Other commonly used measures of distress, which are less austerely concise but still brief (more than five items), include the Hospital Anxiety and Depression Scale (HADS; Bjelland,

Dahl, Haug, & Neckelmann, 2002), the Center for Epidemiologic Studies Depression Scale (CES-D; Radloff, 1977), the Patient Health Questionnaire-9 (PHQ-9; Kroenke, Spitzer, & Williams, 2001), the Generalized Anxiety Questionnaire-7 (Spitzer et al., 2006), the Brief Symptom Inventory-18 (Derogatis, 2000), and the Beck Depression Inventory-II (BDI-II; Beck, Steer, & Brown, 1996). A large database has evaluated the psychometric properties of these instruments, and cutoff values are available to facilitate interpretation of scores. Each has strengths and limitations in screening cancer patients.

Other brief measures have been used to assess a wider array of physical and emotional symptoms. These include the Edmonton Symptom Assessment System (ESAS; Bruera et al., 1991) and the M.D. Anderson Symptom Inventory (MDASI; Cleeland et al., 2000). These tools can be helpful in flagging problems in need of follow-up from various members of the multidisciplinary team (e.g., uncontrolled pain that requires the attention of the palliative care physician, elevated distress that needs to be assessed by the psychologist, etc.). Evidence supports the psychometric adequacy of these instruments, and cutoff scores have been established to guide screening decisions.

Some instruments provide a richer, more focused assessment of a single symptom, such as fatigue (e.g., FACT-Fatigue scale; Yellen et al., 1997), pain (Brief Pain Inventory; Cleeland, 1989), or sleep disturbance (e.g., Insomnia Severity Index; Savard, Savard, Simard, & Ivers, 2005). Others are designed to assess broader, multidimensional aspects of quality of life, including physical, functional, emotional, and social dimensions (FACIT-Pal; Lyons et al., 2009; EORTC QLQ-C15-PAL; Groenvold et al., 2006). Quality-of-life measures often employ a modular approach, in which a core instrument, which addresses concerns common to many types of cancer, is supplemented by a module that captures problems specific to a particular disease site (e.g., ovarian cancer), type of treatment (e.g., bone marrow transplantation), or phase of care (e.g., palliative care). Norms are available to assist interpretation.

How to Further Assess if a Screen Returns Positive

There has been growing interest in the development of models of stepped care in oncology (e.g., Butow et al., 2015; Krebber et al., 2012; Simonton & Sherman, 2000; Turner et al., 2011). In our cancer center, pathways to psychosocial care may include screening, self-referral, or referral from another member of the medical team. Services are open to patients as well as family members. Treatment begins with an appropriate clinical assessment by a psychologist or licensed clinical social worker. A careful evaluation enables the clinician to assess the chronicity and severity of difficulties, explore vulnerabilities and resources, inform patients/families about available resources, and tailor interventions to their particular needs and wishes. Some stepped-care models bypass an initial assessment and propose that all patients who screen positive (Krebber et al., 2012), or those with low levels of distress (Turner et al., 2011), proceed directly to watchful waiting or low-intensity interventions (e.g., educational materials, self-help guides). Although this approach may be viable in some settings, in our view it may result in some patients or families receiving unhelpful resources that are poorly aligned with their actual needs and desires, leading to delays in appropriate care or disillusioned withdrawal from services.

When to Refer

Psychosocial interventions are viewed as one strand within a broader tapestry of support services, which may be offered by psychology, social work, pastoral care, psychiatry, volunteer services, and support groups (in conjunction with palliative care, nutrition, and physical therapy). For ambulatory patients with advanced cancer, who have sufficient functional status to make use of outpatient resources, a clinical assessment can help determine which interventions available within a spectrum of multidisciplinary services might be most useful. Of course, smaller primary care or oncology practices often are unable to provide access to diverse resources on-site, and there is a stronger need for clinicians to be aware of relevant services available within the community (e.g., in-person or online support groups, religious leaders, psychiatry clinics, etc.).

Following an assessment, patients who present with a high level of acuity (e.g., suicidality, delirium) or those with more chronic or extensive psychiatric difficulties (e.g., psychotic symptoms, intractable major depression, unregulated bipolar disorder, debilitating anxiety disorders, active addiction, severe character pathology) can be triaged to an appropriate level of extended care. For patients with more moderate or circumscribed psychosocial difficulties, a range of brief interventions might be helpful. We turn to these next. At the same time, if other needs are identified that have not yet been recognized by the medical team, appropriate referrals can be provided (e.g., pastoral counselors for religious questions, palliative care for poorly controlled pain, treating physician for first- or second-line antidepressant trials, or psychiatry for complex psychopharmacological coverage).

Stepped Care and Brief Psychotherapeutic Approaches

Major goals of brief treatment commonly include reduced distress, enhanced coping and self-care, increased mobilization of support, and assistance with some of the affective and existential difficulties that are inherent in living with advanced disease. Clinicians have a number of widely used therapeutic approaches upon which to draw. These generally incorporate supportive, cognitive-behavioral, affective, and existential treatment strategies, but the relative emphasis on these elements varies across different models. All of the approaches considered below have some level of empirical support, but some have been studied less extensively among advanced cancer patients than among those with early-stage disease.

Supportive Contact and Educational Material

Brief, supportive contact may provide considerable relief for some patients or family caregivers (e.g., Kornblith et al., 2006). They may perceive few opportunities to share their fears and concerns elsewhere, as patients are reluctant to burden their families and as family members in turn seek to avoid undermining the patient's "positive attitude." A safe forum in which to express feelings, and to discover that their reactions are normative, may be highly welcome and reassuring. The assessment interview followed by one or two follow-up sessions with a clinician may be sufficient to meet these needs.

Referrals to support groups or provision of self-management materials may be helpful as well. A wide variety of educational resources are available online or in print from the American Cancer Society (e.g., *Keeping Well in Mind, Body, and Spirit*, *When Cancer Comes Back*, *Nearing the End of Life*), the National Cancer Institute (e.g., *Coping with Cancer*, *Advanced Cancer*), and other disease-specific organizations. Online educational programs (e.g., American Cancer Society's *I Can Cope*) and support networks (e.g., *csn.cancer.org*) can also be useful.

For some patients or family members, these resources serve as a springboard for the other more specialized approaches discussed below. Often these involve four to ten sessions with a mental health specialist. Response to treatment is carefully monitored, and more extended interventions are provided as needed. Traditionally these services have been offered in face-to-face individual, family, or group modalities. However, growing attention has been directed to administering some of these interventions by phone or synchronously online, which may increase access and enhance cost-effectiveness. Evidence for the efficacy of phone or web-based formats for advanced cancer patients is limited as yet (Okuyama et al., 2015), but work in this area is expanding rapidly (e.g., Janssen et al., 2016), and there seems little doubt that these formats will become more common features of the landscape in the years to come.

Cognitive-Behavioral Approaches

Cognitive-behavioral interventions can be helpful in enhancing coping resources (Hart et al., 2012). Self-regulation strategies (e.g., relaxation training, meditation, self-hypnosis) can be particularly useful in managing anxiety and stress, which are common problems for those facing advanced cancer. More broadly, these self-regulation strategies may also provide a tool for self-soothing and help restore a sense of control. Relaxation strategies or other mind-body approaches (e.g., yoga, Tai Chi) may also help patients reestablish a more favorable relationship with their bodies, as a source of comfort instead of fear or betrayal (Simonton & Sherman, 2000). Cognitive coping strategies can be quite useful as well (Savard et al., 2006), by helping patients or caregivers identify reflexive, rigid perceptions that amplify distress and exploring more flexible responses.

Cognitive-behavioral approaches are also useful adjuncts in symptom management. For example, well-established strategies are available to assist with sleep disturbance. Typically these include assistance with relaxation training, stimulus control, sleep hygiene, and sleep restriction—strategies that sometimes are offered in combination with cognitive coping skills (Langford, Lee, & Miakowski, 2012). Other cognitive-behavioral approaches may be helpful in managing pain (Sheinfeld Gorin et al., 2012), nausea, or procedure-related phobias (e.g., fears of MRIs, CTs, or blood draws).

Supportive-Expressive Approaches

Supportive-expressive therapy (Classen et al., 2001; Kissane et al., 2007) offers another approach well-suited to the needs of advanced cancer patients. With roots in existential and interpersonal group therapy, the original treatment model involved a long-term, manualized group intervention offered over the course of a year for women with metastatic breast cancer. Currently, this approach is often construed more broadly as encompassing a variety of briefer individual and group interventions that have not been as extensively studied, but that similarly focus on expressing and processing emotional experience and addressing existential difficulties. Patients are supported in the open, authentic expression of their fears and concerns regarding living with life-threatening illness ("speaking the unspeakable"), without the forced cheerleading or admonitions to stay strong that they sometimes perceive from family or friends. The therapist helps provide a safe holding environment and judicious pacing so that patients can begin to process and integrate their experiences. Reordering priorities in the face of an uncertain future, expanding social support, and enhancing coping are also important areas of focus.

Existential Approaches

A new generation of short-term treatments offers additional models for addressing existential concerns (e.g., Breitbart et al., 2015; Chochinov et al., 2011; Steinhauser et al., 2008). Meaning-centered psychotherapy draws on Viktor Frankl's work and was specifically designed to enhance a sense of meaning, peace, and purpose among patients with advanced cancer. Manualized individual (seven sessions; Breitbart et al., 2012) and group (eight sessions; Breitbart et al., 2015) interventions help participants consider questions of legacy, evaluate personal attitudes toward suffering, and explore important sources of meaning in life. Recently, life review interventions also have gained growing attention. These brief therapies are designed for palliative care patients who are closer to the end of life (i.e., more acutely terminal). The best known example of these is dignity therapy (Chochinov et al., 2011), in which patients are invited to reflect on a series of core questions regarding aspects of their lives that have been most valued or messages that they would like to convey to loved ones. The particular questions addressed are tailored according to patient preferences. The responses are transcribed and edited into a "generativity document" by the therapist, who then reviews the document with the patient in a subsequent session and invites further editing, resulting in a final product that the patient may share with others if desired. Thus far, evaluations of dignity therapy (e.g., Chochinov et al., 2011; Julião et al., 2014) and other life review models (e.g., Ando et al., 2010) have yielded uneven results, but this remains an active area of investigation.

Mindfulness-Based Approaches

Mindfulness-based interventions have garnered significant interest in oncology settings (Piet, Wurtzen, & Zachariae, 2012). Mindfulness involves intentional, nonjudgmental awareness of experience in the current moment. The intervention is intended to diminish deeply ingrained, habitual responses to stress, enhance symptom control, and foster a sense of open acceptance and appreciation for day-to-day experience. Manualized programs for cancer patients have been adapted from the mindfulness-based stress reduction model, which was developed initially for use in primary care (Kabat-Zinn, 1990). These programs usually include 6–8-weekly group sessions, sometimes offered in conjunction with a full-day workshop, which focus on cultivating mindfulness in daily life through training in mindfulness meditation and gentle hatha yoga. Alternatives to the group format, such as individual or Internet-based interventions, are being evaluated as well (e.g., Zernicke et al., 2014). Another adaptation is mindfulness-based cognitive therapy, which incorporates cognitive strategies; originally crafted for use with depressed patients, it has been employed to address other symptoms as well (e.g., cancer pain; Johannsen et al., 2016). There is growing empirical support for use of mindfulness-based treatments for cancer patients with early-stage disease or those in the posttreatment survivorship phase (Piet, Wurtzen, & Zachariae, 2012). Thus far, this approach has received little study among patients or families facing advanced disease (van den Hurk et al., 2015); nonetheless, mindfulness approaches and conceptually related interventions such as Acceptance and Commitment Therapy (Arch & Mitchell, 2016) seem promising for these individuals, given their struggles with uncertainty, limited control, and high symptom burden.

End-of-Life Planning

Mental health clinicians may also play a helpful role in facilitating end-of-life care planning. Patients and their families often have an inaccurate understanding of prognosis (Weeks et al., 2012), harboring unrealistic expectations for recovery, and have a limited recognition of the actual goals of treatment (Teno et al., 2002), mistaking palliative treatment for curative efforts. Communication about the patient's treatment preferences is often poor (Wright et al., 2008). Many patients continue to receive aggressive treatments through their final days, undergo invasive life support, and die in the intensive care unit or elsewhere in the hospital, despite preferences to the contrary (Wright et al., 2008; Teno et al., 2002).

There is wide recognition of the need to improve communication among oncologists, patients, and family members and to plan for end-of-life care proactively instead of waiting for a medical crisis, at which point such discussions may become appreciably more complicated or impossible. However, traditionally oncologists received limited training in communication about end-of-life care; they also face time constraints and competing demands in a busy clinic and may worry about distressing the patient by addressing evocative issues. Psychosocial clinicians can help patients and families explore these concerns, which often evolve over time. They may assess the patient/family's understanding of prognosis and goals of care, examine the importance they ascribe to shared decision-making and receipt of medical information, help them explore personal or cultural values that might be important at the end of life, and facilitate clear communication with the medical team. In addition, these clinicians sometimes serve as consultants to oncologists regarding how best to structure advance care planning conversations or sit in on oncologists' meetings with the family to assist the discussion.

What Does Not Work

Obviously, a brief treatment model may not necessarily resolve all concerns experienced by the patient or family; in many cases it provides helpful resources so that participants can better manage on their own. However, response to treatment and unmet needs should be monitored periodically, with transition to altered or more extended treatment services as clinically indicated. Stepped care dissolves without continued assessment.

As in any treatment setting, the role of the therapist should be consistent with the contours of the treatment model and the needs of the participant. For example, the use of cognitive interventions with cancer patients requires clinicians to be thoughtful in distinguishing recurrent biases in information processing (which are a focus for cognitive restructuring) from "negative thinking" (which often is not). Clearly, patients with advanced cancer have plenty to think negatively about—they may feel discounted, guilty, or resentful if simplistically implemented treatment strategies are insensitive to the reality of their circumstances.

Meaning-focused interventions are highly attuned to the possibilities for personal growth—the discovery of positive changes such as a heightened appreciation for life, a deeper spirituality, or a capacity to live more richly and fully. However, clinicians who strive too assiduously to inculcate these changes rather than listen for them, who convey expectation instead of curiosity, may burden patients with a sense of failure or disillusionment; patients may feel that somehow they have not lived up to oppressive cultural injunctions regarding overcoming adversity and securing happy endings.

For supportive interventions, it may be important for clinicians to be sufficiently receptive and nondirective to allow the patients' or families' concerns to emerge organically. Excessive efforts to provide education, advice, or reassurance may leave little space for the participants' exploration. Supportive-expressive or existential interventions present additional challenges when implemented in a brief therapy model. Clinicians may need to be mindful of not stirring up highly charged material that cannot be adequately metabolized or worked through within the course of short-term treatment. Assisting patients in processing and integrating difficult emotional reactions, particularly those which seem unsafe or unwelcome in other settings, is not the same as a relentless "mining" for affect or unrestrained confrontation of defenses or coping mechanisms.

Role of the Medical Team

Psychosocial problems are notably underdetected in oncology. Rates of referral for psychosocial services are low (Lee et al., 2016), and uptake of services for those with identified needs is limited (Tuinman et al., 2015). Evidence suggests that discussion of psychosocial concerns is usually initiated by the patient rather than by the oncologist (Pollak et al., 2007).

Oncologists, primary care clinicians, and nurses play a central role in ensuring that treatment for advanced cancer is patient-centered and holistic. An important step involves inquiring routinely about psychosocial difficulties during medical visits and normalizing the use of support services to improve quality of life. Patients who screen positive for distress merit more careful inquiry by the physician or nurse. Moreover, follow-up to determine whether psychosocial services were actually received is apt to have an appreciable impact on the uptake of referrals. Finally, coordination of care between physicians and psychosocial clinicians may help ensure timely sharing of important information and minimize redundancy of services or inadequate symptom control. Each of these strategies (i.e., identifying needs, linking patients with psychosocial resources, tracking whether care was received, and coordination of care) is among the prominent recommendations advocated by the Institute of Medicine (2008).

Quality Improvement Processes

Guidelines for quality care are still evolving. Several organizations have issued standards or position statements for psychosocial care in oncology (e.g., National Comprehensive Cancer Network, 2008; American Society of Clinical Oncology/Oncology Nursing Society, Neuss et al., 2013). Most notably, the American College of Surgeons Commission on Cancer (2012) requires accredited cancer centers to provide on-site screening and referral for psychosocial concerns. To implement this requirement, the American Psychosocial Oncology Society (Lazenby, Tan, Pasacreta, Ercolano, & McCorkle, 2015) has recommended a five-step process, which is consistent with the care pathways we outlined earlier. These recommendations include:

1. Brief screening at nodal intervals (e.g., using one of the standardized instruments discussed above)
2. Evaluation for those who screen positive (e.g., assessing the scope of distress, current symptoms, mental health history, suicidal ideation, medication use, etc.)
3. Referral based on assessment findings (e.g., linking participants to mental health services, social work, pastoral care, etc.)
4. Follow-up (e.g., ensuring that patients who screen positive receive appropriate assessment, that those who are referred for services actually receive them, and that outcomes are monitored for any needed modifications in care)
5. Documentation of each of these steps in the medical record

Quality improvement initiatives can track these indicators (e.g., proportion of patients screened, proportion of positive screens that are followed by an assessment, proportion of those assessed who receive referral), to identify processes that require further attention or revision (Lazenby, Ercolano, et al., 2015).

Quality improvement projects might also track administration of outcome measures to help assess treatment response. Of course, outcome assessments should be consistent with the goals of the intervention; they should also be sensitive to change. Given the diverse range of concerns for which patients or family members seek help, it is unlikely that a single measure will be appropriate for all purposes (e.g., depression, existential concerns, family problems, spiritual uncertainties, etc.). Some programs may wish to establish a preferred toolkit of relevant outcome assessments, which encompass the most common presenting problems.

Conclusions

Advanced cancer patients and their families face considerable demands. They confront an uncertain future and difficult changes in many facets of day-to-day life. Mental health clinicians can offer vital contributions. The importance of psychosocial services in oncology has gained growing recognition, formalized in an expanding number of health-care standards and practice guidelines. A range of interventions, varying in intensity and tailored to individual needs, are available to assist patients and their families as they transition through the challenges of progressive illness and end-of-life care. In the coming years, we anticipate continued innovation in the structure of these services and greater integration within routine multidisciplinary cancer care.

References

American College of Surgeons. (2012). *Cancer program standards 2012: Ensuring patient-centered care*. Chicago, IL. Retrieved from http://www.facs.org/cancer/coc/cocprogramstandards2012.pdf

Ando, M., Morita, T., Akechi, T., & Okamoto, T. (2010). Efficacy of short-term life-review interviews on the spiritual well-being of terminally ill cancer patients. *Journal of Pain and Symptom Management, 39*, 993–1002.

Arch, J. J., & Mitchell, J. L. (2016). An acceptance and commitment therapy (ACT) group intervention for cancer survivors experiencing anxiety at re-entry. *Psycho-Oncology, 25*, 610–615.

Beck, A. T., Steer, R. A., & Brown, G. K. (1996). *Manual for the Beck depression inventory-II*. San Antonio, TX: Psychological Corporation.

Bjelland, I., Dahl, A. A., Haug, T. T., & Neckelmann, D. (2002). The validity of the hospital anxiety and depression scale: An updated literature review. *Journal of Psychosomatic Research, 52*, 69–77.

Breitbart, W., Poppito, S., Rosenfeld, B., Vickers, A. J., Li, Y., Abbey, J., … Cassileth, B. R. (2012). Pilot randomized controlled trial of individual meaning-centered psychotherapy for patients with advanced cancer. *Journal of Clinical Oncology, 30*, 1304–1309.

Breitbart, W., Rosenfeld, B., Pessin, H., Applebaum, A., Kulikowski, J., & Lichtenthal, W. G. (2015). Meaning-centered group psychotherapy: An effective intervention for improving psychological well-being in patients with advanced cancer. *Journal of Clinical Oncology*, *33*, 749–754.

Bruera, E., Kuehn, N., Miller, M. J., Selmser, P., & Macmillan, K. (1991). The Edmonton Symptom Assessment System (ESAS): A simple method for the assessment of palliative care patients. *Journal of Palliative Care*, *7*, 6–9.

Butow, P., Price, M. A., Shaw, J. M., Turner, J., Clayton, J. M., Grimison, P., … Kirsten, L. (2015). Clinical pathway for the screening, assessment, and management of anxiety and depression in adult cancer patients: Australian guidelines. *Psycho-Oncology*, *24*, 987–1001.

Carlson, L. E., Waller, A., Groff, S. L., Zhong, L., Bultz, B. D. (2012). Online screening for distress, the 6th vital sign, in newly diagnosed oncology outpatients: Randomised controlled trial of computerised vs. personalised triage. *British Journal of Cancer*, *107*, 617–625.

Chochinov, H. M., Kristjanson, L. J., Breitbart, W., McClement, S., Hack, T. F., Hassard, T., & Harlos, M. (2011). Effect of dignity therapy on distress and end-of-life experience in terminally ill patients: A randomised controlled trial. *Lancet Oncology*, *12*, 753–762.

Classen, C., Butler, L. D., Koopman, C., Miller, E., DiMiceli, S., Giese-Davis, J., … Spiegel, D. (2001). Supportive-expressive group therapy and distress in patients with metastatic breast cancer: A randomized clinical intervention trial. *Archives of General Psychiatry*, *58*, 494–501.

Cleeland, C. S. (1989). Measurement of pain by subjective report. In C. R. Chapman & J. D. Loeser (Eds.), *Issues in pain measurement* (pp. 391–403). New York: Raven Press.

Cleeland, C. S., Mendoza, T. R., Wang, X. S., Chou, C., Harle, M. T., Morrissey, M., & Engstrom, M. C. (2000). Assessing symptom distress in cancer patients. *Cancer*, *89*, 1634–1646.

Coyne, J. C. (2013). Benefits of screening cancer patients for distress still not demonstrated. *British Journal of Cancer*, *108*, 736–737.

Delgado-Guay, M., Parsons, H. A., Li, Z., Palmer, J. L., & Bruera, E. (2009). Symptom distress in advanced cancer patients with anxiety and depression in the palliative care setting. *Supportive Care in Cancer*, *17*, 573–579.

Derogatis, L. R. (2000). *The Brief-Symptom-Inventory-18 (BSI-18): Administration, scoring and procedures manual*. Minneapolis, MN: National Computer Systems.

DiMatteo, M. R., Lepper, H. D., & Croghan, T. W. (2000). Depression is a risk factor for noncompliance with medical treatment: Meta-analysis of the effects of anxiety and depression on patient adherence. *Archives of Internal Medicine*, *160*, 2101–2107.

Dudgeon, D., King, S., Howell, D., Green, E., Gilbert, J., Hughes, E., … Sawka, C. (2012). Cancer Care Ontario's experience with implementation of routine physical and psychological symptom distress screening. *Psycho-Oncology*, *21*, 357–364.

Fallowfield, L., Ratcliffe, D., Jenkins, V., & Saul, J. (2001). Psychiatric morbidity and its recognition by doctors in patients with cancer. *British Journal of Cancer*, *84*, 1011–1015.

Garssen, B., & de Kok, E. (2008). How useful is a screening instrument? *Psycho-Oncology*, *17*, 726–728.

Groenvold, M., Petersen, M. A., Aaronson, N. K., Arraras, J. I., Blazeby, J. M., Bottomley, A., … EORTC Quality of Life Group. (2006). The development of the EORTC QLQ-C15-PAL: A shortened questionnaire for cancer patients in palliative care. *European Journal of Cancer*, *42*, 55–64.

Hart, S. L., Hoyt, M. A., Diefenbach, M., Anderson, D. R., Kilbourn, K. M., Craft, L. L., … Stanton, A. L. (2012). Meta-analysis of efficacy of interventions for elevated depressive symptoms in adults diagnosed with cancer. *Journal of the National Cancer Institute*, *104*, 990–1004.

Hodges, L. J., Humphris, G. M., & Macfarlane, G. (2005). A meta-analytic investigation of the relationship between the psychological distress of cancer patients and their carers. *Social Science and Medicine*, *60*, 1–12.

Institute of Medicine. (2008). *Cancer care for the whole patient: Meeting psychosocial health needs*. Washington, D.C.: National Academy Press.

Janssen, A., Shaw, T., Nagrial, A., Pene, C., Rabbets, M., Carlino, M., … Harnett, P. (2016). An online learning module to increase self-efficacy and involvement in care for patients with advanced lung cancer: Research protocol. *Journal of Medical Internet Research Research Protocols*, *5*, e147.

Johannsen, M., O'Connor, M., O'Toole, M. S., Jensen, A. B., Højris, I., & Zachariae, R. (2016). Efficacy of mindfulness-based cognitive therapy on late post-treatment pain in women treated for primary breast cancer: A randomized controlled trial. *Journal of Clinical Oncology*, *34*, 3390–3399.

Julião, M., Oliveira, F., Nunes, B., Vaz Carneiro, A., & Barbosa, A. (2014). Efficacy of dignity therapy on depression and anxiety in Portuguese terminally ill patients: A phase II randomized controlled trial. *Journal of Palliative Medicine*, *17*, 688–695.

Kabat-Zinn, J. (1990). *Full catastrophe living: Using the wisdom of your body and mind to face stress, pain, and illness*. New York: Delacorte Press.

Kissane, D. W., Grabsch, B., Clarke, D. M., Smith, G. C., Love, A. W., Bloch, S., … Li, Y. (2007). Supportive-expressive group therapy for women with metastatic breast cancer: Survival and psychosocial outcome from a randomized controlled trial. *Psycho-Oncology*, *16*, 277–286.

Kitagawa, R., Yasui-Furukori, N., Tsushima, T., Kaneko, S., & Fukuda, I. (2011). Depression increases the length of hospitalization for patients undergoing thoracic surgery: A preliminary study. *Psychosomatics, 52*, 428–432.

Kornblith, A. B., Dowell, J. M., Herndon, J. E., II, Engelman, B. J., Bauer-Wu, S., Small, E. J., … Holland, J. C. (2006). Telephone monitoring of distress in patients aged 65 years or older with advanced stage cancer. *Cancer, 107*, 2706–2714.

Krebber, A.-M., Leemans, C. R., de Bree, R., van Straten, A., Smit, F., Smit, E. F., … Verdonck-de Leeuw, I. M. (2012). Stepped care targeting psychological distress in head and neck and lung cancer patients: A randomized clinical trial. *BioMed Central Cancer, 12*, 173.

Kroenke, K., Spitzer, R. L., & Williams, J. B. W. (2001). The PHQ-9: Validity of a brief depression severity measure. *Journal of General Internal Medicine, 9*, 606–613.

Kroenke, K., Spitzer, R. L., & Williams, J. B. (2003). The Patient Health Questionnaire-2: Validity of a two-item depression screener. *Medical Care, 41*, 1284–1292.

Langford, D. J., Lee, K., & Miakowski, C. (2012). Sleep disturbance interventions in oncology patients and family caregivers: A comprehensive review and meta-analysis. *Sleep Medicine Reviews, 16*, 397–414.

Lazenby, M., Ercolano, E., Grant, M., Holland, J. C., Jacobsen, P. B., & McCorkle, R. (2015). Supporting commission on cancer-mandated psychosocial distress screening with implementation strategies. *Journal of Oncology Practice, 11*, e413–e420.

Lazenby, M., Tan, H., Pasacreta, N., Ercolano, E., & McCorkle, R. (2015). The five steps of comprehensive psychosocial distress screening. *Current Oncology Reports, 17*, 22.

Lee, J.-Y., Jung, D., Kim, W.-H., Lee, H.-J., Noh, D.-Y., & Ham, B.-J. (2016). Correlates of oncologist-issued referrals for psycho-oncology services: What we learned from the electronic voluntary screening and referral system for depression (eVSRS-D). *Psycho-Oncology, 25*, 170–178.

Lyons, K. D., Bakitas, M., Hegel, M. T., Hanscom, B., Hull, J., & Ahles, T. A. (2009). Reliability and validity of the Functional Assessment of Chronic Illness Therapy-Palliative care (FACIT-Pal) scale. *Journal of Pain and Symptom Management, 37*, 23–32.

Mercadante, S., Vitrano, V., & Catania, V. (2010). Sexual issues in early and late stage cancer: A review. *Supportive Care in Cancer, 18*, 659–665.

Mitchell, A. J. (2007). Pooled results from 38 analyses of the accuracy of Distress Thermometer and other ultra-short methods for detecting cancer-related mood disorders. *Journal of Clinical Oncology, 25*, 4670–4681.

Mitchell, A. J., Chan, M., Bhatti, H., Halton, M., Grassi, L., Johansen, C., & Meader, N. (2011). Prevalence of depression, anxiety, and adjustment disorder in oncological, haematological, and palliative-care settings: A meta-analysis of 94 interview-based studies. *Lancet Oncology, 12*, 160–174.

Mitchell, A. J., Meader, N., Davies, E., Clover, K., Carter, G. L., Loscalzo, M. J., … Zabora, J. (2012). Meta-analysis of screening and case finding tools for depression in cancer: Evidence based recommendations for clinical practice on behalf of the Depression in Cancer Care consensus group. *Journal of Affective Disorders, 140*, 149–160.

National Comprehensive Care Network. (2008). *Distress Management. NCCN Clinical Practice Guidelines in Oncology National Comprehensive Cancer Network.* Retrieved from https://www.nccn.org/professoinals/physician_gls/pdf/distress.pdf

Neuss, M. N., Polovich, M., McNiff, K., Esper, P., Gilmore, T. R., LeFebvre, K. B., … Jacobson, J. O. (2013). 2013 updated American Society of Clinical Oncology/Oncology Nursing Society chemotherapy administration safety standards including standards for the safe administration and management of oral chemotherapy. *Journal of Oncology Practice, 9*(2 Suppl), 5s–13s.

Okuyama, S., Jones, W., & Tran, Z. V. (2015). Psychosocial telephone interventions for patients with cancer and survivors: A systematic review. *Psycho-Oncology, 24*, 857–870.

Parker, K. P., Bliwise, D. L., Ribeiro, M., Jain, S. R., Vena, C. I., Kohles-Baker, M. K., … Harris, W. B. (2008). Sleep/Wake patterns of individuals with advanced cancer measured by ambulatory polysomnography. *Journal of Clinical Oncology, 26*, 2464–2472.

Piet, J., Würtzen, H., & Zachariae, R. (2012). The effect of mindfulness-based therapy on symptoms of anxiety and depression in adult cancer patients and survivors: A systematic review and meta-analysis. *Journal of Consulting and Clinical Psychology, 80*, 1007–1020.

Pollak, K. I., Arnold, R. M., Jeffreys, A. S., Alexander, S. C., Olsen, M. K., Abernethy, A. P., … Tulsky, J. A. (2007). Oncologist communication about emotion during visits with patients with advanced cancer. *Journal of Clinical Oncology, 25*, 5748–5542.

Qaseem, A., Snow, V., Shekelle, P., Casey, D. E., Jr., Cross, J. T., Jr., Owens, D. K., … Shekelle, P. (2008). Evidence-based interventions to improve the palliative care of pain, dyspnea, and depression at the end of life: A clinical practice guideline from the American College of Physicians. *Annals of Internal Medicine, 148*, 141–146.

Radloff, L. S. (1977). The CESD scale: A self report scale for research in the general population. *Applied Psychological Measurement, 1*, 385–401.

Ryan, D. A., Gallagher, P., Wright, S., & Cassidy, E. M. (2012). Sensitivity and specificity of the Distress Thermometer and a two-item depression screen (Patient Health Questionnaire-2) with a "help" question for psychological distress and psychiatric morbidity in patients with advanced cancer. *Psycho-Oncology, 21*, 1275–1284.

Savard, M.-H., Savard, J., Simard, S., & Ivers, H. (2005). Empirical validation of the insomnia severity index in cancer patients. *Psycho-Oncology, 14*, 429–441.

Savard, J., Simard, S., Giguère, I., Ivers, H., Morin, C. M., Maunsell, E., … Marceau, D. (2006). Randomized clinical trial on cognitive therapy for depression in women with metastatic breast cancer: Psychological and immunological effects. *Palliative and Supportive Care*, *4*, 219–237.

Seow, H., Barbera, L., Sutradhar, R., Howell, D., Dudgeon, D., Atzema, C., … Earle, C. (2011). Trajectory of performance status and symptom scores for patients with cancer during the last six months of life. *Journal of Clinical Oncology*, *29*, 1151–1158.

Sheinfeld Gorin, S. S., Krebs, P., Badr, H., Janke, E. A., Jim, H. S. L., Spring, B., … Jacobsen, P. B. (2012). Meta-analysis of psychosocial interventions to reduce pain in patients with cancer. *Journal of Clinical Oncology*, *30*, 539–547.

Sherman, A. C., Merluzzi, T. V., Pustejovsky, J. E., Park, C. L., George, L., Fitchett, G., … Salsman, J. M. (2015). A meta-analytic review of religious or spiritual involvement and social health among cancer patients. *Cancer*, *121*, 3779–3788.

Sherman, A. C., & Simonton, S. (2001). Coping with cancer in the family. *The Family Journal*, *9*, 193–200.

Simonton, S., & Sherman, A. (2000). An integrated model of group treatment for cancer patients. *International Journal of Group Psychotherapy*, *50*, 487–506.

Spitzer, R. L., Kroenke, K., Williams, J. B., & Löwe, B. (2006). A brief measure for assessing generalized anxiety disorder: The GAD-7. *Archives of Internal Medicine*, *166*, 1092–1097.

Steinhauser, K. E., Alexander, S. C., Byock, I. R., George, L. K., Olsen, M. K., & Tulsky, J. A. (2008). Do preparation and life completion discussions improve functioning and quality of life in seriously ill patients? Pilot randomized controlled trial. *Journal of Palliative Medicine*, *11*, 1234–1240.

Teno, J. M., Fisher, E. S., Hamel, M. B., Coppola, K., & Dawson, N. V. (2002). Medical care inconsistent with patients' treatment goals: Association with 1-year Medicare resource use and survival. *Journal of the American Geriatric Society*, *50*, 496–500.

Tuinman, M. A., Van Nuenen, F. M., Hagedoorn, M., & Hoekstra-Weebers, J. E. H. M. (2015). Distress, problems and referral wish of cancer patients: Differences according to relationship status and life phase. *Psycho-Oncology*, *24*, 699–704.

Turner, J., Kelly, B., Clarke, D., Yates, P., Aranda, S., Jolley, D., … McFadyen, L. (2011). A randomized trial of a psychosocial intervention for cancer patients integrated into routine care: The PROMPT study (promoting optimal outcomes in mood through tailored psychosocial therapies). *BioMed Central Cancer*, *11*, 48.

van den Hurk, D. G., Schellekens, M. P., Molema, J., Speckens, A. E., & van der Drift, M. A. (2015). Mindfulness-based stress reduction for lung cancer patients and their partners: Results of a mixed methods pilot study. *Palliative Medicine*, *29*, 652–660.

Wadhwa, D., Burman, D., Swami, N., Rodin, G., Lo, C., & Zimmermann, C. (2013). Quality of life and mental health in caregivers of outpatients with advanced cancer. *Psycho-Oncology*, *22*, 403–410.

Weeks, J. C., Catalano, P. J., Cronin, A., Finkelman, M. D., Mack, J. W., Keating, N. L., … Schrag, D. (2012). Patient's expectations about effects of chemotherapy for advanced cancer. *New England Journal of Medicine*, *267*, 1616–1625.

Wright, A. A., Zhang, B., Ray, A., Mack, J. W., Trice, E., Balboni, T., … Prigerson, H. G. (2008). Associations between end-of-life discussions, patient mental health, medical care near death, and caregiver bereavement adjustment. *Journal of the American Medical Association*, *300*, 1665–1673.

Yellen, S. B., Cella, D. F., Webster, K., Blendowski, C., & Kaplan, E. (1997). Measuring fatigue and other anemia-related symptoms with the Functional Assessment of Cancer Therapy (FACT) measurement system. *Journal of Pain and Symptom Management*, *13*, 63–74.

Zernicke, K. A., Campbell, T. S., Speca, M., McCabe-Ruff, K., Flowers, S., & Carlson, L. E. (2014). A randomized wait-list controlled trial of feasibility and efficacy of an online mindfulness-based cancer recovery program: The eTherapy for cancer applying mindfulness trial. *Psychosomatic Medicine*, *76*, 257–267.

4 Alcohol and Other Substance Misuse

John M. Ray and Michael A. Cucciare

A Brief Description of the Problem

Recently, the American Psychiatric Association (APA) published the fifth edition of the *Diagnostic and Statistical Manual of Mental Disorders (DSM-5)* with simplified diagnostic criteria for alcohol use disorder (AUD) and substance use disorder (SUD), eliminating the terms "abuse" and "dependence" and providing for a general estimate of severity, from mild to severe, based on the number of symptom criteria endorsed by the patient (American Psychiatric Association, 2013). As this change in criteria is relatively new, it is not yet widely reflected in how alcohol and drug use disorders are defined in the literature. Much of the current research on alcohol and other drug use is based on diagnostic criteria from the fourth edition of the DSM (American Psychiatric Association, 2000), which defined substance abuse as a maladaptive pattern of substance use leading to clinically significant impairment or distress occurring within a 12-month period, as manifested by one or more criteria related to negative consequences of use, including negative impact on major life roles, use in dangerous situations (e.g., driving), legal problems, and social and interpersonal problems. Dependence is defined in the DSM-IV as a maladaptive pattern of substance use leading to clinically significant impairment or distress occurring within a 12-month period, as manifested by three or more criteria including tolerance, withdrawal, using more or for longer than intended, and a persistent desire to use or unsuccessful efforts to cut down. The relationship between DSM-IV and DSM-5 disorders is not exact, but substance abuse is comparable to substance use disorder, mild subtype, whereas substance dependence is similar to the moderate to severe subtype.

According to the most recent data from the National Survey on Drug Use and Health (NSDUH), which uses DSM-IV criteria, approximately 12.3% of young adults aged 18–25, and 5.9% of adults aged 26 or older, had an alcohol use disorder in the past year. These numbers represent approximately 4.3 and 12 million people in the USA, respectively. The percentage of those reporting an illicit drug use disorder was 6.6% for young adults and 1.9% for adults aged 26 or older, representing 2.3 and 3.9 million people in the USA, respectively. Approximately 2.6% of

J.M. Ray, Ph.D. (✉) • M.A. Cucciare, Ph.D.
Center for Mental Healthcare and Outcomes Research, Central Arkansas Veterans Affairs Healthcare System, North Little Rock, AR, USA

Department of Psychiatry, University of Arkansas for Medical Sciences, Little Rock, AR, USA

VA South Central Mental Illness Research, Education, and Clinical Center, Central Arkansas Veterans Healthcare System,
North Little Rock, AR, USA
e-mail: john.ray2@va.gov; Michael.cucciare@va.gov

A. Maragakis, W.T. O'Donohue (eds.), *Principle-Based Stepped Care and Brief Psychotherapy for Integrated Care Settings*, https://doi.org/10.1007/978-3-319-70539-2_4

young adults and 0.7% of adults aged 26 and older met criteria for both alcohol and substance use disorder. Many people use alcohol or other drugs in a way that places them at risk for use-related problems and disorder, even though they may not currently meet diagnostic criteria for a disorder. The APA's focus on severity for DSM-5 underscores the importance of recognizing that alcohol and drug use falls along a spectrum, the range of which includes use that does not meet criteria for use disorder but may nonetheless be unhealthy.

Broadly, the phrase "substance misuse" is frequently used to refer to a spectrum, ranging from unhealthy substance use to use that meets diagnostic criteria for SUD, whereas terms referring to the use of specific substances vary by substance type.

Regarding alcohol, the National Institute on Alcohol Abuse and Alcoholism (NIAAA) recommends no more than two standard drinks (12 oz. beer or wine cooler; 5 oz. of wine; 1.5 oz. of spirits) per day for men and no more than one for women, a pattern of use they define as moderate (National Institute of Alcohol Abuse and Alcoholism, 2016). Low-risk drinking is defined as no more than 14 drinks per week and no more than 4 per occasion for men, while for women, low-risk drinking is defined as no more than 7 per week and no more than 3 per occasion. Heavy drinking includes that which exceeds the definition of low-risk drinking. Binge drinking is defined as drinking five or more drinks for men and four or more for women on a single occasion. People who drink heavily and those who binge drink have a significantly higher risk of experiencing negative alcohol-related health and life consequences. For the purposes of this chapter, alcohol consumption that is greater than low-risk but does not meet diagnostic criteria for an AUD is termed "unhealthy drinking," whereas drinking that meets DSM-IV criteria for abuse or dependence, or DSM-5 criteria for alcohol use disorder, is referred to as AUD.

In terms of drug use, there is no recommended level of use. Rather, the term "substance misuse" may be used to signify drug use that falls outside of its intended purpose, such as in the case of prescription drugs. For the purposes of this chapter, drug use that does not meet diagnostic criteria is termed "unhealthy substance use," whereas use that meets DSM-IV criteria for abuse or dependence, or DSM-5 criteria for a drug use disorder, is referred to as DUD.

Effective Ways to Screen for Substance Misuse in the Primary Care Setting

The US Preventive Services Task Force (USPSTF) recommends that primary care clinicians screen adults for alcohol misuse, which it defines as a range of drinking behaviors that includes risky or hazardous alcohol use, harmful alcohol use, and alcohol abuse or dependence (Moyer, 2013). The task force does not recommend for or against such screening practices for adolescents, citing insufficient research evidence for its effectiveness with this population, though research is ongoing. The USPSTF recommends three alcohol misuse screening instruments for primary care settings, which are described below followed by a brief selection of other commonly used screeners.

The most recent USPSTF review of primary care screening for illicit drug use made no recommendation for or against screening for drug misuse in primary care, citing insufficient evidence that the practice improves outcomes (Polen, Whitlock, Wisdom, Nygren, & Bougatsos, 2008). Researchers stress that absence of evidence does not mean evidence of absence and that exploration of drug use with patients in primary care should remain a priority as research continues to develop and test new screening methods for unhealthy drug use (Hingson & Compton, 2014). Given the high prevalence of drug misuse and associated morbidity in primary care populations, and because primary care physicians are in a unique position to recognize patients with problematic use and intervene when appropriate, screening in this setting may be justified.

Ideally, a screening instrument should be brief, easy to administer, and psychometrically sound, to include being both reliable and valid.

For example, validity concerns an instrument's ability to measure what it purports to measure and for a screener is often measured by comparing its results to those of a thorough diagnostic assessment and obtaining the sensitivity (probability that the screening test will be positive among those who have the disorder) and specificity (probability that the screening test will be negative among those who do not have the disorder) of the screener. A valid instrument works as a function of both sensitivity and specificity. Though a highly sensitive screener will identify most or all subjects who have the disorder, it may also identify some without the disorder as having it (false positive).

Screening for Alcohol Misuse

The Alcohol Use Disorder Identification Test (AUDIT). The AUDIT was developed by the World Health Organization (WHO) for healthcare practitioners as a simple screener for unhealthy drinking (Babor, Higgins-Biddle, Saunders, & Monteiro, 2001). The AUDIT has been adapted to a wide range of purposes, including as a screen for hazardous drinking and a potential indicator of alcohol dependence. It is a ten-item instrument that can be administered as a questionnaire or as an interview. The content of the AUDIT consists of items assessing for alcohol consumption (e.g., quantity and frequency), indicators of alcohol dependence (e.g., difficulty controlling drinking), and alcohol-related problems (e.g., drinking-related guilt or remorse). Items are scored on a 0–4 scale, where 0 equals "never" and 4 equals "daily or almost daily" for most items. Total scores of 8 or greater are considered to be indicative of hazardous or harmful drinking, although the AUDIT manual recommends that the cutoff be chosen by the clinician based on national and cultural standards, as well as clinical judgment.

The AUDIT is psychometrically sound (Reinert & Allen, 2007), yielding test-retest reliability in the 0.70–0.89 range using a cutoff score of 8 to dichotomously classify respondents as positive or negative for hazardous drinking. The AUDIT has strong validity, with adequate to excellent sensitivity and specificity across a range of studies. A recent review of the research (de Meneses-Gaya, Zuardi, Loureiro, & Crippa, 2009) found that the measure appears to be appropriate for various subgroups, with a few caveats. For example, it has yielded lower sensitivities and higher specificities among women than men, leading to the recommendation that a lower cutoff of 5 be used for female respondents. Studies of adolescents have suggested that a lower cutoff of 2–3 be used for this subgroup. Among older adults (i.e., ≥65), the AUDIT does not appear to be accurate, leading researchers to recommend a multi-method approach to screening for at-risk and harmful drinking in older adults. The AUDIT appears to perform well among varying ethnic groups, although it may be affected by level of acculturation among Hispanics. Finally, the AUDIT appears to function effectively among people with severe mental illness, including as a means of distinguishing patients with a primary diagnosis of alcohol use disorder from those with primary psychiatric diagnoses.

At ten items, the AUDIT can be burdensome in some settings, leading to the development of the AUDIT-C, so named because it is comprised solely of the AUDIT's three consumption items. The AUDIT-C is scored the same way as the full measure, with a total possible score of 12, hazardous drinking cutoff scores of 4 for men and 3 for women, and a score of 8 or greater suggesting high probability of alcohol dependence (Rubinsky et al., 2012). It appears to perform well among those with comorbid psychiatric disorders and across ethnicities, and like the full measure, less well among the elderly, although there is a need for more research on the AUDIT-C to clarify its utility among subgroups.

Single-item screening questions (SISQ). The USPSTF also recommends single-item screening questions (SISQ), which have adequate sensitivity and specificity across the alcohol misuse spectrum and can be delivered very quickly. For example, NIAAA recommends a single-item screen for unhealthy alcohol use, which asks, "How many times in the past year have you had

X or more drinks in a day?" (where X is 5 for men and 4 for women, and a response of ≥1 is considered positive). A validation study (Smith, Schmidt, Allensworth-Davies, & Saitz, 2009) of this single-item screener, as delivered by an interviewer, yielded moderate sensitivity (87.9%) for AUD, but low to moderate specificity (66.8%). The item performed less well in terms of sensitivity (81.8%) for unhealthy use, but better in terms of specificity (79.3%).

There are reasons a primary care setting may warrant a self-administered SISQ, as opposed to interview, including threat to fidelity when delivered outside the research context, difficulty of incorporating the interview mode in the clinical environment, and the potential for patient discomfort answering SUD-related questions face-to-face with a provider. A recent study (McNeely & Saitz, 2015) examined the utility of the NIAAA alcohol SISQ, as well as a version modified to screen for drug use, delivered as a self-administered instrument on a touchscreen tablet computer and found modest decrements in sensitivity (73.3–87.8% for alcohol, 71.3–85.1% for drugs) and comparable specificity (74.2–84.7% for alcohol, 86.0–94.3% for drugs), when compared to an in-person interview. The authors argued that the small decrease in accuracy should be considered against the potential benefits of the self-administered version of the SISQ, including pre-encounter screening, maintenance of fidelity, and more open disclosure.

The CAGE. Although not specifically recommended by the USPSTF, the most well-known and commonly used screener for unhealthy alcohol use is the CAGE instrument. It is simple and straightforward, and considered to have adequate psychometric properties, making it a popular choice among primary care physicians as an initial step before more complex assessment. The CAGE consists of four questions, each focused on a drinking-related problem. The first letter of the problem addressed by each item comprises the acronym for which the instrument is named: (1) "Have you ever felt you ought to **C**ut down on your drinking?"; (2) "Have people **A**nnoyed you by criticizing your drinking?"; (3) "Have you ever felt bad or **G**uilty about your drinking?"; and (4) "Have you ever had a drink in the morning to steady your nerves or get rid of a hangover (**E**ye opener)?". Limitations of the CAGE include poor psychometrics among women and college students, as well as heavier drinkers, for whom the AUDIT appears to be better suited.

Screening for Drug Use and Misuse

As noted above, to date, there remains a debate as to whether brief interventions, such as Screening, Brief Intervention, and Referral to Treatment, are effective for reducing drug use (Gryczynski et al., 2015; Roy-Byrne et al., 2014; Saitz et al., 2015). However, for clinics interested in screening for drug misuse, the National Institute on Drug Abuse (NIDA) recommends a single-item screener, "How many times in the past year have you used an illegal drug or used a prescription medication for nonmedical reasons?". This item has been validated in primary care (Smith, Schmidt, Allensworth-Davies, & Saitz, 2010), yielding high sensitivity (100%) and moderate specificity (73.5%) for the detection of a DUD. The item performed well for current drug use, as well, yielding 92.9% sensitivity and 94.1% specificity. A positive response to the single-item drug use screen places the patient in an at-risk category and indicates the need for a follow-up assessment, including identification of specific drugs used, quantity and frequency of use, and extent of problems related to use.

The ten-item Drug Abuse Screening Test (DAST 10). A still brief but more comprehensive screening instrument, such as the abbreviated Drug Abuse Screening Test (DAST 10) can help determine whether a DUD diagnosis is warranted. The DAST 10 is a briefer version of the 28-item DAST, which was designed as a variation of the Michigan Alcoholism Screening Test based on the observation of similarities between alcohol and drug abusers. It is scored similarly, using dichotomous (yes/no) responses but without weighting, so that items endorsed in the direction of elevated drug use problems are rated as a 1 for a total summed score range of 0–10. A score of 1–2 is indicative of hazardous use, suggesting monitoring and reassessment at a later date. A score of 3–5 suggests harmful use and warrants further investigation. Scores on the DAST of 6 or greater indicate a need for more intensive assessment to determine whether a DUD is present. Psychometric studies of the DAST and its alternate versions have found the measure to be sound, yielding internal consistency between 0.74 and 0.94 and test-retest reliability in the 0.71–0.89 range using the recommended cutoff of six (Yudko, Lozhkina, & Fouts, 2007). In terms of validity, the DAST has also fared well, yielding adequate to good sensitivity (81–96%) and specificity (71–94%) across a range of studies and populations, including adults seeking drug treatment, psychiatric inpatients and outpatients, female inmates, union members, and adolescents admitted to a crisis intervention unit.

The Alcohol, Smoking and Substance Involvement Screening Test—Drug Version (ASSIST-Drug). The ASSIST-Drug is a two-item instrument for drug use screening based on a revision of items from the Alcohol, Smoking and Substance Involvement Screening Test (ASSIST). The ASSIST was developed in response to a call by the World Health Organization for a screener similar to the AUDIT that could be used for a wide range of substances. Although the ASSIST has been recommended by both NIDA and Substance Abuse and Mental Health Services Administration, it has not been widely adopted in primary care settings, likely because it is relatively lengthy and may be difficult to administer in busy primary care clinics (Ali, Meena, Eastwood, Richards, & Marsden, 2013). The ASSIST-Drug's first item asks about frequency of drug use: "How many days in the past 12 months have you used drugs?". A response of 2 or more days meets criterion for drug use disorder (94.1% sensitive, 89.6% specific), in which case the second question is not needed. The second question asks about consequences: "How many days in the past 12 months have you had a strong desire or urge to use drugs?". A response of 5 or more days is indicative of drug use-related negative consequences (89.8% sensitive, 91.9% specific). Strengths of the ASSIST-Drug include reliability, comparable validity to longer measures (e.g., the ASSIST), the use of a time frame consistent with DSM and ICD, brevity and ease of scoring, and the measure's continuous response format, which allows the adjustment of cut points, and thus the sensitivity and specificity of the instrument, to match the needs of the clinical setting.

How to Further Assess for SUDs if a Screen Returns Positive

In the event of a positive screen, a careful clinical interview should follow. A more intensive assessment may not be feasible for clinics with few resources, in which case referral may be the most appropriate option (see below for a discussion of referral). For clinics with the necessary resources (e.g., a colocated mental health provider is on the premises), a comprehensive assessment should include detailed lifetime and current alcohol or drug use history, symptoms of AUD or DUD based on either DSM-5 or ICD10 criteria, use of other substances, and instances of alcohol-related harm to physical or mental health, including social, interpersonal, and work-related consequences. Practitioners should also assess the patient's level of insight into the role of alcohol or drug use consumption in the problems reported, as well as his or her motivation to change their substance use. Information about past and current mental health symptoms, diagnoses, and treatment should also be obtained, including previous treatment for SUDs or other past disorders and outcomes. Physical examination may also be warranted, for example, when the provider suspects acute intoxication (e.g., slurred speech, ataxia) or withdrawal (e.g., anxiety, agitation, hallucination, hand tremors). In the latter case, medical detoxification for substance use may be needed prior to treatment. In severe cases, a neurological examination can help to identify Wernicke's encephalopathy (confusion, tremors, involuntary eye movements) or acute intracranial lesion (e.g., pupillary asymmetry). A mental status examination can help to identify cognitive signs of alcohol use disorder, such as impaired orientation and short-term memory.

Evidence-Based Stepped Care and Brief Psychotherapeutic Approaches for Substance Misuse

The following sections describe commonly used evidence-based interventions for substance misuse, ranging from least to most resource intensive. Stepped care, from initiation to adjustment to maintenance, will be guided not only by patient and provider factors but also by resources available at the clinic. Typically, changes will be made from one intensity level to another, although changes within intensity level also may be warranted. If a patient and provider determine that a current treatment is ineffective, a move to a different but equally intensive treatment may be chosen. For instance, a decision may be made for a patient to participate in a mutual self-help group such as AA, and he or she may then later decide that while mutual self-help is the appropriate level of treatment, the patient would like to switch to one that does not focus on a higher power.

Psychoeducation. The least resource intensive intervention available is psychoeducation, in which a patient might receive basic advice to reduce their substance use from a provider. Research shows that many people recover from problem alcohol and drug use after receiving feedback related to harmful effects of use, identification of use-related problems, relation to social norms, and information on available treatments and their effectiveness (O'Donnell et al., 2014). The patient should be asked to keep track of agreed-upon indices of use, such as quantity and frequency, to communicate these to the provider on future visits, and to make contact earlier if the patient sees the need due to, for example, increased use or related problems. Indeed, there is evidence to suggest that the simple act of recording one's use patterns can be enough to facilitate change (Michie et al., 2012). If the patient successfully reduces use to non-risky levels, continued check-ins at regular health appointments may be sufficient for monitoring substance use. Should the patient's use behavior remain unchanged or increase, a recommendation should be made to step up treatment to a more intensive level. Such decisions should be made collaboratively, based upon clear outcomes (e.g., days abstinent, number of drinks consumed), and take into account multiple factors, including research evidence, provider resources, and patient preferences.

Self-help and mutual-help groups. Mutual-help groups represent a low-resource, low-intensity intervention option that is known and acceptable to a wide range of potential patients. Many of these mutual-help groups, like AA and NA, follow 12-step approaches that focus on abstinence, as opposed to harm reduction, and involve a real or implied religious or spiritual component. Other mutual-help groups (e.g., SMART Recovery) are more closely aligned with evidence-based treatments such as CBT. Consideration of patient preference, then, is important in the recommendation of mutual-help groups, particularly since people who attend but do not embrace the central tenets of a mutual-help group are less likely to benefit from them (Moos & Timko, 2008). Thus, an assessment of patient motivation to change and to attend the mutual-help groups regularly, as well as an open discussion of the available options in the patient's community and information about how to learn more about them, can help to ensure a good fit. As with advice alone, the provider and patient should agree on clear goals with regard to changes in use behavior that can be discussed and evaluated for progress at future appointments.

Guided self-help. Bibliotherapy involves providing the patient with printed self-help materials to facilitate changes in alcohol or drug use. Some patients may benefit from having self-help materials provided to them in the clinic, which may alleviate some barriers to care related to motivation and access to materials (e.g., Internet) or logistics (e.g., transportation to meetings or libraries), among others. Such materials often utilize aspects of evidence-based therapies, such as monitoring use, developing relapse prevention plans, and identifying and tracking triggers for substance use. A meta-analysis of bibliotherapy interventions for drinking found that self-referred problem drinkers who received self-help materials reduced their drinking more than controls who received no materials and at least as much as individuals who participated in long-term face-to-face therapy (Apodaca & Miller, 2003). The VA's Bibliotherapy Resource Guide includes several resources related to substance use and abuse (available at http://www.mirecc.va.gov/docs/VA_Bibliotherapy_Resource_Guide.pdf).

Guided self-help can also be delivered via computer, allowing for the added benefit of real-time individual feedback from a program. Examples include AlcoholEdu (everfi.com/higher-education-old/alcoholedu), Check Your Drinking (checkyourdrinking.net), and NIAAA's Rethinking Drinking (rethinkingdrinking.niaaa.nih.gov). Most of the research on low-intensity computer- or Internet-based interventions has been conducted with university or student populations, and so care must be taken when applying these interventions to other populations. However, findings on the effectiveness of guided-self-help interventions suggest they be helpful for patients who use substances at a low to moderate level (White et al., 2010).

Screening, brief intervention, and referral to treatment. More intensive interventions may be warranted for the patient for whom lower-intensity approaches have not been successful. Screening, brief intervention, and referral to treatment, or SBIRT, is a public health approach to the identification of individuals who have developed or are at risk of developing SUD and may benefit from early intervention and treatment or referral to specialty programs, in the case of those with higher severity disorders. Intended to bridge the gap between primary prevention and more intensive specialty treatment, SBIRT's flexible design has allowed for its adaptation to a range of settings, including primary care, community-based clinical practices, and hospital emergency departments. The screening component of SBIRT involves brief assessment of substance use (as described above), after which a brief intervention or referral to treatment may follow, depending on severity of use and resources available. A discussion follows of some common brief intervention and referral approaches, along with measurement instruments and methods.

Motivational interviewing (MI). Motivational interviewing (MI) and motivational enhancement therapy (MET) are among the most well-known and studied brief interventions for alcohol and drug misuse. A primary goal of MI is to elicit and resolve ambivalence toward change in substance use (Miller & Rollnick, 2012). The focus of the MI approach is on establishing strong rapport by listening reflectively, asking open-ended questions to elicit the client's own motivations for change, affirming change-related statements and efforts (i.e., "change talk"), eliciting recognition of the gap between current behavior and desired life goals, asking permission before providing information or advice, "rolling with resistance," encouraging the client's self-efficacy for change, and developing an action plan to which the client is willing to commit. Advantages of MI include its brevity (as few as 1 session) and that it can be delivered over the phone (VanBuskirk & Wetherell, 2014). MET is a structured application of MI that includes patient-specific assessment, feedback, and change plans over a four-session course, although it is designed to be flexible with regard to number of sessions needed and can be offered as an extended treatment for patients who do not realize initial goals identified with a brief MI session.

Guided self-change. Guided self-change (GSC; Sobell & Sobell, 2005) is a brief intervention for substance use that combines MI with CBT. GSC can be delivered individually or in a group format, is patient-centered (number of sessions can be adjusted based on need), and allows patients to define treatment goals (abstinence or harm reduction). Patients who use substances but are not experiencing severe consequences or withdrawal symptoms are appropriate for GSC, which facilitates self-change through the application of motivational strategies such as advice-giving, removing barriers to change, and decreasing the attractiveness of drinking or drug use. One study found that a single brief session of GSC advice was as effective as four sessions of GSC in terms of alcohol-related outcomes, but that the four-session group reported significantly higher patient satisfaction (Andreasson, Hansagi, & Osterlund, 2002).

Relapse prevention. Relapse prevention is an intervention approach that can be integrated into any SUD treatment and which focuses on maintaining change over time for the individual who has made the decision to reduce or abstain from substance use. The most commonly used models of relapse prevention (Witkiewitz & Marlatt, 2004) help reduce the risk of relapse by identifying and addressing precipitants of relapse and developing a relapse intervention plan. Rather than a traditional view of relapse as failure, relapse is viewed as a natural dynamic process that can be learned from to reduce future relapse. Strategies used for reducing the risk of relapse include identifying cravings and triggers and using this information to plan for situations that may increase the likelihood of a relapse.

Medication/Pharmacotherapy. Pharmacotherapy is an evidence-based intervention for SUDs (excluding stimulants; Preti, 2007) and is considered to be a higher step in the stepped care model due to it being relatively invasive, costly, and because it carries a high risk of side effects. Medication, however, may be indicated for some primary care patients for the treatment of SUDs. For example, patients with a high degree of craving may benefit from medications that reduce these, such as bupropion for nicotine (Fiore et al., 2000) and methadone or buprenorphine for opiates (Mattick, Breen, Kimber, & Davoli, 2009). Evidence suggests naltrexone is safe, effective, and feasible for treatment of alcohol dependence in the primary care clinic, though it appears to be most effective as a response to relapse rather than in maintaining abstinence and should be administered in conjunction with counseling (Mann, 2004).

How to Make Decisions About "Stepping Up" Care

The general stepped care model is one in which, once identification of a clinical issue has occurred, patients are offered the least restrictive treatment option available and performance-based (i.e., treatment goal) progress is monitored. If satisfactory progress is not made, then the patient is bumped up to a more intensive treatment modality. As with all good treatment planning, the selection of treatment is a collaborative decision between the patient and provider in consideration of a range of important variables, including severity of symptomatology, preferences and motivation of the patient, and resources available. In this context it becomes clear that the most appropriate treatment for a patient may not be the least restrictive. At the same time, patients for whom a less restrictive approach is appropriate initially may experience changes in their presentation that necessitate updated assessment and consideration of a different tier of care, underscoring the importance of ongoing assessment and treatment goal progress monitoring. Regular contact with the patient allows for ongoing data collection to inform decisions about if and when to increase treatment intensity. A range of data sources can be used for this purpose, including those assessed at the screening and comprehensive evaluation (e.g., consumption indices, diagnostic symptom criteria, presence and severity of use-related consequences, and clinical judgment). Breslin et al. (1998) found that within-treatment drinking predicted drinking at 6 months posttreatment better than clinician prognoses did, emphasizing the important role of within-treatment drinking data in informing the decision to step up care to a more intense level of treatment.

Which Approaches Are Not Recommended

Unfortunately, the research on brief interventions for drug use is consistent with that on screening in that it lacks sufficient evidence to recommend either for or against its use (Roy-Byrne et al., 2014; Saitz, Cheng, Allensworth-Davies, Winter, & Smith, 2014). Rather, as with screening, the use of brief interventions for patients who screen positive for drug use in primary care is suggested to continue providing care or referral as the research tries to catch up and make a definitive recommendation (Hingson & Compton, 2014).

When to Refer to Specialty SUD Treatment

Instances in which referral to specialty SUD care may be indicated will vary by patient and clinic needs but will typically reflect the need for more intensive treatment than the primary care clinic can provide. For example, VA Clinical Practice Guidelines (Veterans Affairs/Department of Defense, 2009) recommend that the primary care team should offer referral to specialty SUD care if the patient is willing to engage in specialty care and may benefit from additional assessment or intervention that the primary care clinic is unable to provide, has been diagnosed with alcohol or SUD or has an AUDIT-C score greater than 8, and has significant medical or mental health comorbidities. Basic referral decision rules will be determined by the individual clinic's scope of practice, as well as the resources available. Many primary care clinical teams may refer any patient whose substance use exceeds a definition of at-risk use. Alternatively, providers may decide that, as opposed to use level, a patient's required level of intervention will determine whether referral is necessary. For example, a patient who exhibits problem drinking, high motivation, and the necessary coping skills to support change may respond to a brief intervention, whereas another patient with the same use level may not have these attributes or may have a history of unsuccessful brief intervention that suggests referral to a specialty clinic may be warranted. When referral is made will depend on both the level of care needed (e.g., lower level unsuccessful) and the expertise of providers in the clinic. When a patient crosses the threshold (e.g., fails to change use behavior, incurs continued consequences, or meets dependence in a clinic that isn't prepared to treat it), referral should be made.

Care should be taken with regard to referral from primary care to specialty SUD treatment. For instance, a recent meta-analysis of primary care screening, brief intervention, and referral to treatment found no evidence that the practice increases utilization of substance use treatment services (Glass et al., 2015). The authors noted the need for guidance for primary care clinics on referring patients to specialized SUD care. Patient and provider factors, such as stigma and lack of knowledge about treatment options, are potential barriers to the effective transition from primary care to SUD treatment. Research points to the potential for more intensive provider support to facilitate the transition. Evidence-based practices exist that could be utilized according to the clinic's level of available resources (Cucciare, Coleman, & Timko, 2015). As an example of low-intensity referral practice, Veterans Affairs practice guidelines recommend brief substance use counseling followed by discussion of the patient's preferences and expectations for treatment, education on available services, determination of readiness to change, and where feasible, collaborative care, including participation of colocated mental healthcare providers. Brief motivational interviewing may also facilitate transition. More intensive support might also be of benefit where appropriate, ranging from telephone monitoring to intensive case management.

The Role of the Primary Care Provider/Medical Team in Treatment

As outlined above, the primary care physician and medical team play a critical role in screening of and brief intervention for patients at risk for SUD and treatment or referral for patients with more serious problems and/or SUD. In addition, primary care providers should strive to foster a clinical environment conducive to factors that facilitate screening and brief interventions, such as the inclusion of mentors that can provide invaluable guidance in the often complex process of identifying and treating substance use in a medical setting. Effective primary care teams will be able to educate patients on available treatment options and support the patient in making appropriate treatment decisions, including transition (i.e., "the warm hand-off") to more intensive mental health or substance use treatment when necessary. Making sure the treatment team is knowledgeable about the logistics of substance use disorders, such as the intricacies of insurance and reimbursement issues, is also important.

It is essential to ensure that providers get appropriate training in screening, brief intervention, and referral. This may mean, for example, providing clinicians with paid time to attend training via local workshops that focus on skills training through the use of "hands-on" exercises such as role-playing with "standardized patients." Primary care clinics should be knowledgeable about and work closely with local specialty addiction treatment providers to ensure successful care transitions. A common barrier to effective transition from primary care to substance use treatment involves the referring provider's knowledge about availability and potential efficacy of the treatment to which the patient is referred (Cucciare et al., 2015). Primary care clinical teams' familiarity with available treatment resources for patients with use disorders will help ensure the referral is made with confidence, which in turn can help reduce stigma and doubt on the part of the patient. Knowing about available treatment resources, including those tailored for special populations, such as patients with comorbid chronic health conditions, and having a clear plan to access services, will facilitate patients' access to the system (Cucciare & Timko, 2015).

How to Assess Impact on Care/ Quality Improvement Processes

The process of assessing the impact of stepped care for substance misuse in primary care is challenging but not insurmountable. A recent review of recovery from substance use and mental disorders (Rapporteur, 2016) noted a wide variety of definitions of recovery ranging from simple yes/no assessment of abstinence to biological markers indicating continued use. The authors concluded that the most useful measures of substance misuse intervention effectiveness are comprehensive and multidimensional assessments that accurately capture a patient's place along the dynamic trajectory of recovery (e.g., abstinence or reduction of use, degree and frequency of relapse, improved quality of life). Whereas no validated measure currently exists that both meets these criteria and is feasible for the busy clinic (i.e., brief and easily administered), primary care providers can nonetheless take a multidimensional approach to assessing substance-related outcomes in the clinic.

To do this, providers might consider first defining the outcomes of interest based on the clinic's mission and its goals and the patient's needs. For example, in addition to patient consumption (i.e., quantity and frequency), primary clinics may also be interested in whether patients are following up on referrals and engaging in more intensive care when warranted. Additionally, because the substance use focus of primary care patients may be secondary to comorbid physical or mental health conditions, providers may also wish to assess change in the symptomatology of co-occurring disorders. The primary clinic will need to determine which measurement strategy is feasible for their staff and patient population. For example, a clinic with more resources may administer intensive outcome assessments across the treatment course, including a long-term follow-up, to allow for longitudinal measurement, while others with limited resources may focus on a few targeted self-reported substance consumption questions. How the data is to be utilized by the clinic will help determine the nature and extent of outcome assessed.

References

Ali, R., Meena, S., Eastwood, B., Richards, I., & Marsden, J. (2013). Ultra-rapid screening for substance-use disorders: The Alcohol, Smoking and Substance Involvement Screening test (ASSIST-Lite). *Drug and Alcohol Dependence*, *132*, 352–361.

American Psychiatric Association. (2000). *DSM-IV-TR: Diagnostic and statistical manual of mental disorders* (4th ed., text revision, pp. 739–799). Washington, DC: American Psychiatric Association.

American Psychiatric Association. (2013). *Diagnostic and statistical manual of mental disorders* (5th ed.). Arlington, VA: American Psychiatric Association.

Andreasson, S., Hansagi, H., & Osterlund, B. (2002). Short-term treatment for alcohol-related problems: Four-session guided self-change versus one session of advice—a randomized, controlled trial. *Alcohol*, *28*, 57–62.

Apodaca, T. R., & Miller, W. R. (2003). A meta-analysis of the effectiveness of bibliotherapy for alcohol problems. *Journal of Clinical Psychology, 59*, 289–304.

Babor, T. F., Higgins-Biddle, J. C., Saunders, J. B., & Monteiro, M. G. (2001). *AUDIT: The alcohol use disorders identification test: Guidelines for use in primary care: Department of Mental Health and Substance Dependence*. World Health Organization.

Breslin, F. C., Sobell, M. B., Sobell, L. C., Cunningham, J. A., Sdao-Jarvie, K., & Borsoi, D. (1998). Problem drinkers: Evaluation of a stepped-care approach. *Journal of Substance Abuse, 10*, 217–232.

Cucciare, M. A., Coleman, E. A., & Timko, C. (2015). A conceptual model to facilitate transitions from primary care to specialty substance use disorder care: A review of the literature. *Primary Health Care Research & Development, 16*, 492–505.

Cucciare, M. A., & Timko, C. (2015). Bridging the gap between medical settings and specialty addiction treatment. *Addiction, 110*, 1417–1419.

de Meneses-Gaya, C., Zuardi, A. W., Loureiro, S. R., & Crippa, J. A. (2009). Alcohol Use Disorders Identification Test (AUDIT): An updated systematic review of psychometric properties. *Psychology & Neuroscience, 2*, 83.

Fiore MC, Bailey WC, Cohen SJ, et al. Treating Tobacco Use and Dependence. Clinical Practice Guideline. Rockville, MD: U.S. Department of Health and Human Services. Public Health Service. June 2000.

Glass, J. E., Hamilton, A. M., Powell, B. J., Perron, B. E., Brown, R. T., & Ilgen, M. A. (2015). Specialty substance use disorder services following brief alcohol intervention: A meta-analysis of randomized controlled trials. *Addiction, 110*, 1404–1415.

Gryczynski, J., Mitchell, S. G., Gonzales, A., Moseley, A., Peterson, T. R., Ondersma, S. J., … Schwartz, R. P. (2015). A randomized trial of computerized vs. in-person brief intervention for illicit drug use in primary care: Outcomes through 12 months. *Journal of Substance Abuse Treatment, 50*, 3–10.

Hingson, R., & Compton, W. M. (2014). Screening and brief intervention and referral to treatment for drug use in primary care: Back to the drawing board. *The Journal of the American Medical Association, 312*, 488–489.

Mann, K. (2004). Pharmacotherapy of alcohol dependence. *CNS Drugs, 18*, 485–504.

Mattick, R. P., Breen, C., Kimber, J., & Davoli, M. (2009). Methadone maintenance therapy versus no opioid replacement therapy for opioid dependence. *Cochrane Database of Systematic Reviews*, (3), CD002209.

McNeely, J., & Saitz, R. (2015). Appropriate screening for substance use vs. disorder. *JAMA Internal Medicine, 175*, 1997–1998.

Michie, S., Whittington, C., Hamoudi, Z., Zarnani, F., Tober, G., & West, R. (2012). Identification of behaviour change techniques to reduce excessive alcohol consumption. *Addiction, 107*, 1431–1440.

Miller, W. R., & Rollnick, S. (2012). *Motivational interviewing: Helping people change*. Guilford Press.

Moos, R., & Timko, C. (2008). Outcome research on twelve-step and other self-help programs. In M. Galanter, & H. O. Kleber (Eds.), *Textbook of substance abuse treatment* (4th ed. pp. 511–521). Washington, DC: American Psychiatric Press.

Moyer, V. A. (2013). Screening and behavioral counseling interventions in primary care to reduce alcohol misuse: US preventive services task force recommendation statement. *Annals of Internal Medicine, 159*, 210–218.

National Institute of Alcohol Abuse and Alcoholism. (2016). Rethinking drinking: Alcohol and your health (NIH Publication No. 09–3770). Retrieved from http://rethinkingdrinking.niaaa.nih.gov/

O'Donnell, A., Anderson, P., Newbury-Birch, D., Schulte, B., Schmidt, C., Reimer, J., & Kaner, E. (2014). The impact of brief alcohol interventions in primary healthcare: A systematic review of reviews. *Alcohol and Alcoholism, 49*, 66–78.

Polen, M. R., Whitlock, E. P., Wisdom, J. P., Nygren, P., & Bougatsos, C. (2008). *Screening in primary care settings for illicit drug use: Staged systematic review for the United States Preventive Services Task Force.*

Preti, A. (2007). REVIEW: New developments in the pharmacotherapy of cocaine abuse. *Addiction Biology, 12*, 133–151.

Rapporteur, K. M. (2016). *Measuring recovery from substance use or mental disorders: Workshop summary*. Washington D.C.: The National Academies Press.

Reinert, D. F., & Allen, J. P. (2007). The alcohol use disorders identification test: An update of research findings. *Alcoholism, Clinical and Experimental Research, 31*, 185–199.

Roy-Byrne, P., Bumgardner, K., Krupski, A., Dunn, C., Ries, R., Donovan, D., … Zarkin, G. A. (2014). Brief intervention for problem drug use in safety-net primary care settings: A randomized clinical trial. *The Journal of the American Medical Association, 312*, 492–501.

Rubinsky, A. D., Sun, H., Blough, D. K., Maynard, C., Bryson, C. L., Harris, A. H., … Bradley, K. A. (2012). AUDIT-C alcohol screening results and postoperative inpatient health care use. *Journal of the American College of Surgeons, 214*, 296–305.

Saitz, R., Cheng, D. M., Allensworth-Davies, D., Winter, M. R., & Smith, P. C. (2014). The ability of single screening questions for unhealthy alcohol and other drug use to identify substance dependence in primary care. *Journal of Studies on Alcohol and Drugs, 75*, 153–157.

Saitz, R., Kim, T., Bernstein, J., Cheng, D. M., Samet, J., Lloyd-Travaglini, C., … German, J. (2015). Does screening and brief intervention for drug use in primary care increase receipt of substance use disorder treatment? *Addiction Science & Clinical Practice, 10*, 1.

Smith, P. C., Schmidt, S. M., Allensworth-Davies, D., & Saitz, R. (2009). Primary care validation of a single-question alcohol screening test. *Journal of General Internal Medicine, 24*, 783–788.

Smith, P. C., Schmidt, S. M., Allensworth-Davies, D., & Saitz, R. (2010). A single-question screening test for drug use in primary care. *Archives of Internal Medicine, 170*, 1155–1160.

Sobell, M. B., & Sobell, L. C. (2005). Guided self-change model of treatment for substance use disorders. *Journal of Cognitive Psychotherapy, 19*, 199–210.

VanBuskirk, K. A., & Wetherell, J. L. (2014). Motivational interviewing with primary care populations: A systematic review and meta-analysis. *Journal of Behavioral Medicine, 37*, 768–780.

Veterans Affairs/Department of Defense. (2009). Clinical practice guidelines. Retrieved 9-4-2016 from http://www.healthquality.va.gov/

White, A., Kavanagh, D., Stallman, H., Klein, B., Kay-Lambkin, F., Proudfoot, J., … Young, R. (2010). Online alcohol interventions: A systematic review. *Journal of Medical Internet Research, 12*, e62.

Witkiewitz, K., & Marlatt, G. A. (2004). Relapse prevention for alcohol and drug problems: That was Zen, this is Tao. *American Psychologist, 59*, 224.

Yudko, E., Lozhkina, O., & Fouts, A. (2007). A comprehensive review of the psychometric properties of the Drug Abuse Screening Test. *Journal of Substance Abuse Treatment, 32*, 189–198.

Attention Deficit Hyperactivity Disorder (ADHD) 5

Steven G. Little, Margaret T. Gopaul, and Angeleque Akin-Little

Attention deficit hyperactivity disorder (ADHD) is believed to be the most frequently diagnosed childhood mental health disorder in the world (Furman, 2005). A recent meta-analysis investigating worldwide ADHD prevalence in children age 18 and under found an overall pooled estimate of 7.2% (Thomas, Sanders, Doust, Beller, & Glasziou, 2015). The prevalence rate in the USA is even higher. Pastor, Reuben, Duran, and Hawkins (2015) found that 9.5% of children in the USA aged 4–17 years had been diagnosed with ADHD. That means that approximately two million children in the USA exhibit symptoms of ADHD, ADHD ranks first in terms of referrals to primary care physicians (Barkley, 2006), and ADHD presents a significant challenge to educational systems (Forness & Kavale, 2002).

S.G. Little (✉) • M.T. Gopaul
Department of Psychology, Walden University, Malone, NY, USA
e-mail: stevenlittlephd@yahoo.com; margaret.gopaul@waldenu.edu

A. Akin-Little
Akin-Little and Little Behavioral Psychology Consultants, Malone, NY, USA
e-mail: dr.angeleque@yahoo.com

What Is ADHD?

Attention deficit hyperactivity disorder (ADHD) is a neurodevelopmental disorder occurring in children and adults that presents with a persistent pattern of inattention and/or hyperactivity-impulsivity that impedes day-to-day living or typical development (American Psychiatric Association (APA), 2013). ADHD may present challenges with sustaining attention, working memory, and executive function, whereby the brain's capability to initiate, organize, and manage tasks may be impaired. There are three presentations of ADHD included in the DSM-5: (1) inattention, (2) hyperactivity-impulsivity, and (3) combined inattentive and hyperactive-impulsive (APA, 2013). Inattention is exhibited by behaviors such as digressing off task, poor task persistence, difficulties in sustaining attention, and disorganization. Excessive inappropriate motor activity is the primary feature of hyperactivity. Common behaviors include fidgeting, repetitive tapping, and talkativeness. Impulsivity consists of behaviors that occur with little prior reflection or thought and may have the capability of harming the individual (e.g., darting out into traffic). Behaviors such as excessive interruption and making quick decisions without thought of long-term outcomes are common (APA, 2013).

In order to be diagnosed with ADHD, the individual (child, adolescent, or adult) must meet clearly defined criteria presented in the *Diagnostic*

A. Maragakis, W.T. O'Donohue (eds.), *Principle-Based Stepped Care and Brief Psychotherapy for Integrated Care Settings*, https://doi.org/10.1007/978-3-319-70539-2_5

and Statistical Manual of Mental Disorders (DSM-5) or the *International Classification of Diseases (ICD-10)*. The ICD-10 defines ADHD as a hyperkinetic disorder and requires hyperactivity, impulsivity, and inattention for a diagnosis. These limiting ICD-10 diagnostic criteria result in a lower prevalence rate compared to the more common DSM criteria (Döpfner et al., 2008). The DSM-5 essentially groups symptoms that hinder either development or functioning into two broad areas, inattention or hyperactivity-impulsivity (APA, 2013). These inattention and/or hyperactivity-impulsivity symptoms typically occur in two or more settings, such as home, work, or school, with relatives or friends or in other situations with direct negative effect on academic, occupational, or social functioning. The DSM-5's criteria for an ADHD evaluation include:

Inattention Symptoms

Six or more of the following symptoms must be present for 6 or more months (APA, 2013).

- Regularly disorganized
- Difficulty organizing task
- Lack of focus or inability to attend to activities or directions
- Forgetful
- Habitually misplaces personal belongings, toys, or tools and frequently unprepared
- Difficulty staying on tasks and challenged to follow through with activities
- Appears not to listen, even when directly addressed
- Difficulty paying attention to details with careless mistakes (school and work)
- Avoids activities involving sustained mental effort or concentration

Hyperactivity-Impulsivity Symptoms

Six or more of the following symptoms must be present for 6 or more months although in individuals 17 and older, only five or more of these symptoms are required (APA, 2013).

- Excessively talkative (home, school, or work)
- Difficulty staying seated
- Inappropriately runs or climb (children). Feeling restless (adolescents and adults)
- Frequently fidgets or moves around
- Challenged to play quietly (children) or quietly engaging in activities (teens and adults)
- Seems constantly driven and on the "go"
- Difficulty waiting for a turn
- Interrupts others' dialogues or games
- Shouts out answers before the completion of the question

Clinicians should also state whether the individual with ADHD is in "partial remission" and indicate the present level of severity (mild, moderate, or severe). Partial remission is specified if full criteria were previously met, and partial ADHD criteria have been present for the past 6 months with symptoms continuing to result in limitations in academic, occupational, or social functioning (APA, 2013).

Distinctively, ADHD symptoms should not occur exclusively with schizophrenia or additional psychotic disorder (APA, 2013). Also, it should not be described by another mental disorder (anxiety, mood, personality, dissociative disorder, substance use, or withdrawal). Additionally, autism spectrum disorder (ASD) is not an exclusionary criterion. Therefore, an individual may be diagnosed with ADHD and ASD (APA, 2013).

Effective ADHD Screening in Primary Care Setting

According to the American Academy of Pediatrics (AAP, 2001), primary care offices function as the primary access point for the diagnosis of ADHD for children although psychiatrists and psychologists also perform a significant percentage of ADHD diagnosis (Handler & DuPaul, 2005). Regardless of the setting, having effective ADHD screening is crucial for timely treatment and interventions. The first step to screening for ADHD in a primary care setting involves identifying if the individual's behaviors warrant a more comprehensive ADHD assessment. This can be done as simply as reviewing DSM-5 (APA, 2013) criteria to determine if there are sufficient behavioral reports from the referral source to suggest that ADHD is a possibility. Leslie (2002) also suggests that ADHD-specific scales can also be helpful in initial screening. It should be noted that the use of broad behavior rating scales (e.g., CBCL or BASC-3) are premature at this time but may be a useful component of a more comprehensive assessment with a focus on intervention planning. Common ADHD-specific rating scales for children and adolescent include:

- *ADHD Rating Scale—5 for Children and Adolescents* (DuPaul, Power, Anastopoulos, & Reid, 2016). Includes parent questionnaires on home behaviors (English and Spanish) and teacher questionnaires on for ADHD with each scale taking approximately 5 min to complete.
- *NICHQ Vanderbilt ADHD Parent and Teacher Rating Scales* (VADPRS and VADTRS; Wolraich et al., 2003). Includes parent and teacher questionnaires and offers free download from http://www.nichq.org/childrens-health/adhd/resources/vanderbilt-assessment-scales.
- *Pediatric Attention Disorders Diagnostic Screener* (PADDS; Pedigo et al., 2008). This is a computer administered test of attention and executive functioning for children between the ages of 6 and 12.

Common ADHD-specific rating scales for adults include:

- *Adult ADHD Self-Report Scale* (ASRS; Adler et al., 2006). Is an adult self-report measure consisting of 18 questions based on the TSM-IV-TR criteria. While the screen is based on a previous version of the DSM, it may still be useful in screening. It is available for a free download from https://add.org/wp-content/uploads/2015/03/adhd-questionnaire-ASRS111.pdf.
- *Brown Attention-Deficit Disorder Scale for Adults* (Brown, 2001). The adult version of the Brown scales consists of 40 items that assess 5 clusters of ADHD-related executive function impairments.
- *ADHD Rating Scale* (ADHD-RS) with Adult Prompts (DuPaul et al., 2016). This self-report scale rates the frequency and severity of ADHD symptoms and consists of 18 items (9 inattentive symptoms and 9 hyperactive-impulsive symptoms).
- *Vanderbilt Behavioral Questionnaire-Adult Version* (Wolraich et al., 2003). This 18-item self-report symptom checklist is available for free download at https://add.org/wp-content/uploads/2015/03/adhd-questionnaire-ASRS111.pdf.

How to Further Assess if Screen Returns Positive

Further assessment based on a positive screen may necessitate a discussion with the individual or family of the utility of psychological tests and possible direct observations to fully evaluate and diagnosis ADHD. Psychological testing may be beneficial in ruling (in or out) the existence of intellectual challenges or learning disorders as related conditions in positive ADHD screens (Barkley, 2012a). When working with either a child or adult, the provider needs to ascertain to what extent the individual's symptoms are influencing moods, behavior, productivity, and lifestyle routines as well rule out other conditions. Providers should take the following steps in the assessment of ADHD looking at the different domains, age of onset, period of symptoms, and level of functional impairment:

1. *Clinical examination:* To identify other disorders with overlapping symptoms of ADHD
2. *Interview:* With individual, parents, caregivers, spouse, teachers, or friends to determine:
   (a) Perceptions of ADHD symptoms
   (b) Observations of symptoms or behaviors in different settings
   (c) Medical, psychiatric, and developmental history
   (d) Related family functional challenges

   (e) The existence of any comorbidities
   (f) Patterns of ADHD or related comorbidities shown in the family
3. *Note age when behaviors started*: Children, on average, are usually first diagnosed during the early elementary school years; however, symptoms are usually clear by the age of 4 (APA, 2013). As ADHD is considered a neurodevelopmental disorder, the DSM-5 specifies in adult diagnosis that symptoms should have occurred prior to age 12 years.
4. *Observation:* Direct personal observation is helpful to confirm symptoms reported in interviews. If direct observation is not possible, observational data from teachers, parents, spouses, and adults siblings are helpful. If feasible it is also helpful to obtain behavior reports, report cards, and samples of schoolwork from the child's teacher (Watson & Watson, 2009).
5. *Appropriate screening questionnaires or rating scales*: To evaluate general behavior and psychosocial functioning, ADHD symptomatology and comorbidities from at least two sources [typically parent(s) or caregiver(s) and the teacher(s)] (NICE, 2008). While the screen may include ADHD-specific rating scales, they are also very useful as part of a comprehensive ADHD evaluation. Screens will most likely consist of self- and/or parent-report questionnaires. At the time of a more comprehensive evaluation, it is suggested that behavior rating scales be completed by multiple individuals in the individual's life. This would include both parents, teachers, and possibly siblings for children and spouse/significant other and possibly parents for adults. Having adults complete a child behavior rating scale retrospectively on an adult is one way to establish a developmental history of the disorder. Examples of comprehensive behavior rating scales include the Child Behavior Checklist (CBCL; Achenbach, 2001), Conners' Parent and Teacher Rating Scales (CPRS-R and CTRS-R; Conners, 2001), and the Behavior Assessment System for Children (BASC-3; Reynolds & Kamphaus, 2015).

In addition, a comprehensive assessment specific to the needs of the individual or for intervention planning may be warranted. These measures may include:

1. Rating scales of executive function deficits connected with ADHD:
   (a) *The Barkley Deficits in Executive Functioning Scale—Children and Adolescents* (BDEFS; Barkley, 2012a). This scale is designed to measure dimensions of child and adolescent executive functioning consisting of time management, organization and problem solving, self-restraint, self-motivation, and self-regulation of emotions. There are a parent long form (10–15 min) and a parent short form (3–5 min).
   (b) *Barkley Deficits in Executive Functioning Scale* (BDEFS for Adults; Barkley, 2011). This scale is designed to measure dimensions of adult executive functioning in daily life including time management, organization and problem solving, self-restraint, self-motivation, and self-regulation of emotions.
   (c) *Behavior Rating Inventory of Executive Functioning* (BRIEF; Gioia, Isquith, Guy, & Kenworthy, 2000). This scale assesses executive function behaviors in the school and home environments with parent and teacher questionnaires.
2. Adaptive behavior may be assessed when it is deemed necessary to evaluate an individual's functioning in daily life: vocationally, socially, educationally, etc.:
   (a) *Vineland Adaptive Behavior Scales, Third Edition* (Sparrow, Cicchetti, & Saulnier, 2016).
   (b) *Adaptive Behavior Assessment System, Third Edition* (Harrison & Oakland, 2017).
3. Impairment in major domains of life activities may be assessed:
   (a) *Barkley Functional Impairment Scale—Children and Adolescents* (Barkley, 2012b). This parent-completed report form provides comprehensive coverage of

domains of psychosocial impairment in 15 domains of everyday activities for children and adolescents.

4. Pervasiveness and severity of behaviors across domains (home and public) may be assessed:
   (a) *Home Situations Questionnaire* (HSQ; Barkley & Murphy, 2006). This parent-completed form assesses how ADHD symptoms disrupt children in normal home situations such as meal time or completing chores.
5. Continuous performance tasks are useful in assessing an individual's performance in the areas of inattentiveness, impulsivity, sustained attention, and vigilance:
   (a) *Conners' Continuous Performance Test, 3rd Edition* (Conners, 2014)
   (b) *Test of Variables of Attention* (T.O.V.A.; Leark, Greenberg, Kindschi, Dupuy, & Hughes, 2007)

Evidence-Based Stepped Care and Brief Psychotherapeutic Approaches

Psychoeducation may be one of the first approaches used in ADHD intervention. The goal of psychoeducation is to help parents, teachers, and the individual to better understand ADHD, its symptoms, and behavior management. The rationale being that if the individual and others in his/her life can become more knowledgeable about ADHD, they can better manage their symptoms and any proposed treatment. A first step could be a bibliotherapy approach. Russell Barkley, Clinical Professor of Psychiatry at the Medical University of South Carolina, is one of the most respected ADHD researchers in the world. He has authored books for laypeople for both childhood and adult ADHD. These include *When an Adult You Love Has ADHD: Professional Advice for Parents, Partners, and Siblings* (Barkley, 2016) and *Taking Charge of ADHD, Revised Edition: The Complete, Authoritative Guide for Parents* (Barkley, 2013). Both books also include an appendix offering suggestions for further reading. Either of these could be used independently as a first step in the psychoeducation process or a component of parent training and or treatment.

Ferrin et al. (2014) implemented a psychoeducation program for parents of children and adolescents with ADHD and found significantly reduced levels of inattention, an improvement in prosocial behaviors, and an overall improved impression regarding the severity of symptoms. Bai, Wang, Yang, and Niu (2015) evaluated a psychoeducation program for parents of children with ADHD in enhancing adherence to pharmacological treatment and improving clinical symptoms. Results indicated that medication adherence increased significantly, and ADHD rating scale scores were lower following psychoeducation. In addition, increases in parents' knowledge about ADHD were observed. The results of these and other studies suggest that psychoeducation may be a useful first step in ADHD intervention or a supplement to other more long-term interventions such as parent training.

In addition to psychoeducation, brief psychosocial treatments, particularly cognitive behavior therapy, have also been shown to produce improvement in adults with ADHD (Safren, Otto et al., 2005). Psychodynamic, or other "traditional" psychotherapeutic methods, however, have not been shown to be effective approaches in individuals who present to outpatient psychiatric clinics (Ramsay, 2010). For example, using an abbreviated, eight-session version of the Safren, Perlman, Sprich, and Otto (2005) *Mastering Your Adult ADHD* protocol in college-aged students, Eddy, Canu, Broman-Fulks, and Michael (2015) found it to be a useful short-term treatment option. They noted, however, that improvement of core ADHD symptoms was generally modest. Other research with children, however, has not yielded positive results over those already attained by methylphenidate (van der Oord, Prins, Oosterlaan, & Emmelkamp, 2007).

Pelham et al. (2016) evaluated behavioral and pharmacological treatments in an attempt to determine the optimal sequencing of interventions in the treatment of ADHD in children (age 5–12). Children were randomly assigned to groups who received either (a) behavioral parent training (eight group sessions) and brief teacher consultation to establish a daily report card or (b) extended-release methylphenidate as an initial treatment. Results indicated that the group beginning with behavioral treatment displayed significantly lower rates of classroom rule violations and had fewer out-of-class disciplinary events. In addition, adding medication after initial behavioral treatments resulted in better parent/teacher ratings of oppositional behavior than in those who began treatment in the methylphenidate group.

Consistent with the Pelham et al. (2016) findings, the American Academy of Pediatrics (2011) guidelines advocate that the first choice of treatment for pre-school-aged children (4–5 years of age) with ADHD should be behavior therapy, and physicians are urged to prescribe this treatment option first. The efficacy of parent training in behavior therapy has been well established, and it is also a tool that can be used in classrooms by teachers and childhood caregivers. In 2010, the Agency for Health Care Research and Quality (AHRQ) reviewed treatment choices available for children with ADHD under 6 years of age (Charach et al., 2011). The meta-review reported empirical evidence to support the use of parent training in behavior therapy as evidence-based and an effective choice of care for children (under 6 years) with ADHD symptoms. The following parent training in behavior therapy programs were deemed by the AHRQ review as effective in reducing ADHD symptoms in young children (Note: Pharmacological interventions are added here but were not addressed by the AHRQ review):

- Triple P (Positive Parenting Program)
- Incredible Years Parenting Program
- Parent-Child Interaction Therapy (PCIT)
- New Forest Parenting Program (specifically for parents of children with ADHD)
- Pharmacological Interventions

The following sections provide more detail on these programs:

Triple P (Positive Parenting Program)

Triple P (Positive Parenting Program) has been shown to be one of the most effective evidence-based programs across various family structures, socioeconomic groups, and cultures (Pickering & Sanders, 2016). It has over 30 years of continuous research and is presently used in 25 countries (Triple P—Positive Parenting Program, 2015). Triple P providers can obtain the Selected Triple P Provider Training Course to attain competency in the program so that they may offer parenting information seminars for parents with children (aged 0–12 years). The interventions can be offered in various settings but are usually done via primary care services (family or general physicians, mental health services, daycare sites, and schools). The approach ideally offers brief presentations of information to groups of parents. According to the Triple P—Positive Parenting Program (2015), the typical Triple P Selected Seminar Series consists of three seminars lasting 2 h each that cover the following:

- Positive Parenting
- Raising confident and competent children
- Raising resilient children

Incredible Years Parenting Program

The Incredible Years is a series of interlocking, evidence-based programs for parents, children, and teachers. The goal is to prevent and treat young children's behavior problems and promote their social, emotional, and academic competence. For example, the Incredible Years (IY) Teacher Classroom Management program is a universal intervention designed to strengthen teachers' classroom management skills and enable them to work with all children including those with disruptive behaviors such as those common with children with ADHD. In addition, the program emphasizes effective parent/teacher collaboration (Webster Stratton & Reid, 2003).

Research has, for the most part, supported the efficacy of Incredible Years with both parents and teachers (Weeland et al., 2017). In a recent meta-analysis, Weeland et al. found that Incredible Years decreased parent reports of child externalizing behavior ($d = 0.20$ at posttest, $d = 0.08$ at follow-up), increased both parent reports of ($d = 0.49$, $d = 0.45$) and direct observations of ($d = 0.06$, $d = 0.02$) positive parenting behavior, and decreased parent-reported negative parenting behavior ($d = 0.29$, $d = 0.25$). They did not, however, find support for increases in reported or observed child prosocial behavior, observed child externalizing behavior, or observed negative parenting behavior. Another recent study questioned the efficacy of the Incredible Years Classroom Management Program. Noting that the vast majority of research support for Incredible Years comes from the USA, Kirkhaug et al. (2016) investigated the Incredible Years Teacher Classroom Management program in a Norwegian primary school setting. They concluded that it is not sufficient as a stand-alone program for students with severe externalizing problems with those students needing "more comprehensive and tailored interventions" (p. 2).

Parent-Child Interaction Therapy (PCIT)

Parent-Child Interaction Therapy (PCIT) was developed by Sheila Eyberg in the 1970s as an intervention for children (aged 2–7) with disruptive behavior disorders. PCIT consists of two phases: Child-Directed Interaction (CDI) and Parent-Directed Interaction (PDI). CDI is designed to improve the quality of the parent-child relationship while strengthening attention and reinforcement for positive child behavior. This is accomplished by letting the child take the lead in play while attending to positive behaviors while ignoring minor inappropriate behaviors. Parents are taught to use PRIDE: praise, reflection, imitation, description, and enthusiasm. In PDI parents learn to lead their child's activity. This includes effective instruction giving, using consistent consequences, and the application of praise for compliance and the use of time-out for noncompliance (Funderburk & Eyberg, 2011). Wagner and McNeil (2007) concluded that "research and evidence suggests that PCIT may be effective for young children with ADHD" (p. 231). In addition, PCIT is listed on the National Registry of Evidence-Based Programs and Practices (NREPP), receiving an overall rating of 3.8 on a four point scale (http://legacy.nreppadmin.net/ViewIntervention.aspx?id=23).

New Forest Parenting Program

The New Forest Parenting Program is a parenting training course for the parents of children age 3–11 with ADHD. Developed in the UK, the program consists of eight weekly visits by professions to the family's home. The goal of the visits is to teach parents strategies for managing their children's behavior and difficulties with attention. It was given an effectiveness rating of 3 out of 4 by the Early Intervention Foundation in the UK (http://eif.org.uk/wp-content/uploads/2014/07/New-Forest-Parenting-Programme.pdf). Abikoff et al. (2015) found that while the program improved parent ratings of child behavior, those reported gains were not corroborated by teacher ratings or objective observations. Other studies (e.g., Daley & O'Brien, 2013; Thompson et al., 2009), however, have provided strong support for the efficacy of the program.

Pharmacological Interventions

It is clear that medication (e.g., methylphenidate, dextroamphetamine) can help diminish ADHD symptoms, particularly in those with the most severe ADHD characteristics; however, there is evidence to suggest that they may help everyone lessen even mild ADHD-like behaviors (Shah & Morton, 2013). Psychostimulants, especially methylphenidate, are globally the most prescribed drug for the treatment of ADHD (Swanson, 2003) with an estimated global consumption of 2.4 billion daily doses of methylphenidate in 2013 (International Narcotics Control Board, 2015). It is therefore impossible to discuss interventions for ADHD without addressing pharmacological approaches. Studies have shown that methylphenidate is effective in the treatment of childhood ADHD (e.g., Schachter, Pham, King, Langford, & Moher, 2001) and that, when controlled for placebo effects, it has beneficial effects for about 70% of children with ADHD (Spencer et al., 1996). However, even though pharmacological interventions may be effective in the short term as the sole treatment approach, international guidelines advise that pharmacological treatment should always be part of a comprehensive treatment program that includes psychoeducation including parent- and teacher-administered behavioral interventions and parent training (Subcommittee on Attention-Deficit/Hyperactivity Disorder, Steering Committee on Quality Improvement and Management, 2011) if short-term gains are to be maintained.

What Does Not Work

A number of interventions have been proposed over the years to address etiological, biological, and environmental variables and their hypothesized effect on inattention and hyperactivity. Not all have data to support their efficacy however. The following summarizes some of the more popular intervention approaches with little or questionable empirical support.

Working memory training has been proposed as an intervention to improve an individual's level of sustained attention. It involves the training of working memory, using a computerized task designed to be consistent with the person's skill level and becoming progressively more difficult as training progresses (Klingberg et al., 2005). A meta-analysis performed by Hodgson, Hutchinson, and Denson (2014) resulted in a −0.02 effect size indicating no support for the intervention. Hodgson also evaluated self-monitoring as an intervention for ADHD symptoms and found an even worse effect with an effect size of −5.91 for self-monitoring as a stand-alone approach. Self-monitoring involves regular completion of a checklist of the behaviors one has, or has not, engaged in over time. While self-monitoring may be a useful component in a multimodal treatment approach, it does not appear to be an efficacious intervention when used independently.

Stevenson et al. (2014) conducted a review of meta-analyses on dietary treatments for ADHD and found mixed results. They examined the efficacy of three different diet-related interventions focusing on studies using randomized controlled trials: restricted elimination diets (RED), artificial food color elimination (AFCE), and supplementation with free fatty acids (SFFA). Their results indicated small effect sizes for each (RED, mean effect size = 0.40; AFCE, mean effect size = 0.35; SFFA, mean effect size = 0.31). The authors concluded, however, that more research is needed before firm conclusions can be drawn, partly due to methodological concerns with the existing research. Similar conclusions were made by Rytter et al. (2015) who stated "more thorough investigations will be necessary to decide whether they are recommendable as part of ADHD treatment" (p. 1). Finally, one of the more persistent misconceptions about ADHD etiology and treatment is that there is a direct relationship between sugar consumption and activity level. Research, however, indicates that there is no significant association between total volume of simple sugar intake from snacks and ADHD development (Kim & Chang, 2011).

When to Refer to External Specialty Mental Health

As was mentioned previously, the American Academy of Pediatrics (2011) guidelines advocate that the first choice of treatment for children with ADHD should be behavior therapy. Beginning with low-intensity behavior modification compared to intervention beginning with medication has been found to be both superior and more cost effective (Page et al., 2016). It is therefore recommended that referral be made to a psychiatrist (children or adults) or a pediatrician (children) for possible pharmacological intervention only when behavioral interventions have not been effective.

The Role of Primary Care Provider/ Medical Team in Treatment

As was previously mentioned, ADHD ranks first in terms of referrals for mental health issues to primary care physicians (Barkley, 2006). It is therefore likely that the primary care provider will have initial patient contact. He/she may prescribe medication without making a referral to a psychologist or other behavioral specialist. If, however, referral is made from the school or parents to a psychologist, the primary care provider may be consulted with respect to medication and or physical examination to rule out or identify any comorbid medical conditions.

How to Assess Impact on Care/ Quality Improvement Processes

In discussing the importance of measuring target behaviors before and during treatment, Cooper, Heron, and Heward (2007) identify two preventable mistakes that can occur when frequent measurement of behavior is not obtained and attended to. These are (a) continuing an ineffective treatment when no real behavior change has occurred or (b) discontinuing an effective treatment because subjective judgment detects no improvement. They further point out the following to illustrate the importance of frequent measurement (pp. 74–75):

- Measurement helps practitioners optimize their effectiveness.
- Measurement enables practitioners to verify the legitimacy of treatments touted as "evidence-based."
- Measurement helps practitioners identify and end the use of treatments based on pseudoscience, fad, fashion, or ideology.
- Measurement enables practitioners to be accountable to clients, consumers, employers, and society.
- Measurement helps practitioners achieve ethical standards.

The question is therefore what measures to use to adequately assess progress in individuals diagnosed with ADHD. While direct behavioral observation of identified target behaviors may be ideal, it is not always possible to directly observe behaviors as they occur (Watson & Watson, 2009). Having a third-party (e.g., parents, teacher) record behavior is a possibility, but it is difficult to verify the accuracy of those observations and they may be subject to various biases. Checklists and ratings scales such as those mentioned in the diagnosis section (e.g., ADHD Rating Scale—5 for Children and Adolescents, BASC-2, CBCL, CPRS-R, CTRS-R, Conners-Wells' Adolescent Self-Report Scale, VADPRS, VADTRS, PADDS) can also be used, but they too are subject to bias. A final way to mentor progress is through the use of outcome variables. For example, in schools a child who increases their level of attention will be more likely to turn in assignments. Measuring the quantity and quality of academic output is one way to infer treatment effectiveness. As individuals with ADHD may also engage in externalizing behaviors, a reduction in disciplinary actions in school may be expected. Using multiple effectiveness measures such as direct observation, checklists and questionnaires, and outcome measures would, however, would allow the practitioner to draw the most reliable conclusions on treatment effectiveness.

References

Abikoff, H. B., Thompson, M., Laver-Bradbury, C., Long, N., Forehand, R. L., Miller Brotman, L., … Sonuga-Barke, E. (2015). Parent training for preschool ADHD: A randomized controlled trial of specialized and generic programs. *Journal of Child Psychology and Psychiatry*, *56*, 618–631. https://doi.org/10.1111/jcpp.12346

Achenbach, T. (2001). *Child behavior checklist for ages 6-18*. Burlington, VT: ASEBA, University of Vermont.

Adler, L. A., Spencer, T., Faraone, S. V., Kessler, R. C., Howes, M. J., Biederman, J., & Secnik, K. (2006). Validity of pilot adult ADHD self-report scale (ASRS) to rate adult ADHD symptoms. *Annals of Clinical Psychiatry.*, *18*, 145–148. https://doi.org/10.1080/10401230600801077

American Academy of Pediatrics. (2001). Clinical practice guidelines: Treatment of the school aged child with attention-deficit/hyperactivity disorder. *Pediatrics, 108*, 1033–1044.

American Academy of Pediatrics. (2011). ADHD: Clinical practice guideline for the diagnosis, evaluation, and treatment of Attention-Deficit/Hyperactivity Disorder in children and adolescent. *Pediatrics, 128*, 1007–1022. https://doi.org/10.1542/peds.2011-2654

American Psychiatric Association. (2013). *Diagnostic and statistical manual of mental disorders* (5th ed., text revision). Washington, DC: American Psychiatric Association.

Bai, G., Wang, Y., Yang, L., & Niu, W. (2015). Effectiveness of a focused, brief psychoeducation program for parents of ADHD children: Improvement of medication adherence and symptoms. *Neuropsychiatric Disease and Treatment, 11*, 2721–2735.

Barkley, R. A. (2006). *Attention deficit hyperactivity disorder: A handbook for diagnosis and treatment* (3rd ed.). New York, NY: Guilford Press.

Barkley, R. A. (2011). *The Barkley deficits in executive functioning scale for adults*. New York, NY: Guilford Press.

Barkley, R. A. (2012a). *The Barkley deficits in executive functioning scale—Children and adolescents*. New York, NY: Guilford Press.

Barkley, R. A. (2012b). *The Barkley functional impairment scale—Children and adolescents*. New York, NY: Guilford Press.

Barkley, R. A. (2013). *Taking charge of ADHD, revised edition: The complete, authoritative guide for parents*. New York: Guilford.

Barkley, R. A. (2016). *When an adult you love has ADHD: Professional advice for parents, partners, and siblings*. Washington, DC: APA Books.

Barkley, R. A., & Murphy, K. R. (2006). *Attention-deficit hyperactivity disorder: A clinical workbook* (3rd ed.). New York, NY: Guilford Press.

Brown, T. E. (2001). *Brown attention-deficit disorder scales*. San Antonio: Pearson Assessment.

Charach, A., Dashti, B., Carson, P., Booker, L., Lim, C. G., Lillie, E., … Schachar, R. (2011). *Attention deficit hyperactivity disorder: Effectiveness of treatment in at-risk preschoolers; long-term effectiveness in all ages; and variability in prevalence, diagnosis, and treatment*. Rockville, MD: Agency for Healthcare Research and Quality.

Conners, C. K. (2001). Development of the CRS-R. In C. K. Conners (Ed.), *Conners' rating scales-revised*. North Tonawanda, NY: Multi-Health Systems.

Conners, C. K. (2014). *Conners continuous performance test* (3rd ed.). North Tonawanda, NY: Multi-Health Systems.

Cooper, J. O., Heron, T. E., & Heward, W. L. (2007). *Applied behavior analysis* (2nd ed.). Upper Saddle River, NJ: Pearson Prentice Hall.

Daley, D., & O'Brien, M. (2013). A small-scale randomized controlled trial of the self-help version of the New Forest Parent Training Programme for children with ADHD symptoms. *European Child & Adolescent Psychiatry, 22*, 543–552. https://doi.org/10.1007/s00787-013-0396-8

Döpfner, M., Breuer, D., Wille, N., Erhart, M., Ravens-Sieberer, U., & BELLA Study Group. (2008). How often do children meet ICD-10/DSM-IV criteria of attention deficit/hyperactivity disorder? Parent-based prevalence rates in a national sample: Results of the BELLA study. *European Child and Adolescent Psychiatry, 17*, 59–70. https://doi.org/10.1007/s00787-008-1007-y

DuPaul, G. J., Power, T. J., Anastopoulos, A. D., & Reid, R. (2016). *ADHD Rating Scale--5 for children and adolescents: Checklists, norms, and clinical interpretation* (Revised Edition). New York, NY: The Guilford Press.

Eddy, L. D., Canu, W. H., Broman-Fulks, J. J., & Michael, K. D. (2015). Brief cognitive behavioral therapy for college students with ADHD: A case series report. *Cognitive and Behavioral Practice, 22*, 127–140. https://doi.org/10.1016/j.cbpra.2014.05.005

Ferrin, M., Moreno-Granados, J. M., Salcedo-Marin, M. D., Ruiz-Veguilla, M., Perez-Ayala, V., & Taylor, E. (2014). Evaluation of a psychoeducation programme for parents of children and adolescents with ADHD: Immediate and long-term effects using a blind randomized controlled trial. *European Child & Adolescent Psychiatry, 23*, 637–647. https://doi.org/10.1007/s00787-013-0494-7

Forness, S., & Kavale, K. (2002). Impact of ADHD on school systems. In P. Jensen & J. Gooper (Eds.), *Attention deficit hyperactivity disorder: State of the science practices* (pp. 24-1–24-20). Kingston, NJ: Givic Research Institute.

Funderburk, B. W., & Eyberg, S. (2011). Parent-child interaction therapy. In J. C. Norcross & D. K. Freedheim (Eds.), *History of psychotherapy: Continuity and change* (2nd ed., pp. 415–420). Washington, DC: American Psychological Association.

Furman, L. (2005). What is attention-deficit hyperactivity disorder (ADHD)? *Journal of Child Neurology, 20*, 994–1003. https://doi.org/10.1177/08830738050200121301

Gioia, G. A., Isquith, P. K., Guy, S. C., & Kenworthy, L. (2000). *BRIEF: Behavior rating inventory of executive function: Professional manual*. Odessa, FL: Psychological Assessment Resources, Inc..

Handler, M. W., & DuPaul, G. J. (2005). Assessment of ADHD: Differences across psychology specialty areas. *Journal of Attention Disorders, 9*, 402–412. https://doi.org/10.1177/1087054705278762

Harrison, P., & Oakland, T. (2017). *Adaptive behavior assessment system, Third Edition (ABAS)*. Torrance, CA: WPS.

Hodgson, K., Hutchinson, A. D., & Denson, L. (2014). Nonpharmacological treatments for ADHD: A meta-analytic review. *Journal of Attention Disorders, 18*, 275–282. https://doi.org/10.1177/1087054712444732

International Narcotics Control Board. (2015). *Annual report*. New York: United Nations.

Kim, Y., & Chang, H. (2011). Correlation between attention deficit hyperactivity disorder and sugar consumption, quality of diet, and dietary behavior in school children. *Nutrition Research and Practice*, *5*, 236–245. https://doi.org/10.4162/nrp.2011.5.3.236

Kirkhaug, B., Drugli, M. B., Handegård, B. H., Lydersen, S., Åsheim, M., & Fossum, S. (2016). Does the Incredible Years Teacher Classroom Management Training programme have positive effects for young children exhibiting severe externalizing problems in school?: A quasi-experimental pre-post study. *BMC Psychiatry*, *16*, 1–12.

Klingberg, T., Fernell, E., Olesen, P. J., Johnson, M., Gustafsson, P., Dahlström, K., … Westerberg, H. (2005). Computerized training of working memory in children with ADHD—A randomized, controlled trial. *Journal of the American Academy of Child & Adolescent Psychiatry*, *44*, 177–186. https://doi.org/10.1097/00004583-200502000-00010

Leark, R. A., Greenberg, L. M., Kindschi, C. L., Dupuy, T. R., & Hughes, S. J. (2007). *Test of variables of attention continuous performance*. Los Alamitos, CA: The Tova Company.

Leslie, L. K. (2002). The role of primary care physicians in attention deficit hyperactivity disorder (ADHD). *Pediatric Annuls*, *31*, 475–484. https://doi.org/10.3928/0090-4481-20020801-07

NICE. (2008). Attention deficit hyperactivity disorder: Diagnosis and management. Retrieved from https://www.nice.org.uk/guidance/CG72

Page, T. F., Pelham, W. E., III, Fabiano, G. A., Greiner, A. R., Gnagy, E. M., Hart, K. C., … Pelham, W. E., Jr. (2016). Comparative cost analysis of sequential, adaptive, behavioral, pharmacological, and combined treatments for childhood ADHD. *Journal of Clinical Child and Adolescent Psychology*, *45*, 416–427. https://doi.org/10.1080/15374416.2015.1055859

Pastor, P. N., Reuben, C. R., Duran, C. R., & Hawkins, L. D. (2015). *Association between diagnosed ADHD and selected characteristics among children aged 4-17 years: United States, 2011-2013. NCHS Data Brief, 201*. Hyattsville, MD: National Center for Health Statistics.

Pedigo, T. K., Pedigo, K. L., Scott, V. B., Jr., Swanson, J. M., Nolan, W., & Pelham, W. E. (2008). *Pediatric attention disorders diagnostic screener*. Atascadero, CA: SenseLabs.

Pelham, W. E., Fabiano, G. A., Waxmonsky, J. G., Greiner, A. R., Gnagy, E. M., Pelham, W. E., … Murphy, S. A. (2016). Treatment sequencing for childhood ADHD: A multiple-randomization study of adaptive medication and behavioral interventions. *Journal of Clinical Child and Adolescent Psychology*, *45*, 396–415. https://doi.org/10.1080/15374416.2015.1105138

Pickering, J. A., & Sanders, M. R. (2016). Reducing child maltreatment by making parenting programs available to all parents: A case example using the Triple P-Positive Parenting Program. *Trauma, Violence, and Abuse*, *17*, 398–407. https://doi.org/10.1177/1524838016658876

Ramsay, J. R. (2010). *Nonmedication treatments for adult ADHD*. Washington, DC: American Psychological Association.

Reynolds, C., & Kamphaus, R. (2005). *Behavioral assessment system for children - 3*. San Antonio, TX: Pearson Assessment.

Rytter, M. J. H., Andersen, L. B. B., Houmann, T., Bilenberg, N., Hvolby, A., Mølgaard, C., … Lauritzen, L. (2015). Diet in the treatment of ADHD in children: A systematic review of the literature. *Nordic Journal of Psychiatry*, *69*, 1–18. https://doi.org/10.3109/08039488.2014.921933

Safren, S. A., Otto, M. W., Sprich, S., Winett, C. L., Wilens, T. E., & Biederman, J. (2005). Cognitive-behavioral therapy for ADHD in medication-treated adults with continued symptoms. *Behavior Research and Therapy*, *43*, 831–842. https://doi.org/10.1016/j.brat.2004.07.001

Safren, S. A., Perlman, C. A., Sprich, S., & Otto, M. W. (2005). *Mastering your adult ADHD: A cognitive behavioral treatment program: Therapist guide*. New York, NY: Oxford University Press.

Schachter, H. M., Pham, B., King, J., Langford, S., & Moher, D. (2001). How efficacious and safe is short-acting methylphenidate for the treatment of attention-deficit disorder in children and adolescents? A meta-analysis. *Canadian Medical Association Journal*, *165*, 1475–1488.

Shah, P. J., & Morton, M. J. S. (2013). Adults with attention-deficit hyperactivity disorder—Diagnosis or normality? *The British Journal of Psychiatry*, *203*, 317–319. https://doi.org/10.1192/bjp.bp.113.126474

Sparrow, S. S., Cicchetti, D. V., & Saulnier, C. A. (2016). *Vineland adaptive behavior scales* (3rd ed.). San Antonio, TX: Pearson Assessment.

Spencer, T., Biederman, J., Wilens, T., Harding, M., O'Donnel, D., & Griffin, S. (1996). Pharmacotherapy of attention-deficit hyperactivity disorder across the life cycle. *Journal of the American Academy of Child and Adolescent Psychiatry*, *35*, 409–432.

Stevenson, J., Buitelaar, J., Cortese, S., Ferrin, M., Konofal, E., Lecendreux, M., … Sonuga-Bark, E. (2014). Research review: The role of diet in the treatment of attention-deficit/hyperactivity disorder—An appraisal of the evidence on efficacy and recommendations on the design of future studies. *Journal of Child Psychology and Psychiatry*, *55*, 416–427. https://doi.org/10.1111/jcpp.12215

Subcommittee on Attention-Deficit/Hyperactivity Disorder, Steering Committee on Quality Improvement and Management. (2011). ADHD: Clinical practice guideline for the diagnosis, evaluation, and treatment of attention-deficit/hyperactivity disorder in children and adolescents. *Pediatrics*, *128*, 1007–1022. https://doi.org/10.1542/peds.2011-2654

Swanson, J. (2003). Compliance with stimulants for attention-deficit/hyperactivity disorder. *CNS Drugs, 17*, 117–131.

Thomas, R., Sanders, S., Doust, J., Beller, E., & Glasziou, P. (2015). Prevalence of attention-deficit/hyperactivity disorder: A systematic review and meta-analysis. *Pediatrics, 135*, 994–1001. https://doi.org/10.1542/peds.2014-3482

Thompson, M. J. J., Laver-Bradbury, C., Ayres, M., Le Poidevin, E., Mead, S., Dodds, C., … Sonuga-Barke, E. J. S. (2009). A small-scale randomized controlled trial of the Revised New Forest Parenting Programme for preschoolers with attention deficit hyperactivity disorder. *European Child & Adolescent Psychiatry, 18*, 605–616. https://doi.org/10.1007/s00787-009-0020-0

Triple P—Positive Parenting Program. (2015). Triple P takes the guesswork out of parenting. Retrieved from http://www.triplep.net/glo-en/home/

van der Oord, S., Prins, P. J. M., Oosterlaan, J., & Emmelkamp, P. M. G. (2007). Does brief, clinically based, intensive multimodal behavior therapy enhance the effects of methylphenidate in children with ADHD? *European Child Adolescent Psychiatry, 16*, 48–57. https://doi.org/10.1007/s00787-006-0574-z

Wagner, S. M., & McNeil, C. B. (2007). Parent-Child Interaction Therapy for ADHD: A conceptual overview and critical literature review. *Child & Family Behavior Therapy, 30*, 231–256. https://doi.org/10.1080/07317100802275546

Watson, T. S., & Watson, T. S. (2009). Behavioral assessment in the schools. In A. Akin-Little, S. G. Little, M. A. Bray, & T. J. Kehle (Eds.), *Behavioral interventions in schools: Evidence-based positive strategies* (pp. 27–41). Washington, DC: American Psychological Association.

Webster Stratton, C., & Reid, M. J. (2003). The incredible years parents, teachers, and children training series. In A. E. Kazdin & J. R. Weisz (Eds.), *Evidence based psychotherapies for children and adolescents* (pp. 194–210). New York: Guilford Press.

Weeland, J., Chhangur, R. R., van der Giessen, D., Matthys, W., de Castro, B. O., & Overbeek, G. (2017). Intervention effectiveness of the incredible years: New insights into sociodemographic and intervention-based moderators. *Behavior Therapy, 48*, 1–18. https://doi.org/10.1080/15374416.2015.1038823

Wolraich, M., Lambert, W., Doffing, M., Bickman, L., Simmons, T., & Worley, K. (2003). Psychometric properties of the Vanderbilt ADHD Diagnostic Parent Rating Scale in a referred population. *Journal of Pediatric Psychology, 28*, 559–567. https://doi.org/10.1093/jpepsy/jsg046

6 Avoidant Restrictive Food Intake Disorder

Melissa L. González, Thomas D. Mulderink, and Peter A. Girolami

Avoidant Restrictive Food Intake Disorder in Pediatric Populations

Oral consumption of food and drink is often viewed as a basic behavior that is present immediately following birth with advancements in intake of variety, volume, texture of foods, and overall independence occurring following a developmental trajectory. However, learning to eat is a complex process. For many children, this natural progression of feeding development is delayed and/or is disrupted by medical complications, structural or anatomical abnormalities, neurodevelopmental disabilities, conditioned aversion, or other environmental factors (Berlin, Lobato, Pinkos, Cerezo, & LeLeikos, 2011).

Avoidant restrictive food intake disorder (ARFID) is a diagnosis that was introduced in the *Diagnostic and Statistical Manual of Mental Disorders* (5th ed.; DSM-5; American Psychiatric Association, 2013) that is a reformulation of the *DSM-IV feeding disorder of infancy or early childhood* (Eddy et al., 2015). ARFID is defined by a failure to meet adequate caloric and nutritional intake which is associated with one or more of the following: (1) weight loss or failure to meet appropriate weight gain, (2) nutritional deficiencies or health-related issues, (3) dependence on enteral feedings or supplements, or (4) interference with psychosocial functioning. Symptoms are characterized by an apparent lack of interest in eating, avoidance of certain foods based on sensory characteristics (e.g., appearance, color, smell, texture, taste, temperature, or brand), or concern about the aversive consequences of eating. This occurs despite having available food and is not associated with a culturally sanctioned practice, and symptoms are not better accounted for a concurrent medical condition or another mental disorder. This diagnosis allows for the identification of feeding/eating problems in individuals of varying ages as well as those within normal weight and overweight ranges (Eddy et al., 2015). Given the varied criteria, ARFID can take the form of *total food refusal* where the child is dependent on enteral sources for most or all of their nutrition. Alternatively, this disorder can take the form of *partial food refusal* or *food selectivity* where the child consumes preferred foods orally while refusing the

M.L. González (✉)
Pediatric Development and Therapy Center, Our Lady of the Lake Physicians Group, Baton Rouge, Louisiana 70806, USA
e-mail: Melissa.Gonzalez@fmolhs.org

T.D. Mulderink
Pediatric Feeding Disorders Program, St. Vincent, Evansville, IN 47714, USA
e-mail: Thomas.Mulderink@ascension.org

P.A. Girolami
Department of Behavior Psychology, Kennedy Krieger Institute, Johns Hopkins University School of Medicine, Baltimore, MD, USA
e-mail: Girolami@kennedykrieger.org

A. Maragakis, W.T. O'Donohue (eds.), *Principle-Based Stepped Care and Brief Psychotherapy for Integrated Care Settings*, https://doi.org/10.1007/978-3-319-70539-2_6

majority of other foods or drinks based on the appearance, type, brand, or texture of the food (Bandini et al., 2010).

While the majority of clinical cases of ARFID described in the literature are young children and/or the onset of the condition was early in development (Fischer, Luiselli, & Dove, 2015; Williams et al., 2015), ARFID may also be presented in older individuals (Eddy et al., 2015; Wildes, Zucker, & Marcus, 2012). The most common etiology described for ARFID is medical complications that either make eating more difficult, unsuccessful, or otherwise aversive for an individual. Commonly reported medical complications associated with feeding problems are gastrointestinal (GI) in nature such as functional motility (e.g., reflux, constipation), malabsorption, or inflammatory disorders (González & Stern, 2016; Williams, Field, & Seiverling, 2010). Allergy and immune disorders (e.g., food allergy or eosinophilic esophagitis) are also frequently associated with refusal of oral intake. Discomfort associated with these conditions is repeatedly paired with eating to create a conditioned aversion. When the medical condition is resolved, treated, or the diet is appropriately modified, the aversion may persist due to the past association of pain with eating. Other early-life complications including disorders of the central nervous system (e.g., autism spectrum disorder, ASD, Down syndrome, cerebral palsy), oral-motor difficulties (vocal cord paralysis, cleft palate/lip), pulmonary and renal disorders, and prematurity-related complications (e.g., intubation) may also set the stage for difficulty with oral intake creating an aversion to eating or drinking.

For many, due to persistent decreased intake and insufficient weight gain, enteral feedings (i.e., nasogastric feeding or gastrostomy tube feedings) are initiated. With ongoing continued aversion to oral intake, opportunities to practice and develop skills in eating may be minimized. Thus, the child may miss opportunities to develop age-appropriate eating skills, further disrupting the developmental eating process. Environmental factors such as caregiver responses to cope with refusal during feedings often play a role in the maintenance of the feeding issues overtime (Piazza, Fisher et al., 2003). For example, the presentation of food may evoke refusal in the form of crying, attempts to push away feeder/spoon, turning of the head, blocking the mouth, and in some cases, running away from table, aggression, and/or self-injury. The child may learn that specific behaviors (i.e., turning the head, crying, blocking the mouth) during mealtime (or otherwise) are associated with different responses from caregivers such as a variation in the amount or quality of caregiver attention provided (i.e., coaxing or comforting) or the demands that are placed (i.e., amount or type of food presented or duration of the meal; Borrero, Woods, Borrero, Masler, & Lesser, 2010; Piazza, Fisher et al., 2003).

Clinically, the present authors have seen a number of older children and adolescents who have acute-onset ARFID immediately following an illness associated with GI discomfort, vomiting, and/or an episode of constipation. These patients eat typically prior to the onset of the illness. Similar to the clinical course described above, the avoidant responses that are conditioned (i.e., pain associated with eating) persist following the resolution of the illness and are reinforced overtime. That is, these patients may avoid eating in an attempt to prevent symptom relapse or other discomfort and may become hypersensitive to bodily sensations that further reinforce food avoidance.

Given the relatively new diagnostic criteria, current prevalence rates of ARFID offer crude estimates within clinical populations. For instance, retrospective studies evaluating prevalence rates in children aged 8–18, report that 2–14% of patients in specialty clinics (e.g., pediatric gastroenterology or eating disorder clinics) meet criteria for ARFID (Eddy et al., 2015; Fisher et al., 2014; Norris, Spettigue, & Katzman, 2016; Williams et al, 2015), in a retrospective clinical review of 422 children referred for pediatric feeding problems (ages ranging from 4 months to 18 years), found that at least 32% of the sample would qualify for a diagnosis of ARFID. Though these may be conservative estimates, as the retrospective nature of the study made it difficult to determine in some cases if the food refusal was above and beyond, one might expect for the concurrent medical condition. Previous literature suggest that feeding problems are common in young children with typical development and occur at significantly higher rates in children with developmental disabilities (Field, Garland, & Williams, 2003; Ledford & Gast, 2006; Williams et al., 2010). Those with diagnoses of ARFID are likely to have comorbid psychiatric and/or medical conditions (Williams et al., 2010, 2015).

Difficulties with feeding not only have the potential to impact the child's growth and development but also the opportunities for socialization and community participation (i.e., school placement, peer interactions, cultural, and family rituals/holidays; Bandini et al., 2010; Milnes & Piazza, 2013). These difficulties often set the stage for increased caregiver stress (Greer, Gulotta, Masler, & Laud, 2008; Jones & Bryant-Waugh, 2012; Sharp, Burrell, & Jaquess, 2013) and may have implications on caregiver perception of their child and/or impact caregiver-child interactions outside of the meal context (González & Stern, 2016; Johnson et al., 2014).

Screening in Primary Care

Symptom presentation may range greatly in type of concern and in severity. This is further complicated by the varied ages in which symptoms may be reported and the individuals' ability to self-report symptoms or cause of concern. More severe symptoms may include a total refusal to eat or drink as evidence by significant weight loss, failure to gain appropriate weight, and/or dehydration. While these may be obvious signs of a problem across any age, less severe signs may not be as readily identified in younger children including refusal to sit at a table, grazing (i.e., eating small amounts continually throughout the day), limited variety of intake, lack of interest in eating or rarely requesting food, tantrums, refusal, or aggression during meals and long meal durations. Older patients may present as anxious or fearful of specific foods; restrict intake to avoid pain, nausea, or risk of choking, vomiting, or other somatic complaints; or have an aversion to specific tastes or textures.

While a diagnosis of ARFID does not require that the individual be underweight, one of the most commonly reported concerns and an obvious reason for referral for further evaluation and treatment is when the individual, not following his or her growth curve, has reached status of failure to thrive or is otherwise dependent on enteral or supplemental nutrition. *Failure to thrive* means a failure to gain weight or grow when compared to other children of their age group due to inadequate nutritional intake. Specifically, failure to thrive may be diagnosed when weight-for-height or body mass index (BMI; Kg/m^2) is at or below the third to fifth percentile compared to others in his/her age group or when there is a significant decrease in weight across two major growth percentiles (Cole & Lanham, 2011). On the other hand, some children with ARFID, particularly those with limited dietary variety and food selectivity, may present as overweight or obese (Shmaya, Eilat-Adar, Leitner, Reif, & Gabis, 2015). A second common indicator of possible ARFID is dehydration or limited methods for hydration. A commonly reported example is a child who will only drink juice out of a specific cup. This is concerning as it restricts methods for taking in liquid and if this method is no longer effective or available, the individual will be at risk for dehydration. Finally, variety of dietary intake, physical examination, or laboratory testing may be used as indicators of risk for nutritional deficiencies (Williams et al., 2015). There are a variety of screening measures available for children with feeding difficulties and subpopulation (i.e., autism and feeding difficulties) that may be helpful. In a self-study survey conducted by Silverman (2016) among professionals working within the area of feeding difficulties who are participating in a professional consortium of feeding programs, the most frequently used screening measures for feeding difficulties reported were *Behavioral Pediatrics Feeding Assessment Scale* (BPFAS), *Children's Eating Behavior Inventory* (CEBI), *Mealtime Behavior Questionnaire* (MBQ), *About Your Child's Eating* (AYCE), *Brief Autism Mealtime Inventory* (BAMBI), *Brief Assessment of Mealtime Behavior in Children* (BAMBIC), and *Parent Mealtime Action Scale* (PMAS). Further, Sanchez, Spittle, Allinson, and Morgan (2015) systematically reviewed standardized caregiver report questionnaires on feeding abilities and behavior in preschool children. They identified five commercially available measures specific to feeding behavior that were appropriate for children ages 2–5 years; these included BPFAS, CEBI, *Children's Feeding Assessment Questionnaire* (CFAQ), MBQ, and *Montreal Children's Hospital Feeding Scale* (MCH Feeding Scale). Of these, these authors concluded that the BPFAS was the most psychometrically robust parent qeustionnaire available for measuring feeding disorders in preschool children. During the screening, it is often helpful to observe the child and the caregiver during prearranged "snack." This may allow the clinician to get a better idea of the challenges associated with mealtime or the presentation of a specific food.

Differential diagnosis. With younger children, a physician will likely have to determine if the restrictive eating is different from "picky eating" that is often part of a normal developmental trajectory and often observed in children ages 2–6 years. While there is no standard definition of "picky eating," it is generally defined as occurring in children with normal weight but who consume an inadequate variety of foods. Common characteristics of "picky eating" is limiting the variety of foods he/she is willing to eat, unwilling to try new foods (i.e., food neophobia), or rejection of foods of a particular texture, consistency, or smell (Norris et al., 2016). What distinguishes "picky eating" from ARFID is the level of intake restriction as well as the health and social implications and/or impairments that occur as a result.

For older children and adolescents, the physician may consider symptoms and a differential diagnosis with more traditional eating disorders such as anorexia nervosa (AN) and bulimia nervosa (BN). The main distinguishing feature is those with ARFID do not have weight and body-image concerns that are commonly associated with AN and BN. These individuals do not fear weight gain and are not dissatisfied with their body weight, shape, or size (Norris et al., 2016). Recent studies have found that those individuals diagnosed with ARFID were more likely to be male and younger and had a longer duration of illness compared to those with other forms of eating disorders (Forman et al., 2014; Nicely, Lane-Loney, Masciulli, Hollenbeak, & Ornstein, 2014).

Associated conditions. Feeding problems are very common in children with developmental delays. Specifically, food selectivity is often reported among children with autism spectrum disorders (ASD; Bandini et al., 2010; Johnson et al., 2014). Factors that complicate ARFID in those with ASD are that a medical impetus is not always apparent, and the child may add or eliminate food overtime. Longitudinal studies within the ASD population suggest that selectivity does not improve over time without treatment (Suarez, Nelson, & Curtis, 2014). Co-occurring anxiety disorders are also commonly observed in those with ARFID (Eddy et al., 2015; Fischer et al., 2015; Fisher et al., 2014; Nicely et al., 2014).

Further Assessment Prior to Intervention

Patients' needs might differ depending on their age/developmental level and what factors are contributing to the condition (Norris et al., 2016). Given the complexity of feeding problems, it is important that appropriate evaluations and rule-outs are completed prior to treatment. In many cases, concerns related to nutritional status and hydration may need to be addressed immediately via nasogastric tube feeding or other supplemental feedings (i.e., high-calorie formula or calorie booster such as Carnation® Breakfast Essentials) as a short-term course of action while treatment is initiated. Clinically, this will allow for the individual to obtain the proper nutrition and hydration and also decrease the time pressure to achieve the treatment goal(s). For many individuals, successful treatment involves gradual increases in volume or variety of foods; these concerns will likely not be resolved immediately at the onset of treatment.

Given the frequent comorbidity of GI-related and allergy-related issues, it is best practice for those who are restricting intake to first see a gastroenterologist and an allergist to rule out possible untreated medical issues (i.e., reflux, eosinophilic esophagitis, food allergies) precipitating or exacerbating the food refusal. Attempts to treat food refusal will likely be unsuccessful if an active medical issue is undetected/untreated since pain or discomfort will continue to be paired with eating. For individuals who have a history of consuming very little or have a history of lung disease and/or pneumonia, consult an oral motor specialist to evaluate the safety of the swallow to determine if a modified barium swallow (MBS) study or another form of evaluation may be needed.

Evidence-Based Stepped Care and Therapeutic Approaches

Treatments of pediatric feeding disorders vary widely in regard to their theoretical foundations and use across disciplines. Interestingly, some of the most commonly used approaches to address feeding problems in children offer little peer-reviewed support for their effectiveness. To date, the interventions with the most empirical support for the treatment of pediatric feeding disorders come from the applied behavioral analysis (ABA) literature and are often implemented in specialty clinics and in intensive treatment programs (Kerwin, 1999). These interventions are typically based on the identified or hypothesized behavioral function (i.e., factors that are maintaining refusal overtime). Piazza, Fisher et al. (2003), and subsequent studies provide data supporting that the overwhelming majority of children's inappropriate mealtime behavior is maintained by escape from mealtime demands (i.e., negative reinforcement) or some combination of escape and access to attention or tangibles (i.e., negative and positive reinforcement). Thus, many of the empirically supported treatments described below are aimed at disrupting the association of refusal or inappropriate mealtime behavior (i.e., IMB) with a break from eating and/or contingent access to caregiver attention (e.g., comforting statements, coaxing, or reprimands) or preferred toys or activities. It is important to note that many of the following approaches are often used in combination, rather than as isolated treatments. Behavioral caregiver training is also an essential part of the treatment process for this population, particularly with those of younger ages (Kozlowski, Taylor, González, & Girolami, 2015). This training usually involves psychoeducation, developmentally appropriate nutrition education, as well as instruction in the specific intervention involving written description, modeling, behavioral rehearsal, and performance feedback.

The following intervention procedures are empirically supported and would be appropriate in an integrated, brief care clinic. While many offices may not allow food in their conference rooms, it would be beneficial to have a dedicated space for evaluation and intervention of feeding difficulties that is free from interruptions or distractions and equipped with necessary materials (i.e., napkins, age-appropriate table and chair/booster/highchair, sink, etc.). It is not uncommon for children to be sensitive environmental interruptions that may decrease the validity of the observation or effectiveness of the intervention.

Simultaneous presentation. Theoretically based on flavor-flavor learning (Holman, 1975), simultaneous presentations of food has been demonstrated to be effective in increasing acceptance of non-preferred foods for children with feeding problems (Ahearn, 2003; Piazza et al., 2002). A simultaneous presentation involves the feeder presenting bites of a non-preferred food either embedded in, placed next to, or on top of a preferred food item (Ahearn, 2003; Buckley & Newchok, 2005; Piazza et al., 2002). Volkert and Piazza (2012) identify simultaneous presentation as a promising treatment, noting that many of the studies involving simultaneous presentation also incorporate other components in a comprehensive package. Thus, research is necessary to identify the effectiveness of this intervention independent of other treatment elements. This approach may be effective for individuals with mild forms of food selectivity; however, it is not advisable with individuals who have very few foods within their repertoire as a potential negative outcome may be that the individual no longer is willing to eat the previously preferred foods that is presented with the non-preferred food, thus further limiting his or her diet.

High-probability instructional sequence. Another promising approach to increasing acceptance of foods is high-probability instructional sequence, wherein the feeder delivers a series of verbal instructions that the child is likely to produce followed by an instruction to complete the target behavior (e.g., take a bite of a novel or non-preferred food; Piazza, Milnes, & Shalev, 2015). The high-probability instruction is most effective when it is tied to the target behavior such as providing instructions to consume a bite of a highly preferred food prior to a bite of non-preferred food (Penrod, Gardella, & Fernand, 2012). Again, this will likely be most effective with individuals with mild food selectivity who are likely to comply with requests and/or otherwise motivated toward the treatment goal.

Stimulus/demand/texture fading. Stimulus fading, the process by which a stimulus (e.g., texture, food, utensil) is gradually faded to the target stimulus. Kozlowski et al. (2015) identified several studies in which children transitioned from spoon to cup drinking, liquids to solids, and preferred to non-preferred foods. They similarly identified demand fading (gradually increasing mealtime demands) as an effective intervention to increase food volume and variety, though this procedure is often paired with other treatment components as part of a treatment package. Essentially, the initial treatment goal is one that is considered highly achievable (e.g., accepting an empty spoon, familiar food, or very small amount) and following consistent success; the target is gradually modified to more closely approximate the end goal (e.g., novel food, spoonful). This strategy is frequently used alone and in combination with other procedures and could be used in a brief, integrated stepped care setting. This approach will likely be most effective with individuals who comply with requests and/or otherwise motivated toward the treatment goal.

Differential reinforcement. Differential reinforcement of an alternative behavior (DRA) is a procedure in which a reinforcer is delivered for a behavior that serves as an appropriate alternative to the behavior targeted for reduction and withheld following instances of problem behavior. For example, praise/preferred toy may be provided when a child accepts a bite of a novel food; whereas, the praise/preferred toy is withheld following nonacceptance. Differential reinforcement has shown promise as an intervention to increase appropriate feeding behaviors (Casey, Cooper-Brown, Wacker, & Rankin, 2006; Koegel et al., 2012; Riordan, Iwata, Wohl, & Finney, 1980). Specifically, Kerwin (1999) identified differential attention ("positive attention for appropriate feeding behavior and ignoring inappropriate behavior" p. 196) as a well-established treatment for feeding problems (Luiselli, 1994; Riordan, Iwata, Finney, Wohl, & Stanley, 1984). A reinforcement-based intervention is ideal for clinicians and caregivers alike, as the likelihood that the child will experience distress during protocol meals is significantly reduced. Numerous studies have demonstrated that differential reinforcement (reinforcement delivered contingent upon a target response) and noncontingent reinforcement (reinforcement is delivered based on a fixed time schedule, irrespective of the child's behavior) are beneficial for some children alone but most effective when paired with other interventions. Use of these procedures may reduce the occurrence of inappropriate mealtime behaviors and negative vocalizations during meals to manageable levels and otherwise increase motivation for compliance (Piazza, Patel, Gulotta, Sevin, & Layer, 2003).

Noncontingent escape. Noncontingent reinforcement is a treatment that is aimed to decrease problem behavior by disrupting the association of problem behavior with the reinforcing variables such as escape or attention (Cooper, Heron, & Heward, 2007). Escape is commonly found to be a maintaining variable or reinforcer for food refusal. In this case, one goal of treatment is to have the child learn that refusal does not result in escape or termination of the meal. One easily implemented strategy to achieve this is to terminate the meal based on set time period rather than the occurrence of refusal or IMB. That is, the caregiver can set a timer for a relatively brief period of time and let the child know that the meal will end when the food is gone or when the time elapses, whichever comes first. This is a strategy often recommended in outpatient settings to help dissociate refusal/IMB with escape from eating, and can be effective when used with other interventions (e.g., differential reinforcement) as described above.

To summarize, within an integrated care setting, the following recommendations may be helpful and appropriate for children with ARFID:

1. Be strategic when introducing new foods, start with something familiar (i.e., a different brand of yogurt or spread), and/or pair it with something familiar.
2. Structure food introduction separate from meals or supplemental feedings as "taste" or "homework sessions." Keep these sessions brief and successful.
3. Start small. Ask the child to only try a small amount of something new. As he or she is successful, the amount of the new food presented can be gradually increased.
4. Provide praise and/or other rewards to increase the child's motivation and reinforce compliance with trying new foods.
5. End the meal or "taste session" based on a fixed time rather than contingent upon the child's refusal or IMB.

Escape extinction. Numerous studies have demonstrated that escape extinction is an effective intervention for reducing inappropriate mealtime behavior, increasing oral intake, and weight (Hoch, Babbitt, Coe, Krell, & Hackbert, 1994; Kerwin, 1999). Extinction is discontinuing reinforcement of a previously reinforced behavior (Cooper et al., 2007). In many cases, refusal maintains overtime due to the child learning that refusal eventually results in the removal of the bite or escape from the meal (i.e., negative reinforcement). Escape extinction involves continued presentation of the avoidance-producing stimulus (i.e., food). Thus, emitting refusal or IMB does not terminate the presentation of the food. The most common form of escape extinction for this population involves nonremoval of the spoon wherein the feeder places the utensil at the child's lips where it remains until the feeder can deposit the food into the child's mouth (Ahearn, Kerwin, Eicher, Shantz, & Swearingin, 1996). Volkert and Piazza (2012) identified escape extinction as a well-established treatment for feeding problems in children, and is often the essential component of many treatment packages utilized in the literature and in practice. However, due to increases in the intensity and frequency of problem behaviors when escape extinction is first implemented (i.e., *extinction burst*), implementing these procedures with some form of differential or noncontingent reinforcement may be appropriate (Kozlowski et al., 2015). Given the technical training needed and potential varied responses (i.e., increases in IMB, expels or spitting out food, or holding food in cheek) that may occur when implementing, it is essential that the expertise and resources are available from a feeding specialist who is highly trained and experienced in this treatment to ensure proper implementation and a successful outcome. Thus, while this strategy is effective and empirically supported, it is not recommended for use in settings or professionals who do not have appropriate and sufficient training in the use of these procedures.

Treatment Approaches with Limited Empirical Evidence

As noted above, there are many unique approaches to treating feeding disorders that are applied in clinical practice; however, the literature is not currently available to substantiate the effectiveness of many approaches.

Hunger provocation. Clinical hunger provocation has been used as a method of increasing oral feeding in children and infants exclusively fed by tube (e.g., gastrostomy, nasogastric). One such example of hunger provocation involves a brief intensive, multidisciplinary approach in which children receiving their caloric intake via tube have their feedings cut initially to 50% of their preadmission intake (Hartdorff et al., 2015). After 2 days of significant and continued tube reductions, oral feeding occasions are presented 4–5 times daily in which oral feeding was reinforced. Authors reported that of all 21 patients, 18 patients were successfully weaned with hunger provocation based on their criteria. These results are similar to those presented for other clinical hunger provocation programs, with Dunitz-Scheer et al. (2009) reporting 91.9% of tube-dependent patients being successfully weaned for patients treated over a duration of 7 years. While these results are promising, there is insufficient peer-reviewed evidence to support these results. Those studies supporting the effectiveness of clinical hunger provocation lack procedural rigor and replication across sites. Specifically, there is no comparison to an established treatment and lack of data related to important outcome measures including growth parameters such as height and BMI, information on the occurrence and frequency of mealtime problem behaviors during and after discharge, type and/or variety of foods consumed, and calorie intake. Additionally, the data reported by Hartdorff et al. (2015) suggest that 86% of patients were able to generally maintain their preadmission weight at a 6-month follow-up; however, given the mean age of the participants (M = 19.8 months), when a continued rate of weight gain would be expected, it would be critical to include patient height or a metric such as weight-to-height percentile as a preadmission/follow-up measure for growth. Though promising, further research is required to assess the success and viability of a clinical hunger provocation program for treatment of pediatric feeding disorders.

Sensory integration. Many of the evidence-based interventions reviewed thus far have approached mealtime difficulties from a theoretically behavioral perspective, such that they are viewed as learned behaviors resulting from environmental influences. In practice, many interventionists follow a sensory-based theoretical framework. Within a sensory integration framework, behaviors such as gagging, spitting, or refusing foods are viewed to be the result of hypo- or hyper-reactivity to sensory information that arise due to difficulties in modulating sensory information. Treatment often involves a sensory diet in which sensory input is provided to aid the individual in organizing sensory information effectively (Kimball, 1999). Unfortunately, limited research is available on the sensory integrative approach to the treatment of feeding disorders despite this approach being commonly used in practice. Results of a study comparing a sensory integrative approach to a behavioral approach in the treatment of two individuals with pediatric feeding disorders (specifically, escape extinction paired with noncontingent reinforcement), were in favor of the ABA-based approach in increasing food acceptance and reduction of IMB (Addison et al., 2012). At this time, not enough evidence is available to confidently recommend this approach to remediate severe feeding problems.

Sequential-oral-sensory (SOS) approach. Another sensory-based approach is the sequential-oral-sensory (SOS) approach, a treatment that uses systematic desensitization within a hierarchy of skills necessary for appropriate eating (Toomey, 2007). Specifically, through this approach, the child progresses through six major categories including tolerating, interacting, smelling, touching, tasting, and eating. The child is to relax or play with the food as they progress through these categories, with the food being removed if the child displays distress at any stage after which the therapist returns to a lower stage in the hierarchy to reduce the level of stress (Boyd, 2008). Benson, Parke, Gannon, and Muñoz (2013) reviewed the charts of 34 children exposed to the SOS approach to feeding. Their results suggest that 16 of the 34 children did not show advancement despite prolonged exposure to this treatment approach. According to the results of a study attempting to compare a modified version of the SOS approach (for purposes of direct comparison of the two approaches) to an applied behavior analytic approach (ABA) including elements of escape extinction (nonremoval of the spoon), continuous interaction, and re-presentation of expelled bites, the ABA treatment was more effective in increasing acceptance and decreasing IMB (Peterson, Piazza, & Volkert, 2016). Based on their findings, participants who received approximately 17–21 h of the modified SOS treatment had no increases in acceptance or swallowing relative to their peers who, while receiving the ABA-based treatment, had 80% or greater levels of acceptance and swallowing for their first food within 16 min to 4 h of treatment. It is important to note that many practitioners of the SOS approach caution interpretation of these findings, as the modified SOS approach was not conducted exactly as prescribed by Toomey (2007) in order to create a more conceptually sound research design. Additionally, Peterson et al. note that the goals of SOS therapy may be focused on aiding the child to complete the steps of the SOS process and less so on the end goal of a feeding intervention, which is ultimately acceptance and consumption of food. These findings suggest that, while the SOS approach may be effective in producing increases in tolerance of certain aspects of interacting with food for some children, alternate treatments should be considered when the goals of treatment are to increase consumption and reduce inappropriate behaviors during mealtimes. Further evaluation and comparison of this approach to other empirically supported treatments are needed.

When to Refer to External Specialty

It is important to consider the individuals' developmental level, experience, social/family expectations, and the skills (i.e., drinking from a cup, clearing a spoon efficiently, chewing skills, self-feeding skills) he or she may need to acquire before increasing intake. Similarly, if physical limitations are present, adaptive equipment may be considered in order to best support the individuals' success with feeding. With the increased levels of family stress and psychosocial and/or behavioral concerns that may co-occur with ARFID (e.g., extinction bursts during treatment or other behavioral concerns outside of meals; Greer et al., 2008; González & Stern, 2016), it is important to consider if the child may be better served by a referral for treatment to clinicians who are familiar with and/or specialize in working with feeding issues, have adequate resources and expertise available to address ongoing concerns, and are able to collaborate, communicate, and coordinate care across providers.

The Role of Primary Care Provider/ Medical Team in Treatment

With an increased emphasis on healthy eating and more awareness of the long-term impact of a nutritious diet upon development and growth, the first stop for caregivers concerned about their children's mealtime behavior is often their primary care physician/provider (PCP). Typically, the PCP is in a position to determine growth parameters and to identify more obvious atypical eating patterns (and other comorbid developmental conditions). However, given the paucity of research and training opportunities related to ARFID, some primary care providers may feel ill-equipped to address some of eating/mealtime concerns. Because some children's intake does improve over time with limited intervention, some providers may tend to downplay the parents reports of problems and follow the "children will grow out of it" rule to dealing with the issue (Zucker et al., 2015). For those children requiring additional intervention, downplaying parental concerns may end up making things worse, leading to additional stress on family members and problematic interactions at home.

If a practitioner identifies someone that may require specialized services, it's imperative that they have access to appropriate referral sources. Ideally, these resources should be able to provide a continuum of care model that provides a level of frequency or intensity that matches the presenting problem. Referral sources should also be able to provide some empirical support regarding effectiveness of their treatment and parental satisfaction. As we learn more about this population, there needs to be further development of appropriate guidelines for referrals or recommendations that can be disseminated to the frontline practitioners.

How to Assess Impact on Care/ Quality Improvement Processes

Identifying and treating individuals diagnosed with ARFID can be a complex process, so efforts should be made to ensure that families are being provided adequate guidance to navigate the path from initial evaluation through eventual discharge and long-term follow-up. Caregiver feedback on the effectiveness of these interventions and their satisfaction will play a key role in evaluating quality of care. In addition, there should be a concerted effort for practitioners to keep each other updated regarding patient outcomes/satisfaction, progress, recommendations, and wait times for service. Periodic correspondence between professionals will help ensure a more efficient use of clinic time, consistency of recommendations, and more clarity for caregivers. Ultimately, assessment of progress should include the collection of relevant outcome data including growth measures, levels of refusal, meal duration, volume and variety/type/texture of foods consumed, and caregiver satisfaction across the course of treatment. This information should be published and presented at national conferences so that other healthcare professionals can subsequently share with caregivers.

References

Addison, L. R., Piazza, C. C., Patel, M. R., Bachmeyer, M. H., Rivas, K. M., Milnes, S. M., & Oddo, J. (2012). A comparison of sensory integrative and behavioral therapies as treatment for pediatric feeding disorders. *Journal of Applied Behavior Analysis, 45*, 455–471.

Ahearn, W. H. (2003). Using simultaneous presentation to increase vegetable consumption in a mildly selective child with autism. *Journal of Applied Behavior Analysis, 36*(3), 361–365.

Ahearn, W. H., Kerwin, M. E., Eicher, P. S., Shantz, J., & Swearingin, W. (1996). An alternating treatments comparison of two intensive interventions for food refusal. *Journal of Applied Behavior Analysis, 29*, 321–332.

American Psychiatric Association. (2013). *Diagnostic and statistical manual of mental disorders* (5th ed.). Washington, DC: Author.

Bandini, L. G., Anderson, S. E., Curtin, C., Cermak, S., Evans, E. W., Scampini, R., … Must, A. (2010). Food selectivity in children with autism spectrum disorders and typically developing children. *The Journal of Pediatrics, 157*(2), 259–264. https://doi.org/10.1016/j.jpeds.2010.02.013

Benson, J. D., Parke, C. S., Gannon, C., & Muñoz, D. (2013). A retrospective analysis of the Sequential Oral Sensory feeding approach in children with feeding difficulties. *Journal of Occupational Therapy, Schools, & Early Intervention, 6*, 289–300.

Berlin, K. S., Lobato, D. J., Pinkos, B., Cerezo, C. S., & LeLeikos, N. S. (2011). Patterns of medical and developmental comorbidities among children presenting with feeding problems: A latent class analysis. *Journal of Developmental and Behavioral Pediatrics, 32*(1), 41–47. https://doi.org/10.1097/DBP.0b013e318203e06d

Borrero, C. S. W., Woods, J. N., Borrero, J. C., Masler, E. A., & Lesser, A. D. (2010). Descriptive analyses of pediatric food refusal and acceptance. *Journal of Applied Behavior Analysis, 43*(1), 71–88. https://doi.org/10.1901/jaba.2010.43-71

Boyd, K. L. (2008). *The effectiveness of the sequential oral sensory approach group feeding program* (Unpublished doctoral dissertation). Colorado School of Professional Psychology, Colorado Springs, CO.

Buckley, S. D., & Newchok, D. K. (2005). An evaluation of simultaneous presentation and differential reinforcement with response cost to reduce packing. *Journal of Applied Behavior Analysis, 38*(3), 405–409.

Casey, S. D., Cooper-Brown, L. J., Wacker, D. P., & Rankin, B. E. (2006). The use of descriptive analysis to identify and manipulate schedules of reinforcement in the treatment of food refusal. *Journal of Behavioral Education, 15*(1), 39–50.

Cole, S. Z., & Lanham, J. S. (2011). Failure to thrive: An update. *American Family Physician, 83*, 829–834.

Cooper, J. O., Heron, T. E., & Heward, W. L. (2007). *Applied behavior analysis* (2nd ed.). Upper Saddle River, NJ: Pearson/Merril-Prentice Hall.

Dunitz-Scheer, M., Levine, A., Roth, Y., Kratky, E., Beckenbach, H., Braegger, C., … Scheer, P. J. (2009). Prevention and treatment of tube dependency in infancy and early childhood. *Infant, Child, and Adolescent Nutrition, 1*(2), 73–82.

Eddy, K. T., Thomas, J. J., Hastings, E., Edkins, K., Lamont, E., Nevins, C., … Becker, A. E. (2015). Prevalence of DSM-5 avoidant/restrictive food intake disorder in a pediatric gastroenterology healthcare network. *International Journal of Eating Disorders, 48*, 464–470.

Field, D., Garland, M., & Williams, K. (2003). Correlates of specific childhood feeding problems. *Journal of Paediatrics and Child Health, 39*(4), 299–304. https://doi.org/10.1046/j.1440-1754.2003.00151.x

Fischer, A. J., Luiselli, J. K., & Dove, M. B. (2015). Effects of clinic and in-home treatment on consumption and feeding-associated anxiety in an adolescent with avoidant/restrictive food intake disorder. *Clinical Practice in Pediatric Psychology, 3*, 154–166.

Fisher, M. M., Rosen, D. S., Ornstein, R. M., Mammel, C. A., Katzman, D. K., Rome, E. S., … Walsh, B. T. (2014). Characteristics of avoidant/restrictive intake disorder in children and adolescents: A "new disorder" in DSM-5. *Journal of Adolescent Health, 55*, 49–52.

Forman, S. F., McKenzie, N., Hehn, R., Monge, M. C., Kapphahn, C. J., Mammel, K. A., … Woods, E. R. (2014). Predictors of outcome at 1 year in adolescents with DSM-5 restrictive eating disorders: Report of the national eating disorders quality improvement collaborative. *Journal of Adolescent Health, 55*, 750–756.

González, M. L., & Stern, K. (2016). Co-occurring behavioral difficulties in children with severe feeding problems: A descriptive study. *Research in Developmental Disabilities, 58*, 45–54. https://doi.org/10.1016/j.ridd.2016.08.009

Greer, A. J., Gulotta, C. S., Masler, E. A., & Laud, R. B. (2008). Caregiver stress and outcomes of children with pediatric feeding disorders treated in an intensive interdisciplinary program. *Journal of Pediatric Psychology, 33*, 612–620. https://doi.org/10.1093/jpepsy/jsm116

Hartdorff, C. M., Kneepkens, C. M. F., Stok-Akerboom, A. M., van Dijk-Lokkart, E. M., Engels, M. A. H., & Kindermann, A. (2015). Clinical tube weaning supported by hunger provocation in fully-tube-fed children. *Journal of Pediatric Gastroenterology and Nutrition, 60*(4), 538–543.

Hoch, T. A., Babbitt, R. L., Coe, D. A., Krell, D. M., & Hackbert, L. (1994). Contingency contacting: Combining positive reinforcement and escape extinction procedures to treat persistent food refusal. *Behavior Modification, 18*(1), 106–128.

Holman, E. W. (1975). Immediate and delayed reinforcers for flavor preferences in rats. *Animal Learning & Behavior, 6*, 91–100.

Johnson, C. R., Turner, K., Stewart, P. A., Schmidt, B., Shui, A., Macklin, E., … Courtney, P. M. (2014). Relationships between feeding problems, behavioral characteristics and nutritional quality in children with ASD. *Journal of Autism and Developmental Disorders, 44*, 1–10. https://doi.org/10.1007/s10803-014-2095-9

Jones, C., & Bryant-Waugh, R. (2012). Development and pilot of a group skills-and-support intervention for mothers of children with feeding problems. *Appetite, 58*(2), 450–456. https://doi.org/10.1016/j.appet.2011.12.017

Kerwin, M. E. (1999). Empirically supported treatments in pediatric psychology: Severe feeding problems. *Journal of Pediatric Psychology, 24*(3), 193–214.

Kimball, J. G. (1999). Sensory integration frame of reference: Postulates regarding change and application to practice. In P. Kramer & J. Hinojosa (Eds.), *Frames of reference for pediatric occupational therapy* (pp. 169–204). Philadelphia, PA: Lippincott.

Koegel, R. L., Bharoocha, A. A., Ribnick, C. B., Ribnick, R. C., Bucio, M. O., Fredeen, R. M., & Koegel, L. K. (2012). Using individualized reinforcers and hierarchical exposure to increase food flexibility in children with autism spectrum disorders. *Journal of Autism and Developmental Disorders, 42*(8), 1574–1581.

Kozlowski, A. M., Taylor, T., González, M. L., & Girolami, P. A. (2015). Feeding Disorders. In J. L. Matson & M. L. Matson (Eds.), *Comorbid conditions in individuals with intellectual disabilities* (pp. 109–143). Cham: Springer International Publishing.

Ledford, J. R., & Gast, D. L. (2006). Feeding problems in children with autism spectrum disorders a review. *Focus on Autism and Other Developmental Disabilities, 21*(3), 153–166. https://doi.org/10.1177/10883576060210030401

Luiselli, J. K. (1994). Oral feeding treatment of children who are deaf and blind. *Behavior Modification, 17*, 457–473.

Milnes, S. M., & Piazza, C. C. (2013). Feeding disorders. *International Review of Research in Developmental Disabilities, 44*, 143–166. https://doi.org/10.1016/B978-0-12-401662-0.00005-1

Nicely, T. A., Lane-Loney, S., Masciulli, E., Hollenbeak, C. S., & Ornstein, R. M. (2014). Prevalence and characteristics of avoidant/restrictive food intake disorder in a cohort of young patients in day treatment for eating disorders. *Journal of Eating Disorders, 2*, 21. https://doi.org/10.1186/s40337-014-0021-3

Norris, M. L., Spettigue, W. J., & Katzman, D. K. (2016). Update on eating disorders: Current perspectives on avoidant/restrictive food intake disorder in children and youth. *Neuropsychiatric Disease and Treatment, 12*, 213–218.

Penrod, B., Gardella, L., & Fernand, J. (2012). An evaluation of a progressive high-probability instructional sequence combined with demand fading in the treatment of food selectivity. *Journal of Applied Behavior Analysis, 45*, 527–537.

Peterson, K. M., Piazza, C. C., & Volkert, V. M. (2016). A comparison of a modified sequential oral sensory approach to an applied behavior-analytic approach in the treatment of food selectivity in children with autism spectrum disorders. *Journal of Applied Behavior Analysis, 49*, 1–27.

Piazza, C. C., Fisher, W. W., Brown, K. A., Shore, B. A., Patel, M. R., Katz, R. M., … Blakely-Smith, A. (2003). Functional analysis of inappropriate mealtime behaviors. *Journal of Applied Behavior Analysis, 36*, 187–204.

Piazza, C. C., Milnes, S. M., & Shalev, R. A. (2015). A behavior-analytic approach to the assessment and treatment of pediatric feeding disorders. In H. S. Roane, J. L. Ringdahl, & T. S. Falcomata (Eds.), *Clinical and organizational applications of applied behavior analysis* (pp. 69–91). London: Elsevier Inc..

Piazza, C. C., Patel, M. R., Gulotta, C. S., Sevin, B. M., & Layer, S. A. (2003). On the relative contributions of positive reinforcement and escape extinction in the treatment of food refusal. *Journal of Applied Behavior Analysis, 36*(3), 309–324.

Piazza, C. C., Patel, M. R., Santana, C. M., Goh, H. L., Delia, M. D., & Lancaster, B. M. (2002). An evaluation of simultaneous and sequential presentation of preferred and nonpreferred food to treat food selectivity. *Journal of Applied Behavior Analysis, 35*(3), 259–270.

Riordan, M. M., Iwata, B. A., Finney, J. W., Wohl, M. K., & Stanley, A. E. (1984). Behavioral assessment and treatment of chronic food refusal in handicapped children. *Journal of Applied Behavior Analysis, 17*, 327–341.

Riordan, M. M., Iwata, B. A., Wohl, M. K., & Finney, J. W. (1980). Behavioral treatment of food refusal and selectivity in developmentally disabled children. *Applied Research in Mental Retardation, 1*(1), 95–112.

Sanchez, K., Spittle, A. J., Allinson, L., & Morgan, A. (2015). Parent questionnaires measuring feeding disorders in preschool children: A systematic review. *Developmental Medicine & Child Neurology, 57*, 798–807. https://doi.org/10.1111/dmcn.12748

Sharp, W. G., Burrell, T. L., & Jaquess, D. L. (2013). The Autism MEAL Plan: A parent-training curriculum to manage eating aversions and low intake among children with autism. *Autism, 18*(6), 712–722. https://doi.org/10.1177/1362361313489190

Shmaya, Y., Eilat-Adar, S., Leitner, Y., Reif, S., & Gabis, L. (2015). Nutritional deficiencies and overweight prevalence among children with autism spectrum disorders. *Research in Developmental Disabilities, 38*, 1–6. https://doi.org/10.1016/j.ridd.2014.11.020

Silverman, A. (2016). *Feeding programs self-study*. Report for Feeding Programs Consortium Business meeting in Cincinnati, OH.

Suarez, M. A., Nelson, N. W., & Curtis, A. B. (2014). Longitudinal follow-up factors associated with food selectivity in children with autism spectrum disorders. *Autism, 18*, 924–932. https://doi.org/10.1177/1362361313499457

Toomey, K. (2007, July). An introduction to the SOS approach to feeding. *Pediatric Feeding and Dysphagia Newsletter, 8*(1), 2–10.

Volkert, V. M., & Piazza, C. C. (2012). Empirically supported treatments for pediatric feeding disorders. In P. Sturmey & M. Hersen (Eds.), *Handbook of evidence based practice in clinical psychology* (Vol. 1, pp. 456–481). Hoboken, NJ: Wiley.

Wildes, J. E., Zucker, N. L., & Marcus, M. D. (2012). Picky eating in adults: Results of a web-based survey. *International Journal of Eating Disorders, 45*, 575–582. https://doi.org/10.1002/eat.20975

Williams, K. E., Field, D. G., & Seiverling, L. (2010). Food refusal in children: A review of the literature. *Research in Developmental Disabilities, 31*(3), 625–633.

Williams, K. E., Hendy, H. M., Field, D. G., Belousov, Y., Riegel, K., & Harclerode, W. (2015). Implications of avoidant/restrictive food intake disorder (ARFID) on children with feeding problems. *Children's Health Care, 44*, 307–321. https://doi.org/10.1080/02739615.2014.921789

Zucker, N., Copeland, W., Franz, L., Carpenter, K., Keeling, L., Angold, A., & Egger, H. (2015). Psychological and psychosocial impairment in preschoolers with selective eating. *Pediatrics, 136*, e582–e590. https://doi.org/10.1542/peds.2014-2386

Bereavement

7

Martha Zimmermann and Anthony Papa

A Brief Description of the Disorder or Problem

The loss of a loved one is an inevitable part of the human experience. Normal grieving may be characterized by an acute, time-limited experience of yearning, emotional distress, and intrusive thoughts related to the deceased that tends to remit within 4–6 months of the loss (Bonanno, 2005). Normal grieving may be also characterized by brief, transient distress, continuing to experience and express positive emotion, and a quick return to functioning (Bonanno et al., 2002; Bonanno, Papa, Lalande, Westphal, & Coifman, 2004). Regardless of level of intensity, grief is typically a transitory experience in which a person either continues to function or returns to previous function after a period of time. Despite a return to functioning, many individuals still report sadness when reminded of the deceased throughout the lifetime. As such, categorizing grief as a mental disorder has often been considered controversial for fear of pathologizing a normal human phenomenon. While most bereaved individuals experience a wide range of responses that are considered healthy and normal, research suggests that for a certain group of individuals, the experience of losing a loved one can result in significant levels of unrelenting distress and impairment that may benefit from clinical intervention. These reactions can include a number of issues that require clinical evaluation and monitoring including pathological grief (see below), major depressive disorder (MDD), posttraumatic stress disorder (PTSD), poor sleep, substance abuse, suicidal ideation, physical disease, poor health behaviors, underutilization of mental health services, and an overall reduction in quality of life and social isolation (e.g., Lannen, Wolfe, Prigerson, Onelov, & Kreicbergs, 2008; Lee, 2015; Lichtenthal et al., 2011; Papa, Lancaster, & Kahler, 2013; Prigerson et al., 1995; Simon et al., 2007; Stahl & Schulz, 2014). These risks indicate an important need for clinical intervention given the considerable impact they may have on quality of life, health behaviors, and functional impairment in important domains such as social relationships and occupational functioning. However, interventions for grief when pathological grief is not present have been shown to be ineffective and potentially iatrogenic (Schut & Stroebe, 2005). Thus, effectively distinguishing normal reactions to loss from those that require treatment is imperative in an integrated care setting.

Pathological grief has been conceptualized differently in the two main nosological systems.

M. Zimmermann, B.A. (✉) • A. Papa, Ph.D.
Department of Psychology, University of Nevada, Reno, Reno, NV, USA
e-mail: mzimmermann@nevada.unr.edu; apapa@unr.edu

A. Maragakis, W.T. O'Donohue (eds.), *Principle-Based Stepped Care and Brief Psychotherapy for Integrated Care Settings*, https://doi.org/10.1007/978-3-319-70539-2_7

The ICD-11 will include a conceptualization of pathological grief based on the criteria developed for Prolonged Grief Disorder (PGD). This consist of significant impairment due to chronic yearning, longing, preoccupation about the deceased, and/or emotional pain that had endured for more than 6 months accompanied by feeling shocked, angry, and/or numb from the loss; diminished sense of self and meaning; trouble accepting their loss, trusting others, and moving on; and avoidance of reminders (see Prigerson et al., 2009). Estimates of the prevalence of PGD in normative population samples range from 3.7 to 4.8 in Western European countries (Forstmeier & Maercker, 2007; Kersting, Brähler, Glaesmer, & Wagner, 2011; Newson, Boelen, He, Hofman, & Tiemeier, 2011) and 1.6–2.4% in Japan (Fujisawa, Miyashita, Nakajima, Ito, Kato, & Kim, 2010; Mizuno, Kishimoto, & Asukai, 2012). Importantly, those symptoms that are unique to pathological grief predict impairment and dysfunction over and above MDD or PTSD alone, as well as differential responses to therapeutic intervention (Prigerson, 2009; Shear et al., 2011).

While it is clear that pathological grief is both significantly impairing to warrant clinical intervention and also characterized by unique symptoms that differ from MDD and PTSD, its definition as a distinct disorder has not yet been recognized by the *DSM*. The inclusion of pathological grief in the *DSM-5* was considered by the Trauma and Stress Disorders Work Group. Ultimately, the *DSM* Work Group determined that persistent complex bereavement disorder (PCBD; APA, 2013) should be proposed as a new potential disorder for future study. PCBD criteria were constructed via literature review, expert consultation, and consensus discussion. This conceptualization shares characteristics of PGD but has been extend to include more symptoms. PCBD has not been validated in clinical populations at the time of this writing. To date, a number of studies have validated PGD in clinical samples, and as such, its use as diagnostic criteria is recommended when screening for pathological grief reactions (Lee, 2015; Prigerson et al., 2009).

Effective Ways to Screen for it in the Primary Care Setting

Self-report questionnaires can be used to indicate the presence of pathological grief. The most well validated is the Prolonged Grief Disorder (PG-13) Scale (Prigerson & Maciejewski, 2008) which may also be used to indicate the presence of pathological grief. To meet criteria, the individual must have experienced the loss of a loved one, be experiencing yearning or emotional pain at least daily 6 months after the loss, and be experiencing at least five cognitive, emotional, and behavioral symptoms that result in significant impairment in some important area of functioning. In addition to the PG-13 scale, the Brief Grief Questionnaire (Shear & Essock, 2002) is less well validated but only consists of five items, lending itself to an integrated care setting. It assesses trouble accepting the death, how much grief interferes with daily life, trouble with images or thoughts related to the death, trouble engaging with or avoiding important pre-death activities, and social isolation. A score of five or more may indicate the presence of pathological grief.

In addition to screening for pathological grief, a thorough evaluation of bereavement-related difficulties should include an evaluation of loss including mood or anxiety reactions, suicidal ideation, substance abuse, and other adverse health behaviors. Preexisting psychiatric comorbidities should also be assessed, as the existence of psychopathology prior to the loss is associated with greater grief symptom severity.

This task can be difficult as MDD, PTSD, PGD, and other problems rend to be highly comorbid. Pathological grief is distinct from PTSD or MDD in particularly in the yearning, feeling stunned, shocked or dazed by the loss, and difficulty accepting the loss symptoms (Papa, Lancaster, & Kahler, 2014). While exposure to death through loss may constitute a criterion A stressor for PTSD, symptoms that tend to be unique to PTSD include emotional reactivity, physical reactivity, cognitive avoidance of distressing thoughts and emotions, irritability or anger, and hypervigilance. Characteristics that tend to be more unique to MDD but not pathological grief include loss of interest in daily activities, low mood, fatigue or low energy, and changes in appetite. In previous iterations of the *DSM*, bereavement was considered a life event that excluded the diagnoses of a major depressive episode. The bereavement clause was thought to prevent pathologizing grief by considering depressive symptoms as a result of bereavement not formally depression. Further study, however, suggested that bereavement-related depression does not differ from a standard depressive episode in a meaningful way (Zisook & Kendler, 2007). As such, this exclusion criterion was removed in the *DSM-5*, and MDD may be diagnosed following bereavement and treated accordingly. Assessment procedures and interventions for MDD and PTSD should follow non-loss-related protocols as described in this book.

Increases in pathological grief symptoms are associated with increased psychiatric comorbidity, suggesting that the presence of PTSD and MDD may interact with pathological grief to produce greater symptom severity. Onset of mood or anxiety disorders before the loss in particular is associated with greater likelihood of the development of pathological grief (Simon et al., 2007). Thus, a determination should be made as to whether or not pathological grief, or another clinical problem, is primary and preceded other clinical problems. If 6 months has not passed and the individual meets criteria for another disorder, the comorbid disorder should be addressed first without specific intervention aimed at pathological grief symptoms. Preexisting psychopathology should be assessed, as the presence of a psychiatric disorder prior to the loss is associated with increased severity of pathological grief, which in turn is associated with greater functional impairment (Simon et al., 2007).

In addition to assessing the presence of MDD and PTSD, suicidal ideation and substance abuse should be assessed following a loss, as both are more likely to occur following bereavement. Substance abuse, particularly alcohol and tobacco use, is more common among bereaved individuals than their non-bereaved counterparts. Widowers, in particular, may be more prone to alcohol use, and elderly widowers are at a much higher risk for suicide than any other group indicating that these groups should be carefully monitored (McIntosh, Santos, Hubbard, & Overholser, 1994; Prigerson et al., 1997; Stroebe, Schut, & Stroebe, 2007; Szanto, Prigerson, & Reynolds, 2001). Suicidality and substance abuse should be assessed and treated as per recommendation in this book.

Risk factors associated with increased likelihood of developing pathological grief should be evaluated. These factors include the nature of the relationship to the deceased as well as the circumstances of the death. Closeness to the deceased is associated with more risk, as relationships characterized as overly dependent may confer more risk. Conversely, relationships marked by conflict or abuse are also associated with an increased risk of the development of pathological grief responses. Dementia or HIV+ caregivers are associated with more risk (Bonanno, Moskowitz, Papa, & Folkman, 2005; Schulz, Boerner, Shear, Zhang, & Gitlin, 2006). Caregiver burden may be associated with increased risk after a loss as it is more likely to create disruption to the bereaved individual's daily life and access to rewards in his or her environment. The loss of a child is associated with more risk (Kersting et al., 2011), as is perinatal loss, particularly for bereaved mothers. Sudden, violent death is associated with more risk (Dyregrov, Nordanger, & Dyregrov, 2003).

A number of demographic characteristics have been determined to increase risk for pathology. Childhood experiences such as history of childhood abuse or adversity such as the death of a parent (Silverman, Johnson, & Prigerson, 2001), childhood separation anxiety (Vanderwereker, Jacobs, Park, & Prigerson, 2001), insecure attachment style (Johnson, Zhang, Greer, & Prigerson, 2007), history of childhood abuse and serious neglect (e.g., Silverman et al., 2001), and significant loss of financial and material resources due to the loss (Balk et al., 2004) are all associated with increased risk. Greater number of prior bereavement should also be evaluated as a potential risk factor. Access to resources may also play a role in functioning after loss. Individuals of low socioeconomic status or those who experience a significant loss of financial or material resources as a result of the loss may be at a higher risk of experiencing pathological grief in the wake of a death.

In terms of resilience factors, perceptions of preparedness for a loss are associated with reduced risk of pathological grief (Barry, Kasl, & Prigerson, 2002). Engaging with a social support network has been found to be a protective factor against the onset of pathological grief, PTSD, and MDD following a loss as well as an increased quality of life (Vanderwerker & Prigerson, 2004). Continuing to experience positive emotions may be an important component of maintaining social connectedness and is considered a protective factor (Bonanno & Keltner, 1997).

How to Further Assess if a Screen Returns Positive

Time since loss and severity of distress and impairment are the key domains that should be assessed if a screen for pathological grief is positive. The time since loss is an important determinant in whether or not an individual's symptoms warrant clinical intervention. Because acute symptoms within the range of normal grieving are difficult to distinguish from pathological grief, it is suggested that pathological grief should not be diagnosed or treated until 6 months following the loss (Prigerson, 2009). This criterion reduces the likelihood of a false-positive diagnosis of pathological grief. Importantly, early symptom severity does not indicate subsequent functional impairment, and clinical intervention without pathological grief may be iatrogenic.

As such, watchful waiting is suggested before 6 months has passed in order to identify those who may be at high risk of developing the disorder as well as those who develop associated risks as a result of the loss (e.g., suicidality, substance abuse, etc.). Resilient or recovered individuals likely demonstrate lower symptom levels as soon as 2–3 months following the loss (Bonanno, 2005; Lichtenthal et al., 2011). Watchful waiting should include addressing comorbidities such as adverse reactions to the loss (e.g., MDD, PTSD), preexisting psychopathology, suicidal ideation, and substance use.

A positive result from these screening tools should be accompanied by an assessment of distress severity and functional impairment to determine whether or not the bereaved individual should be treated in primary care or specialty mental health. Assessment of distress should include assessment of perceptions of loss and the circumstances surrounding the loss. Trauma and grief may have a synergistic effect. As such, if the person is bereaved as a result of a traumatic event, such as homicide or suicide, or perceives the death as sudden and violent, this may be suggestive of greater distress and impairment (Neria & Litz, 2004). If the bereaved individual was exposed to death, then perceptions of helplessness, fear, or horror should be examined as indicators of distress severity.

Functional impairment should be assessed by evaluating the individual's ability to participate and function in key life domains. Pathological grief is associated with significant changes in activities, including decreased contact with social relationships, more missed meals, starting work later, and decreased engagement in outdoor activities and exercise (Monk, Houck, & Shear, 2006). Activities may change to avoid social interaction and engage in more solitary activities.

Social relationships in particular should be monitored, as perceived social support has been shown to be both a protective factor against the development of pathological grief, MDD, and PTSD (Vanderwerker & Prigerson, 2004), as well as an area functioning impacted strongly by PGD, MDD, and PTSD. Thus, the individual's report of helpful social relationships may be an important construct to assess early on following a loss. General perceptions of social support can be measured using the 12-item Interpersonal Support Evaluation List (ISEL; Cohen & Hoberman, 1983). This measure assesses several aspects of the individual's perceived social support and relationship quality. Low scores on this index may suggest that intervention directed at helpful support may be warranted. Measurement of general social functioning could include items 20 and 32 from the Medical Outcomes Study 36-item Short Form Health Survey (SF-36; Ware & Sherbourne, 1992) which measured the degree that physical and emotional difficulties impacted normal social activities. More molecular-specific assessment of which social roles or relationship functioning are problematic could include the 14-item Social Adjustment Scale Self-Report – Screener Version (Gameroff, Wickramaratne, & Weissman, 2012) which measures work, social and leisure, extended family, family unit, primary relationship, and parental roles.

The extent to which the individual's life has been disrupted should be evaluated. For example, if the person was a caretaker for the deceased, the impact on the individual's daily life may be substantial (e.g., the "role limitations due to emotional problems" scale of the SF-36). This assessment may include determining the quality of the relationship, potential conflict, and level of dependency. The individual's age at the time of the loss may also have bearing on factors related to distress and impairment. If the bereaved individual is an older adult, support resources such as family, degree of physical and functional dependency on deceased, health status, and cognitive ability may be relevant indicators of distress or impairment (Stroebe et al., 2007). If the bereaved is a child or adolescent, support systems such as family and caregiver mental health status and behaviors should be taken into consideration. Additional stressors more common among children or adolescents include conduct problems, irritability, anxiety symptoms, and fear of death (Luecken & Roubinov, 2012). Difficulties in these areas may be associated with greater severity of pathological grief.

Evidence-Based Stepped Care and Brief Psychotherapeutic Approaches

Mental Health Literacy/Psychoeducation

Little is known about mental health literacy and pathological grief development and outcomes. A number of websites are available that provide information about grief. While not studied via randomized controlled trial, Internet and e-mail use has been associated with decreased grief symptoms. The protective factors associated with Internet use may relate to a reduction in social isolation gained from interacting with a larger community (Vanderwerker & Prigerson, 2004).

However, it is likely that information provided about common reactions to grief and helpful ways of coping may help bereaved individuals to know what is considered normal grieving. Particularly, it may be important to dispel lay beliefs about the stages of grief that are necessary to "work through" grief, such that individuals who are undergoing normal grief reactions are not pathologized. "Grief work" is a popular lay belief that stems from a psychoanalytic interpretation of grief. In this view, the bereaved individual must confront and process the loss in a way that leads to the end of attachment to the deceased. This interpretation has led to a widely held idea that all bereaved individuals must "work through" negative thoughts related to bereavement. This idea, however, is not supported by empirical investigation. While it may be that confronting the loss is an important component for the small minority of bereaved individuals who go on to develop pathological grief, no empirical evidence suggests that all bereaved individuals must confront the loss or that a search for meaning must follow the loss (Stroebe, Schut, & Stroebe, 2005). As such, there appears to be no "right" way to grieve following the loss of a loved one. Another myth that often is discussed in the public domain and might need to be addressed is the idea of delayed grief (the idea that individuals who did not immediately display distress following bereavement are abnormal and will experience grief later), which also has not found empirical support (Bonanno & Kaltman, 2001; Bonanno & Field, 2001).

Education in this area should emphasize the wide variety of reactions that constitute normal and resilient grief trajectories may be helpful in normalizing reactions to loss. Psychoeducation has been examined as a component of interventions and typically focuses on describing characteristics of normal grief and pathological grief, including typical symptoms, course, and associated risks (Rosner, Lumbeck, & Geissner, 2011). Preliminary evidence also indicates that psychoeducation with a specific focus on developing helpful interpersonal relationships may be particularly useful (Nam, 2016).

Bibliotherapy

Bibliotherapy has demonstrated efficacy as a stand-alone treatment for many clinical problems and may be used as an adjunct to psychotherapy in order to reduce treatment time (Floyd, 2003). However, while many resources related to grief are available for purchase, their use for the treatment of pathological grief has not been empirically examined. Given this lack of evidence at this time, no existing literature can be recommended for the improvement of pathological grief symptoms.

Computer-Based Interventions/e-Health

This modality may be particularly useful for this population as the use of the computer may obviate stigma and shame associated with treatment. Computer-based interventions are beneficial in that they are more accessible to individuals with physical disability and thus may be particularly useful among older adults. Further, the majority of patients report feeling treatment for pathological grief is acceptable without face-to-face contact and found that using the computer was a pleasant experience (Wagner, Knaevelsrud, & Maercker, 2006).

Computer-assisted behavioral activation has demonstrated efficacy in the treatment of those with pathological grief. *Healthy Experiences After Loss* (HEAL) is a cognitive-behavioral intervention for individuals with pathological grief. This therapist-assisted intervention uses behavioral activation strategies to target disengagement from the present including yearning and intrusive thoughts regarding the deceased (Litz et al., 2014). Behavioral activation delivered via the Internet should include psychoeducation and rationale for this treatment. Patients are assigned homework to record activities for 1 week, indicating the pleasantness and importance of each activity. Following homework assignments should continue to track activities while identifying values that could be meaningful connected to the introduction of new pleasurable activities. These assignments would serve to increase the frequency with which the bereaved individual contacted natural reinforcers in his or her new environment without the deceased (Eisma et al., 2015).

Behavioral Health Interventions for Primary Care Settings

While randomized controlled trials are limited, preliminary evidence indicates that at present, behavioral activation principles may be the most likely to be effective in an integrated care setting. Because behavioral activation can be flexibly adapted to different settings such as primary care, these principles constitute the best available intervention that can be applied across all levels of a stepped care approach to treating pathological grief. Moreover, these techniques can be applied by primary care providers of all levels of training from professional to paraprofessional (e.g., Ekers, Richards, McMillan, Bland, & Gilbody, 2011).

Behavioral activation is theoretically well-suited to the treatment of pathological grief, and preliminary evidence supports this conclusion (Acierno et al., 2012; Eisma et al., 2015; Litz et al., 2014; Papa, Sewell, Garrison-Diehn, & Rummel, 2013). Bereavement leads to changes in an individual's environment that may drastically alter important components of the individual's daily life such as changing social status, handling challenges related to the death such as making funeral arrangements and the possessions of the deceased, and navigating a new social reality. Pathological grief is characterized by environmental disengagement, avoidance, and rumination that may result from disruption of essential aspects of individual's way of life and identity that are vital to effective engagement with one's environment. Behavioral activation intervenes on social and behavioral disengagement by identifying activities that reinforce adaptive behaviors and scheduling these activities. This process aims to increase the frequency with which the individual contacts natural reinforcers in the environment following the loss, to help ameliorate behavioral patterns maintaining symptoms, and to facilitate reengagement with one's life after loss (Papa et al., 2013).

Rumination is also seen as a key process that is associated with distress, grief symptoms, and behavioral withdrawal. Both depressive rumination and frequent thinking about the deceased or the death have been conceptualized as an avoidance strategy in that it may substitute for confrontation of painful emotions, cognitions, and environmental reminders of the loss. By exposing the person to feared loss-related stimuli, this intervention works to decrease the amount of time spent engaging in rumination (Eisma et al., 2015). Behavioral activation may also serve to reduce rumination by replacing it with more adaptive behaviors. It is important to note that interventions are indicated only in the presence of pathological grief and should not be implemented for most bereaved individuals.

Medication

Given the available evidence, there is little evidence for the use of psychotropic medication in the treatment for individuals experiencing PGD. Well-designed and adequately powered studies have yet to be conducted examining the efficacy of pharmacological interventions for pathological grief. Small, preliminary studies suggest that tricyclic antidepressants may alleviate depression-related symptoms but not symptoms specific to pathological grief. One study to date has shown that the administration of SSRIs may reduce both grief symptoms and depressive symptoms, but more research is needed in this area to reach a conclusive recommendation (Bui, Nadal-Vicens, & Simon, 2012).That said, use of psychotropic medications in the treatment of non-PGD reactions to loss (e.g., MDD) and other comorbid disorders should follow the guidelines specific to those disorders.

What Does Not Work

It is well supported in the literature that clinical intervention is only warranted for a minority of bereaved individuals who demonstrate abnormally persistent and impairing reactions to the loss of a loved one. Broad-based primary prevention programs (bereavement groups for all recently bereaved) or specialty care for those who have not been adequately screened for PGD or other disorders has been found to be unhelpful and at times iatrogenic. Thus, restraint from clinical intervention for those who either show an acute distress response or little grief response is recommended.

Support Groups

Support groups can be a useful source of information about how other people who are experiencing grief deal with issues such as what to do with the deceased's possessions, are they feeling normal, etc. This may be especially important for people who feel isolated or alone in their reactions to the death or the circumstances leading top or following the loss. However, in terms of recommending a person, seeking a support group is one that should be exercised with caution. Groups vary widely on the focus (peer or professional lead, religiosity, type of loss, etc.) such that it may be hard to find a good match and may emphasize the person's sense of isolation. Also, there is very little research supporting the effectiveness of these programs. What research that does exist suggests that programs associated with (1) extensive outreach efforts or (2) use as early intervention have been associated with worse outcomes (see Currier, Neimeyer, & Berman, 2008; Levy, Derby, & Martinkowski, 1993; Schut, Stroebe, van den Bout, & Terheggen, 2001).

When to Refer to External Specialty Mental Health

More extended and intensive interventions may be required for individuals suffering from pathological grief and may be warranted in the case of non-response to stepped or brief interventions outlined above. Low motivation for treatment is also associated with poorer outcomes, suggesting that more time with a mental health specialist may be necessary (Boelen, de Keijser, van den Hout, & van den Bout, 2011). Specialty mental health should also be considered if there are cases of high symptom severity, suicidal ideation, severe substance abuse, and significant functional impairment or if severe PTSD-related re-experiencing symptoms are present.

Specialty mental healthcare may include cognitive-behavioral therapy (CBT) techniques that are used in individual psychotherapy in conjunction with homework to reduce symptoms of grief. Both cognitive restructuring and exposure therapy alone and in tandem have been effective in this aim. Sessions are typically 45 min for at least 12 weeks. Cognitive-behavioral therapy (CBT) for pathological grief has consistently demonstrated success in the reduction of grief symptoms for individuals experiencing pathological grief (Wittouck, Van Autreve, De Jaegere, Portzky, & van Heeringen, 2011). Loss-related negative cognitions and avoidance of loss-related cues are thought to be the mechanisms of change that should be specifically targeted by clinical intervention to produce improvement in pathological grief symptoms (Boelen et al., 2011). To this effect, CBT typically consists of psychoeducation, cognitive restructuring of distorted thinking related to the loss, exposure to loss-related cues, and behavioral activation targeting behavioral isolation and social disengagement that characterizes pathological grief.

Cognitive techniques include teaching health behaviors, identification and modification of irrational self-relevant beliefs related to the loss, and differentiating between moving on and forgetting the loved one. While negative thoughts may be accurate appraisals of a situation in the case of bereavement, it may be that idiosyncratic meanings attached to the loss contribute to difficulties. Most common among bereaved individuals include assumptions about the world that have been violated. Cognitive restructuring may target these assumptions by focusing on incorporating the loss into a new set of assumptions about the world by reframing the individual as a "coper" or "survivor." This strategy would also include the development of more nuanced beliefs about the world to target all-or-nothing thinking (e.g., "The world is always bad"). Another target of cognitive techniques would be counterfactual thinking, in which the individual generates alternative courses of events that may have prevented the death. This type of thinking may be examined and intervened upon to shape a more adaptive, accurate appraisal of the individual's causal role in the death (Fleming & Robinson, 2001).

While individual behavioral activation for pathological grief has yet to be examined in an integrated care setting, the state of the available evidence would suggest the use of this intervention. Individual sessions may include the use of *Overcoming Depression One Step at a Time* (Addis & Martell, 2004), a self-guided workbook that can be used to facilitate the use of behavioral activation in the individual psychotherapy context. While this protocol was developed for the treatment of depression, it may be adapted for use in the treatment of pathological grief by providing the patient with the appropriate rationale for the use of this protocol. The rationale should include that the changing environmental context related to the loss can lead to social and occupational disengagement in ways that contribute to pathological grief, that avoidance and rumination may be ways to cope that can also lead to maladaptive functioning, and, finally, that the treatment stresses a goal-oriented way of becoming more active in the face of grief-related distress (Papa et al., 2013). Pathological grief symptoms are conceptualized as avoidance and disengagement from the environment. Patients are asked to describe how their life was different before the loss and how they might imagine a life without the deceased if they were not experiencing grief symptoms. Activity monitoring and activity scheduling are then used as the key procedures to target avoidance and disengagement. Activities should be chosen if they serve to reconnect the individual with rewards in his or her environment that may have been disrupted by the loss or construct new ways for the individual to come into contact with rewards. For example, a bereaved spouse who used to go on walks with her deceased husband might look for ways to incorporate physical activity into her life in a new way, such as joining a walking group. While individual behavioral activation typically consists of 12–16 1-h sessions over the course of 12 weeks, preliminary evidence suggests that it may be adapted for integrated care settings and completed with significant benefit in just 4–5 sessions including over the phone sessions (Acierno et al., 2012; Gros & Haren, 2011).

Evidence suggests the use of leader-facilitated groups for individuals with pathological grief symptoms. Existing research supports the use of group techniques such as psychoeducation, skills training, and emotion-focused support. Skills trainings include coaching on confronting problems and fostering positive health behaviors. Emotion-focused support consists of sharing experiences, reframing some negative aspects of the loss, and receiving emotional support (Murphy et al., 1998). It may also be useful for groups to be tailored to specific populations. For example, bereaved HIV+ caregivers may benefit from skills tailored to living with HIV and psychoeducation relevant to this community (Sikkema et al., 2006).

While the efficacy of behavioral activation groups specifically has yet to be examined for pathological grief, behavioral activation is likely an effective group treatment for the use in an integrated care setting. Behavioral activation delivered in a group format has demonstrated efficacy in the treatment of depression in community mental health and managed care (Porter, Spates, & Smitham, 2004). Importantly, while support groups are widely used and accepted among the public, the efficacy of group interventions has only been demonstrated for those individuals who are experiencing pathological levels of grief. Thus, broad-based group therapy for bereaved individuals who do not necessarily meet criteria for pathological grief is likely to reduce effectiveness.

The Role of the Primary Care Provider/Medical Team in Treatment

The chronic stress associated with bereavement has been shown to result in decrements in associated domains including autonomic, neuroendocrine, and immune systems, in addition to sleep quality (e.g., Cohen, Granger, & Fuller-Thomson, 2015). While consequences of an acute stressor as can be seen are common after a loss, these symptoms remit within months following the loss for most individuals. For some individuals, physiological changes in their neuroendocrine and immune systems persist after the loss (Hall & Irwin, 2001). Further, physical illnesses including cancer, cardiovascular disease, stroke, and high blood pressure have all been associated with pathological grief. As such, overall physical well-being should be assessed, particularly for those individuals at greater risk of developing pathological grief. It is likely that these physiological changes are mediated by behavioral responses to bereavement, including health behaviors such as smoking, changes in eating, decreases in social support, maladaptive coping, and sleep difficulties (Hall & Irwin, 2001; Prigerson et al., 1997).

Sleep in particular should be monitored, as grief has been associated with disturbances in sleep, both in difficulty falling asleep and staying asleep and overall sleep quality. Grief symptom severity is associated with a greater likelihood of experiencing insomnia. Sleep disturbances related to grief are also associated with impaired functioning and substance dependence. Intrusive thoughts and rumination associated with the deceased are associated both with insomnia and pathological grief (Hardison, Neimeyer, & Lichstein, 2005). Traumatically bereaved individuals in particular are more likely to suffer from insomnia. Increased risk of insomnia has also been associated with spousal bereavement, as the loss of a spouse may represent the loss of a zeitgeber that interferes with circadian rhythms (Brown et al., 1996). Sleep disruption is an important outcome to monitor, as it is associated with increased mortality.

Medication is sometimes prescribed to target the insomnia associated with bereavement. However, medication should be prescribed with particular caution for older adults, for whom the risk nighttime falling and injury is much greater. CBT for insomnia (CBT-I) may be a useful alternative in this case, as it has demonstrated similar efficacy with longer effects without the risk of side effects. Further, CBTI-I can be conducted in between one and four sessions by a master's level practitioner or nurse (Monk, Germain, & Reynolds, 2008).

How to Assess Impact on Care/ Quality Improvement Processes

Clearly, changes in symptom-specific measures, such as the Prolonged Grief Disorder (PG-13) Scale, can help determine whether or not efforts to impact symptom severity are effective. These can be supplemented by measures of suicidal behaviors and ideation, substance use, and other adverse health behavior engagement. Measures of physical, social, and emotional functioning in general (such as the MOS SF-36) can be used to track overall well-being as well as inform care in the case of bereavement but also index efficacy of integrated health delivery models in general. Given the impact of pathological grief on health, general healthcare, medication compliance, and the frequency with which the individual utilizes medical services should also be assessed to determine the impact of care.

References

Acierno, R., Rheingold, A., Amstadter, A., Kurent, J., Amella, E., Resnick, H., … Lejuez, C. (2012). Behavioral activation and therapeutic exposure for bereavement in older adults. *American Journal of Hospice and Palliative Medicine*, *29*(1), 13–25.

Addis, M. E., & Martell, C. R. (2004). *Overcoming depression one step at a time*. Oakland, CA: New Harbinger.

American Psychiatric Association. (2013). *Diagnostic and statistical manual of mental disorders: DSM-5*. Washington, DC: American Psychiatric Association.

Balk, D., Cook, A. S., Doka, K., Hall, M., Hansson, R. O., Klass, D., & Shapiro, E. R. (2004). Report on bereavement and grief research. *Death Studies*, *28*(6), 491–575.

Barry, L. C., Kasl, S. V., & Prigerson, H. G. (2002). Psychiatric disorders among bereaved persons: The role of perceived circumstances of death and preparedness for death. *The American Journal of Geriatric Psychiatry*, *10*(4), 447–457.

Boelen, P. A., de Keijser, J., van den Hout, M. A., & van den Bout, J. (2011). Factors associated with outcome of cognitive–behavioural therapy for complicated grief: A preliminary study. *Clinical Psychology & Psychotherapy*, *18*(4), 284–291.

Bonanno, G. A. (2005). Resilience in the face of potential trauma. *Current Directions in Psychological Science*, *14*(3), 135–138.

Bonanno, G. A., & Field, N. P. (2001). Examining the delayed grief hypothesis across 5 years of bereavement. *American Behavioral Scientist*, *44*(5), 798–816.

Bonanno, G. A., & Kaltman, S. (2001). The varieties of grief experience. *Clinical Psychology Review*, *21*, 705–734.

Bonanno, G. A., & Keltner, D. (1997). Facial expressions of emotion and the course of conjugal bereavement. *Journal of Abnormal Psychology*, *106*(1), 126.

Bonanno, G. A., Moskowitz, J. T., Papa, A., & Folkman, S. (2005). Resilience to loss in bereaved spouses, bereaved parents, and bereaved gay men. *Journal of Personality and Social Psychology*, *88*, 827–843.

Bonanno, G. A., Papa, A., Lalande, K., Westphal, M., & Coifman, K. (2004). The importance of being flexible the ability to both enhance and suppress emotional expression predicts long-term adjustment. *Psychological Science*, *15*(7), 482–487.

Bonanno, G. A., Wortman, C. B., Lehman, D. R., Tweed, R. G., Haring, M., Sonnega, J., … Nesse, R. M. (2002). Resilience to loss and chronic grief: A prospective study from preloss to 18-months postloss. *Journal of Personality and Social Psychology*, *83*(5), 1150.

Brown, L. F., Reynolds, C. F., Monk, T. H., Prigerson, H. G., Dew, M. A., Houck, P. R., … Kupfer, D. J. (1996). Social rhythm stability following late-life spousal bereavement: Associations with depression and sleep impairment. *Psychiatry Research*, *62*(2), 161–169.

Bui, E., Nadal-Vicens, M., & Simon, N. M. (2012). Pharmacological approaches to the treatment of complicated grief: Rationale and a brief review of the literature. *Dialogues in Clinical Neuroscience*, *14*(2), 149–157.

Cohen, M., Granger, S., & Fuller-Thomson, E. (2015). The association between bereavement and biomarkers of inflammation. *Behavioral Medicine*, *41*(2), 49–59.

Cohen, S., & Hoberman, H. M. (1983). Positive events and social supports as buffers of life change stress. *Journal of Applied Social Psychology, 13*(2), 99–125.

Currier, J. M., Neimeyer, R. A., & Berman, J. S. (2008). The effectiveness of psychotherapeutic interventions for bereaved persons: A comprehensive quantitative review. *Psychological Bulletin, 134*, 648–661.

Dyregrov, K., Nordanger, D., & Dyregrov, A. (2003). Predictors of psychosocial distress after suicide, SIDS and accidents. *Death Studies, 27*, 143–165.

Eisma, M. C., Boelen, P. A., van den Bout, J., Stroebe, W., Schut, H. A., Lancee, J., & Stroebe, M. S. (2015). Internet-based exposure and behavioral activation for complicated grief and rumination: A randomized controlled trial. *Behavior Therapy, 46*(6), 729–748.

Ekers, D., Richards, D., McMillan, D., Bland, J. M., & Gilbody, S. (2011). Behavioural activation delivered by the non-specialist: Phase II randomised controlled trial. *The British Journal of Psychiatry, 198*(1), 66–72.

Fleming, S., & Robinson, P. (2001). Grief and cognitive-behavioral therapy. In M. S. Stroebe, R. O. Hansson, W. E. Stroebe, & H. E. Schut (Eds.), *Handbook of bereavement research: Consequences, coping, and care* (pp. 647–669). Washington, DC: American Psychological Association.

Floyd, M. (2003). Bibliotherapy as an adjunct to psychotherapy for depression in older adults. *Journal of Clinical Psychology, 59*(2), 187–195.

Forstmeier, S., & Maercker, A. (2007). Comparison of two diagnostic systems for complicated grief. *Journal of Affective Disorders, 99*(1), 203–211.

Fujisawa, D., Miyashita, M., Nakajima, S., Ito, M., Kato, M., & Kim, Y. (2010). Prevalence and determinants of complicated grief in general population. *Journal of Affective Disorders, 127*(1), 352–358.

Gameroff, M. J., Wickramaratne, P., & Weissman, M. M. (2012). Testing the short and screener versions of the social adjustment scale-self-report (SAS-SR). *International Journal of Methods in Psychiatry Research, 21*(1), 52–65.

Gros, D. F., & Haren, W. B. (2011). Open trial of brief behavioral activation psychotherapy for depression in an integrated veterans affairs primary care setting. *The Primary Care Companion to CNS disorders, 13*(4). pii: PCC.11m01136.

Hall, M., & Irwin, M. (2001). Physiological indices of functioning in bereavement. In M. S. Stroebe, R. O. Hansson, W. E. Stroebe, & H. E. Schut (Eds.), *Handbook of bereavement research: Consequences, coping, and care* (pp. 473–492). Washington, DC: American Psychological Association.

Hardison, H. G., Neimeyer, R. A., & Lichstein, K. L. (2005). Insomnia and complicated grief symptoms in bereaved college students. *Behavioral Sleep Medicine, 3*(2), 99–111.

Johnson, J. G., Zhang, B., Greer, J. A., & Prigerson, H. G. (2007). Parental control, partner dependency, and complicated grief among widowed adults in the community. *The Journal of Nervous and Mental Disease, 195*(1), 26–30.

Kersting, A., Brähler, E., Glaesmer, H., & Wagner, B. (2011). Prevalence of complicated grief in a representative population-based sample. *Journal of Affective Disorders, 131*(1), 339–343.

Lannen, P. K., Wolfe, J., Prigerson, H. G., Onelov, E., & Kreicbergs, U. C. (2008). Unresolved grief in a national sample of bereaved parents: Impaired mental and physical health 4 to 9 years later. *Journal of Clinical Oncology, 26*(36), 5870–5876.

Lee, S. A. (2015). The Persistent Complex Bereavement Inventory: A measure based on the DSM-5. *Death Studies, 39*(7), 399–410.

Levy, L. H., Derby, J. F., & Martinkowski, K. S. (1993). Effects of membership in bereavement support groups on adaptation to conjugal bereavement. *American Journal of Community Psychology, 21*, 361–381.

Lichtenthal, W. G., Nilsson, M., Kissane, D. W., Breitbart, W., Kacel, E., Jones, E. C., & Prigerson, H. G. (2011). Underutilization of mental health services among bereaved caregivers with prolonged grief disorder. *Psychiatric Services, 62*(10), 1225–1229.

Litz, B. T., Schorr, Y., Delaney, E., Au, T., Papa, A., Fox, A. B., … Prigerson, H. G. (2014). A randomized controlled trial of an internet-based therapist-assisted indicated preventive intervention for prolonged grief disorder. *Behaviour Research and Therapy, 61*, 23–34.

Luecken, L. J., & Roubinov, D. S. (2012). Pathways to lifespan health following childhood parental death. *Social and Personality Psychology Compass, 6*(3), 243–257.

McIntosh, J. L., Santos, J. F., Hubbard, R. W., & Overholser, J. C. (1994). *Elder suicide: Research, theory, and treatment*. Washington, DC: American Psychological Association.

Mizuno, Y., Kishimoto, J., & Asukai, N. (2012). A nationwide random sampling survey of potential complicated grief in Japan. *Death Studies, 36*(5), 447–461.

Monk, T. H., Germain, A., & Reynolds, C. F. (2008). Sleep disturbance in bereavement. *Psychiatric Annals, 38*(10), 671–675.

Monk, T. H., Houck, P. R., & Shear, K. M. (2006). The daily life of complicated grief patients—What gets missed, what gets added? *Death Studies, 30*(1), 77–85.

Murphy, S. A., Johnson, C., Cain, K. C., Das Gupta, A., Diamond, M., Lohan, J., & Baugher, R. (1998). Broad-spectrum group treatment for parents bereaved by the violent deaths of their 12-to 28-year-old children: A randomized controlled trial. *Death Studies, 22*(3), 209–235.

Nam, I. S. (2016). Effects of psychoeducation on helpful support for complicated grief: A preliminary randomized controlled single-blind study. *Psychological Medicine, 46*(1), 189–195.

Neria, Y., & Litz, B. T. (2004). Bereavement by traumatic means: The complex synergy of trauma and grief. *Journal of Loss and Trauma, 9*(1), 73–87.

Newson, R. S., Boelen, P. A., Hek, K., Hofman, A., & Tiemeier, H. (2011). The prevalence and characteristics of complicated grief in older adults. *Journal of Affective Disorders, 132*(1), 231–238.

Papa, A., Lancaster, N. G., & Kahler, J. (2014). Commonalities in grief responding across bereavement and non-bereavement losses. *Journal of Affective Disorders, 161*, 136–143.

Papa, A., Sewell, M. T., Garrison-Diehn, C., & Rummel, C. (2013). A randomized open trial assessing the feasibility of behavioral activation for pathological grief responding. *Behavior Therapy, 44*(4), 639–650.

Porter, J. F., Spates, C. R., & Smitham, S. (2004). Behavioral activation group therapy in public mental health settings: A pilot investigation. *Professional Psychology: Research and Practice, 35*(3), 297–301.

Prigerson, H. G., Bierhals, A. J., Kasl, S. V., Reynolds, C., Shear, M. K., Day, N., … Jacobs, S. (1997). Traumatic grief as a risk factor for mental and physical morbidity. *American Journal of Psychiatry, 154*, 616–623.

Prigerson, H. G., Frank, E., Kasl, S. V., Reynolds, C. F., Anderson, B., Zubenko, G. S., … Kupfer, D. J. (1995). Complicated grief and bereavement-related depression as distinct disorders: Preliminary empirical validation in elderly bereaved spouses. *American Journal of Psychiatry, 152*(1), 22–30.

Prigerson, H. G., Horowitz, M. J., Jacobs, S. C., Parkes, C. M., Aslan, M., Goodkin, K., … Bonanno, G. (2009). Prolonged grief disorder: Psychometric validation of criteria proposed for DSM-V and ICD-11. *PLoS Medicine, 6*(8), e1000121.

Prigerson, H., & Maciejewski, P. (2008). *Prolonged grief disorder (PG-13) scale*. Boston, MA: Dana-Farber Cancer Institute.

Rosner, R., Lumbeck, G., & Geissner, E. (2011). Effectiveness of an inpatient group therapy for comorbid complicated grief disorder. *Psychotherapy Research, 21*(2), 210–218.

Schulz, R., Boerner, K., Shear, K., Zhang, S., & Gitlin, L. N. (2006). Predictors of complicated grief among dementia caregivers: A prospective study of bereavement. *The American Journal of Geriatric Psychiatry, 14*(8), 650–658.

Schut, H., Stroebe, M. S., van den Bout, J., & Terheggen, M. (2001). The efficacy of bereavement interventions: Determining who benefits. In M. S. Stroebe, R. O. Hansson, W. Stroebe, & H. Schut (Eds.), *Handbook of bereavement research: Consequences, coping, and care* (pp. 705–737). Washington, DC: American Psychological Association.

Shear, K., & Essock, S. (2002). *Brief grief questionnaire*. Pittsburgh, PA: University of Pittsburgh.

Shear, M. K., Simon, N., Wall, M., Zisook, S., Neimeyer, R., Duan, N., … Gorscak, B. (2011). Complicated grief and related bereavement issues for DSM-5. *Depression and Anxiety, 28*(2), 103–117.

Sikkema, K. J., Hansen, N. B., Ghebremichael, M., Kochman, A., Tarakeshwar, N., Meade, C. S., & Zhang, H. (2006). A randomized controlled trial of a coping group intervention for adults with HIV who are AIDS bereaved: Longitudinal effects on grief. *Health Psychology, 25*(5), 563.

Silverman, G. K., Johnson, J. G., & Prigerson, H. G. (2001). Preliminary explorations of the effects of prior trauma and loss on risk for psychiatric disorders in recently widowed people. *The Israel Journal of Psychiatry and Related Sciences, 38*(3/4), 202.

Simon, N. M., Shear, K. M., Thompson, E. H., Zalta, A. K., Perlman, C., Reynolds, C. F., … Silowash, R. (2007). The prevalence and correlates of psychiatric comorbidity in individuals with complicated grief. *Comprehensive Psychiatry, 48*, 395–399.

Stahl, S. T., & Schulz, R. (2014). Changes in routine health behaviors following late-life bereavement: A systematic review. *Journal of Behavioral Medicine, 37*(4), 736–755.

Stroebe, M., & Schut, H. (2005). To continue or relinquish bonds: A review of consequences for the bereaved. *Death Studies, 29*(6), 477–494.

Stroebe, W., Schut, H., & Stroebe, M. S. (2005). Grief work, disclosure and counseling: Do they help the bereaved? *Clinical Psychology Review, 25*(4), 395–414.

Stroebe, M., Schut, H., & Stroebe, W. (2007). Health outcomes of bereavement. *The Lancet, 370*(9603), 1960–1973.

Szanto, K., Prigerson, H. G., & Reynolds, C. F., III. (2001). Suicide in the elderly. *Clinical Neuroscience Research, 1*(5), 366–376.

Vanderwerker, L. C., Jacobs, S. C., Parkes, C. M., & Prigerson, H. G. (2006). An exploration of associations between separation anxiety in childhood and complicated grief in later life. *The Journal of Nervous and Mental Disease, 194*(2), 121–123. https://doi.org/10.1097/01.nmd.0000198146.28182.d

Vanderwerker, L. C., & Prigerson, H. G. (2004). Social support and technological connectedness as protective factors in bereavement. *Journal of Loss and Trauma, 9*(1), 45–57.

Wagner, B., Knaevelsrud, C., & Maercker, A. (2006). Internet-based cognitive-behavioral therapy for complicated grief: A randomized controlled trial. *Death Studies, 30*(5), 429–453.

Ware, J. E., Jr., & Sherbourne, C. D. (1992). The MOS 36-item short-form health survey (SF-36): I. Conceptual framework and item selection. *Medical Care, 30*, 473–483.

Wittouck, C., Van Autreve, S., De Jaegere, E., Portzky, G., & van Heeringen, K. (2011). The prevention and treatment of complicated grief: A meta-analysis. *Clinical Psychology Review, 31*(1), 69–78.

Zisook, S., & Kendler, K. S. (2007). Is bereavement-related depression different than non-bereavement-related depression? *Psychological Medicine, 37*(6), 779–794.

Borderline Personality Disorder 8

Eamonn Arble and Laura Krasean

A Brief Description of Borderline Personality Disorder

Borderline personality disorder (BPD) is a chronic and severe form of character pathology defined by fluctuating affect, unstable interpersonal relationships, a poor sense of identity, and frequently comorbid mood disorders. One of the hallmark features of BPD is a strained history of interpersonal relationships; patients with the diagnosis will frequently describe a persistently unmet need for emotional support, resulting in a sense of emptiness and solitude. For the individual with BPD, these interpersonal frustrations are more than mere annoyances, they represent a fundamental sense of unreliability in the external world, and this is often paralleled by the individual's unstable and fragile sense of self (Berenson et al., 2016). This disorder also consists of negative affectivity; individuals with the diagnosis will often experience abrupt and potent shifts in mood, with feelings of anger, sadness, and anxiety being the most common outcomes. The emotional instability of the borderline patient is often coupled with notable behavioral disinhibition; patients with BPD often engage in risky impulses, the extent to which can range from financial (e.g., excessive spending) to life-threatening (e.g., self-directed violence). This impulsivity is perhaps the most concerning aspect of the pathology, as individuals with BPD are at an elevated risk for self-injurious behavior, substance abuse, and suicide (Oldham, 2006).

BPD represents one of the most challenging clinical presentations and can prove particularly burdensome in the arena of primary care. A growing body of research has identified the frequent utilization of healthcare services by individuals suffering from BPD (Sansone, Farukhi, & Wiederman, 2011). The rate of BPD within a primary care context is significantly higher than among the general population, and many individuals seeking services for a less complicated clinical issue, such as depression, may in fact carry the diagnosis (Riihimaki, Vuorilehto, & Isometsa, 2014). Notably, when compared to other primary care patients, individuals with BPD demonstrate more frequent office visits, more frequent telephone contact, higher rates of referrals to specialists, and higher rates of prescriptions (Sansone et al., 2011). BPD has also been found to correlate with more frequent hospitalizations, longer inpatient stays, and more frequent emergency room visits (Ansell, Sanislow, McGlashan, & Grilo, 2007).

E. Arble, Ph.D. (✉)
Psychology, Eastern Michigan University, Ypsilanti, MI, USA
e-mail: earble2@emich.edu

L. Krasean, Ph.D.
Rainbow Rehabilitation Centers, Livonia, MI, USA
e-mail: krasean@uwindsor.ca

A. Maragakis, W.T. O'Donohue (eds.), *Principle-Based Stepped Care and Brief Psychotherapy for Integrated Care Settings*, https://doi.org/10.1007/978-3-319-70539-2_8

Effective Ways to Screen for BPD in the Primary Care Setting

A central challenge in the diagnosis of BPD is its resemblance to, and frequent comorbidity with, related psychiatric diagnoses. However, with the use of appropriate measures, a thorough clinical interview, and comprehensive behavioral observations, a firm diagnostic picture may be established. To that end, initial screening information will likely come from three primary sources: significant elevations on broad measures of pathology, treatment history, and behavioral/interpersonal observations.

Standard measures of mood and affective functioning, such as the Beck Depression Inventory (BDI; Beck, Ward, Mendelson, Mock, & Erbaugh, 1961) and the Patient Health Questionnaire-9 (PHQ-9; Kroenke & Spitzer, 2002), can provide an initial insight into the potential presence of BPD. Symptoms of affective distress, particularly items concerning self-injurious behavior and suicidal ideation, will be of obvious importance for the sake of patient safety but may also indicate the presence of personality pathology. Clarification of the extent and duration of these symptoms may help to determine if the noted symptoms are better conceptualized as transient mood states or as part of a more consistent personality style such as BPD.

The patient's reported treatment history will likely provide additional insight into the likelihood of a BPD diagnosis. Specifically, as compared to other primary care patients, individuals with BPD are more likely to have requested the services of specialists, requested psychiatric consults, and reported a lengthy history of various psychological treatments. Should the patient report a lengthy and complicated history of various disorders and numerous referrals, the presence of BPD should be considered (National Collaborating Centre for Mental Health, 2009). Given the prominence of self-injurious behavior for BPD, a history of emergency room visits is particularly worthy of further inquiry.

Finally, BPD, as with any personality disorder, can in part be identified by the patient's interpersonal style. The challenging nature of patients with BPD has been long recognized (e.g., Magill & Garrett, 1987), with numerous clinicians and practitioners commenting on the demanding, inconsistent, and frustrating interpersonal style of patients with the diagnosis. Indeed, the diagnostic criteria of mood changes, hypersensitivity, neediness, and conflicted relationships all emerge as barriers to treatment. What another patient may experience as a minor annoyance (e.g., having an appointment time delayed) may be experienced by an individual with BPD as greatly injurious, and an individual with BPD may have a reaction to the experience that, from the clinician's perspective, is surprisingly intense. Reports from staff, the medical record, or the treating practitioner that identify this style of impaired interpersonal functioning and negative affectivity all offer preliminary evidence of a borderline character organization.

However, it should be noted that BPD is not to be regarded as shorthand for unpleasantness. There are other diagnoses, situational factors, and personality dispositions that can lead one to be experienced as demanding or hostile, and negative reactions to a patient are far from sufficient to arrive at a firm diagnosis. Nonetheless, a clinician's reaction to a patient, as well as observations of the patient's interpersonal style, can provide important clues that merit further investigation.

How to Further Assess if a Screen Returns Positive

Should a consideration of the previous factors suggest a potential diagnosis of BPD, a more detailed investigation is required. Fortunately, several self-report measures assessing borderline personality disorder are now available. The 10-item McLean Screening Instrument for BPD (MSI-BPD; Zanarini et al., 2003) has proven useful across numerous age groups and several languages (the scale is reproduced within the cited article). A similarly useful, albeit lengthier, measure is the Borderline Personality Questionnaire (BPQ; Poreh et al., 2006; available for download at: https://www.researchgate.net/publication/236111181_BPQ_English_formatted), an 80-item measure that has demonstrated strong psychometric properties (Chanen et al., 2008). Finally, the Personality Diagnostic Questionnaire-4 BPD (PDQ-4 BPD; Hyler, 1994) is a fairly popular screening instrument for BPD (available for purchase at: http://www.pdq4.com), though some research has questioned its utility (de Reus, van den Berg, & Emmelkamp, 2011).

Given the prominence of self-injurious behavior within BPD, a careful assessment of the extent of prior suicide attempts, suicidal ideation, and non-suicidal self-injury will represent a central aspect of the diagnostic process. A clinician should ask about aspects of suicidal thinking, including frequency, intensity, and duration of thoughts, about any specific plans, access to means, rehearsal or preparatory behaviors, and intent or plan to engage in self-directed violence. Completing an assessment of previous suicidal behaviors is also of import (Hunter, Goodie, Oordt, & Dobmeyer, 2009). To that end, screening measures such as the 22-item Self-Harm Inventory (SHI; Sansone, Wiederman, & Sansone, 1998) can prove useful (the scale is reproduced in Sansone & Sansone, 2010, available at: https://www.ncbi.nlm.nih.gov/pmc/articles/PMC2877617/). Designed to provide a patient's history of self-injury and provide evidence of borderline pathology, the SHI appears to be highly predictive of BPD symptomatology in primary care settings (Sansone & Wiederman, 2015).

While these self-report measures provide an important initial step in the diagnosis of BPD, they should not be relied upon solely. Large-scale and meta-analytic investigations suggest only a moderate correlation between self-report questionnaires and clinical interviews in regard to BPD symptoms (e.g., Hopwood et al., 2009; Samuel & Widiger, 2008). This difficulty is not unique to the assessment of BPD and likely reflects the limitations of mono-method assessment, as opposed to a fundamental weakness of the noted measures. Nonetheless, there is reason to suggest that individuals with BPD are not entirely accurate in their ability to report on their own symptoms, particularly in regard to mood instability and their role in interpersonal conflict (Hasler, Hopwood, Brandle, & Schute-Vels, 2014).

A thorough clinical interview thus provides a necessary supplement to the aforementioned measures. The *Diagnostic and Statistical Manual of Mental Disorders*, Fifth Edition (*DSM-5; American Psychiatric Association, 2013*), requires the presence of at least five of the diagnostic criteria noted in Table 8.1. In order to identify the presence of these symptoms, and distinguish these symptoms from

Table 8.1 Borderline personality disorder diagnostic criteria

A. Significant impairments in personality functioning manifest by:
1. Impairments in self-functioning (a or b):
(a) Identity: Markedly impoverished, poorly developed, or unstable self-image, often associated with excessive self-criticism; chronic feelings of emptiness; dissociative states under stress
(b) Self-direction: Instability in goals, aspirations, values, or career plans
2. Impairments in interpersonal functioning (a or b):
(a) Empathy: Compromised ability to recognize the feelings and needs of others associated with interpersonal hypersensitivity (i.e., prone to feel slighted or insulted); perceptions of others selectively biased toward negative attributes or vulnerabilities
(b) Intimacy: Intense, unstable, and conflicted close relationships, marked by mistrust, neediness, and anxious preoccupation with real or imagined abandonment; close relationships often viewed in extremes of idealization and devaluation and alternating between overinvolvement and withdrawal
B. Pathological personality traits in the following domains:
1. Negative affectivity, characterized by:
(a) Emotional liability: Unstable emotional experiences and frequent mood changes; emotions that are easily aroused, intense, and/or out of proportion to events and circumstances
(b) Anxiousness: Intense feelings of nervousness, tenseness, or panic, often in reaction to interpersonal stresses; worry about the negative effects of past unpleasant experiences and future negative possibilities; feeling fearful, apprehensive, or threatened by uncertainty; fears of falling apart or losing control
(c) Separation insecurity: Fears of rejection by—And/or separation from—Significant others, associated with fears of excessive dependency and complete loss of autonomy

(continued)

Table 8.1 (continued)

(d) Depressivity: Frequent feelings of being down, miserable, and/or hopeless; difficulty recovering from such moods; pessimism about the future; pervasive shame; feeling of inferior self-worth; thoughts of suicide and suicidal behavior
2. Disinhibition, characterized by:
(a) Impulsivity: Acting on the spur of the moment in response to immediate stimuli; acting on a momentary basis without a plan or consideration of outcomes; difficulty establishing or following plans; a sense of urgency and self-harming behavior under emotional distress
(b) Risk taking: Engagement in dangerous, risky, and potentially self-damaging activities, unnecessarily and without regard to consequences; lack of concern for one's limitations and denial of the reality of personal danger
3. Antagonism, characterized by:
(a) Hostility: Persistent or frequent angry feelings; anger or irritability in response To minor slights and insults

those of another disorder, a thorough psychosocial history must be conducted. The consistent presence of the noted difficulties, as opposed to a cycle of emergence and dissipation, will help to clarify if the noted symptoms are better conceptualized as part of a mood disorder, such as bipolar disorder.

During this clinical interview, particular attention should be given to clinical presentation of BPD that is somewhat unique to the primary care setting. In a review of the symptom presentation of BPD in primary care settings, Sansone and Sansone (2015) identified the presence of unsubstantiated physical complaints as frequent diagnostic indicator, elaborating that these symptoms could be categorized into two main clusters: pain sensitivity and multiple somatic symptoms. The same analysis identified that self-injury in the primary care context was often manifested as an exaggeration of one's functional deficits, with patients with BPD often failing to engage in necessary day-to-day activities (e.g., reporting that they are unable to maintain employment due to experiencing pain), in contrast to the self-injurious behavior observed in other settings (e.g., cutting of one's skin). Finally, the intentional disruption of medical treatments and procedures was also characteristic of patients with BPD.

When operating under significant time restraints, it is recommended that the practitioner rely upon self-report measures for a broad overview of the patient's symptoms. Clinical interviews can then focus upon safety assessment, clarification of symptom severity and history, and consideration of the patient's interpersonal style. Should safety issues present a significant concern, designation of appropriate follow-up and plan of care will likely dominate this time. Nonetheless, a relatively short clinical interview, if combined with self-report data, staff behavioral observations, and medical record review, can provide a strong diagnostic picture.

Evidence-Based Stepped Care Approaches

The goal of behavioral health providers in the primary care setting is to provide brief, evidenced-based, targeted interventions (Hunter et al., 2009). Maintaining a brief appointment slot (e.g., 15–30 min) can be especially challenging when working with patients with BPD, as they often present in acute physical and/or emotional distress and pull for more time and attention compared to other patients within primary care. Patients with BPD often present with comorbid-presenting concerns, including mood disorders and post-traumatic stress disorder (PTSD), and experience high emotional reactivity and instability. In general, patients seen for behavioral health treatment are seen for a limited number of sessions (e.g., one to six), but the average number of appointments may vary from setting to setting. While the long-term treatment of severe personality disorders, including BPD, is beyond the scope of the primary care setting, patients with BPD may benefit from psychoeducation about their disorder, as well as several skill-based interventions detailed below.

Relevant psychoeducation begins with the introduction of the diagnosis itself. When a clinician is making a diagnosis of BPD, it is important to use clear, nonclinical language to explain how BPD can present in individuals and what this diagnosis means. Presenting this information in a way that communicates empathy, patience, thoughtfulness, and nonjudgment is also recommended, noting that an individual is not to blame for their diagnosis, as it arises from a combination of genetic and environmental risk factors (Distel et al., 2009). Individuals presenting for treatment within primary care may have had a wide range of experiences with mental health care, and the patient's understanding of the meaning of the diagnosis and its treatment implications is critical to establish. Asking about an individual's perception of prior treatments, if any, can be a useful starting point. It may also help to explain to the client how and why a diagnosis of BPD can develop and normalize that they are not alone.

It can also be useful and motivating to ask about what potential benefits a patient might experience, if any, if he or she were to gain skills to assist with emotional instability or negative affectivity. These types of questions, designed to work collaboratively with the patient to elicit their own motivation and commitment to change, are based on the principles of motivational interviewing (Rollnick, Miller, & Butler, 2008). Instilling hope is also of import, providing psychoeducation about how effective evidenced-based treatments have been developed specifically to address BPD, and with time, energy, and a lot of hard work, improvements in symptoms are possible. The installation of hope can be a powerful clinical tool, and providing individuals both a context for this disorder and a possible direction forward can assist with clinical engagement. Motivational enhancement, particularly as a precursor to making a referral, can be critical (Ben-Porath, 2004).

Individuals with BPD often present with depressive symptomatology, including anhedonia, reduced energy and interest, inappropriate guilt, attention and concentration concerns, psychomotor slowing, and changes in sleep and appetite. Comorbid rates of BPD and major depressive disorder have been found to range from 19.9 to 35.7% (Grant et al., 2009; Gross et al., 2002); identifying depressive symptomatology in a BPD patient is especially important given that the presence of comorbid diagnoses has been associated with an increase in both the number and seriousness of suicide attempts (Soloff, Lynch, Kelly, Malone, & Mann, 2000).

Brief, targeted treatments of depression have been shown to be effective in reducing depressive symptoms. A frontline intervention, behavioral activation, involves assisting the patient with reengagement in previously enjoyed activities as a way to improve mood; goals are developed collaboratively and should be specific and realistic for the patient, in order to increase the chances of successful implementation (Hunter et al., 2009). A behavioral activation approach can target essential factors that can contribute to depressed mood: dimensions in a patient's life that need modification in order to improve mood and the ways that withdrawal and avoidance from others and daily activities maintain or increase depression (Dimidjian, Martell, Addis, & Herman-Dunn, 2008).

A similar brief intervention is problem-solving therapy, which involves working collaboratively with the patient to identify a present issue of concerns, brainstorm possible solutions, consider the pros and cons of engaging in each possible solution, determining an appropriate course of action, and evaluating the outcome after a solution has been put in place in order to determine if an alternative solution is needed (Nezu, Nezu, & D'Zurilla, 2013). Other empirically validated treatments for depression, including cognitive restructuring and training in relaxation techniques, have been shown to be effective in reducing symptoms of depression and can be implemented within the structure of the primary care setting (Hunter et al., 2009).

Individuals with BPD may also present with long-standing interpersonal concerns and may identify anger as a contributing factor. Helping a patient develop awareness regarding how he/she experiences anger, expresses anger, and the consequence of this anger may be beneficial, along with training in empirically supported anger management skills. Relaxation-based interventions, including diaphragmatic breathing and cue-controlled relaxation, teach patients to use relaxation coping skills; skills are developed using both within-session practice and between-session homework. These interventions focus on emotional and physiological components of anger, and research has demonstrated their effectiveness (Deffenbacher, Oetting, and DiGisueppe, 2002). Related CBT-based interventions teach patients to identify cues and triggers that lead to feelings of anger and hostility, alter their perception of those situations, and consider alternative responses using cognitive and behavioral coping strategies (Morland et al., 2010). Providing patients with brief assertiveness training, which allows patients to communicate thoughts and feelings in a respectful and healthy, rather than aggressive, manner, may also be of assistance to patients (Hunter et al., 2009).

Individuals with BPD may also experience symptoms of anxious mood, characterized by difficulty controlling anxiety and worry, feelings of restlessness, irritability, fatigue, difficulty with attention and concentration, muscle tension, and disrupted sleep. Behavioral treatments, which focus on reducing the physiological symptoms of anxiety, can be an effective starting point for treatment with primary care. These strategies, including relaxation training, involve teaching one or more of the following skills: progressive muscle relaxation, guided imagery, diaphragmatic breathing, and cue-controlled relaxation (Bourne, 2005). Training can be introduced in the therapy session, either guided by the clinician or using media designed specifically for this purpose (e.g., a CD or web-based video clip) which helps guide the patient through the relaxation exercise process. Patients are further encouraged to set a specific time each day to engage in practice, and/or link this practice to an activity that they engage in daily, to increase the probability of task completion. Providing psychoeducation about what differentiates "problem-solving" from "worry" (e.g., anxious rumination) can also be of benefit to patients. This discussion will likely include a reminder that the goal of psychotherapy is not to eliminate worry, but rather reduce the frequency and intensity of worry to a more manageable level (Hunter et al., 2009). Cognitive strategies, including the use of a worry log or the establishment of "worry time" (e.g., the creation of a specific time and place to engage in worry), can also be effective.

The topic of mindfulness, a core skill in dialectical behavior therapy (Linehan, 1993), can also be introduced to the patient. Mindfulness, or the ability to be aware of one's thoughts, emotions, bodily sensations, and actions in the present moment, without engaging in judgment of the experience, has been found to significantly dampen the experience of anxiety (McKay, Wood, & Brantley, 2007).

What Does Not Work

The severity of BPD, combined with its interpersonal correlates, presents a unique clinical challenge. Provided below are several pitfalls for the clinical practitioner to avoid.

- *Not remaining emotionally neutral*: Practitioners should recognize that they may have a negative reaction to patients with BPD and that failure to recognize and manage these reactions can lead to poor clinical decisions and worse patient outcomes.
- *Failure to address the limits of primary care treatment*: Patients with BPD often have histories of trauma and abandonment and can be highly sensitive to perceived rejection. If the time-limited nature of primary care treatment and the likelihood of referral are not promptly discussed, the patient may experience feelings of rejection when referral sources are mentioned.
- *Establishing poor boundaries*: Structure is a key aim when working with patients with BPD. Expectations of appropriate topics of focus (e.g., discussing present-focused concerns and/or specific symptom management, rather than delving into a discussion of previous traumas) and what the consequences of

violating those expectations are should be collaboratively discussed with the patient. Following referral to external specialty mental health, these boundaries may take the form of reminding the patient, "This sounds like a topic that would be useful to address when you transition into your therapy."

- *Poor coordination*: Patients may, at times, find themselves receiving a referral to a community mental health program, having occasional contact with independent crisis hotlines, and receiving in-house psychiatric care. Therefore, it is essential that there is adequate communication among all relevant parties regarding treatment progress, patient safety, and therapeutic outcomes.
- *Diagnostic errors*: The challenges of diagnosing BPD have already been discussed. However, it is equally important that comorbid diagnoses are not neglected (e.g., substance abuse, PTSD, bipolar disorder, depression), as these may affect subsequent treatment decisions.
- *Offering nonspecific referrals*: BPD is often challenging to treat, particularly if the symptoms are severe. Many facilities that are typically strong referral resources may lack the training and capacity to treat the disorder. Thus, referral sources should be carefully examined for their suitability. This will also prevent the patient from experiencing the painful feeling of rejection if a referral site, after an intake, reports that the patient is not appropriate for treatment at their facility.
- *Incomplete risk assessment*: Patients with BPD are at an elevated risk for self-injury and suicide, making the careful assessment of risk factors a central priority. Failure to conduct a comprehensive risk assessment, or to recognize features associated with greater risk (e.g., previous suicide attempts, reports of hopelessness, comorbid depression; Black, Blum, Pfohl, & Hale, 2004), places the patient at risk.

When to Refer to External Specialty Mental Health

Due to the severity of the disorder, and the need for intensive and specialized treatment, referral to external specialty mental health is to be regarded as a frontline option. Despite the disorder's complexity, a number of empirically supported interventions have been developed to treat BPD, including dialectical behavior therapy (Linehan, 1993), transference-focused psychotherapy (Yoemans, Clarkin, & Kernberg, 2002), and mentalization-based treatment (Bateman & Fonagy, 2010). All of these treatment protocols provide cause for optimism regarding the treatment of borderline personality features; however, each is a highly specialized form of intervention, requiring a length of time that is likely beyond the scope of the primary care practitioner. As such, if BPD is conceptualized as a core clinical issue, referral to a specialized practitioner is an immediate recommendation.

The nature of the borderline character pathology introduces a particular difficulty into the referral process. The interpersonal deficits that are central to the disorder are often manifested in the testing of boundaries and the experience of painful rejections. Individuals with BPD, despite being referred to treatment elsewhere, may seek to pull for more individual time from their primary care provider and may cite the unique ability of the primary care practitioner to help them while characterizing the referred practitioner as incompetent. This idealizing of some while demonizing others is a process known as splitting and can present unique challenges in a primary care setting where many individuals are involved in a patient's treatment. Furthermore, if a primary care practitioner is seen as "dismissing" or "abandoning" the patient via referral, the patient may become irate and engage in disruptive behavior in the primary care setting or in the referred treatment facility. Such an outcome will likely prove disruptive for all parties involved. Accordingly, boundary setting will be a key aspect of successful treatment. If BPD is the determined diagnosis, the limitations of the primary care facility must be communicated quickly and firmly. The borderline character pathology makes individuals highly sensitive to perceived slights, and if the boundaries of treatment are not clearly communicated, the patient may create unreasonable expectations that become a source of future disappointment. Early referral to external specialty mental health is thus a priority.

The Role of the Primary Care Provider/Medical Team in Treatment

Given that referral to external specialty mental health is the primary aim of intervention with BPD, the role of the primary care team will be highly variable. In some instances, the primary care role will be one of psychopharmacology. The extant literature does not support the use of medications as the primary means of intervention for BPD; of the limited trials conducted, the results have been inconsistent and hampered by small sample sizes and methodological issues (Stoffers et al., 2010). Although popular, the use of selective serotonin reuptake inhibitors does not appear viable as a frontline treatment option (Stoffers & Lieb, 2015). Nonetheless, the use of medications to address specific symptoms of BPD (e.g., mood stabilizers) may be justified. In these instances, the primary care team may serve as an important adjunct to ongoing psychological interventions. In such a case, careful monitoring of patient medication use is necessary, as the aforementioned impulsivity of BPD makes potential medication abuse, and potential for overdose, legitimate and realistic concerns.

Beyond the use of medications, the importance of providing structure for patients with BPD is essential. Every member of the primary care team, whether clinicians or staff, can prove helpful in establishing a consistent and understandable set of structures and boundaries for patient. With a disorder that is largely relational in nature, interpersonal exchanges within the office setting can serve as a kind of treatment. It need be remembered that individuals suffering from BPD have developed maladaptive coping and help-seeking strategies; the extent to which primary care interactions reinforce these patterns is a matter of some importance. Indeed, part of the challenge of personality disorders in general is the patient's ability to draw others, including treatment providers, into maladaptive patterns.

For example, the patient may be highly sensitive to injury and greatly fear rejection. However, primary care professionals may experience this patient's interpersonal presentation as demanding and irritating, thus leading team members to approach him/her in an annoyed and cold way. In this manner, the patient with BPD now experiences the very rejection that was feared and has justification to withdraw from treatment—an unfortunately common occurrence (De Panfilis et al., 2012). In a similar fashion, the patient with BPD may demonstrate extreme outbursts or boundary-testing behaviors—for example, demanding immediate appointments every week due to new crises. If these requests are met, then these undesirable behaviors are positively reinforced and will continue. Because of this, members of the primary care team must be collaborative and unified in their approach to working with this difficult population. As such, it is absolutely vital to have frequent communication regarding the patient's requests and treatment and present the patient with a clear sense of boundaries and limits. Setting and maintaining clear boundaries and limits reduces the chance that the patient will engage in splitting among members of the treatment team.

The importance of boundary setting will also serve as a protective factor against the emergence of legal and ethical complications. Some research has suggested that patients with BPD may be more likely to initiate legal proceedings (Reid, 2009), though other research has questioned the accuracy of these concerns (Sansone, Leung, & Wiederman, 2012). Nonetheless, careful consideration of legal vulnerability is recommended given that individuals with the BPD diagnosis may experience rage in the face of disappointment, are prone to feeling victimized, and are at risk for numerous dangerous outcomes (e.g., suicide). Thus, involving the entire primary care team in *clear boundary setting* and *careful documentation* can communicate a sense of clarity to the patient, will help maintain active *collaboration and consultation* around legal and ethical matters, and will offer evidence of a coherent and demonstrable approach to patient care and safety (Gutheil, 2004).

Practitioners must also reflect on their own role in clinical interactions, retaining enough awareness and introspection to recognize if they are being drawn into the maladaptive interpersonal patterns and/or are reinforcing a maladaptive behavior pattern due to poor limit setting. Examples of poor limit setting include offering a prescription of dubious worth to avoid conflict with an angry patient or acquiescing to the patient's aggressive demands to be seen much earlier than the scheduled appointment time. Even if not the source of formal psychological treatment, the primary care team can provide an important resource for the borderline patient by providing a consistent source of source of empathy, motivational enhancement, and structure.

How to Assess Impact on Care/ Quality Improvement Process

In the case of BPD, the assessment of clinical improvement should follow from the initial screening and diagnostic results. In other words, the characteristics that inform the diagnosis of BPD should be the characteristics assessed to measure improvement.

The broad measures of mood, such as the BDI and the PHQ-9, should demonstrate a downward trend in scores as the affective distress is alleviated. These measures, combined with the SHI, should provide an essential assessment of ongoing patient safety. With successful treatment, the experience of suicidal ideation and self-injury should decrease. Additionally, repeated administration of borderline-specific measures, such as the MSI-BPD and the BPQ, will provide an assessment of the client's changing characterological pathology. Although treatment of BPD can be slow and difficult, research suggests that patients with the diagnosis can improve over time (Zanarini, 2009).

Some researchers have suggested that particular attention should be paid to the changing interpersonal style of patients with BPD as a measure of symptom improvement (e.g., Sinnaeve, Van Den Bosch, & Van Steenbergen-Weijenburg, 2015). Over the course of successful treatment, the patient's style of interacting with others, including those in the primary care setting, should demonstrate some improvement. Research in this area is in its nascent stages, but some studies have found that treatment can lead to improvement in these domains (e.g., Bellino, Rinaldi, & Bogetto, 2010). Examples of improved interpersonal functioning may be observed by the primary care team. For instance, a patient may demonstrate a decrease in boundary-testing behaviors or demonstrate fewer instances of aggressive verbal outbursts toward staff. These types of changes provide an important sense of the patient's improvement. Indeed, the appropriate use of referral sources (e.g., psychotherapy referral), in contrast to continued overuse of primary care appointments, may reflect significant improvement. However, more systematic evaluation of interpersonal functioning can also be of benefit. Measures such as the Inventory of Interpersonal Problems Circumplex (IIP-C; Alden, Wiggins, & Pincus, 1990) provide a nuanced view of a patient's interpersonal functioning. However, it should be noted that the extent to which interventions for BPD are likely to affect the scores on such measures is uncertain.

References

Alden, L. E., Wiggins, J. S., & Pincus, A. L. (1990). Construction of circumplex scales for the inventory of interpersonal problems. *Journal of Personality Assessment, 55*, 521–536.

American Psychological Association. (2013). *Diagnostic and statistical manual of mental disorders* (5th ed.). Washington, DC: Author.

Ansell, E. B., Sanislow, C. A., McGlashan, T. H., & Grilo, C. M. (2007). Psychosocial impairment and treatment utilization by patients with borderline personality disorder, and other personality disorders, mood and anxiety disorders, and a healthy comparison group. *Comprehensive Psychiatry, 48*, 329–336.

Bateman, A., & Fonagy, P. (2010). Mentalization based treatment for borderline personality disorder. *World Psychiatry, 9*, 11–15.

Beck, A. T., Ward, C. H., Mendelson, M., Mock, J., & Erbaugh, J. (1961). An inventory for measuring depression. *Archives of General Psychiatry, 4*, 561–571.

Bellino, S., Rinaldi, C., & Bogetto, F. (2010). Adaptation of interpersonal psychotherapy to borderline personality disorder: a comparison of combined therapy and single pharmacotherapy. *The Canadian Journal of Psychiatry*, *55*(2), 74–81.

Ben-Porath, D. D. (2004). Strategies for securing commitment to treatment from individuals with borderline personality disorder. *Journal of Contemporary Psychotherapy*, *34*(3), 247–263.

Berenson, K. R., Gregory, W. E., Glaser, E., Romirowsky, A., Rafaeli, E., Yang, A., & Downey, G. (2016). Impulsivity, rejection sensitivity, and reactions to stressors in borderline personality disorder. *Cognitive Therapy and Research*, *40*(4), 510–521.

Black, D. W., Blum, N., Pfohl, B., & Hale, N. (2004). Suicidal behavior in borderline personality disorder: Prevalence, risk factors, prediction, and prevention. *Journal of Personality Disorders*, *18*(3), 226.

Bourne, E. J. (2005). *The anxiety and phobia workbook* (4th ed.). New Harbinger: Oakland, CA.

Chanen, A. M., Jovev, M., Djaja, D., McDougall, E., Yuen, H. P., Rawlings, D., & Jackson, H. J. (2008). Screening for borderline personality disorder in outpatient youth. *Journal of Personality Disorders*, *22*(4), 353–364.

De Panfilis, C., Marchesi, C., Cabrino, C., Monici, A., Politi, V., Rossi, M., & Maggini, C. (2012). Patient factors predicting early dropout from psychiatric outpatient care for borderline personality disorder. *Psychiatry Research*, *400*, 422–429.

de Reus, R. J. M., van den Berg, J. F., & Emmelkamp, P. M. G. (2011). Personality diagnostic questionnaire 4+ is not useful as a screener in clinical practice. *Clinical Psychology and Psychotherapy*, *20*, 49–54.

Deffenbacher, J. L., Oetting, E. R., & DiGisueppe, R. A. (2002). Principles of empirically interventions to applied anger management. *The Counseling Psychologist*, *30*, 262–280.

Dimidjian, S., Martell, C. R., Addis, M. E., & Herman-Dunn, R. (2008). Behavioral activation for depression. In D. H. Barlow (Ed.), *Clinical handbook of psychological disorders: A step-by-step treatment manual* (4th ed., pp. 328–364). Guilford Press: New York, NY.

Distel, M. A., Trull, T. J., Willemsen, G., Vink, J. M., Derom, C. A., Lynskey, M., … Boomsma, D. I. (2009). The five-factor model of personality and borderline personality disorder: A genetic analysis of comorbidity. *Biological Psychiatry*, *66*(12), 1131–1138.

Grant, B. F., Chou, S. P., Goldstein, R. B., Huang, B., Stinson, F. S., Saha, T. D., … Ruan, W. J. (2009). Prevalence, correlates, disability and comorbidity of DSM-IV borderline personality disorder: Results from the wave 2 national epidemiologic survey on alcohol and related conditions. *The Journal of Clinical Psychiatry*, *69*, 533–545.

Gross, R., Olfson, M., Gameroff, M., Shea, S., Feder, A., Fuentes, M., … Weissman, M. M. (2002). Borderline personality disorder in primary care. *Archives of Internal Medicine*, *162*, 53–60.

Gutheil, T. G. (2004). Suicide, suicide litigation, and borderline personality disorder. *Journal of Personality Disorders*, *18*(3), 248–256.

Hasler, G., Hopwood, C. J., Brandle, L. S., & Schute-Vels, T. (2014). Patient-reported outcomes in borderline personality disorder. *Dialogues in Clinical Neuroscience*, *16*(2), 255–266.

Hopwood, C. J., Newman, D. A., Donnellan, M. B., Markowitz, J. C., Grilo, C. M., Sanislow, C. A., … Morey, L. C. (2009). The stability of personality traits in individuals with borderline personality disorder. *Journal of Abnormal Psychology*, *118*, 806–815.

Hunter, C. L., Goodie, J. L., Oordt, M. S., & Dobmeyer, A. C. (2009). *Integrated behavioral health in primary care: Step-by-step guidance for assessment and intervention*. Washington, DC: American Psychological Association.

Hyler, S. E. (1994). *PDQ-4+ manual*. New York, NY: NiJo.

Kroenke, K., & Spitzer, R. L. (2002). The PHQ-9: A new depression and diagnostic severity measure. *Psychiatric Annals*, *32*, 509–521.

Linehan, M. (1993). *Cognitive-behavioral treatment of borderline personality disorder*. New York: The Guilford Press.

Magill, M. K., & Garrett, R. W. (1987). Borderline personality disorder. *American Family Physician*, *35*, 187–195.

McKay, M., Wood, J. C., & Brantley, J. (2007). The dialectical behavior therapy skills workbook. Oakland: New Harbinger.

Morland, L. A., Greene, C. J., Rosen, C. S., Foy, D., Reilly, P., Shore, J., … Frueh, B. C. (2010). Telemedicine for anger management therapy in a rural population of combat veterans with posttraumatic stress disorder: A randomized noninferiority trial. *Journal of Clinical Psychiatry*, *71*, 855–863. https://doi.org/10.4088/JCP.09m05604blu

National Collaborating Centre for Mental Health. (2009). *Borderline personality disorder: Treatment and management. National clinical practice guideline number 78*. Leicester: The British Psychological Society and the Royal College.

Nezu, A. M., Nezu, C. M., & D'Zurilla, T. (2013). *Problem-solving therapy: A treatment manual*. New York, NY: Springer.

Oldham, K. M. (2006). Borderline personality disorder and suicidality. *The American Journal of Psychiatry*, *163*, 20–26.

Poreh, A. M., Rawlings, D., Claridge, G., Freeman, J. L., Faulkner, C., & Shelton, C. (2006). The BPQ: A scale for the assessment of borderline personality based on DSM-IV criteria. *Journal of Personality Disorders*, *20*(3), 247–260.

Reid, W. H. (2009). Borderline personality disorder and related traits in forensic psychiatry. *Journal of Psychiatric Practice®*, *15*(3), 216–220.

Riihimaki, K., Vuorilehto, M., & Isometsa, E. (2014). Borderline personality disorder among primary care depressive patients: A five year study. *Journal of Affective Disorders*, *155*, 303–306.

Rollnick, S., Miller, W. R., & Butler, C. C. (2008). *Motivational interviewing in health care: Helping patients change behavior*. New York, NY: The Guilford Press.

Samuel, D. B., & Widiger, T. A. (2008). A meta-analytic review of the relationships between the five-factor model and DSM-IV-TR personality disorders: A facet level analysis. *Clinical Psychology Review, 28*, 1326–1342.

Sansone, R. A., Farukhi, S., & Wiederman, M. W. (2011). Utilization of primary care physicians in borderline personality. *General Hospital Psychiatry, 33*, 343–346.

Sansone, R. A., Leung, J. S., & Wiederman, M. W. (2012). Litigious history and borderline personality symptomatology. *The primary care companion for CNS disorders, 14(6)*.

Sansone, R. A., & Sansone, L. A. (2010). Measuring self-harm behavior with the self-harm inventory. *Psychiatry*, *7*(4), 16–20.

Sansone, R. A., & Sansone, L. A. (2015). Borderline personality in the medical setting. *The Primary Care Companion for CNS Disorders, 17(3)*, https://doi.org/10.4088/PCC.14r01743.

Sansone, R. A., & Wiederman, M. W. (2015). The self-harm inventory: A meta-analysis of its relationship to the personality diagnostic questionnaire-4 as a measure of borderline personality disorder. *International Journal of Psychiatry in Clinical Practice*, *19*(4), 44–293. https://doi.org/10.3109/13651501.2015.1074708

Sansone, R. A., Wiederman, M. W., & Sansone, L. A. (1998). The self-harm inventory (SHI): Development of a scale for identifying self- destructive behaviors and borderline personality disorder. *Journal of Clinical Psychology*, *54*, 973–983.

Sinnaeve, R., Bosch, L., & Steenbergen-Weijenburg, K. M. (2015). Change in interpersonal functioning during psychological interventions for borderline personality disorder—a systematic review of measures and efficacy. *Personality and mental health*, *9*(3), 173–194..

Soloff, P. H., Lynch, K. G., Kelly, T. M., Malone, K. M., & Mann, J. J. (2000). Characteristics of suicide attempts of patients with major depressive episode and borderline personality disorder: A comparative study. *American Journal of Psychiatry*, *157*, 601–608.

Stoffers, J. M., & Lieb, K. (2015). Pharmacotherapy for borderline personality disorde—Current evidence and recent trends. *Current Psychiatry Reports*, *17*, 534.

Stoffers, J., Vollm, B. A., Rucker, G., Timmer, A., Huband, N., & Lieb, K. (2010). Pharmacological interventions for borderline personality disorder. *Cochrane Database of Systematic Reviews*.

Yoemans, F. E., Clarkin, J. F., & Kernberg, O. F. (2002). *A primer for transference focused psychotherapy for the borderline patient*. Northvale, NJ: Jason Aronson.

Zanarini, M. C. (2009). Psychotherapy of borderline personality disorder. *Acta Psychiatrica Scandinavica*, *120*, 373–377.

Zanarini, M. C., Vujanovic, A. A., Parachini, E. A., Boulanger, J. L., Frankenburg, F. R., & Hennen, J. (2003). A screening measure for borderline personality disorder: The McLean screening instrument for BPD (MSI-BPD). *Journal of Personality Disorders*, *17*, 568–573.

Cancer-Related Eating Problems

9

Kate Happel Krautbauer and Claudia Drossel

A Brief Description of the Presenting Problem

While survival times have increased and investigations of long-term quality of life have become more common, many people with current or past cancer diagnoses undergo changes in their eating patterns. Avoidance of specific foods and generally reduced food consumption can increase the risk of malnutrition. Malnutrition has been linked to decreased response to treatment, increased risk of infection, and overall survival. Complications related to malnutrition and involuntary weight loss include cancer cachexia (Fearon et al., 2011), a multifactorial metabolic disturbance involving a progressive loss of lean body mass that is the cause of death of approximately 20% of patients with cancer, and Wernicke-Korsakoff syndrome secondary to thiamine deficiency, which recently has been reported to be more common than expected (Isenberg-Grzeda, Rahane, DeRosa, Ellis, & Nicolson, 2016). Of note, once it occurs, cachexia is rarely systematically managed, at least partially due to a lacking evidence base, and it further decreases the tolerability of cytotoxic treatments.

In addition to the effects of cancer itself, necessary chemotherapy and radiation therapies may generate impairments in physiological functions vital to eating by compromising motoric or sensory processes. These processes must be considered before assessing the role of behavioral processes—related to avoidance learning as well as the social properties of food preparation and consumption—in food intake.

Impairment in Physiological Functions Vital to Eating

Cytotoxic chemotherapy and radiation disrupt digestive and metabolic processes, which already may have been compromised by the cancer, and can cause tissue damage. In addition to mucositis, further loss of appetite, nausea and vomiting, gastrointestinal discomfort or pain, diarrhea, constipation, and early satiety are common. Nausea and vomiting can occur immediately after each treatment (i.e., within 24 h) or after a delay of up to 7 days. In head or neck cancers, difficulties opening the mouth, chewing, and swallowing are frequent: for example, swallowing difficulties affect most patients within 1 month of chemo- and radiation therapies.

Individuals receiving cytotoxic cancer treatments are at risk of taste and smell alterations, which often outlast the acute treatment phase (Thorne, Olson, & Wismer, 2015), and may

K.H. Krautbauer (✉) • C. Drossel
Eastern Michigan University, Ypsilanti, MI, USA
e-mail: khappel@emich.edu

A. Maragakis, W.T. O'Donohue (eds.), *Principle-Based Stepped Care and Brief Psychotherapy for Integrated Care Settings*, https://doi.org/10.1007/978-3-319-70539-2_9

extend into adulthood after childhood cancer treatment (Cohen et al., 2014). Tissue damage from irradiation for head and neck cancers and neurotoxic properties of chemotherapies can change sensory functioning in a variety of ways: patients may have altered taste perception (i.e., sweet, sour, bitter, salty, or umami), taste detection and recognition may be globally impaired, or detection of "phantom" tastes that overshadow others (e.g., persistent metallic taste). In terms of olfaction, here too patients may show difficulties in detecting or recognizing different odors, or they may report heightened sensitivity to some smells. In addition, significantly reduced salivation—temporarily due to chemotherapy or chronically from gland injury secondary to head or neck radiation—reduces the palatability of food. Dry mouth, along with nausea, vomiting, and loss of appetite, is also a common adverse event when opioids are used to manage cancer pain.

During the acute phases of cancer treatment, adjunctive treatments (e.g., antiemetic and dietary interventions, interventions to enhance taste perception) aim to prevent or target these adverse effects to prevent significant weight loss, malnutrition, and related complications (see Roila et al., 2017, for antiemetic guidelines). Furthermore, new antineoplastic agents have been developed that carry a reduced risk of vomiting and nausea. However, management—particularly of nausea—remains difficult. In addition to the direct physical effects of cytotoxic cancer treatments, indirect learning and conditioning processes may further interfere with eating.

Psychological Barriers to Eating: Taste Aversion, Food Avoidance, and Psychosocial Factors

All animals—and humans among them—quickly learn to avoid toxins. When experimenters induce sickness in the presence of specific food cues (e.g., through radiation or toxic drugs), laboratory animals require only a single learning trial to stay away from these foods. From an evolutionary perspective, *conditioned taste aversion* upon retching or vomiting helps protect animals from repeated consumption of naturally occurring poisonous substances that, based upon the animals' experience, have come to signal sickness. However, experimental support for conditioned taste aversion in association with chemotherapy and radiation therapies has been inconsistent. In practice, rather than specific foods, situational cues (e.g., treatment room, nursing staff, angiocatheter) may acquire signaling properties and elicit nausea, retching, or vomiting. Patients usually receive treatment in periodic cycles, with predictable malaise following the appointment and then diminishing by the time of the next administration. Hence, approximately one quarter of patients used to develop *anticipatory nausea and vomiting* by the fourth treatment cycle. Since the 1990s, more effective antiemetic prophylaxis has reduced the incidence of such conditioned anticipatory responses. Risk factors are younger age, female, histories of motion sickness or pregnancy-induced nausea/vomiting, and possibly anxiety (Ahrari, Chow, Goodall, & DeAngelis, 2017; Roscoe, Morrow, Aapro, Molassiotis, & Olver, 2011).

In addition to nausea, which is more difficult to control pharmacologically than vomiting, gastrointestinal discomfort or pain may dominate many patients' experience. Operant learning processes can reduce general food intake regardless of taste when discomfort or pain accompanies or follows eating (*food avoidance learning*).

Changes in appetite and a related decline in nutritional status are also symptoms of depression or anxiety (American Psychiatric Association, 2013): Psychological distress in cancer patients is common, and clinical recommendations for assessing and managing distress have been developed (see Holland et al., 2013). Moreover, recent oncological approaches to prevent or manage cachexia are emphasizing continued engagement in physical activities (but see Grande et al., 2014, who suggest a lack of evidence), to which clinically significant distress may function as a barrier. If, on the other hand, a patient already has been taking psychotropic medications, reduced appetite as a common adverse effect from these psychotropic medications should also be ruled out (Naik, Shetty, & Maben, 2010).

Once difficulties with eating are present, they can disrupt social routines that typically support eating, which in turn may exacerbate existing problems. Patients may avoid the social aspects of eating when they evaluate their eating as bothersome or upsetting to others (e.g., because eating takes longer, chewing is laborious, food selection is cumbersome, or lacking enjoyment of food is perceived as disappointing to others). Patients' changes in eating are worrisome to family care partners: A majority endorsed anxiety related to patients' loss of appetite and reduced eating, suggesting that both patients and their care partners may benefit from interventions addressing eating patterns during or after cancer treatment (Hawkins, 2000). Family conflict over food choices and intake is common and may inadvertently exacerbate eating difficulties.

Finally, cancer survivorship does not preclude continued difficulties with eating. As mentioned earlier, impaired physiological functioning may outlast the acute administration of cytotoxic treatments. Particularly after head or neck cancer, survivors may have continued mechanical difficulties with food intake; furthermore, persistent chemosensory alterations are understudied, although they are common in clinical practice and affect patient's quality of life. Cancer survivorship also may bring about additional challenges, such as weight gain linked to cancer treatment (commonly observed in adult breast cancer, but see endocrine late effects in childhood and adolescent cancer survivors), increased risk of cardiovascular disease, body image concerns, and worries about cancer recurrence or second cancers with concurrent confusion about related "healthy eating" messages. Given the plethora of nutritional advice available on social media or via the internet, cancer survivors may avoid a specific food or restrict overall variety, thereby compromising their nutritional status. Thus, eating-related difficulties may persist, and health behavior change—promoting adherence to individualized nutrition and exercise plans and addressing smoking cessation—should constitute but rarely becomes a part of follow-up care.

Screening

The first step in addressing eating problems related to cancer is to determine the current role of primary care services by reviewing the nature of the cancer diagnosis and patient status: Is cancer acute, is it chronic but not life-threatening, is there advanced cancer, or is the cancer in remission? Are patients newly diagnosed and preparing for treatment, or are they currently receiving cytotoxic treatment? Did they receive cancer treatment in the past and have potential late effects, or are they monitored for chronic cancer with intermittent repeated cycles of treatment when indicated? Knowledge of a patient's oncological status and treatment plan—whether for acute, chronic, or follow-up care—is critical to screening for and addressing eating-related difficulties. Special assessment considerations apply to geriatric patients with cancer (Wildiers et al., 2014). If an oncology team is actively involved in patient care, the team monitors weight and works multimodally, to promote adequate food intake and prevent cachexia via personalized oncology, patient and family education, exercise, nutritional support, and anti-inflammatory agents. Lack of access to prophylactic treatment (e.g., due to insurance barriers) and other factors influencing adherence should be considered. The aim is to detect and address barriers to eating before clinical symptoms of malnutrition emerge, especially as malnutrition increases the risk of cachexia as noted earlier.

Some evidence suggests that specialty providers, focusing on the treatment of life-threatening aspects of malignancies, do not prioritize eating-related difficulties or may accept them as inevitable. Consequently, while eating is one component of cachexia prevention that patients can actively influence, patients may ignore, minimize, or dismiss their eating difficulties as inconsequential during acute cytotoxic treatment and endure preventable or reducible eating-related problems. Further, lack of mental health coverage or stigma surrounding mental health problems may prevent the self-report of any eating-related difficulties linked to learning processes, such as anticipatory nausea and vomiting. While failure to self-report may put patients at risk, obesity may contribute to difficulties detecting clinically significant metabolic changes: about half of patients with cancer are obese, and sarcopenic obesity—the loss of lean body mass in the presence of an elevated body mass index—may be overlooked.

As primary care physicians (PCPs) increasingly share the care of patients during and after cancer treatment to provide patient-centered care in proximity to the patient's home, PCPs—rather than specialty providers—may be the first to hear about eating-related problems from patients. To overcome barriers to the early detection of eating-related difficulties on the providers' and the patients' side, regular screening during cancer treatment is recommended (Huhmann & Cunningham, 2005). As noted earlier, cancer survivorship also warrants attention to changed eating patterns, signaling potentially significant decrements in quality of life.

Prior to an appointment, a brief record review can predetermine any existing evidence of weight loss. Unintentional weight loss—as subtle as 2.5% of body weight—may signal a need for preventive interventions (Lisa et al., 2015), with loss of more than 5% the best indicator of malnutrition (Douglas & McMillan, 2014). A clinical interview can probe for the most common barriers to eating, listed in Table 9.1.

Table 9.1 Common barriers to eating

Barriers
Breathing problems
Changes in the taste of food
Fatigue
Gastrointestinal problems, including:
Bloating
Constipation
Diarrhea
Nausea
Stomach cramps
Vomiting
Loss of appetite
Mood changes, including:
Anxiety (i.e., worry about cancer recurrence, rules about food intake)
Depression
Pain or discomfort, including:
Dry mouth
Muscle aches
Sore mouth, mucositis
Psychosocial factors, including interpersonal conflict
Swallowing difficulties

Screening Measures

Risk of malnutrition

The malnutrition screening tool (MST; Ferguson, Capra, Bauer, & Banks, 1999) is recommended for use with oncology patients in outpatient settings. Two questions assess unintentional weight loss and loss of appetite. Alternatively, the patient-generated subjective global assessment (PG-SGA, available at http://pt-global.org; Ottery, 1996) is a screener whose completion can be initiated by behavioral health providers. It first relies on patient self-report in four domains (weight, food intake, symptoms/barriers, and activities/function) and then is completed by medical staff (physician, nurses, or dietitians) who integrate information related to metabolic demand and nutritional physical exam results (Hurt & McClave, 2016). Both tools can be used for monitoring and suggest action plans dependent on scores. In contrast to the MST, the PG-SGA provides details that are useful if a subsequent detailed assessment is indicated.

Mood and cognition

Measures of quality of life of individuals during and after cancer treatment assess eating-related concerns. Depression and anxiety (including worry about dietary effects on cancer recurrence and potentially counterproductive rules about food intake) are most likely to affect eating. Rough screening tools such as the distress thermometer, developed for use in oncology, may be adopted and administered repeatedly (Holland et al., 2013); standard screening tools for depression and anxiety are also recommended for the detection of risk and of the need for further detailed assessment (Andersen et al., 2014). As neurocognitive decline is more common in late life and cancer treatment may affect cognition regardless of age, cognitive screening is recommended to determine whether cognitive inefficiencies present barriers to coping and whether treatment planning must accommodate cognitive deficits. Of note, the relationship between cognition and malnutrition is bidirectional: While cognitive decline may be a risk factor for malnutrition, nutritional deficits may also affect the cognitive functioning of patients with cancer.

Detailed Assessment

Given the idiosyncratic nature of the barriers to eating difficulties in cancer, assessments must be individualized. First, to confirm potential malnutrition or cachexia, physiological assessments within the purview of the medical providers are necessary (see Fearon et al., 2011, for review). A medical assessment will consider and subsequently address the potential physiological or chemosensory processes interfering with eating. The goal of behavioral health at this point will be to support the patient's interaction with medical providers and to advocate for the patient's voicing and pinpointing difficulties and describing them effectively to initiate medical assessment and intervention.

Regardless whether there is a risk of malnutrition, or confirmed malnutrition or cachexia, the behavioral health specialist should collaborate with nutrition services to support the detailed assessment process (Academy of Nutrition and Dietetics, 2013). Individualized food logs, while relatively labor-intensive, have the greatest utility for identifying current eating patterns and the conditions that affect the likelihood of eating (e.g., time in the cytotoxic therapy cycle, avoidance of a specific food versus an entire food group or preparation style, gastrointestinal symptoms, social context, etc.). When patients are fatigued and reluctant to engage in systematic and continuous self-monitoring, intermittent sampling procedures may be indicated and can be tailored to the specific needs of the patient. For example, a patient may receive a digital prompt to monitor food on randomly selected days. For general principles of self-monitoring, please refer to Humphreys, Marx, and Lexington (2009). Mobile health applications tailored to patients with cancer have been developed and are expected to play a major role in improving care (Odeh, Kayyali, Nabhani-Gebara, & Philip, 2015).

Ideally, logs provide systematic information about food intake, physical activity, and barriers to food intake (see Table 10.1). Because eating difficulties may be associated with a general withdrawal from activities, an overall loss of pleasure, or pervasive hopelessness, activity level and adherence to exercise recommendations during cancer treatment should be assessed (Mustian et al., 2016). Once barriers have been pinpointed, they must be addressed with individually tailored treatment plans.

Evidence-Based Stepped Care/Brief Psychotherapy

In general, patients diagnosed with cancer should receive psychoeducation about potential cancer or cancer treatment-related eating problems and strong encouragement to speak with their physicians about changes in eating patterns, should they emerge. Patient guides to nutritional self-care during and after cancer treatment are available through the American Cancer Society and the National Cancer Institute (see Resources below). They promote prevention of and preparation for eating-related difficulties and provide problem-solving tips for use in advance of, during, and after cancer treatment. Of note, these guides also emphasize that eating-related problems—while frequent—may not affect all patients. If problems have not reached clinical significance and watchful waiting is indicated, a patient—in collaboration with the primary care team—may elect to implement tips and strategies from the patient guides for prevention. In this case, the role of the behavioral health provider focuses on directing the patient to continue self-monitoring to document the use of potential strategies and their perceived effects.

If eating-related difficulties emerge from the record review, interview, or screening measures, potential psychological or skills barriers to patient communication with his or her healthcare provider should be assessed. For some patients, brief in-session role plays may be necessary to facilitate effective communication with their medical providers, whether the PCP or the oncology team.

Interventions that mitigate or address eating-related difficulties in primary care can be divided broadly into three categories: (1) building a patient's distress tolerance, (2) reducing anticipatory nausea and vomiting, and (3) targeting concomitant mood changes and eating difficulties.

Building Distress Tolerance to Minimize the Impact of Adverse Events

Patient self-directed intervention packages to build distress tolerance with minimal provider guidance are available. They easily lend themselves to use in primary care, but they tend not to be specific to cancer. Thus, detailed education about the importance of nutritional status, physiological barriers to eating including taste alterations, and taste aversion or food avoidance learning must be provided separately, and none of the interventions listed below are indicated for targeting nausea or vomiting during acute cancer treatment. Rather, evidence suggests that these interventions might increase general patient comfort and can be used prophylactically to enhance a person's tolerability of adverse events:

(a) Distraction, including guided imagery
(b) Relaxation training, including progressive muscle relaxation (contraindicated when a person is too weak or fatigued)
(c) Cognitive techniques (e.g., restructuring/reframing) to promote eating for health and eliminate or reduce counterproductive rules related to eating or food selection
(d) Mindfulness-based stress reduction (MBSR)

(see Ledesma & Kumano, 2009; O'Donohue, Fisher, & Hayes, 2003). There is insufficient research on early termination of chemotherapies or radiation therapies and nonadherence to oncological recommendations, but it is plausible that these interventions promote adherence by teaching patients how to cope with adverse effects.

Systematic Desensitization to Reduce Anticipatory Nausea and Vomiting

When PCPs are involved in oncology care, the behavioral health provider may monitor patient eating, as described above, and take an active role in promoting non-pharmacological interventions to nausea and vomiting, including training of the oncology team if appropriate and needed. Systematic desensitization—which combines progressive muscle relaxation with imaginary or in vivo exposure—is the only intervention with sufficient evidence to be considered an evidence-based complementary treatment alternative for anticipatory nausea and/or vomiting (Morrow & Morrell, 1982). (Note that there is additional evidence for the use of hypnosis with children.) Counteracting taste aversion learning, patients first learn to implement progressive muscle relaxation and then systematically imagine aversive situations of increasing intensity while fully relaxed (imaginary exposure). Each exposure ends with imagining a complete disappearance of the aversive event. Evidence supports the in vivo implementation of treatment by oncology physicians and nurses in the radiation or chemotherapy setting without administration of treatment (Morrow et al., 1992). Typically, a 2-h intervention is scheduled in the chemotherapy setting outside of the regularly scheduled chemotherapy.

Targeting Mood Changes and Eating Difficulties

During acute cancer treatment, non-pharmacological interventions may be provided within the purview of the oncology care team: Preliminary data are available for two sessions of motivational interviewing (MI) in combination with very brief (10-min) biweekly sessions of MI and cognitive behavioral therapy for depression, cautiously suggesting long-term benefits in nutritional status and improved mortality of patients with moderate to severe depression who underwent radiotherapy for head and neck cancers (Britton et al., 2016). A Cochrane Review of psychological interventions for women with metastatic breast cancer (Mustafa, Carson-Stevens, Gillespie, & Edwards, 2013) found relatively increased survival at 12 months and not at long-term follow-up, but also cited a dearth of available studies.

When assessment has identified depression or anxiety as primary problems, then interventions follow the respective standard protocols for distress management of individuals with cancer (Andersen et al., 2014; Holland et al., 2013) or mood disorders in primary care, depending on a patient's oncological status and idiographic needs. Interventions designed to target restrictive eating may be implemented in primary care when nutritional status does not require specialty intervention, in conjunction with the primary care team, and when food restriction is not better accounted for by the effects of acute treatment or ongoing physiological or medical problems, depression, or anxiety. Evidence-based cognitive behavioral therapy protocols (e.g., Fairburn, 2008) are available for adaptation in primary care settings.

What Does Not Work

Cancer-related eating difficulties—while they may significantly affect a patient's quality of life in the short and long term—are understudied. Thus, other than systematic desensitization for anticipatory nausea and vomiting, there is currently no solid evidence base guiding practitioners in non-pharmacological behavioral health interventions, and most recommendations or guidelines arise from expert consensus. Because of the multifactorial nature and the resulting complexity of cancer-related eating difficulties even in survivorship, idiographic assessment and intervention appear necessary. Fatigue, weakness, and pain should be considered as potential barriers to treatment implementation, and a care partner may have to be present to carry out aspects of the treatment. Moreover, individuals without elevated levels of distress may not benefit from intervention.

When to Refer to Specialty Treatment

Given the important role of nutritional status in cancer treatment, any suspicion of malnutrition, risk for cachexia, or further unintentional weight loss should be addressed by or in conjunction with the specialized oncology team. Referral to specialized behavioral health providers is necessary when significant barriers to health behavior change complicate the presentation, such as preexisting or comorbid mental health diagnoses (e.g., neurocognitive or substance use disorders).

The Role of the PCP and the Team

Traditionally, primary care has been regarded as first contact for patients with cancer who was then referred for specialty services. As noted above, a focus on patient-centered care and patient medical homes has expanded oncology care into other specialties, including primary care. Novel payment and delivery models ideally broaden the behavioral health services reimbursable in primary care (e.g., to include care partner coaching); however, these model changes currently generate a highly variable practice environment. In general, the role of the primary care team is to collaborate with oncology in coordinated service provision closer to the patient's home, including:

- Motivating health behavior change (e.g., maintaining or improving nutritional status and regular exercise, implementing smoking cessation)
- Monitoring adherence
- Detecting and managing cancer- or treatment-related symptoms including eating difficulties in a timely manner to prevent long-term consequences
- Assessing and intervening on cancer-related eating difficulties, coordinating care, or referring patients to mental health providers, to ascertain optimal psychosocial functioning
- Continuing survivorship care

It is expected that individuals with cancer will receive increasingly complex services in primary care settings.

Assessing Impact

Benchmarks for improved care are (a) periodic, repeated screenings of nutritional status and changes in eating behavior, (b) appropriate follow-up when a screening is positive, and (c) provision of brief interventions or appropriate referral. Patients' self-reported quality of life also is an indicator of improved cancer care.

Patient Resources

The National Cancer Institutes published a detailed brochure in 2011 (https://www.cancer.gov/publications/patient-education/eatinghints.pdf) providing suggestions for eating before, during, and after cancer treatment. Patients and loved ones may find this information helpful and easy to understand as they navigate changes in eating related to cancer.

References

Academy of Nutrition and Dietetics. (2013). *Oncology evidence-based nutrition practice guideline*. Chicago, IL: Academy of Nutrition and Dietetics.

Ahrari, S., Chow, R., Goodall, S., & DeAngelis, C. (2017). Anticipatory nausea: Current landscape and further directions. *Annals of Palliative Medicine*, *6*(1), 1–2. 10.21037/apm.2016.10.01

American Psychiatric Association. (2013). *Diagnostic and statistical manual of mental disorders* (5th ed.). Washington, DC: Author.

Andersen, B. L., DeRubeis, R. J., Berman, B. S., Gruman, J., Champion, V. L., Massie, M. J., … Rowland, J. H. (2014). Screening, assessment, and care of anxiety and depressive symptoms in adults with cancer: An American Society of Clinical Oncology Guideline Adaptation. *Journal of Clinical Oncology*, *32*(15), 1605–1619. https://doi.org/10.1200/JCO.2013.52.4611

Britton, B., Baker, A., Clover, K., McElduff, P., Wratten, C., & Carter, G. (2016). Heads up: A pilot trial of a psychological intervention to improve nutrition in head and neck cancer patients undergoing radiotherapy. *European Journal of Cancer Care*. doi: https://doi.org/10.1111/ecc.12502

Cohen, J., Laing, D. G., Wilkes, F. J., Chan, A., Gabriel, M., & Cohn, R. J. (2014). Taste and smell dysfunction in childhood cancer survivors. *Appetite*, *75*, 135–140. https://doi.org/10.1016/j.appet.2014.01.001

Douglas, E., & McMillan, D. C. (2014). Towards a simple objective framework for the investigation and treatment of cancer cachexia: The Glasgow Prognostic Score. *Cancer Treatment Reviews*, *40*(6), 685–691. https://doi.org/10.1016/j.ctrv.2013.11.007

Fairburn, C. (Ed.). (2008). *Cognitive behavior therapy and eating disorders*. New York, NY: Guilford Press.

Fearon, K., Strasser, F., Anker, S. D., Bosaeus, I., Bruera, E., Fainsinger, R. L., … Baracos, V. E. (2011). Definition and classification of cancer cachexia: An international consensus. *The Lancet Oncology*, *12*(5), 489–495. https://doi.org/10.1016/S1470-2045(10)70218-7

Ferguson, M., Capra, S., Bauer, J., & Banks, M. (1999). Development of a valid and reliable malnutrition screening tool for adult acute hospital patients. *Nutrition*, *15*(6), 458–464. https://doi.org/10.1016/S0899-9007(99)00084-2

Grande, A. J., Silva, V., Riera, R., Medeiros, A., Vitoriano, S. G. P., Peccin, M. S., & Maddocks, M. (2014). Exercise for cancer cachexia in adults. *Cochrane Database of Systematic Reviews, (11)*. doi: https://doi.org/10.1002/14651858.CD010804.pub2.

Hawkins, C. (2000). Anorexia and anxiety in advanced malignancy: the relative problem. *Journal of Human Nutrition and Dietetics, 13*(2), 113–117.

Holland, J. C., Andersen, B., Breitbart, W. S., Buchmann, L. O., Compas, B., Deshields, T. L., … Freedman-Cass, D. A. (2013). Distress management. *Journal of the National Comprehensive Cancer Network*, *11*(2), 190–209.

Huhmann, M. B., & Cunningham, R. S. (2005). Importance of nutritional screening in treatment of cancer-related weight loss. *The Lancet Oncology*, *6*(5), 334–343. https://doi.org/10.1016/S1470-2045(05)70170-4

Humphreys, K. L., Marx, B. P., & Lexington, J. M. (2009). Self-monitoring as a treatment vehicle. In W. T. O'Donohue & J. E. Fisher (Eds.), *General principles and empirically supported techniques of cognitive behavior therapy* (pp. 576–583). Hoboken, NJ: John Wiley & Sons.

Hurt, R. T., & McClave, S. A. (2016). Nutritional assessment in primary care. *Medical Clinics of North America*, *100*(6), 1169–1183. https://doi.org/10.1016/j.mcna.2016.06.001

Isenberg-Grzeda, E., Rahane, S., DeRosa, A. P., Ellis, J., & Nicolson, S. E. (2016). Wernicke-Korsakoff syndrome in patients with cancer: A systematic review. *The Lancet Oncology*, *17*(4), e142–e148. https://doi.org/10.1016/s1470-2045(16)00037-1

Ledesma, D., & Kumano, H. (2009). Mindfulness-based stress reduction and cancer: A meta-analysis. *Psycho-Oncology*, *18*(6), 571–579. https://doi.org/10.1002/pon.1400

Lisa, M., Pierre, S., Ioannis, G., Sami, A., Federico, B., Chris, D., … Vickie, E. B. (2015). Diagnostic criteria for the classification of cancer-associated weight loss. *Journal of Clinical Oncology*, *33*(1), 90–99. https://doi.org/10.1200/JCO.2014.56.1894

Morrow, G. R., Asbury, R., Hammon, S., Dobkin, P., Caruso, L., Pandya, K., & Rosenthal, S. (1992). Comparing the effectiveness of behavioral treatment for chemotherapy-induced nausea and vomiting when administered by oncologists, oncology nurses, and clinical psychologists. *Health Psychology*, *11*(4), 250–256.

Morrow, G. R., & Morrell, C. (1982). Behavioral treatment for the anticipatory nausea and vomiting induced by cancer chemotherapy. *New England Journal of Medicine, 307*(24), 1476–1480. https://doi.org/10.1056/nejm198212093072402

Mustafa, M., Carson-Stevens, A., Gillespie, D., & Edwards, A. G. K. (2013). Psychological interventions for women with metastatic breast cancer. *Cochrane Database of Systematic Reviews, (6).* doi: https://doi.org/10.1002/14651858.CD004253.pub4

Mustian, K. M., Cole, C. L., Lin, P. J., Asare, M., Fung, C., Janelsins, M. C., … Magnuson, A. (2016). Exercise recommendations for the management of symptoms clusters resulting from cancer and cancer treatments. *Seminars in Oncology Nursing, 32*(4), 383–393. https://doi.org/10.1016/j.soncn.2016.09.002

Naik, B. S., Shetty, N., & Maben, E. V. S. (2010). Drug-induced taste disorders. *European Journal of Internal Medicine, 21*(3), 240–243. https://doi.org/10.1016/j.ejim.2010.01.017

O'Donohue, W. T., Fisher, J. E., & Hayes, S. C. (Eds.). (2003). *Cognitive behavior therapy: Applying empirically supported techniques in your practice*. Hoboken, NJ: John Wiley & Sons.

Odeh, B., Kayyali, R., Nabhani-Gebara, S., & Philip, N. (2015). Optimizing cancer care through mobile health. *Supportive Care in Cancer, 23*(7), 2183–2188. https://doi.org/10.1007/s00520-015-2627-7

Ottery, F. D. (1996). Definition of standardized nutritional assessment and interventional pathways in oncology. *Nutrition, 12*(1), S15–S19. https://doi.org/10.1016/0899-9007(95)00067-4

Roila, F., Warr, D., Hesketh, P.J., Gralla, R., Herrstedt, J., Jordan, K., Aapro, M., Ballatori, E., & Rapoport, B. (2017). 2016 updated MASCC/ESMO consensus recommendations: Prevention of nausea and vomiting following moderately emetogenic chemotherapy. *Supportive Care in Cancer, 25*(1), 289–294.

Roscoe, J. A., Morrow, G. R., Aapro, M. S., Molassiotis, A., & Olver, I. (2011). Anticipatory nausea and vomiting. *Supportive Care in Cancer, 19*(10), 1533–1538. https://doi.org/10.1007/s00520-010-0980-0

Thorne, T., Olson, K., & Wismer, W. (2015). A state-of-the-art review of the management and treatment of taste and smell alterations in adult oncology patients. *Supportive Care in Cancer, 23*, 2843–2851. https://doi.org/10.1007/s00520-015-2827-1

Wildiers, H., Heeren, P., Puts, M., Topinkova, E., Janssen-Heijnen, M. L. G., Extermann, M., … Hurria, A. (2014). International Society of Geriatric Oncology Consensus on geriatric assessment in older patients with cancer. *Journal of Clinical Oncology, 32*(24), 2595–2603. https://doi.org/10.1200/jco.2013.54.8347

Child Physical Abuse (CPA) 10

Brittany R. Patterson and Brittany M. Hayden

Problem

Over 2 million reports of suspected child maltreatment are investigated by Child Protective Services (CPS) annually (Christian, 2015). Of those, more than 650,000 cases are substantiated requiring intervention, and approximately 149,000 cases in the United States, Puerto Rico, and District of Columbia involve child physical abuse (National Child Traumatic Stress Network; NCTSN, 2009). Sadly, reports and investigations often occur too late or not at all, with at least 1500 cases of abuse and neglect resulting in child death each year.

Perhaps most disturbing is that these data are conservative estimations based on differentiating state guidelines and, of course, do not include unreported incidences. Therefore, identification and treatment of child physical abuse are largely influenced by definitions ascribed to by specific states (Children's Bureau, 2009) and professional familiarity with mandates. At a minimum, child physical abuse occurs when a caretaker "commits an act that results in physical injury to a child or adolescent, even if the injury was unintentional" (NCTSN, 2009). Harmful actions may result in observable injuries such as cuts, welts, bruises, broken bones, muscle sprains, and/or red marks, but physical evidence is not required for reporting in every state. For example, using a closed fist to hit a child is considered physical abuse in the District of Columbia (DC), Minnesota, and Arkansas (NCTSN, 2009).

Other legislative specificities that may vary across states include the use of terminologies such as "substantial risk," "risk of harm," and "severe pain." Reporting thresholds also differ and may require descriptions of objects used, impact sites (e.g., face, arm), and degree of injury before launching an investigation (NCTSN, 2009). Therefore, it is the responsibility of professionals that have frequent contact with children to know and adhere to mandated reporter guidelines of the state. For more information regarding legal definitions, visit www.childwelfare.gov.

B.R. Patterson, Ph.D. (✉)
Department of Psychiatry, University of Maryland School of Medicine, Center for School Mental Health, Baltimore, MD, USA
e-mail: bparham@som.umaryland.edu

B.M. Hayden, Ph.D.
Outpatient Behavioral Health Department, Sarah A. Reed Children's Center, Erie, PA, USA
e-mail: bhayden@sarahreed.org

Impact of Child Physical Abuse

While children of all ages, genders, socioeconomic backgrounds, races, and ethnicities can be exposed to child physical abuse, a few

A. Maragakis, W.T. O'Donohue (eds.), *Principle-Based Stepped Care and Brief Psychotherapy for Integrated Care Settings*, https://doi.org/10.1007/978-3-319-70539-2_10

subcategories are particularly susceptible. Youth aged 4–7 and young adolescents aged 12–15 along with children from low socioeconomic status (SES) backgrounds (Herrenkohl & Herrenkohl, 2007), single-parent homes (Berger, Paxon, & Waldfogel, 2009), and large families (DePanfilis & Zuravin, 1999; Solomon, Morgan, Asberg, & McCord, 2014) are at greater risk of being physically abused. Research also suggests risk factors specific to child and parent characteristics.

Youth risk factors include cognitive deficits, developmental disabilities, mental health challenges, and disruptive behavior disorders (e.g., attention-deficit/hyperactivity disorder, oppositional defiant disorder, conduct disorder; Gokten, Duman, Soylu, & Uzun, 2016; Kolko & Swenson, 2002). Parenting children requiring intensive supports can make caregivers vulnerable to elevated stress which is a variable robustly associated with increased incidences of child physical abuse (Cummings & Berkowitz, 2014).

Another variable is former exposure to physical abuse as a child, and rates of previous abuse as high as 30% have been estimated (Kaufman & Zigler, 1987). However, as the majority of physically abused children are not likely to perpetrate in adulthood, other parent factors such as negative cognitions, emotional regulation problems, coping capacity, and mental health status have been investigated in the maltreatment literature (Kolko & Swenson, 2002). Several studies have identified that attributional biases including rigidity, critical evaluations, and unreasonable expectations related to a child's behavior put parents at risk of implementing more harsh disciplining practices (Kolko & Swenson, 2002; Whipple & Webster-Stratton, 1991). Parents exercising abusive tactics are also more likely than non-abusing counterparts to endorse explosiveness, hostility (Caspi & Elder, 1988), irritability, anxiety, and sadness (Kolko & Swenson, 2002; Simons, Whitbeck, Conger, & Chyi-ni, 1991) as commonly experienced affective states.

Other evidence suggests that deficits in problem-solving skills, basic parent management skills (e.g., monitoring, Premack principle), and utilization of prosocial behaviors (e.g., affection, positive affect, and attention) can contribute to incidences of child abuse (Azar, Robinson, Hekimian, & Twentyman, 1984; Kolko & Swenson, 2002). Associations between parental psychiatric problems, as well as substance use, post-traumatic stress disorder (PTSD), and depression symptoms have also been found (Cummings & Berkowitz, 2014).

Short- and long-term sequelae associated with survival of child physical abuse (CPA) vary dependent upon many child, parent, and family characteristics. The extant research indicates that physically abused youth experience increased incidences of academic failure, including lower math and reading scores as well as higher rates of discipline referrals, suspensions, grade retention, and school dropout than their non-abused counterparts (Kolko & Swenson, 2002). They also have higher rates of delinquency (Kolko & Swenson, 2002; Walker, Downey, & Bergman, 1989), oppositional behavior (Trickett & Kuczynski, 1986), property offences, substance use (Gelles & Straus, 1990; Kaplan et al., 1998), and arrests (Gelles & Straus, 1990). Poor social competence, interpersonal problems, and negative emotional symptoms are additional areas of potential difficulty for victims of child physical abuse. Longitudinal evidence also suggests such deficits can persist throughout childhood (Hoffman-Plotkin & Twentyman, 1984; Howes & Espinosa, 1985) and into adulthood (Springer, Sheridan, Kuo, & Carnes, 2007).

Regarding emotional responses, child physical abuse is associated with a host of negative symptoms including low self-esteem, sadness, fear, and anxiety (Kolko & Swenson, 2002). Hypervigilance, cognitive distortions, and avoidance, symptoms associated with post-traumatic stress disorder (PTSD), are other symptoms commonly endorsed by physically abused youth. In fact, many research studies indicate that being physically abused results in diagnoses of PTSD in approximately one-third of victims (Famularo, Fenton, Augustyn, & Zuckerman, 1996). Furthermore, they are at increased risk of generalized anxiety disorder (GAD), agoraphobia, depression, conduct disorder, and dysthymia (Kazdin, Moser, Colbus, & Bell, 1985).

Other enduring consequences include attachment difficulties and cognitive impairments. In securely attached children, CPA has resulted in regression and development of insecure attachment styles (Cicchetti & Barnett, 1992), increasing victim likelihood of conflict with others, psychological distress, and poor coping capacity (Kolko & Swenson, 2002).

Neurological problems related to brain damage are another potential consequence. Specifically, deficits in reading ability, expressive language (Burke, Crenshaw, Green, Scholosser, & Strocchia-Rivera, 1989), receptive language (McFayden & Kitson, 1996), auditory attention, and verbal fluency (Tarter, Hegedus, Winsten, & Alterman, 1985) are more likely to occur in youth exposed to physical maltreatment as compared to similarly aged counterparts.

Given the significant impact on victim's well-being, it is apparent that child maltreatment is a public health concern warranting evidence-based assessment and intervention efforts in IC settings to ensure effective identification and treatment of physically abused youth.

Screening and Assessment

Distinct from many presenting problems, treatment and referral planning for CPA requires evaluation of both the child and caregiver. Assessment focused on either in isolation will be insufficient as identification of critical risk factors may be neglected (Swenson & Spratt, 1999). The two evaluation modalities for child physical abuse are forensic and clinical assessment (Kolko & Swenson, 2002). The former is intended to investigate the validity of abuse accusations through physical evaluation and typically requires an interview and medical exam to identify abuse specifics. The latter is used to assess child, parent, and/or family symptomology to determine treatment needs and follows completion of a forensic exam confirming that physical abuse occurred. For the purposes of this chapter, it is important to note that comprehensive clinical assessment may not be feasible in the integrated care (IC) setting; however, there are tools that can support identification and treatment of CPA.

Regarding CPA, the traditional approach to assessment would involve a thorough clinical intake integrating multiple respondent interviews (e.g., child, parents, teachers, CPS worker, and other caretakers) with administration of valid/reliable screening and/or assessment tools. More specifically, acquiring information across five domains is recommended by Hoagwood, Jensen, Petti, and Burns (1996) and includes evaluation of symptom severity, functioning across diverse settings, family needs and supports (specific emphasis on abuse risk), child/family stage of change/readiness to engage in services (Prochaska & DiClemente, 1992), and history of accessing mental health care.

Intensive evaluation of the aforementioned domains is not likely feasible in IC settings; therefore, behavioral health providers should target identification of child mental health symptomology and brief assessment of parental stress. Best practice skills including the use of simple language and open-ended questions (Brubacher, Powell, Snow, Skouteris, & Manger, 2016) should also be used during the initial assessment and throughout treatment to encourage accurate responding.

Generally, evidence-based screening and assessment involves the use of reliable and valid tools that evidence specificity (i.e., differentiation between symptoms/disorders) and sensitivity (i.e., identifies changes in symptomology; Connors, Arora, Curtis, & Stephan, 2015); however, it is important to differentiate between screening and assessment. Screening is used to determine what symptoms are present and generally involves administration of a brief measure (i.e., 5–15 min) that evaluates global and/or specific symptoms. Beyond initial identification, psychometrically sound screening tools are used for comprehensive assessment and progress monitoring throughout treatment. Assessment follows indication of positive screens and methodically evaluates endorsed symptoms through involvement of multiple respondents and various modalities including chart review, observation, survey, cognitive/achievement testing, and medical examination (MRI's, CT scan).

The complexities of child physical abuse warrant comprehensive investigation of child symptoms and adult risk factors associated with recidivism. Be that as it may, feasibility of specific measures should be considered in development of assessment batteries applied to IC settings (Swenson & Spratt, 1999). The following screening and assessment tools are evidence-based, demonstrate acceptable reliability and validity, and evidence efficacious evaluation of symptoms associated with CPA. Data gathered during intake should guide and support selection of appropriate screening tools to assess specific social, emotional, behavioral, and psychological domains. Table 10.1 lists brief evidence-based tools used to *screen* for

Table 10.1 Screening tools to assess for global symptoms, anxiety, depression, and PTSD

Tools[a]	Age	Focus Area	Forms	Author(s)[b]
Global				
PSC	3–16	Anxiety, Depression, Disruptive Behavior, Hyperactivity, Inattention	Parent report Youth report (11–17)	Gardner et al. (1999) (17-item)
SDQ	3–17	Emotional Problems, Conduct Problems, Hyperactivity, Inattention, Peer Relationships, Pro social Behavior	Parent report Teacher report Youth report (11–17)	Goodman (1997)
BPC	7–17	Internalizing and Externalizing Problems	Parent report Youth report	Chorpita et al. (2010)
Anxiety				
RCADS	Grades 3–12	Separation and General Anxiety, Social Phobia, Panic Disorder, Obsessive Compulsive Disorder, Major Depressive Disorder	Youth report Parent report	Ebesutani et al. (2011)
SCARED	8–18	Separation and General Anxiety, Social Phobia, School Phobia, Somatization	Youth report Parent report	Birmaher, Khetarpal, Cully, Brent, and McKenzie (1995)
Depression				
CES-DC	6–17	Depression	Youth report	Faulstich, Carey, Ruggiero, Enyart, and Gresham (1986)
DSRS	8–14	Depression	Youth report	Birleson, Hudson, Buchanan, and Wolff (1987)
PHQ-9	13+	Depression	Youth report	Spitzer, Kroenke, and Williams (1999)
Disruptive behavior				
Vanderbilt	6–12	ADHD, CD, ODD	Parent report Teacher report	Wolraich et al. (2003)
DBD-RS	6–17	ADHD, CD, ODD	Parent report Teacher report	Pelham, Gnagy, Greenslade, and Milich (1992)
CADBI	3–18	Oppositionality, Hyperactivity, Impulsivity	Parent report Teacher report	Burns, Taylor, and Rusby (2001)
Trauma				
CPSS	8–18	PTSD, Functional Impairment	Youth report	Foa, Johnson, Feeny, and Treadwell (2001)
TESI-C	3–18	PTSD	Clinician administered interview	Ghosh-Ippen et al. (2002)
PEDS *UCLA PTSD RI*	2–10 6+	Emotional Distress, Anxiety, Fear PTSD	Parent report Youth report	Saylor, Swenson, Reynolds, and Taylor (1999) Steinberg et al. (2013)

[a]For To access full names of the above mentioned tools, downloadable forms, and additional screening measures, visit http://csmh.umaryland.edu

[b]See references for complete list of authors

youth symptoms of anxiety, depression, disruptive behavior disorders, and trauma, which are commonly endorsed by CPA survivors.

How to Further Assess if a Screen Returns Positive

Positive screens guide the selection of additional assessment tools to evaluate identified areas of concern. Findings may warrant further evaluation of abuse history and mental health symptoms (e.g., anxiety, depression, PTSD), as well as behavioral difficulties, social competence, anger and coping, cognitions, and other psychiatric diagnoses (See Table 10.2).

A complete assessment is one in which child symptoms have been explored across settings, and positive findings have been supported by at least one additional tool (e.g., an additional screening or assessment measure). Evaluation of parent abuse history, abuse risk, stress/dysfunction, substance use, mental health, attributions, and parenting skills should occur concurrently, but feasibility will vary based on IC site. See Table 10.3 for applicable assessment tools.

Observation of parent, child, and family interactions is an additional assessment modality that can be utilized. Informal documentation of interaction styles may prove useful for treatment purposes, but structured and semi-structured observation schedules are available to provide

Table 10.2 Assessment tools for abuse history, behavior difficulties, cognitions, and psychiatric disorders

Tools[a]	Focus Area	Forms	Author(s)
Abuse history			
BATE	Physical abuse specifics, screens for other traumas	Clinician administered	Lipovsky and Hanson (1992)
ADI	Physical and sexual abuse severity	Clinician administered	Chaffin, Wherry, Newlin, Crutchfield, and Dykman (1997)
ROME	Frequency data on experienced traumas, constructive parenting practices	Parent report Youth report	McGee, Wolfe, and Wilson (1997)
Behavioral difficulties			
CBCL	Internalizing (anxiety, depression) externalizing behaviors(ADHD, ODD, CD), social competence, adaptive behavior	Parent report Teacher report	Achenbach (1991); Achenbach and Edelbrock (1983)
CBCL-YSR	Internalizing (anxiety, depression), externalizing (ADHD, ODD, CD) Social competence, adaptive behavior	Youth report	Achenbach (1991)
CCI	Parent-child conflict	Clinician administered parent report	Frankel and Weiner (1990)
CHI	Youth aggression	Parent report Youth report	Kazdin, Rodgers, Colbus, and Siegel (1987)
Cognitions			
CAPS	Personal attributions for negative events, interpersonal trust, perceived credibility, feeling different from peers	Youth report	Mannarino, Cohen, and Berman (1994)
Cites-R	Self-blame, stigma, severity of associations	Youth report	Wolfe, Gentile, Michienzi, Sas, and Wolfe (1991)
Other psychiatric			
Kiddie-SADS	Affective disorders, schizophrenia	Interview	Kaufman, Birmaher, Brent, Rao, and Ryan (1996)
DISC	Affective disorders	Interview	Shaffer et al. (1996)

[a]See references for complete names of measures.

Table 10.3 Tools for assessment of parental abuse history, abuse risk, stress, and attributions

Tools[a]	Focus Area	Author(s)
Abuse history		
CANIS-R	Various forms of maltreatment (e.g., sexual, neglect, physical)	Ammerman, Hersen, Van Hasselt, Lubetsky, and Sieck (1994)
MCS	Abuse history	Barnett, Manly, and Cicchetti (1993)
ADI	Physical and sexual abuse, incident severity	Chaffin et al. (1997)
Abuse risk		
CAPI	Risk of physical abuse includes validity scales	Milner (1986)
CTSPC	Frequency of parental violence, specific tactics (e.g., slapping, knife, gun), nonviolent discipline, physical assault, neglect and sexual abuse	Straus, Hamby, Finkelhor, Moore, and Runyan (1998)
WRAI	Brief, severity of parental anger, parental use of threats or physical force/discipline, severity of family problems	Kolko (1996)
Parental stress/dysfunction		
PSI	Child stress, parental stress, life stress	Abidin (1997)
BSI	Parental psychological distress, dysfunction	Derogatis and Melisaratos (1983)
BDI	Depressive symptoms	Beck, Ward, Mendelson, Mock, and Erbaugh (1961)
Parental Attributions/distortions		
POQ	Expectations of child	Azar et al. (1984)
PAT	Parental expectations, success/failure responsibility	Bugental, Mantyla, and Lewis (1989)
APQ	Parenting practices, discipline, consequences, follow through	Shelton, Frick, and Wootton (1996)
PS	Disciplining practices	Arnold, O'Leary, Wolfe, and Acker (1993)
PPI	Child report, positive and negative interactions with parent	Hazzard, Christensen, and Margolin (1983)

[a]See references for complete names of measures.

objective data. Suggested observation schedules include the Dyadic Parent Child Interaction Coding System (DPICS; Eyberg & Robinson, 1983), Family Interaction Global Coding System (FIGCS; Heatherington, Hagan, & Eisenberg, 1990), and the Mother-Child Interaction Scale (MCIS; Tuteur, Ewigman, Peterson, & Hosokawa, 1995). More information regarding the aforementioned can be found in Kolko and Swenson (2002) and Hansen, Sedlar, and Warner-Rogers (1999).

Evidence-Based Stepped Care and Brief Psychotherapeutic Approaches

IC settings allow for brief, 20–30 min sessions over the course of three to five visits; thus, implementaion of an intensive therapeutic intervention is not often feasible. This may appear problematic considering the potentially complex dynamics of families presenting for care related to CPA. Fortunately, IC settings have undergone rigorous evaluation, and findings suggest it to be well positioned to provide effective, holistic care (Kolko & Perrin, 2014).

Treatment programs employed must be targeted and efficient to fit the standard structure and can be achieved through utilization of common evidence-based elements and modularized content (Kolko & Perrin, 2014). Common elements refer to general skills and specific strategies implemented across intervention curricula for diverse behavioral health concerns. General crosscutting themes include psychoeducation, modeling, practice, problem-solving, and homework. A host of specific evidence-based techniques are also evident across treatment programs, a few of which are relaxation training, cognitive restructuring/coping, and parenting strategies. Coupled with support from modularized programs, routine structure for facilitation of procedures, the aforementioned themes are applicable to treatment of CPA in IC settings.

Limits of Confidentiality and Psychoeducation. Initial treatment sessions should prioritize rapport building and increasing family knowledge regarding target concerns, while later sessions are focused on skill development and maintenance. Assessment findings assist with identification and targeting of family educational needs and also influence treatment dosage (i.e., time allotted to specific skills). The following interventions target skill deficits most frequently found in children and caregivers presenting for treatment of CPA (e.g., anxiety, parental stress, parental expectations).

The first session across treatment settings is typically dedicated to rapport building and review of standard treatment laws such as Health Insurance Portability and Accountability Act (HIPAA) and limits of confidentiality. In cases involving CPA, this session must also include a review of abuse reporting procedures (Kolko & Swenson, 2002). That being said, clinicians must be familiar with legal requirements and are encouraged to reference state policies regarding specific protocols.

In general, families should be informed that the clinician is a mandated reporter responsible for disclosing suspicions of child abuse (e.g., physical, sexual, neglect, and psychological) to higher authorities, including Child Protective Services (CPS; Kolko & Swenson, 2002). Factors that may contribute to a clinician's suspicion should also be discussed, including observed marks/injuries and child or parent report of abuse. Further, physical abuse should be defined in concrete terms that enable the family to understand what parental/family tactics are considered illegal and reportable. Examples from the clinical intake and assessment can be integrated to improve understanding. Additionally, requirements to breach confidentiality in instances of suicidal and/or homicidal ideation need to be explained (Kolko & Swenson, 2002). Providing written explanation of limits of confidentiality and mandated reporting is recommended, and time should be allotted for answering related questions.

Psychoeducation is another integral feature of treatment that typically occurs at the outset but is frequently integrated throughout sessions. Content related to CPA minimally includes the purpose and parameters of abuse laws, differentiation between discipline and abuse, and common consequences associated with child maltreatment (Kolko & Swenson, 2002). Integration of psychoeducation based on clinical assessments (e.g., impact of parental stress, symptoms of anxiety) is encouraged. For example, if screening yields elevated symptoms of hypervigilance in the youth, normalizing endorsed symptoms as common reactions to traumatic experiences can be therapeutic and empowering for the victim (Kolko & Swenson, 2002).

Relaxation. Symptoms of anxiety are common among youth exposed to CPA (Kolko & Swenson, 2002) and can be treated using a variety of CBT strategies. They are additionally beneficial for caregivers, particularly for managing elevated levels of parental stress (Lundahl, Nimer, & Parsons, 2006; Solomon et al., 2014). In fact, research considers treatment of parental distress paramount in effective intervention with CPA (Jouriles et al., 2010; Solomon et al., 2014). Relaxation training, an evidence-based technique used for treatment of various diagnoses and negative symptomology (e.g., anxiety, depression, PTSD, stress), can be implemented to support the victim and perpetrator of physical abuse in an IC setting. Controlled breathing, progressive muscle relaxation (PMR), and guided imagery (Solomon et al., 2014) are skills that emphasize awareness of physiological stress and employment of strategies to achieve a calm, relaxed state following physical arousal.

Relevant modularized programs can provide structure for implementation of relaxation training (Kolko & Swenson, 2002). Brief cognitive behavioral therapy (BCBT) is an exemplary adaptation of an intensive treatment program used to treat anxiety problems (Crawley et al.,

2013; Kendall & Hedtke, 2006). Precise directions are provided regarding how to teach application of relaxation techniques through modeling, practice (e.g., role-play), and homework assignments. Scripts for teaching these techniques are also readily available online for use with various developmental levels (i.e., children, adolescents, adults; http://childrenwithanxiety.com).

Parenting Practices. The relationship between poor discipline tactics and child maltreatment is well documented and consistently highlights the critical importance of building parenting efficacy (Turner and Sanders, 2006). However, caregiver coping ability, expectations of children, and parenting skills often underpin employed practices and mediate feelings of parental isolation, stress, and depressive symptoms (Patterson, Dishion, & Chamberlain, 1993; Turner and Sanders, 2006). Caregivers receiving treatment for CPA should learn specific parenting skills and related strategies for this reason, precisely targeting abovementioned domains (Solomon et al., 2014).

Promoting positive parenting (Triple P; Sanders, 1999) is a behavioral family intervention (BFI) that acknowledges the bi-directional and mutually reciprocal qualities of parent-child interactions and seeks to arm caregivers with positive parenting skills to improve youth emotional, behavioral, and social outcomes (Turner and Sanders, 2006). A brief, four-session version emphasizing consistent discipline strategies, realistic expectations, and managing emotions is available and can support treatment in an IC setting. For example, the modules provide a detailed rationale for learning positive parenting practices to encourage caregiver amenability during treatment. Various teaching modalities (e.g., DVD, fact sheet, role-play) are used to facilitate parent learning of evidence-based practices including praise, planned ignoring, effective requests, behavior charts, and the use of consistent consequences (i.e., reward and punishment; Kolko & Swenson, 2002).

Parent-child interaction training (PCIT; Eyberg, Boggs, & Algina, 1995) is another evidence-based intervention program that can be used to support parent training needs with the added benefit of explicit child-caregiver problem-solving and interaction training (Kolko & Perrin, 2014). Implementation of the evidence-based four-session program in primary care settings yielded maintenance of increased parenting skills, decreased stress, and improved child behavior at 6-month follow-up in a study by Berkovits, O'Brien, Carter, and Eyberg (2010). Combined with other modularized CBT curricula such as PracticeWise MATCH-ADTC (Chorpita & Weisz, 2009), a manual with 33 modules to treat depression, disruptive behavior, and anxiety, the aforementioned programs can support a range of diverse child and family problems.

Treating children exposed to physical abuse and their caregivers using a one-size-fits-all approach is ill-advised. The heterogeneous presentation of this population necessitates a flexible assessment and treatment procedure supported by implementation of common element practices. Given the potential for content flexibility aligned with unique youth and family clinical presentations, modularized adherence to the CBT format (e.g., psychoeducation, practice, problem-solving, homework) across programs enables consistency in delivery of evidence-based strategies.

Maintenance and Termination. Latter sessions are dedicated to maintenance of learned skills and termination, which could result in referral to a more intensive treatment setting. Re-administration of relevant screening tools helps to evaluate changes in symptomology, areas of patient growth, and potential need for supplementary support. If subclinical levels are evident, plans for maintenance may include increasing social supports and help-seeking through PCP as needed. The clinician may also direct the family to additional resources such as bibliotherapy (i.e., books, readings) and prevention groups. However, some cases will require referral to intensive treatment of interconnected CPA-related variables, and, in these instances, the notion of effective screening and assessment remains paramount.

Other Intervention Tools. Varying resources for learning should be offered to support brief in-person treatment. Bibliotherapy is a stepped care strategy used for treatment of many clinical concerns, including CPA, and is associated with positive outcomes. In youth experiencing abuse, bibliotherapy increased feelings identification skills, improved problem-solving capacity, and taught cognitive restructuring skills. Pardeck (1990) provides a list of children's books addressing child maltreatment including *Michael's Story* (Anderson & Finne, 1986a), *Robin's Story* (Anderson & Finne, 1986b), *The Pinballs* (Byars, 1977), *The Lottery Rose* (Hunt, 1976), *Like the Lion's Tooth* (Kellogg, 1972), *The War on Villa Street* (Mazer, 1978), *Gunner's Run* (Orr, 1980), *Don't Hurt Laurie* (Roberts, 1978), and *Tough Chauncey* (Smith, 1974). The paper also comments on procedures for integrating these resources into treatment.

Bibliotherapy can be similarly beneficial for adults and/or caregivers that perpetrate abuse. Books such as *The Body Keeps the Score* (van der Kolk, 2014) and *The Whole-Brain Child* (Siegel and Bryson, 2011) provide complementary information, one covering the impact of child maltreatment on developing youth and the other educating on the benefits of positive caregiver-parent interactions through an engaging workbook. Additional resources, including fact sheets and suggested readings ranging from child mental health to parental stress management, are free and available through the National Child Traumatic Stress Network (nctsn.org). PCPs and behavioral health specialists may also refer families with various presenting needs to parentsanonymous.org and circleofparents.org, general self-help websites with access to webinars, parent resources, and blogs.

What Does Not Work

The effects of child physical abuse are based on duration, severity, intensity, and child perception of caregiver-perpetrated maltreatment. Parent-focused therapy has been the traditional modality of CPA treatment, while child-only treatment is less common. Be that as it may, both are insufficient models as either in isolation neglects potentially important variables mediating and moderating incidences of CPA (Swenson & Spratt, 1999). Comprehensive treatment, simultaneous intervention with the victim and perpetrator, is regarded as best practice.

Along similar lines, treating only the physical evidence of CPA disregards the emotional, behavioral, and psychological impact of child maltreatment (Swenson & Spratt, 1999). Primary care providers (PCPs) need training on identification of symptomology attributable to CPA enabling appropriate referral to behavioral health specialists.

As discussed above, approaching all families presenting for CPA with a standard assessment and intervention process will prove ineffective. Also, relying solely on intervention services from CPS will often fail to meet the needs of youth and their families. First, not all instances are substantiated due to sub-threshold or uncorroborated findings; therefore, supports will not be activated for families that would benefit from common treatment elements (e.g., psychoeducation, parenting skills). Second, the literature is sparse concerning the effectiveness of CPS interventions warranting the arrangement of supplementary supports (Kolko, 2000).

When to Refer to External Specialty Mental Health

As is the recurrent theme, evidence-based screening and assessment should be used as the foundation of treatment and referral procedures because it contributes to data-informed decision-making, improves quality of care, and increases accountability for services provided (Connors et al., 2015). Therefore, decisions regarding treatment appropriateness and referral needs should follow clinical assessment. Brief CBT has proven effective for treatment of anxiety, depression, trauma, and disruptive behavior disorders (Kolko & Perrin, 2014). It is evident that youth with easily targeted, uncomplicated symptomology are appropriate and will benefit from brief treatment in IC settings. In other cases, families are best served by assessment feedback and referral to appropriate programs. Endorsement of significant symptomology across multiple domains in the child (e.g., anxiety, depression, psychiatric disorder) and caregiver (e.g., psychiatric disorder, parental distress, severely distorted cognitions) is not conducive to brief, time-limited therapy due to the potential impact of confounding problems (Cully & Teten, 2008).

Additionally, families reporting chronic, severe physical abuse and/or out-of-home placement would likely benefit from intensive services such as Parent-Child Interaction Therapy, Alternatives for Families: A Cognitive Behavioral Therapy (AF-CBT), Multisystemic Therapy for Child Abuse and Neglect (MST-CAN), and Combined Parent-Child Cognitive Behavioral Therapy (CPC-CBT), all of which are evidence-based programs for treatment of child maltreatment (Cummings & Berkowitz, 2014). Based on predetermined areas of needs, clinicians may refer patients to professionals trained in a specific treatment modality.

Families should also be referred when significant symptoms persist after treatment. Effective treatment of families deemed appropriate for an IC can be negatively influenced by factors such as client engagement (e.g., readiness to change), developmental level, and instances of recidivism. Barriers created by such variables may impede client progress and require referral at the conclusion of treatment.

The Role of the Primary Care Provider/Medical Team in Treatment

Identification and treatment of CPA is not easy, but the process is often improved with collaboration between behavioral health and medical staff (Swenson & Spratt, 1999). PCPs and the medical team may be involved in identification, assessment, treatment, and ongoing monitoring of CPA. Specifically, medical staff can lead forensic assessments. In children younger than 2 years old, for example, skeletal surveys are mandatory, but imaging decisions in older youth are based on clinical indications and may involve magnetic resonance imaging (MRI) or computed tomography (CT; Swenson & Spratt, 1999). Medical staff are particularly poised to provide guidance on appropriate actions and conduct diagnostic assessments.

Children and caregivers presenting with elevated levels of anxiety, depression, and other psychiatric conditions may also benefit from consultation with the primary care provider about the role of psychopharmacological approaches to treatment. Although psychopharmacologic intervention with post-traumatic stress disorder (PTSD) has limited support prior to engagement in psychotherapy (Cummings & Berkowitz, 2014), concurrent treatment may be optimal for specific clinical presentations. For example, ameliorating symptoms of comorbid ADHD and autism spectrum disorder (ASD) may improve client ability to engage in treatment for CPA.

PCPs may also function as conduits of ongoing progress monitoring and maintenance of treatment gains. Following brief therapy, PCPs remain in contact with families and could feasibly administer screening tools used for initial identification and assessment. Results can initiate referrals to support resources, brief treatment, or intensive specialty clinics.

How to Assess Impact on Care/Quality Improvement Processes

Effective screening tools achieve several goals: initial identification of need, support comprehensive assessment, and can be utilized for progress monitoring. Therefore, utilization of evidence-based global screening tools should be considered as a means to assess impact of care. For example, the pediatric symptom checklist is a brief, validated, easy-to-use, and cost-effective (i.e., free) tool that does not require specialized training to administer and could serve as a universal measure of treatment effectiveness. The PSC, along with the Brief Problems Checklist (BPC) and Strength and Difficulties Questionnaire (SDQ), has been successfully employed in IC settings (Kolko & Perrin, 2014). The Child Conflict Index (CCI), Parenting Scale (PS), and Parent Perception Inventory (PPI) may be additionally helpful in determining changes in child-caregiver interactions upon termination (Kolko & Swenson, 2002).

In terms of quality improvement, the National Commission on Quality Assurance (NCQA) offers standards to improve quality of care including data tracking of patient access, employment of tracking measures, data-driven diagnoses, provision of self-management supports, test result monitoring and tracking, referral tracking, treatment impact assessment, and interdisciplinary collaboration tracking (Talen & Valeras, 2013). However, the NCQA does not offer a specific recommendation as to appropriate screening tools for child maltreatment due to the heterogeneity of the population. Providers should consider the abovementioned screening and assessment tools and whether they fit into the larger IC context.

References

Abidin, R. (1997). Parenting stress index: A measure of the parent-child system. In C. P. Zalaquett & R. J. Wood (Eds.), *Evaluating stress: A book of resources* (pp. 277–291). Lanham, MD: Scarecrow Press.

Achenbach, T. M. (1991). *Manual for the child behavior checklist/4-18 and 1991 profile* (p. 288). Burlington, VT: Department of Psychiatry, University of Vermont.

Achenbach, T. M., & Edelbrock, C. S. (1983). *Manual for the child behavior checklist and revised behavior profile*. Burlington: University of Vermont Department of Psychiatry.

Ammerman, R. T., Hersen, M., Van Hasselt, V. B., Lubetsky, M. J., & Sieck, W. R. (1994). Maltreatment in psychiatrically hospitalized children and adolescents with developmental disabilities: Prevalence and correlates. *Journal of the American Academy of Child & Adolescent Psychiatry, 33*(4), 567–576.

Anderson, D., & Finne, M. (1986a). *Michael's story*. Minneapolis, MN: Dillon Press.

Anderson, D., & Finne, M. (1986b). *Robin's story*. Minneapolis, MN: Dillon Press.

Arnold, D. S., O'Leary, S. G., Wolff, L. S., & Acker, M. M. (1993). *The Parenting Scale: A measure of dysfunctional parenting in discipline situations*. Psychological Assessment, *5*(2), 137–144.

Azar, S. T., Robinson, D. R., Hekimian, E., & Twentyman, C. T. (1984). Unrealistic expectations and problem-solving ability in maltreating and comparison mothers. *Journal of Consulting and Clinical Psychology, 52*, 687–691.

Barnett, D., Manly, J. T., & Cicchetti, D. (1993). Defining child maltreatment: The interface between policy and research. *Child Abuse, Child Development, and Social Policy, 8*, 7–73.

Beck, A. T., Ward, C. H., Mendelson, M., Mock, J., & Erbaugh, J. (1961). An inventory for measuring depression. *Archives of General Psychiatry, 4*, 561–571.

Berger, L., Paxon, C., & Waldfogel, J. (2009). Mothers, mean and child protective service involvement. *Child Maltreatment, 14*(3), 263–276.

Berkovits, M. D., O'Brien, K. A., Carter, C. G., & Eyberg, S. M. (2010). Early identification and intervention for behavior problems in primary care: A comparison of two abbreviated versions of parent-child interaction therapy. *Behavior Therapy, 21*(3), 375–387.

Birleson, P., Hudson, I., Buchanan, D. G., & Wolff, S. (1987). Clinical evaluation of a self-rating scale for depressive disorder in childhood (depression self-rating scale). *Journal of Child Psychology and Psychiatry, 28*(1), 43–60.

Birmaher, B., Khetarpal, S., Cully, M., Brent, D., & McKenzie, S. (1995). *Screen for child anxiety related disorder (SCARED)*. Pittsburgh: Western Psychiatric Institute & Clinic, University of Pittsburgh.

Brubacher, S. P., Powell, M. B., Snow, P. C., Skouteris, H., & Manger, B. (2016). Guidelines for teachers to elicit detailed and accurate narrative accounts from children. *Children and Youth Services Review, 63*, 83–92.

Bugental, D. B., Mantyla, S. M., & Lewis, J. (1989). Parental attributions as moderates of affective communication to children at risk for hysical abuse. In D. Cicchetti & V. Carlson (Eds.), *Child maltreatment: Theory and research on the causes and consequences of child abuse and neglect* (pp. 254–279). New York: Cambridge University Press.

Burke, A. E., Crenshaw, D. A., Green, J., Scholosser, M. A., & Strocchia-Rivera, L. (1989). Influence of verbal ability on the expression of aggression in physically abused children. *Journal of the American Academy of Child Psychiatry, 28*, 215–218.

Burns, G. L., Taylor, T. K., & Rusby, J. C. (2001). Child and adolescent disruptive behavior inventory 2.3: Parent version. Pullman: Washington State University, Department of Psychology.

Byars, B. (1977). *The pinballs*. New York: Harper and Row.

Caspi, A., & Elder, G. H. (1988). Emergent family patterns: The intergenerational construction of problem behavior and relationships. In R. A. Hinde & J. Stevenson-Hinde (Eds.), *Relationships with families: Mutual influences* (pp. 218–240). Oxford: Clarendon.

Chaffin, M., Wherry, J. N., Newlin, C., Crutchfield, A., & Dykman, R. (1997). The abuse dimensions inventory initial data on a research measure of abuse severity. *Journal of Interpersonal Violence, 12*(4), 569–589.

Children's Bureau. (2009, February). Definitions of child abuse and neglect: Summary of state laws. Retrieved from http://www.childwelfare.gov/systemwide/laws_policies/statutes/define.cfm

Chorpita, B. F., Reise, S., Weisz, J. R., Grubbs, K., Becker, K. D., & Krull, J. L. (2010). Evaluation of the brief problem checklist: Child and caregiver interviews to measure clinical progress. *Journal of Consulting and Clinical Psychology, 78*(4), 526.

Chorpita, B. F., & Weisz, J. R. (2009). *MATCH-ADTC: Modular approach to therapy for children with anxiety, depression, trauma, or conduct problems*. Satellite Beach, FL: PracticeWise.

Christian, C. W. (2015). The evaluation of suspected child physical abuse. *Pediatrics, 135*(5), 1–21.

Cicchetti, D., & Barnett, D. (1992). Attachment organization in maltreated preschoolers. *Development and Psychopathology, 3*, 397–411.

Connors, E. H., Arora, P., Curtis, L., & Stephan, S. H. (2015). Evidence-based assessment in school mental health. *Cognitive and Behavioral Practice, 22*(1), 60–73.

Crawley, S. A., Kendall, P. C., Benjamin, C. L., Brodman, D. M., Wei, C., Beidas, R. S., … Mauro, C. (2013). Brief cognitive-behavioral therapy for anxious youth: Feasibility and initial outcomes. *Cognitive and Behavioral Practice, 20*(2), 123–133.

Cully, J. A., & Teten, A. L. (2008). *A therapist's guide to brief cognitive behavioral therapy*. Houston, TX: South Central Mental Illness Research, Education, and Clinical Center.

Cummings, M., & Berkowitz, S. J. (2014). Evaluation and treatment of childhood physical abuse and neglect: A review. *Current Psychiatry Reports, 16*(1), 1–10.

DePanfilis, D., & Zuravin, S. (1999). Predicting child maltreatment recurrences during treatment. *Child Abuse & Neglect, 23*(8), 729–743.

Derogatis, L. R., & Melisaratos, N. (1983). The brief symptom inventory: An introductory report. *Psychological Medicine, 13*(3), 595–605.

Ebesutani, C., Chorpita, B. F., Higa-McMillan, C. K., Nakamura, B. J., Regan, J., & Lynch, R. E. (2011). A psychometric analysis of the revised child anxiety and depression scales—Parent version in a school sample. *Journal of Abnormal Child Psychology, 39*(2), 173–185.

Eyberg, S. M., Boggs, S. R., & Algina, J. (1995). Parent-child interaction therapy: A psychosocial model for the treatment of young children with conduct problem behavior and their families. *Psychopharmacology Bulletin, 3*(1), 83–91.

Eyberg, S. M., & Robinson, E. A. (1983). Conduct problem behavior: Standardization of a behavioral rating. *Journal of Clinical Child & Adolescent Psychology, 12*(3), 347–354.

Famularo, R., Fenton, T., Augustyn, M., & Zuckerman, B. (1996). Persistence of pediatric post traumatic stress disorder after two years. *Child Abuse & Neglect, 20*, 1245–1248.

Faulstich, M. E., Carey, M. P., Ruggiero, L., Enyart, P., & Gresham, F. (1986). Assessment of depression in childhood and adolescence: An evaluation of the Center for Epidemiological Studies Depression Scale for children (CES-DC). *American Journal of Psychiatry, 143*, 1024–1027.

Foa, E. B., Johnson, K. M., Feeny, N. C., & Treadwell, K. R. (2001). The child PTSD symptom scale: A preliminary examination of its psychometric properties. *Journal of Clinical Child Psychology, 30*(3), 376–384.

Frankel, F., & Weiner, H. (1990). The child conflict index: Factor analysis, reliability, and validity for clinic-referred and Nonreffered children. *Journal of Clinical Child Psychology, 19*(3), 239–248.

Gardner, W., Murphy, M., Childs, G., Kelleher, K., Pagano, M., Jellinek, M., … Chiappetta, L. (1999). The PSC-17: A brief pediatric symptom checklist with psychosocial problem subscales. A report from PROS and ASPN. *Ambulatory Child Health, 5*, 225–225.

Gelles, R. J., & Straus, M. A. (1990). The medical and psychological costs of family violence. In M. A. Straus & R. J. Gelles (Eds.), *Physical violence in American families: Risk factors and adaptations to violence in 8,145 families* (pp. 431–470). New Brunswick, NJ: Transaction.

Ghosh-Ippen, C., Ford, J., Racusin, R., Acker, M., Bosquet, K., Rogers, C., & Edwards, J. (2002). *Trauma events screening inventory-parent report revised*. San Francisco: The Child Trauma Research Project of the Early Trauma Network and The National Center for PTSD Dartmouth Child Trauma Research Group.

Gokten, E. S., Duman, N. S., Soylu, N., & Uzun, M. E. (2016). Effects of attention-deficit/hyperactivity disorder on child abuse and neglect. *Child Abuse & Neglect, 62*, 1–9.

Goodman, R. (1997). The strengths and difficulties questionnaire: A research note. *Journal of Child Psychology and Psychiatry, 38*(5), 581–586.

Hansen, D. J., Sedlar, G., & Warner-Rogers, J. E. (1999). Child physical abuse. In R. T. Ammerman & M. Hersen (Eds.), *Assessment of family violence: A clinical and legal sourcebook* (pp. 127–156). New York: John Wiley.

Hazzard, A., Christensen, A., & Margolin, G. (1983). Children's perceptions of parental behaviors. *Journal of Abnormal Child Psychology, 11*(1), 49–59.

Heatherington, E. M., Hagan, M. S., & Eisenberg, N. (1990). *Coping with marital transitions (monographs of the Society for Research in child development)*. Chicago: University of Chicago Press.

Herrenkohl, T. I., & Herrenkohl, R. C. (2007). Examining the overlap and prediction of multiple forms of child maltreatment, stressors, and socioeconomic status: A longitudinal analysis of youth outcomes. *Journal of Family Violence, 22*(7), 553–562.

Hoagwood, K., Jensen, P. S., Petti, T., & Burns, B. J. (1996). Outcomes of mental health care for children and adolescents: I. A comprehensive conceptual model. *Journal of the American Academy of Child & Adolescent Psychiatry, 35*(8), 1055–1063.

Hoffman-Plotkin, D., & Twentyman, C. T. (1984). A multimodal assessment of behavioral and cognitive deficits in abused and neglected preschoolers. *Child Development, 55*, 794–802.

Howes, C., & Espinosa, M. P. (1985). The consequences of child abuse for the formation of relationships with peers. *Child Abuse & Neglect, 9*, 397–404.

Hunt, I. (1976). *The Lottery Rose*. New York, NY: Charles Scribner's.

Jouriles, E. N., McDonald, R., Rosenfield, D., Norwood, W. D., Spiller, L., Stephens, N., … Ehrensaft, M. (2010). Improving parenting in families referred for child maltreatment: A randomized controlled trial examining effects of project support. *Journal of Family Psychology, 24*(3), 328.

Kaplan, S. J., Pelcovitz, D., Salzinger, S., Weiner, M., Mandel, F. S., Lesser, M. L., & Labruna, V. E. (1998). Adolescent physical abuse: Risk for adolescent psychiatric disorders. *American Journal of Psychiatry, 155*(7), 954–959.

Kaufman, J., Birmaher, B., Brent, D., Rao, U., & Ryan, N. (1996). *KIDDIE-SADS-present and lifetime version (K-SADS-PL)*. Instrument developed at Western Psychiatric Institute and Clinic, Pittsburgh, PA.

Kaufman, J., & Zigler, E. (1987). Do abused children become abusive parents? *American Journal of Orthopsychiatry, 57*, 186–192.

Kazdin, A. E., Moser, J., Colbus, D., & Bell, R. (1985). Depressive symptoms among physically abused and psychiatrically disturbed children. *Journal of Abnormal Psychology, 94*(3), 298–307.

Kazdin, A. E., Rodgers, A., Colbus, D., & Siegel, T. (1987). Children's hostility inventory: Measurement of aggression and hostility in psychiatric inpatient children. *Journal of Clinical Child Psychology, 16*, 320–328.

Kellogg, M. (1972). *Like the lion's tooth*. New York, NY: Farrar, Straus, and Giroux.

Kendall, P. C., & Hedtke, K. A. (2006). *Cognitive-behavioral therapy for anxious children: Therapist manual*. Ardmore: Workbook.

Kolko, D. (1996). Clinical monitoring of treatment course in child physical abuse: Child and parent reports. *Child Abuse & Neglect, 20*, 23–43.

Kolko, D. (2000). Treatment research in child maltreatment: Clinical and research directions. *Journal of Aggression, Maltreatment & Trauma, 4*(1), 139–164.

Kolko, D. J., & Perrin, E. (2014). The integration of behavioral health interventions in children's health care: services, science, and suggestions. *Journal of Clinical Child & Adolescent Psychology, 43*(2), 216–228.

Kolko, D., & Swenson, C. C. (2002). *Assessing and treating physically abused children and their families: A cognitive-behavioral approach*. Thousand Oaks, CA: SAGE Publications.

Lipovsky, J.A., Hanson, R.F. (1992, October). *Multiple traumas in the histories of child/adolescent psychiatric inpatients*. Paper presented at the annual meeting of the International Society for Traumatic Stress Studies, Los Angeles, CA.

Lundahl, B. W., Nimer, J., & Parsons, B. (2006). Preventing child abuse: A meta-analysis of parent training programs. *Research on Social Work Practice, 16*(3), 251–262.

Mannarino, A. P., Cohen, J. A., & Berman, S. R. (1994). The Children's Attributions and Perceptions Scale: A new measure of sexual abuse-related factors. *Journal of Clinical Child Psychology, 23*(2), 204–211.

Mazer, H. (1978). *The war on villa street*. New York, NY: Delacorte.

McFayden, R. G., & Kitson, W. J. H. (1996). Language comprehension and expression among adolescents who have experienced childhood physical abuse. *Journal of Child Psychology and Psychiatry and Allied Disciplines, 37*(5), 551–562.

McGee, R. A., Wolfe, D. A., & Wilson, S. K. (1997). Multiple maltreatment experiences and adolescent behavior problems: Adolescents' perspectives. *Development and Psychopathology, 9*(1), 131–149.

Milner, J. S. (1986). Assessing physical child abuse risk: The child abuse potential inventory. *Clinical Psychology Review, 14*, 547–583.

National Child Traumatic Stress, & Network, physical abuse collaborative group. (2009). *Child physical abuse fact sheet*. Los Angeles, CA: National Center for Child Traumatic Stress.

Orr, R. (1980). *Gunner's run*. New York, NY: Harper and Row.

Pardeck, J. T. (1990). Children's literature and child abuse. *Child Welfare: Journal of Policy, Practice, and Program, 69*(1), 83–88.

Patterson, G. R., Dishion, T. J., & Chamberlain, P. (1993). Outcomes and methodological issues relating to treatment of antisocial children. In *Handbook of effective psychotherapy* (pp. 43–88). New York: Springer.

Pelham, W. E., Gnagy, E. M., Greenslade, K. E., & Milich, R. (1992). Teacher ratings of DSM-III-R symptoms for the disruptive behavior disorders. *Journal of the American Academy of Child & Adolescent Psychiatry, 31*(2), 210–218.

Prochaska, J. O., & DiClemente, C. C. (1992). Stages of change in the modification of problem behaviors. *Progress in Behavior Modification, 28*, 183.

Roberts, W. (1978). *Don't hurt Laurie*. New York, NY: Atheneum.

Sanders, M. R. (1999). Triple P-positive parenting program: Towards an empirically validated multilevel parenting and family support strategy for the prevention of behavior and emotional problems in children. *Clinical Child and Family Psychology Review, 2*(2), 71–90.

Saylor, C. F., Swenson, C. C., Reynolds, S. S., & Taylor, M. (1999). The pediatric emotional distress scale: A brief screening measure for young children exposed to traumatic events. *Journal of Clinical Child Psychology, 28*(1), 70–81.

Shaffer, D., Fisher, P., Dulcan, M. K., Davies, M., Piacentini, J., Schwab-Stone, M. E., … Canino, G. (1996). The NIMH Diagnostic Interview Schedule for Children Version 2.3 (DISC-2.3): Description, acceptability, prevalence rates, and performance in the MECA study. *Journal of the American Academy of Child & Adolescent Psychiatry, 35*(7), 865–877.

Shelton, K. K., Frick, P. J., & Wootton, J. (1996). Assessment of parenting practices in families of elementary school-age children. *Journal of Clinical Child Psychology, 25*(3), 317–329.

Siegel, D. J., & Bryson, T. P. (2011). *The whole-brain child: 12 revolutionary strategies to nurture your child's developing mind.* New York: Random House Digital.

Simons, R. L., Whitbeck, L. B., Conger, R. D., & Wu, C.-i. (1991). Intergenerational transmission of harsh parenting. *Developmental Psychology, 17*, 762–765.

Smith, D. (1974). *Tough Chauncey.* New York, NY: William Morrow.

Solomon, D., Morgan, B., Asberg, K., & McCord, D. (2014). Treatment implications based on measures of child abuse potential and parent mental health: Are we missing an intervention opportunity. *Children and Youth Services Review, 43*, 153–159.

Spitzer, R. L., Kroenke, K., & Williams, J. B. W. (1999). Patient health questionnaire study group. Validity and utility of a self-report version of prime-md: The PHQ primary care study. *JAMA, 282*, 1737–1744.

Springer, K. W., Sheridan, J., Kuo, D., & Carnes, M. (2007). Long-term physical and mental health consequences of childhood physical abuse: Results from a large population-based sample of men and women. *Child Abuse & Neglect, 31*(5), 517–530.

Steinberg, A. M., Brymer, M. J., Kim, S., Ghosh, C., Ostrowski, S. A., Gulley, K., … Pynoos, R. S. (2013). Psychometric properties of the UCLA PTSD reaction index: Part 1. *Journal of Traumatic Stress, 26*, 1–9.

Straus, M. A., Hamby, S. L., Finkelhor, D., Moore, D. W., & Runyan, D. (1998). Identification of child maltreatment with the Parent-Child Conflict Tactics Scales: Development and psychometric data for a national sample of American parents. *Child Abuse & Neglect, 22*(4), 249–270.

Swenson, C. C., & Spratt, E. G. (1999). Identification and treatment of child physical abuse through medical and mental health collaborations. *Children's Health Care, 28*(2), 123–139.

Talen, M. R., & Valeras, A. B. (Eds.). (2013). *Integrated behavioral health in primary care.* New York, NY: Springer.

Tarter, R. E., Hegedus, A. M., Winsten, N. E., & Alterman, A. I. (1985). Intellectual profiles and violent behavior in juvenile delinquents. *The Journal of Psychology, 119*, 125–128.

Trickett, P. K., & Kuczynski, L. (1986). Children's misbehaviors and parental discipline strategies in abusive and nonabusive families. *Developmental Psychology, 22*, 115–123.

Turner, K. M. T., & Sanders, M. R. (2006). Help when it's needed first: A controlled evaluation of brief, preventive behavioral family intervention in a primary care setting. *Behavior Therapy, 37*(2), 131–142.

Tuteur, J. M., Ewigman, B. E., Peterson, L., & Hosokawa, M. C. (1995). The Maternal Observation Matrix and the Mother-Child Interaction Scale: Brief observational screening instruments for physically abusive mothers. *Journal of Clinical Child Psychology, 24*(1), 55–62.

Van Der Kolk, B. (2014). *The body keeps the score.* New York City: Viking.

Walker, E., Downey, G., & Bergman, A. (1989). The effects of parental psychopathology and maltreatment on child behavior: A test of the diathesis-stress model. *Child Development, 60*, 15–24.

Whipple, E. E., & Webster-Stratton, C. (1991). The role of parental stress in physically abusive families. *Child Abuse & Neglect, 15*, 279–291.

Wolfe, V., Gentile, C., Michienzi, T., Sas, L., & Wolfe, D. A. (1991). The Children's impact of traumatic events scale: A measure of post-sexual-abuse PTSD symptoms. *Behavioral Assessment, 13*, 359–383.

Wolraich, M. L., Lambert, W., Doffing, M. A., Bickman, L., Simmons, T., & Worley, K. (2003). Psychometric properties of the Vanderbilt ADHD diagnostic parent rating scale in a referred population. *Journal of Pediatric Psychology, 28*(8), 559–568.

Chronic Obstructive Pulmonary Disease

11

Stefanie Poehacker, Megha Garg, and Claudia Drossel

A Brief Description of Chronic Obstructive Pulmonary Disease

The Global Initiative for Chronic Obstructive Lung Disease (GOLD) defines chronic obstructive pulmonary disease (COPD) as "a common, preventable and treatable disease that is characterized by persistent respiratory symptoms and airflow limitation […] usually caused by significant exposure to noxious particles or gases" (Vogelmeier et al., 2017, p. 576). COPD constitutes an important health challenge, particularly considering long-term exposure to air pollution as a major contributor and aging populations (Vogelmeier et al., 2017). It is a major cause of chronic morbidity and mortality worldwide: While COPD is the fourth leading cause of death in the world and third leading cause of death in the United States, the World Health Organization (WHO) projects an increase in COPD deaths, making it the third leading cause of death in the world by 2030 (Diaz-Guzman & Mannino, 2014).

The most common respiratory symptoms include breathlessness, dyspnea and wheezing, chronic cough, and sputum production (Vogelmeier et al., 2017). As these symptoms are often underreported, COPD remains underdiagnosed (Han et al., 2015); moreover, differential diagnosis of COPD and asthma might be difficult (Postma & Rabe, 2015). In general, and in contrast to asthma, the chronic airflow restrictions that characterize COPD worsen progressively and are not fully reversible (Kruis et al., 2013). However, the clinical presentation and the course of COPD are heterogeneous, and chronic disease progress might be interspersed with periods of acute worsening of symptoms referred to as exacerbations (Vestbo et al., 2014; Vogelmeier et al., 2017). Depending on degree of hypoxia and hypoxemia (Kent, Mitchell, & McNicholas, 2011), functional impairment can range from subtle to severe. As the disease progresses, it changes sleep architecture, appetite and weight, and skeletal muscle functioning, resulting in poor exercise tolerance. COPD can impact physical, work, and self-care activities as well as social, emotional, and cognitive functioning, and impairment may occur in isolated domains or affect functioning in a global manner.

The development of COPD is a complex interplay of a variety of risk factors. As noted in the definition above, COPD is related to long-term exposure to noxious gases, fumes, and particles, the most common of which is tobacco smoking, implicated in 80–90% of cases. Other types of air pollution, such as outdoor, indoor, and occupational exposure to biomass fuels, dust, and

S. Poehacker, M.S. (✉) • M. Garg • C. Drossel
Department of Psychology, Eastern Michigan University, Ypsilanti, MI, USA
e-mail: spoehack@emich.edu; mgarg3@emich.edu; cdrossel@emich.edu

A. Maragakis, W.T. O'Donohue (eds.), *Principle-Based Stepped Care and Brief Psychotherapy for Integrated Care Settings*, https://doi.org/10.1007/978-3-319-70539-2_11

chemicals, are also major risk factors. Genetic factors, age and gender, lung growth and development, socioeconomic status, asthma and airway reactivity, chronic bronchitis, and infections contribute to the development and exacerbation of COPD (Vogelmeier et al., 2017). COPD is highly comorbid with other chronic conditions with similar behavioral health risk factors (Vogelmeier et al., 2017), such as cardiovascular disease, and associated with poor mental health, especially anxiety and depression (Burgess, Kunik, & Stanley, 2005). Given the progressive and irreversible nature of COPD and the associated impairments, prevention, early detection, and early intervention are crucial.

Primary care providers screen for COPD when patients present with reported or recognizable respiratory symptoms, such as dyspnea, chronic cough, chronic sputum production, or recurrent lower respiratory infections. Additionally, the decision to screen may be based on the presence of risk factors, such as a family history of COPD, or childhood factors (Vogelmeier et al., 2017). Medical providers may use brief questionnaires to assess for symptoms as well as risk factors. Depending on the outcome of the self-report measures, high-risk patients then undergo pulmonary function tests.

Once a diagnosis has been established, primary care management of COPD focuses on symptom reduction, prevention of exacerbations, and delay of disease progression. It employs a multicomponent approach consisting of:

- Monitoring. The primary care provider monitors disease progression periodically (e.g., yearly spirometry) and collaborates with secondary care and pulmonary rehabilitation services. When managing COPD, adequacy of symptom control (breathlessness, exercise tolerance, exacerbation frequency) and presence of complications are assessed regularly. While education and nutrition are part of pulmonary rehabilitation (see below), nutritional screening and brief assessment such as simple BMI screens and weight monitoring also may take place in the primary care setting (Bellamy & Smith, 2007).
- Delivering education about COPD as a treatable disease (see Patient Resources).
- Assessing and promoting avoidance of risk factors/exposures, including referral to a behavioral health specialist for smoking cessation. Primary care providers should strongly encourage smoking cessation and reassess the patient's desire to quit or adherence to smoking cessation every 6 months (Bellamy & Smith, 2007). The behavioral health specialist can facilitate patient-provider interactions by training primary care staff to use motivational interviewing techniques for health behavior change (for a review, see Rollnick, Miller, & Butler, 2007).
- Prescribing drugs and vaccines (e.g., bronchodilators, inhaled corticosteroids, anti-inflammatory agents, or a combination thereof); of note, these drugs may alleviate acute symptoms but do not alter disease progression. Systematic monitoring should include drug treatment effects (including potential adverse effects—see below, or tolerance effects), and assessment of inhaler technique (Bryant et al., 2013).
- Prescribing home oxygen therapy for chronic hypoxia. As 15–25% of individuals on home oxygen therapy continue to smoke, patients must receive warnings regarding the fire hazard and their increased risk for smoke inhalation and burn injuries (Sharma et al., 2015).
- Referring to pulmonary rehabilitation, a three-pronged non-pharmacological approach involving education, nutrition (for weight management), and exercise. Exercise, particularly endurance training, is the keystone of pulmonary rehabilitation, to build strength and prevent physical deconditioning (Vogelmeier et al., 2017), and physical strength is a prognostic indicator in patients with moderate to severe COPD (Kent et al., 2011).

Despite the positive impact of comprehensive COPD management on exercise capacity, dyspnea, fatigue, emotional function, and patient sense of control, adherence is poor: Only 10–40% of patients follow through with their treatment regimen as prescribed (Sanduzzi et al., 2014). While nonadherence can be an active choice that reflects the patient's deliberate reduction or discontinuation of the prescribed regimen without physician input upon symptom relief, in practice it is mostly non-deliberate and occurs as a function of other factors (Bryant et al., 2013). Barriers to treatment fall into the following five categories (Sabaté, 2003):

1. Socioeconomic (e.g., cost of medications, poor access to transportation)
2. Patient-related (e.g., age, coping repertoire, cognitive functioning, correlated depression and anxiety)
3. Therapy-related (e.g., treatment complexity, such as number of medications or difficulties handling the device)
4. Disease-related (e.g., subtle or mild symptoms, underestimation of disease severity, dyspnea-related exercise avoidance)
5. Healthcare systems or provider-related factors (e.g., fragmented care, lack of evidence-based care, ineffective patient-clinician interactions, poor instruction). For example, Johnston, Young, Grimmer-Somers, Antic, and Frith (2011) found that lack of physician knowledge about pulmonary rehabilitation and the referral process was associated with failure to follow guidelines and refer patients to pulmonary rehabilitation.

Nonadherence has negative effects on disease progression and outcomes, worsening quality of life and increasing healthcare costs. Hence, identifying poor adherence and removing potential barriers are crucial to treating COPD.

Screening for Adherence

To evaluate adherence to COPD management, several indirect and direct assessment methods are available, such as self-reports, inhaler weighing, review of pharmacy records, pill counts, or biological assays (George, Kong, & Stewart, 2007). There is wide variability in how "optimal" adherence is defined and assessed, and there is no gold standard measure for assessing nonadherence among COPD patients.

Self-report measures are often criticized for underreporting and poor reliability, but they are cheap, brief, and easy to administer. They also have the added advantage of identifying potential reasons for nonadherence, particularly when compared with other strategies such as electronic monitoring or biological assays. The use of brief, general adherence questionnaires, such as the Morisky Medication Adherence Scale (Morisky, Ang, Krousel-Wood, & Ward, 2008) or the Beliefs and Behaviour Questionnaire (George, Mackinnon, Kong, & Stewart, 2006), is feasible in primary care settings, and the patient can complete questionnaires in the waiting room (Sanduzzi et al., 2014). Please refer to Chap. 4 and Nguyen, Caze, and Cottrell (2014) for a review of general adherence measures.

Adherence measures have been developed specifically for patients with COPD. For example, the Medication Adherence Rating Scale-COPD (MARS-COPD) adapted from the MARS (Horne, 1996) includes ten statements about inhaler use patterns. The Adherence to Pulmonary Rehabilitation Questionnaire (APRQ; Ayiesah, Leonard, & Chong, 2014) is an 18-item self-report screener that assesses six domains: disease management behavior, perceived treatment benefits, emotion, perceived severity of disease, barriers toward treatment, and coping attitude. Alternatively, Sanduzzi et al. (2014) suggest assessing patient characteristics associated with poor treatment adherence via a brief six-item psycho-socio-economic questionnaire, evaluating number of medications, living situation, and health behaviors and beliefs (psychometric data for this questionnaire are not available).

Detailed Assessment of Adherence

When nonadherence is a concern, a thorough assessment of barriers is crucial to inform intervention efforts. Chart review, clinical interview, administration of questionnaires, or worksheets the patient completes to capture the context of the problematic behavior (e.g., smoking a cigarette), selected to match the presentation of the individual patient, are indicated.

Socioeconomic Factors

Low socioeconomic status (SES) is an independent risk factor for COPD (Grigsby et al., 2016). Low SES also is associated with tobacco smoking at high rates, fewer attempts to quit, and social networks that consist of fellow smokers, thus increasing the risk of secondary exposure (Hitchman et al., 2014). Indicated in the development of COPD, low SES also poses barriers to the management of COPD: Financial difficulties can interfere with medication purchase and attendance of medical services that require a co-payment. Lack of transportation to pulmonary rehabilitation or smoking cessation programs is a concern (Keating, Lee, & Holland, 2011). While the presence of an informal caregiver, who may assist with medication management, transportation, and other instrumental tasks of daily living, may increase adherence (Trivedi, Bryson, Udris, & Au, 2012), living alone predicts poor adherence to pulmonary rehabilitation and the medication regimen (Hayton et al., 2013).

In addition to financial status, the patient's educational level should be considered. Most health information, pamphlets, or brochures require at least a 12th-grade reading level. As about 36% of adults have basic or below-basic health literacy, they are less likely to receive their health information from written materials and tend to use TV or radio broadcasts as their sources. For patients with COPD, poorer health literacy correlates with poorer health status and a greater likelihood of emergency healthcare utilization (Omachi, Sarkar, Yelin, Blanc, & Katz, 2013).

Patient-Related Factors

Age. Individuals older than 65 years of age are at higher risk of poverty and tend to present with comorbid conditions, leading to complex medication regimes. Age is also a risk factor for increased cognitive difficulties (Bourbeau & Bartlett, 2008; George et al., 2007), and cognition can be screened with tools such as the Montreal Cognitive Assessment (MoCA; Nasreddine et al., 2005).

Coping repertoire. Given the difficulties in breathing, withdrawal and disengagement from activities are common yet counterproductive coping strategies. Any patterns that might contribute to sedentary behavior and avoidance of effort should be evaluated. Of note, lack of sleep is associated with increased devaluation of long-term, effortful goals (Libedinsky et al., 2013). Patients with COPD constantly choose between short-term relief (e.g., by sitting down or escaping from physical activities) that makes things worse in the long run and disproportionate effort or discomfort (e.g., related to engaging in physical activity) that will improve their chances of long-term increases in quality of life. Pointing out this circumstance may be important, as many patients—particularly those who have never engaged in systematic physical activity, such as high school sports—may not be in touch with the long-term benefits and instead perceive encouragement and promotion of rehabilitative activities as neglecting or rejecting their difficulties. Correspondingly, a large percentage of patients with COPD indicate that their providers do not acknowledge the negative impact of COPD on their quality of life, and many providers are unequipped to handle their patients' understandable behavioral health concerns (Moreo, Greene, & Sapir, 2016).

It should also be noted that, for some clients, tobacco use may function as a coping mechanism (e.g., it increases vigilance; it allows withdrawal from difficult situations in the form of a "smoke break;" it occasions identification with "strength;" or it facilitates social interactions). To the extent that a patient is participating in smoking cessation, alternative coping and problem-solving strategies should be promoted.

Evaluation of factors related to a patient's choice of short- versus long-term behavioral strategies, such as illness perception, disease attribution, and self-efficacy, can be useful in identifying barriers. In particular, increased illness perception and an internal attribution of the disease are associated with increased disability and lower health-related quality of life (Mewes, Rief, Kenn, Ried, & Stenzel, 2016), while a greater sense of control—measured as higher self-efficacy beliefs—is correlated with adherence to pulmonary rehabilitation and improved functional capacity (Selzler, Rodgers, Berry, & Stickland, 2016).

Mood. When a screener has been positive for depression or anxiety, details of the presentation should be assessed carefully. Anxiety and depression more frequently accompany COPD than other chronic diseases and are associated with worse prognosis, but the relationship among depression, anxiety, and COPD is not clear. There is some evidence that the withdrawal, disengagement, and avoidance behaviors that characterize depression and anxiety might be direct sequelae of chronic hypoxia and inflammation secondary to COPD (Kent et al., 2011). Changing social roles related to a narrowing range of activities may also contribute to depression. Depressed behavior may result in a less active lifestyle and more physical deterioration, yet severity of impairment and decreased quality of life predict depression, and mood symptoms correlate with reduced adherence to COPD management (Turan, Yemez, & Itil, 2014), disease progression, and healthcare utilization (Maurer et al., 2008). Assessment should be ongoing, as worsening of the condition as well as treatment (e.g., pulmonary rehabilitation) might increase reported symptoms and the likelihood of nonadherence. Using data from the National Comorbidity Survey Replication, Goodwin (2011) suggested a link between COPD, suicidal ideation, and suicide attempts. For a proactive problem-solving approach to assessment of suicidality, directly leading to intervention, see Chiles and Strosahl (2005).

Unique to COPD, pulmonary rehabilitation includes exercise regimens that can be associated with short-term breathing difficulties. For this reason, anxiety—often overlapping with symptoms of panic and particularly related to physical movement and exercise—should be evaluated for potential intervention. Individuals with COPD might be at increased risk of developing panic disorders (Pumar et al., 2014), due to potential misinterpretation of physiological changes (e.g., seeing them as more dangerous and harmful than indicated), associated with a history of potential traumatic events (e.g., severe dyspnea during exacerbation) and hyperventilation (e.g., breathing more than actual need). Of note, many of the medications used to alleviate inflammation or airway obstruction can have anxiogenic effects and thus, paradoxically, may contribute to anxiety that might interfere with adherence or predispose patients to panic.

Disease-Related Factors

COPD as a progressive, chronic condition with periods of improvements and exacerbations has been found to lead to changes in disease management depending on the severity of current symptoms (George, Kong, Thoman, & Stewart, 2005). Some patients are likely to stop adhering to treatment when they have reduced symptoms, yet—as noted above—greater functional impairments are also associated with reduced adherence. Assessment of disease-related factors should include the patient's perceptions of his or her disease progression and specific reactions to symptom changes.

Therapy-Related Factors

COPD is a heterogeneous disease with complex sequelae, and many patients demonstrate a profound lack of knowledge about the overall purpose and goals of their treatment regimens (Sanduzzi et al., 2014). Routine assessment of patient's perception of his or her treatment regimen and success is recommended. As noted above, patients often report a lack of perceived benefits as a reason for discontinuation of treatment (Keating et al., 2011). Because improvement only occurs in the long term and may be slow, monitoring techniques and graphic displays of personalized data (e.g., duration of walking, achieved distance) may aid patients in detecting small, incremental change.

Adherence to medication is greatly influenced by regimen complexity (e.g., number of medications, dosage, administrations per day) and improper use of inhalers. Assessment of patient medication knowledge and ability to manage multiple medications should also include observations of proper inhaler use. Additional factors influencing nonadherence to home oxygen therapy may be portability and related lifestyle restrictions and associated stigma (Cullen, 2006).

Healthcare Systems or Provider-Related Factors

Lack of trust in the provider and poor communication between the provider and patient have been found to increase nonadherence to treatment (Bourbeau & Bartlett, 2008). Making room for patient concerns regarding interactions with providers—including the behavioral health specialist—and assessing patient preferences in designing an individualized care plan are important. Table 11.1 provides an overview of relevant factors, sample interview questions, as well as assessment tools.

Table 11.1 Assessing for barriers to COPD adherence

Factors	Sample clinical interview questions	Assessment tools
Socioeconomic	What could get in the way of filling your prescription at the pharmacy? How do you plan to get to and from rehab? What does your living situation look like?	Demographic Questionnaire (e.g., income, household composition, relationship status)
Patient-related	*Cognition and executive functioning*	
	Do you ever have difficulty remembering to take your medication/attend your appointments?	The Montreal Cognitive Assessment (MoCA)[a]
	Coping style	
	What do you usually do when you experience breathing difficulties?	Brief COPE[b]
	Smoking Are you currently smoking? How many cigarettes do you smoke in a day? Have you ever considered quitting smoking? On a scale from 1 to 10, how ready are you to quit smoking?	
	Self-efficacy	
	How confident do you feel in managing your COPD? Do you feel like your health behaviors can affect the progression of COPD?	COPD Self-Efficacy Scale (CSES)[c]
	Depression and anxiety	
	What changes have you seen in your mood? How has your mood been lately? Have you been feeling more down? How often do you feel worried or stressed? Have you ever had thoughts of harming yourself or ending your life? What goes through your mind when you have trouble catching your breath? How do you feel when you are having trouble getting enough air?	Primary Care Evaluation of Mental Disorders (PRIME-MD)[d]; Beck Depression Inventory-II (BDI)-II[e]; Beck Anxiety Inventory (BAI)[f]; Hospital Anxiety and Depression Scale (HADS)[g]; Center for Epidemiologic Studies Depression Scale (CESD)[h]; Geriatric Depression Scale[i]
Disease-related	In what way is COPD interfering with your life? Have you ever stopped taking your medication when you feel better?	Brief Illness Perception Questionnaire[j]; St George's Respiratory Questionnaire (SGRQ)[k]

(continued)

Table 11.1 (continued)

Factors	Sample clinical interview questions	Assessment tools
Treatment-related	*Treatment knowledge and complexity*	
	How many medications are you currently taking? How many times a day do you take your medications? Do ever experience difficulties keeping track of your medications? How many doctors/pharmacists are you seeing to manage your health conditions? Do you ever have too much going on to attend your PR program? Could you show me how you use your inhaler? What is the purpose of each of the medications you are currently taking?	Morisky Medication Adherence Scale (MMAS-8)[l]; MARS-COPD[m]; Bristol COPD Knowledge Questionnaire[n] ; Adherence to Pulmonary Rehabilitation Questionnaire (APRQ)[o]
	Treatment perception	
	Do you think your [symptoms] are improving upon taking your medication/attending PR?	Beliefs about Medicine[p]
Provider-related	On a scale from 1 to 10 – How effective is your provider in helping you manage your COPD? – How much are you involved in making decisions about your treatment? – How much do you feel your provider listens to you and addresses your concerns?	Patient-Doctor Relationship Questionnaire (PDRQ-9)[q]

Note:
[a]Nasreddine et al. (2005)
[b]Carver (1997)
[c]Wigal, Creer, and Kotses (1991)
[d]Spitzer, Kroenke, and Williams (1999)
[e]Beck, Steer, and Brown (1996)
[f]Beck and Steer (1993)
[g]Zigmond and Snaith (1983)
[h]Radloff (1977)
[i]Yesavage et al. (1983)
[j]Broadbent, Petrie, Main, and Weinman (2006)
[k]Jones, Quirk, and Baveystock (1991)
[l]Morisky et al. (2008)
[m]Horne (1996)
[n]White, Walker, Roberts, Kalisky, and White (2006)
[o]Ayiesah et al. (2014)
[p]Horne, Weinman, and Hankins (1999)
[q]Van der Feltz-Cornelis, Van Oppen, Van Marwijk, De Beurs, and Van Dyck (2004)

Evidence-Based Stepped Care/Brief Psychotherapy

Once barriers to adherence have been identified, brief interventions can be employed to increase adherence to all aspects of COPD treatment (smoking cessation, pulmonary rehabilitation, pharmacological treatment) to slow or prevent disease progression. A stepped-care approach allows providers and patients to identify individualized interventions for each patient by starting with the least intrusive, most effective intervention. If a patient does not benefit from one level of care, interventions of increasing intensity are offered. Approaches in primary care may include education, motivational interviewing, problem-solving, skills building, and relapse prevention techniques as indicated (for a description of these techniques applied to adherence, please consult O'Donohue & Levensky, 2006). In some cases, cognitive-behavioral therapy for anxiety or depression may be necessary to promote active engagement with treatment regimens. Of note, while evidence supports particular intervention packages to manage COPD, such as pulmonary rehabilitation, strategies that increase adherence specific to COPD remain to be studied systematically.

Step 1: Psychoeducation and Self-Management

COPD requires a complex treatment regimen including smoking cessation, self-management, pulmonary rehabilitation, and pharmacological treatment. "Adherence," that is, the behavior change that is required from the patient within the collaborative plan of care, is viewed as a process toward a common goal rather than an either-or, all-or-none outcome. To orient patients to all aspects of treatment, psychoeducation is the first step: Knowledge about COPD, its progression, recommended behavior and lifestyle changes, and treatment components helps patients view COPD as an intervenable condition, establishing motivation and a sense of control as a basis for managing the disease.

Patients with high levels of self-efficacy and few barriers will benefit from self-management. Benefits of self-management include better quality of life, early detection of exacerbations, and reductions in hospitalizations and emergency department visits (Koff, Jones, Cashman, Voelkel, & Vandivier, 2009; Rice et al., 2010; Zwerink et al., 2014). Implementation of self-management strategies relies on a collaborative care team that includes the patient and his or her family. According to self-regulatory models, patients are expected to commit to long-term outcomes, schedule and implement activities that will support their respective long-term goals, monitor these activities, evaluate their progress, identify barriers and facilitators, and use self-generated feedback to correct their strategies and make them more effective (Kanfer, 1975). Self-management in COPD presents a mix of approaches that commonly include disease knowledge, medication and nutrition advice, inhaler techniques, pacing of activities ("energy conservation"), structured exercise, breathing techniques, action planning for exacerbations, smoking cessation support, relaxation training, and stress management (Jolly et al., 2016) in group or individual settings. The COPD Breathlessness Manual (Howard & Dupont, 2014) is an example of one of the guides available to promote self-management in primary care. Other materials are listed in Patient Resources.

Step 2: Motivational Interviewing

Motivational interviewing is indicated when commitment to health behavior change is lacking (see Rollnick et al., 2007). It provides a tool to reassess barriers and slowly shape the patient's verbal commitment to taking actions in the service of his or her health. While motivational interviewing can be used to address all aspects of treatment, smoking cessation is used as an example here. As the greatest risk factor for COPD, smoking cessation should be the primary target of intervention, but many individuals with COPD continue smoking. In general, patients with COPD tend to have higher levels of nicotine dependence, a longer pack-per-day history of smoking, distinguishing inhalation patterns, higher levels of depression, and a decreased sense of control over smoking when compared with smokers without COPD (van Eerd, van der Meer, van Schayck, & Kotz, 2016). While motivational interviewing interventions are conducted by the behavioral health specialist, medical staff should have at least some knowledge and training in the basics of motivational interviewing, to prevent an approach to behavior change that could be construed as patronizing or chiding. Instead, motivational interviewing promotes nonjudgmental assessment of the patient's readiness to quit and a constructive and collaborative exploration of ambivalence, normalizing it and using it as a starting point to shape a strong commitment for smoking cessation. Providers should be aware that long-term adherence to smoking cessation programs is generally low (10–30%), and multiple attempts to quit are common. Thus, medical providers should not give up change attempts but assess for smoking cessation regularly, providing steady encouragement.

Step 3: Skills Building and Relapse Prevention Techniques

General issues. When commitment to change is present, patients may need to learn new skills (e.g., interpersonal skills, to address social situations that could sabotage gains; distress tolerance skills to manage cravings; problem-solving skills to access transportation or solve other instrumental problems). Techniques and strategies are available in O'Donohue & Fisher (2008).

Behavioral health providers can communicate that health behavior change truly matters by providing additional support: They may facilitate action plans in session and provide monthly follow-up calls to assess progress, addressing barriers and reinforcing facilitators (Rice et al., 2010). Computer and mobile technologies also promote self-management in the short term, but to date it is unclear whether engagement with technology is sustained over time (McCabe, McCann, & Brady, 2017). Thus, behavioral health specialists play an important role in the assessment of individual barriers to adherence, followed by targeted problem-solving, solicitation of additional resources (e.g., for transportation or caregiving activities), or skills building.

Smoking cessation. High-intensity behavioral support in combination with pharmacological intervention appears to increase quit rates among individuals with COPD (van Eerd et al., 2016). Intensive behavioral support includes the self-management components discussed above, particularly facilitation of action planning and development of a treatment plan, promotion of self-monitoring, strategies for weight control, and promotion of social support (Bartlett, Sheeran, & Hawley, 2014). For those individuals who quit, no conclusive data support any one behavioral strategy for relapse prevention (Hajek et al., 2013).

Given that patients with COPD already have compromised health, they may be more likely to discontinue pharmacotherapy or nicotine replacement for smoking cessation when they experience common adverse effects, such as disrupted sleep and gastrointestinal discomfort, including vomiting, diarrhea or constipation, dry mouth, headache, joint aches, sore throat, blurred vision, or dizziness. Such barriers should be acknowledged, and open dialogue with the prescribing provider should be encouraged—and, if necessary, practiced in a role play—to explore alternatives.

Medication management. The prerequisite skills to manage complex regimens should never be assumed. Pharmacological interventions in COPD include oral medications and inhalers or a combination thereof. Approaches to increasing medication adherence should include simplifying the treatment regimen by reducing doses and selecting the inhaler with which the patient is most comfortable. To emphasize, because patients may have very complex medication regimens and thus have an increased risk of adverse drug effects, monitoring of potential adverse effects and promoting an open dialogue with the prescribing physician, as well as potential consultation from a pharmacist, should occur. Education and hands-on training related to home oxygen, medication, and inhaler use should be provided and proper use monitored (Bryant et al., 2013; Cullen, 2006). Patients can practice inhaler use in session, with direct feedback from the provider. Patients' perception of oxygen use, stigma, and the potential social or instrumental consequences of such use on activities of daily living should be addressed.

Behavioral support with regard to pharmacological interventions should cover the patient's organization of her complex medication regimen, reminders, memory aids, or electronic options. If significant cognitive difficulties with organization, planning, or generally the performance of instrumental activities of daily living are present, caregiver support is indicated.

Step 4: Brief Cognitive-Behavioral Interventions

Behavioral health providers can improve adherence to COPD management by intervening on comorbid mood problems. Depression and anxiety are related to decreased self-management and adherence to pulmonary rehabilitation. Pulmonary rehabilitation is one of the most effective interventions for COPD management and increases health-related quality of life and exercise capacity, relieves dyspnea and fatigue, and improves emotional functioning and self-efficacy (McCarthy et al., 2015). As one of pulmonary rehabilitation's main components, endurance training can induce breathing difficulties with correlated anxiety, which often leads to further exercise avoidance. Brief anxiety reduction techniques (such as relaxation training or guided imagery) and breathing exercises may increase adherence to pulmonary rehabilitation and help clients better cope with exacerbations. Pursed lip breathing and diaphragmatic breathing can be practiced with the client in session (see Patient Resources, COPD Management, for information). Acceptance-based strategies (see O'Donohue & Fisher, 2008) may be helpful, too. Because participation in comprehensive pulmonary rehabilitation has been shown to decrease anxiety and depression (Coventry & Hind, 2007), educating patients about the bidirectional relationship of COPD with depression and anxiety is important to prevent a further narrowing of the range of activities.

Treatments follow standard protocols for brief evidence-based therapies in primary care. Generally, in consultation with the pulmonary rehabilitation team, behavior health specialists should emphasize pacing, carefully shaping increased endurance over time, and monitoring patient progress which may be slow.

When interoceptive exposure or distress tolerance-based techniques are used to reduce anxiety or panic, close collaboration with the medical provider is recommended. Barrera, Grubbs, Kunik, and Teng (2014) listed the contraindicators for interoceptive exposure as pulmonary hypertension with dizziness or fainting, severe and unmanaged congestive heart failure, bone instability due to malignancy, severe fatigue, and stage 4 COPD. Of note, severe dyspnea and panic do not disqualify patients from participating.

Step 5: Medication, Consultation, and Referral

Pharmacological interventions are also indicated to improve adherence. Evidence-based strategies for smoking cessation include pharmacological interventions such as the antidepressant bupropion (Hughes, Stead, Hartmann-Boyce, Cahill, & Lancaster, 2014). Patients may also receive psychotropics for severe depression. Given the usually large medication load of patients with COPD, careful monitoring for sedation or respiratory depression and other side effects or interactions should be initiated, as noted above (Tselebis et al., 2016).

When individuals are on multiple medications, consultation with a pharmacist, specialized in geriatric pharmacology if indicated, may be necessary. Concerns about a decline in organizational skills and difficulties performing stepwise tasks can be addressed through referral to occupational therapists who provide skills-based support to patients and their care partners for effective medication management.

Patients with preexisting and long-standing mental health problems that interfere with adherence or patients who do not adhere to brief primary care interventions for tobacco or other substance use, anxiety, or depression should be referred to specialized psychologists for more intensive or longer-term evidence-based interventions.

What Does Not Work

Delivering COPD education didactically, rather than within an active back-and-forth interaction with the patient, is not recommended. Instead, the self-management strategies discussed earlier should be implemented, preceded by motivational interviewing if a patient is reluctant to engage in treatment. However, motivational interviewing is contraindicated if a patient with COPD is already motivated to begin a smoking cessation program (Bartlett et al., 2014). Bartlett and her colleagues also suggest that the assessment of nicotine dependence might be counterproductive when attempting to engage patients in smoking cessation.

While cognitive behavioral therapy (CBT) for chronic diseases can be adapted to address anxiety, including panic disorder, and depression that accompany COPD, potential pharmacological interventions may have to be altered specifically for COPD: Specifically, recent population-based retrospective studies have raised questions regarding the use of benzodiazepines for insomnia, depression, anxiety, or dyspnea when patients with COPD are older, suggesting a significantly increased risk of serious adverse respiratory events (Vozoris et al., 2014).

Current evidence for non-pharmacological approaches, including CBT, to treat anxiety specifically coexisting with COPD is promising but not conclusive due to small sample sizes and heterogeneity of analytic strategies (Usmani et al., 2017). While breathing exercises improve exercise tolerance, they do not alleviate dyspnea or increase health-related quality of life. Thus, breathing exercises may be part of the behavioral management for adherence to rehabilitation programming but not integral to medical management of COPD (Holland, Hill, Jones, & McDonald, 2012).

Lastly, while the evidence supports both pulmonary rehabilitation and self-management in COPD, the active ingredients of these comprehensive approaches are largely unexamined (Jolly et al., 2016; McCarthy et al., 2015; Zwerink et al., 2014).

When to Refer to Specialty Treatment

Enhancing quality of care for patients with COPD will require primary care providers to obtain knowledge of pulmonary rehabilitation as well as other treatment recommendations (see above). In addition to the referral to pulmonary rehabilitation services, the primary care team directs patients to other available resources and support services (see Patient Resources), provides referrals to mental healthcare and pulmonary specialists, and coordinates care. Referrals to specialty providers are recommended if the onset of COPD is before the age of 40, the patient is experiencing frequent exacerbation or shows rapid decline despite optimal treatment, and there is a family history of alpha-1 antitrypsin deficiency, with onset of comorbid medical conditions and a need for long-term oxygen therapy or surgery (Bellamy & Smith, 2007).

Behavioral health specialists have the advantage of addressing barriers that can interfere with implementation of treatment and improve outcomes in conjunction with the medical team. Referral to specialized mental health is indicated when a history of emotional, behavioral, or cognitive difficulties is exacerbated by or reemerges with chronic disease, when the patient does not benefit from brief treatment and problems require more intensive intervention, or when the patient has concerns that are not amenable to treatment in medical settings (e.g., couples therapy).

The Role of the Primary Care Team

As the first contact, the primary care team plays an important role in COPD management and referral to appropriate services (Vogelmeier et al., 2017). As noted above, targets include spirometric diagnosis of COPD, reduction of exposure including smoking cessation, non-pharmacological interventions (e.g., education, nutrition, and exercise), medication regimens and influenza and pneumococcal vaccinations, and early recognition of acute exacerbations (Vogelmeier et al., 2017).

It is the responsibility of healthcare professionals and care teams to attend continuing education workshops and seminars that focus on evidence-based guidelines. Because of the far-ranging consequences of COPD and the complexity of the treatment regimen, the primary care team should expect barriers to adherence. Team knowledge of motivational interviewing techniques is useful when addressing barriers: Rather than labeling the patient's behavior as "resistant," nonadherence can be understood in the context of the factors noted above. Listening and communication skills that demonstrate understanding and compassion about the effects of COPD can increase patient openness to active problem-solving and promote more accurate reporting of barriers (Moreo et al., 2016). The patient ideally has an active role in treatment decisions and implementation thereof, to allow for stepwise yet lasting health behavior change and setting achievable goals.

Assessing Impact

Suggested outcome measures directly related to the quality of COPD management are regular assessment of symptoms—including spirometry testing and evaluation of anxiety and depression as noted above, tobacco cessation intervention, oxygen saturation assessment, bronchodilator therapy, periodic arterial blood gas measurement, oxygen therapy, and influenza and pneumococcal immunization (O'Donoghue et al., 2006).

From the health behavior specialist's perspective, quality improvement related to adherence to COPD management includes documenting regular assessment and interventions to support self-management; to promote smoking cessation; to remove barriers to care (including anxiety and depression); to increase access to resources, potentially involving caregivers in all aspects of treatment; and to track patient outcome systematically.

Patient Resources

Organizations

- American Lung Association (http://www.lung.org/)
- COPD Foundation (https://www.copdfoundation.org/)
- American Association for Respiratory Care (http://www.aarc.org/)
- National Heart, Lung, and Blood Institute (https://www.nhlbi.nih.gov/health/educational/copd/index.htm)
- National Emphysema Foundation (http://www.emphysemafoundation.org)

COPD Management Resources

- https://www.copdfoundation.org/What-is-COPD/Living-with-COPD/Breathing-Techniques.aspx
- https://www.lung.ca/lung-health/lung-disease/chronic-obstructive-pulmonary-disease-copd/resources includes PDFs for a COPD BreathWorks Plan, pulmonary rehabilitation, and self-management guides.
- COPD Learn More Breathe Better Program
- (https://www.nhlbi.nih.gov/health/educational/copd/lmbb-campaign/index.htm).
- How to Use Inhalers website (http://use-nhalers.com) provides instructions on the use of a wide range of inhalers and may be a useful site for patients or to have available in the office.
- COPD Foundation. Educational video series—for patients and caregivers: COPD 101. Available at http://www.copdfoundation.org/Learn-More/For-Patients-Caregivers/Educational-Video-Series/COPD-101.aspx.

Support Groups

- Lung HelpLine and Tobacco QuitLine 1-800-LUNGUSA.
- Better Breathers Club (http://www.lung.org/support-and-community/better-breathers-club/); call 1-800-LUNGUSA to find a club near you.
- Online support communities:
  - Living with COPD Support Community (https://www.inspire.com/groups/american-lung-association-copd/)
  - Living with Lung Disease Support Community (https://www.inspire.com/groups/american-lung-association-lung-disease/)
  - Freedom from Smoking Community (http://www.lung.org/support-and-community/online-support-communities/join-freedom-from-smoking.html)

– Drive4COPD: 1-866-316-COPD (2673) (http://www.drive4copd.org/)

Financial Assistance

- RXAssist: Help your patients obtain free or low-cost medications and learn more about safety net programs for the uninsured (http://www.rxassist.org/).
- Partnership for Prescription Assistance (http://www.pparx.org/).
- Patient Advocate Foundation: Co-Pay Relief (http://www.copays.org/).
- Patient Access Network Foundation: 1-866-316-PANF (7263) (http://www.panfoundation.org/).

Resources for Caregivers

- Caregiving Support Community (http://www.lung.org/support-and-community/caregiving-support-community/)
- Caregiver Support Community (http://www.copd.com/support/caregiver-support.html)
- Lotsa Helping Hands (http://lung.lotsahelpinghands.com/caregiving/home/)
- National Alliance for Caregiving (http://www.caregiving.org/)

Statistics/Facts

- Centers for Disease Control and Prevention: Chronic Obstructive Pulmonary Disease (COPD) (http://www.cdc.gov/copd/index.html)
- World Health Organization: Chronic Obstructive Pulmonary Disease (COPD) (http://www.who.int/mediacentre/factsheets/fs315/en/)

References

Ayiesah, R., Leonard, J. H., & Chong, C. Y. (2014). Development and validation of non-adherence to pulmonary rehabilitation questionnaire: A clinical tool for patients with chronic obstructive pulmonary diseases. *La Clinica Terapeutica, 165*(3), 123–128. https://doi.org/10.7417/CT.2014.1708

Barrera, T. L., Grubbs, K. M., Kunik, M. E., & Teng, E. J. (2014). A review of cognitive behavioral therapy for panic disorder in patients with chronic obstructive pulmonary disease: The rationale for interoceptive exposure. *Journal of Clinical Psychology in Medical Settings, 21*(2), 144–154. https://doi.org/10.1007/s10880-014-9393-4

Bartlett, Y. K., Sheeran, P., & Hawley, M. S. (2014). Effective behaviour change techniques in smoking cessation interventions for people with chronic obstructive pulmonary disease: A meta-analysis. *British Journal of Health Psychology, 19*(1), 181–203. https://doi.org/10.1111/bjhp.12071

Beck, A. T., & Steer, R. A. (1993). *Beck anxiety inventory manual*. San Antonio, TX: Psychological Corporation.

Beck, A. T., Steer, R. A., & Brown, G. K. (1996). *Manual for the Beck depression inventory-II*. San Antonio, TX: Psychological Corporation.

Bellamy, D., & Smith, J. (2007). Role of primary care in early diagnosis and effective management of COPD. *International Journal of Clinical Practice, 61*(8), 1380–1389. https://doi.org/10.1111/j.1742-1241.2007.01447.x

Bourbeau, J., & Bartlett, S. J. (2008). Patient adherence in COPD. *Thorax, 63*(9), 831–838. https://doi.org/10.1136/thx.2007.086041

Broadbent, E., Petrie, K. J., Main, J., & Weinman, J. (2006). The brief illness perception questionnaire. *Journal of Psychosomatic Research, 60*(6), 631–637. https://doi.org/10.1016/j.jpsychores.2005.10.020

Bryant, J., McDonald, V. M., Boyes, A., Sanson-Fisher, R., Paul, C., & Melville, J. (2013). Improving medication adherence in chronic obstructive pulmonary disease: A systematic review. *Respiratory Research, 14*(1), 109. https://doi.org/10.1186/1465-9921-14-109

Burgess, A., Kunik, M. E., & Stanley, M. A. (2005). Chronic obstructive pulmonary disease: Assessing and treating psychological issues in patients with COPD. *Geriatrics, 60*, 18.

Carver, C. S. (1997). You want to measure coping but your protocol's too long: Consider the brief COPE. *International Journal of Behavioral Medicine, 4*, 92–100. https://doi.org/10.1207/s15327558ijbm0401_6

Chiles, J. A., & Strosahl, K. D. (2005). *Clinical manual for assessment and treatment of suicidal patients*. Arlington, VA: American Psychiatric Publishing.

Coventry, P. A., & Hind, D. (2007). Comprehensive pulmonary rehabilitation for anxiety and depression in adults with chronic obstructive pulmonary disease: Systematic review and meta-analysis. *Journal of Psychosomatic Research, 63*(5), 551–565. https://doi.org/10.1016/j.jpsychores.2007.08.002

Cullen, D. L. (2006). Long term oxygen therapy adherence and COPD: What we don't know. *Chronic Respiratory Disease, 3*(4), 217–222. https://doi.org/10.1177/1479972306070506

Diaz-Guzman, E., & Mannino, D. M. (2014). Epidemiology and prevalence of chronic obstructive pulmonary disease. *Clinics in Chest Medicine*, *35*(1), 7–16. https://doi.org/10.1016/j.ccm.2013.10.002

George, J., Kong, D. C. M., & Stewart, K. (2007). Adherence to disease management programs in patients with COPD. *International Journal of Chronic Obstructive Pulmonary Disease*, *2*(3), 253–262.

George, J., Kong, D. C. M., Thoman, R., & Stewart, K. (2005). Factors associated with medication nonadherence in patients with COPD. *Chest*, *128*(5), 3198–3204.

George, J., Mackinnon, A., Kong, D. C. M., & Stewart, K. (2006). Development and validation of the Beliefs and Behaviour Questionnaire (BBQ). *Patient Education and Counseling*, *64*(1), 50–60. https://doi.org/10.1016/j.pec.2005.11.010

Goodwin, R. D. (2011). Is COPD associated with suicide behavior? *Journal of Psychiatric Research*, *45*(9), 1269–1271. https://doi.org/10.1016/j.jpsychires.2011.01.014

Grigsby, M., Siddharthan, T., Chowdhury, M. A. H., Siddiquee, A., Rubinstein, A., Sobrino, E., … Checkley, W. (2016). Socioeconomic status and COPD among low- and middle-income countries. *International Journal of Chronic Obstructive Pulmonary Disease*, *11*, 2497–2507. https://doi.org/10.2147/COPD.S111145

Hajek, P., Stead, L. F., West, R., Jarvis, M., Hartmann-Boyce, J., & Lancaster, T. (2013). Relapse prevention interventions for smoking cessation. *Cochrane Database of Systematic Reviews*, (8), CD003999. https://doi.org/10.1002/14651858.CD003999.pub4

Han, M. K., Steenrod, A. W., Bacci, E. D., Leidy, N. K., Mannino, D. M., Thomashow, B. M., … Martinez, F. J. (2015). Identifying patients with undiagnosed COPD in primary care settings: Insight from screening tools and epidemiologic studies. *Chronic Obstructive Pulmonary Diseases*, *2*(2), 103–121. 10.15326/jcopdf.2.2.2014.0152

Hayton, C., Clark, A., Olive, S., Browne, P., Galey, P., Knights, E., … Wilson, A. M. (2013). Barriers to pulmonary rehabilitation: Characteristics that predict patient attendance and adherence. *Respiratory Medicine*, *107*(3), 401–407. https://doi.org/10.1016/j.rmed.2012.11.016

Hitchman, S. C., Fong, G. T., Zanna, M. P., Thrasher, J. F., Chung-Hall, J., & Siahpush, M. (2014). Socioeconomic status and smokers' number of smoking friends: Findings from the International Tobacco Control (ITC) Four Country Survey. *Drug and Alcohol Dependence*, *143*, 158–166. https://doi.org/10.1016/j.drugalcdep.2014.07.019

Holland, A. E., Hill, C. J., Jones, A. Y., & McDonald, C. F. (2012). Breathing exercises for chronic obstructive pulmonary disease. *Cochrane Database of Systematic Reviews*, (10), CD008250. https://doi.org/10.1002/14651858.CD008250.pub2

Horne, R. (1996). *The medication adherence report scale*. Brighton: University of Brighton.

Horne, R., Weinman, J., & Hankins, M. (1999). The beliefs about medicines questionnaire: The development and evaluation of a new method for assessing the cognitive representation of medication. *Psychology & Health*, *14*(1), 1–24. https://doi.org/10.1080/08870449908407311

Howard, C., & Dupont, S. (2014). 'The COPD breathlessness manual': A randomised controlled trial to test a cognitive-behavioural manual versus information booklets on health service use, mood and health status, in patients with chronic obstructive pulmonary disease. *NPJ Primary Care Respiratory Medicine*, *24*, 14076. https://doi.org/10.1038/npjpcrm.2014.76

Hughes, J. R., Stead, L. F., Hartmann-Boyce, J., Cahill, K., & Lancaster, T. (2014). Antidepressants for smoking cessation. *Cochrane Database of Systematic Reviews*, (1), CD000031. https://doi.org/10.1002/14651858.CD000031.pub4

Johnston, K. N., Young, M., Grimmer-Somers, K. A., Antic, R., & Frith, P. A. (2011). Why are some evidence-based care recommendations in chronic obstructive pulmonary disease better implemented than others? Perspectives of medical practitioners. *International Journal of Chronic Obstructive Pulmonary Disease*, *6*, 659–667. https://doi.org/10.2147/COPD.S26581

Jolly, K., Majothi, S., Sitch, A. J., Heneghan, N. R., Riley, R. D., Moore, D. J., … Jordan, R. E. (2016). Self-management of health care behaviors for COPD: A systematic review and meta-analysis. *International Journal of Chronic Obstructive Pulmonary Disease*, *11*, 305–326. https://doi.org/10.2147/COPD.S90812

Jones, P. W., Quirk, F. H., & Baveystock, C. M. (1991). The St George's respiratory questionnaire. *Respiratory Medicine*, *85*, 25–31. https://doi.org/10.1016/S0954-6111(06)80166-6

Kanfer, F. H. (1975). Self-management methods. In F. H. Kanfer & A. P. Goldstein (Eds.), *Helping people change*. New York: Pergamon Press.

Keating, A., Lee, A., & Holland, A. E. (2011). What prevents people with chronic obstructive pulmonary disease from attending pulmonary rehabilitation? A systematic review. *Chronic Respiratory Disease*, *8*(2), 89–99. https://doi.org/10.1177/1479972310393756

Kent, B. D., Mitchell, P. D., & McNicholas, W. T. (2011). Hypoxemia in patients with COPD: Cause, effects, and disease progression. *International Journal of Chronic Obstructive Pulmonary Disease*, *6*, 199–208. https://doi.org/10.2147/COPD.S10611

Koff, P. B., Jones, R. H., Cashman, J. M., Voelkel, N. F., & Vandivier, R. W. (2009). Proactive integrated care improves quality of life in patients with COPD. *European Respiratory Journal*, *33*(5), 1031.

Kruis, A. L., Smidt, N., Assendelft, W. J. J., Gussekloo, J., Boland, M. R. S., Rutten-van Mölken, M., & Chavannes, N. H. (2013). Integrated disease management interventions for patients with chronic obstructive pulmonary disease. *Cochrane Database of Systematic Reviews*, (10), CD009437. https://doi.org/10.1002/14651858.CD009437.pub2

Libedinsky, C., Massar, S. A. A., Ling, A., Chee, W., Huettel, S. A., & Chee, M. W. L. (2013). Sleep deprivation alters effort discounting but not delay discounting of monetary rewards. *Sleep, 36*(6), 899–904. https://doi.org/10.5665/sleep.2720

Maurer, J., Rebbapragada, V., Borson, S., Goldstein, R., Kunik, M. E., Yohannes, A. M., & Hanania, N. A. (2008). Anxiety and depression in COPD: Current understanding, unanswered questions, and research needs. *Chest, 134*(4 Suppl), 43S–56S. https://doi.org/10.1378/chest.08-0342

McCabe, C., McCann, M., & Brady, A. M. (2017). Computer and mobile technology interventions for self-management in chronic obstructive pulmonary disease. *Cochrane Database of Systematic Reviews*, (5), CD011425. https://doi.org/10.1002/14651858.CD011425.pub2

McCarthy, B., Casey, D., Devane, D., Murphy, K., Murphy, E., & Lacasse, Y. (2015). Pulmonary rehabilitation for chronic obstructive pulmonary disease. *Cochrane Database of Systematic Reviews*, (2), CD003793. https://doi.org/10.1002/14651858.CD003793.pub3

Mewes, R., Rief, W., Kenn, K., Ried, J., & Stenzel, N. (2016). Psychological predictors for health-related quality of life and disability in persons with chronic obstructive pulmonary disease (COPD). *Psychology & Health, 31*(4), 470–486. https://doi.org/10.1080/08870446.2015.1111369

Moreo, K., Greene, L., & Sapir, T. (2016). Improving interprofessional and coproductive outcomes of care for patients with chronic obstructive pulmonary disease. *BMJ Quality Improvement Reports, 5*(1). https://doi.org/10.1136/bmjquality.u210329.w4679

Morisky, D. E., Ang, A., Krousel-Wood, M., & Ward, H. J. (2008). Predictive validity of a medication adherence measure in an outpatient setting. *The Journal of Clinical Hypertension, 10*(5), 348–354. https://doi.org/10.1111/j.1751-7176.2008.07572.x

Nasreddine, Z. S., Phillips, N. A., Bedirian, V., Charbonneau, S., Whitehead, V., Collin, I., … Chertkow, H. (2005). The Montreal Cognitive Assessment, MoCA: A brief screening tool for mild cognitive impairment. *Journal of the American Geriatrics Society, 53*(4), 695–699. https://doi.org/10.1111/j.1532-5415.2005.53221.x

Nguyen, T.-M.-U., Caze, A. L., & Cottrell, N. (2014). What are validated self-report adherence scales really measuring? A systematic review. *British Journal of Clinical Pharmacology, 77*(3), 427–445. https://doi.org/10.1111/bcp.12194

O'Donoghue, D. L., Gerbert, D., Herman, L., Larson, L., Léger, M., McNellis, R., … van Dyke, E. (2006). Clinical practice guidelines for managing COPD in a primary care setting. *Journal of the American Academy of Physician Assistants, 19*(8), 24–26.

O'Donohue, W. T., & Fisher, J. E. (2008). *Cognitive behavior therapy: Applying empirically supported techniques in your practice* (2nd ed.). Hoboken, NJ: Wiley.

O'Donohue, W. T., & Levensky, E. R. (Eds.). (2006). *Promoting treatment adherence: A practical handbook for health care providers*. Thousand Oaks, CA: Sage Publishing.

Omachi, T. A., Sarkar, U., Yelin, E. H., Blanc, P. D., & Katz, P. P. (2013). Lower health literacy is associated with poorer health status and outcomes in chronic obstructive pulmonary disease. *Journal of General Internal Medicine, 28*(1), 74–81. https://doi.org/10.1007/s11606-012-2177-3

Postma, D. S., & Rabe, K. F. (2015). The asthma–COPD overlap syndrome. *New England Journal of Medicine, 373*(13), 1241–1249. https://doi.org/10.1056/NEJMra1411863

Pumar, M. I., Gray, C. R., Walsh, J. R., Yang, I. A., Rolls, T. A., & Ward, D. L. (2014). Anxiety and depression—Important psychological comorbidities of COPD. *Journal of Thoracic Disease, 6*(11), 1615–1631. https://doi.org/10.3978/j.issn.2072-1439.2014.09.28

Radloff, L. S. (1977). The CES-D scale: A self-report depression scale for research in the general population. *Applied Psychological Measurement, 1*, 385–401. https://doi.org/10.1177/014662167700100306

Rice, K. L., Dewan, N., Bloomfield, H. E., Grill, J., Schult, T. M., Nelson, D. B., … Niewoehner, D. E. (2010). Disease management program for chronic obstructive pulmonary disease: A randomized controlled trial. *American Journal of Respiratory and Critical Care Medicine, 182*(7), 890–896.

Rollnick, S., Miller, W. R., & Butler, C. C. (2007). *Motivational interviewing in health care: Helping patients change behavior*. New York, NY: The Guilford Press.

Sabaté, E. (2003). *Adherence to long-term therapies: Evidence for action*. Geneva: World Health Organization.

Sanduzzi, A., Balbo, P., Candoli, P., Catapano, G. A., Contini, P., Mattei, A., … Stanziola, A. A. (2014). COPD: Adherence to therapy. *Multidisciplinary Respiratory Medicine, 9*(1), 60. https://doi.org/10.1186/2049-6958-9-60

Selzler, A. M., Rodgers, W. M., Berry, T. R., & Stickland, M. K. (2016). The importance of exercise self-efficacy for clinical outcomes in pulmonary rehabilitation. *Rehabilitation Psychology, 61*(4), 380–388. https://doi.org/10.1037/rep0000106

Sharma, G., Meena, R., Goodwin, J. S., Zhang, W., Kuo, Y.-F., & Duarte, A. G. (2015). Burn injury associated with home oxygen use in patients with chronic obstructive pulmonary disease. *Mayo Clinic Proceedings, 90*(4), 492–499. https://doi.org/10.1016/j.mayocp.2014.12.024

Spitzer, R., Kroenke, K., & Williams, J. B. (1999). Validation and utility of a selfreport version of PRIMEMD: The PHQ primary care study. *The Journal of the American Medical Association, 282*(18), 1737–1744. https://doi.org/10.1001/jama.282.18.1737

Trivedi, R. B., Bryson, C. L., Udris, E., & Au, D. H. (2012). The influence of informal caregivers on adherence in COPD patients. *Annals of Behavioral Medicine*, *44*(1), 66–72. https://doi.org/10.1007/s12160-012-9355-8

Tselebis, A., Pachi, A., Ilias, I., Kosmas, E., Bratis, D., Moussas, G., & Tzanakis, N. (2016). Strategies to improve anxiety and depression in patients with COPD: A mental health perspective. *Neuropsychiatric Disease and Treatment*, *12*, 297–328. https://doi.org/10.2147/NDT.S79354

Turan, O., Yemez, B., & Itil, O. (2014). The effects of anxiety and depression symptoms on treatment adherence in COPD patients. *Primary Health Care Research & Development*, *15*(3), 244–251. https://doi.org/10.1017/S1463423613000169

Usmani, Z. A., Carson, K. V., Heslop, K., Esterman, A. J., De Soyza, A., & Smith, B. J. (2017). Psychological therapies for the treatment of anxiety disorders in chronic obstructive pulmonary disease. *Cochrane Database of Systematic Reviews,* (3), CD010673. https://doi.org/10.1002/14651858.CD010673.pub2

Van der Feltz-Cornelis, C. M., Van Oppen, P., Van Marwijk, H. W., De Beurs, E., & Van Dyck, R. (2004). A patient-doctor relationship questionnaire (PDRQ-9) in primary care: Development and psychometric evaluation. *General Hospital Psychiatry*, *26*(2), 115–120. https://doi.org/10.1016/j.genhosppsych.2003.08.010

van Eerd, E. A. M., van der Meer, R. M., van Schayck, O. C. P., & Kotz, D. (2016). Smoking cessation for people with chronic obstructive pulmonary disease. *Cochrane Database of Systematic Reviews*, (8), CD010744. https://doi.org/10.1002/14651858.CD010744.pub2

Vestbo, J., Agusti, A., Wouters, E. F. M., Bakke, P., Calverley, P. M. A., Celli, B., … Tal-Singer, R. (2014). Should we view chronic obstructive pulmonary disease differently after ECLIPSE? A clinical perspective from the study team. *American Journal of Respiratory and Critical Care Medicine*, *189*(9), 1022–1030.

Vogelmeier, C. F., Criner, G. J., Martinez, F. J., Anzueto, A., Barnes, P. J., Bourbeau, J., … Agusti, A. (2017). Global strategy for the diagnosis, management and prevention of chronic obstructive lung disease 2017 report: GOLD executive summary. *Respirology*, *22*(3), 575–601. https://doi.org/10.1111/resp.13012

Vozoris, N. T., Fischer, H. D., Wang, X., Stephenson, A. L., Gershon, A. S., Gruneir, A., … Rochon, P. A. (2014). Benzodiazepine drug use and adverse respiratory outcomes among older adults with COPD. *European Respiratory Journal*, *44*(2), 332. https://doi.org/10.1183/09031936.00008014

White, R., Walker, P., Roberts, S., Kalisky, S., & White, P. (2006). Bristol COPD Knowledge Questionnaire (BCKQ): Testing what we teach patients about COPD. *Chronic Respiratory Disease*, *3*(3), 123–131. https://doi.org/10.1191/1479972306cd117oa

Wigal, J. K., Creer, T. L., & Kotses, H. (1991). The COPD self-efficacy scale. *Chest*, *99*(5), 1193–1196. https://doi.org/10.1378/chest.99.5.1193

Yesavage, J. A., Brink, T. L., Rose, T. L., Lum, O., Huang, V., Adey, M., & Leirer, V. O. (1983). Development and validation of a geriatric depression screening scale: A preliminary report. *Journal of Psychiatric Research*, *17*(1), 37–49. https://doi.org/10.1016/0022-3956(82)90033-4

Zigmond, A. S., & Snaith, R. P. (1983). The hospital anxiety and depression scale. *Acta Psychiatrica Scandinavica*, *67*(6), 361–370. https://doi.org/10.1111/j.1600-0447.1983.tb09716.x

Zwerink, M., Brusse-Keizer, M., van der Valk, P. D., Zielhuis, G. A., Monninkhof, E. M., van der Palen, J., … Effing, T. (2014). Self management for patients with chronic obstructive pulmonary disease. *Cochrane Database of Systematic Reviews*, (3), CD002990. https://doi.org/10.1002/14651858.CD002990.pub3

Chronic Pain 12

Melanie P. Duckworth, Tony Iezzi, and Gwendolyn C. Carlson

Stepped Care for Chronic Pain in Integrated Care Settings

Pain is experienced by almost everyone at some point over the course of a life. Pain is the most common symptom presentation in the emergency room and primary care physician's office, and pain is now recognized as the fifth vital sign in hospital settings. For most persons, the experience of pain is brief and uncomplicated, with pain remitting fully in the absence of medical intervention, but for a significant proportion of the population, the experience of pain will result in a significant impact and precipitate contact with a healthcare provider. Approximately 56% of the American adult population will have some level of pain within a 3-month sampling period (Nahin, 2015). Pain is also expensive, as denoted by the 2010 total cost estimates (i.e., healthcare cost and work loss productivity) that range from 262 to 300 billion dollars, a cost that is greater than the total annual cost for heart disease, cancer, and diabetes (Gaskin & Richard, 2012).

Because pain has a significant impact on function, quality of life, and emotional status, persistent pain will often require the attention of health providers from different medical and allied health disciplines. In the current era of healthcare, with its emphasis on efficient, integrated case management *and* cost containment, stepped and collaborative case management in integrated care settings is becoming the new standard for management of chronic pain. Stepped care models are designed to optimize the match between identified healthcare needs and the interventions deployed to effectively manage those needs, all while minimizing care costs. In the specific context of chronic pain, the stepped care model maximizes patient-provider interactions by using education and activation during the earliest stages of pain management and providing care management and support from other systems when necessary. The stepped care approach to chronic pain management is consistent with best evidence guidelines for pain, which recommend multidisciplinary care and educational and cognitive behavioral strategies (Gatchel & Okifuji, 2006); empirical support for these guidelines is strong and has been demonstrated and summarized in meta-analytic and systematic reviews (Broderick et al., 2016; Thorn, Cross, & Walker, 2007).

The present chapter will describe the stepped care model of chronic pain in integrated care

M.P. Duckworth, Ph.D. (✉) • G.C. Carlson
Department of Psychology,
University of Nevada, Reno, Reno, NV, USA
e-mail: melanied@unr.edu; gcarlson@unr.edu

T. Iezzi
Behavioural Medicine Service,
London Health Sciences Center,
London, ON, Canada
e-mail: tony.iezzi@lhsc.on.ca

A. Maragakis, W.T. O'Donohue (eds.), *Principle-Based Stepped Care and Brief Psychotherapy for Integrated Care Settings*, https://doi.org/10.1007/978-3-319-70539-2_12

settings. Particular emphasis will be placed on the role of the behavioral health specialist (BHS; usually a psychologist or other mental specialist) in providing stepped care to patients with chronic pain.

Description of Chronic Pain

Despite the significant number of persons presenting to primary care and other healthcare providers for evaluation and management of pain, pain is an experience that patients find difficult to communicate and that care providers find difficult to quantify. According to the International Association for the Study of Pain (IASP), pain is defined as "an unpleasant sensory and emotional experience associated with actual or potential tissue damage, or described in terms of such damage" (Merskey & Bogduk, 1994, p. 210). *Acute pain* is commonly defined as pain that does not last longer than 6 months and that remits when the underlying cause of pain has healed. Pain that persists for longer than 6 months is referred to as *chronic pain* (Merskey & Bogduk, 1994). Although the IASP definitions of acute pain and chronic pain are widely recognized and accepted, the acute and chronic pain label are frequently used to capture pain that persists up to 3 months and longer than 3 months, respectively. In general, medical settings, the BHS usually does not tend to become involved with acute pain management, but in a stepped care model of chronic pain, the BHS can play a significant role in early case management and in reducing the likelihood that pain-related impairment and disability will ensue. Timely provision of care, something that is inherent to the stepped care approach, and cost savings due to increased clinical effectiveness and efficiency are outgrowths of this approach.

Effective Ways to Screen for Chronic Pain in the Primary Care Setting

Pain is one of the most common clinical presentations in primary care settings. Pain symptoms may be experienced consequent to injury, in conjunction with various disease conditions, and in the absence of an identifiable cause. Primary care providers (PCPs) are usually the first professionals to be called upon to evaluate a patient's complaint of pain (Gureje, Simon, & Von Korff, 2001). When evaluating a patient's report of pain, the PCP is tasked with establishing the location, duration, intensity, and quality of the patient's pain symptoms and determining the relation of that pain to physical injuries, disease conditions, and/or health behaviors present in the patient's medical history. Information regarding the parameters of pain is usually obtained via the patient's verbal report and physical examination. In addition to determining the basic parameters of the patient's pain symptoms and evaluating possible causes, the PCP works to determine those treatment-related and nontreatment-related factors that seem to be associated with changes in pain intensity and/or quality (e.g., activity level, level of fatigue, medication, and emotional distress) and to establish an intervention plan aimed at full restoration of health and function.

In the context of acute pain management, the initial pain assessment can serve as the PCP's opportunity to provide psychoeducation aimed at supporting timely recovery of function and lessening the likelihood that an acute experience of pain will transition to a chronic circumstance. Although the BHS is considered to be essential to the management of pain-related psychological distress and distress and dysfunction, the BHS can participate in the assessment of different aspects of pain at any point in the patient's pain experience.

Further Assessment of Chronic Pain in the Face of Positive Screening Results

Because the BHS is particularly knowledgeable of those patient-specific factors that influence the progression from an acute pain circumstance to a chronic pain circumstance, the BHS can facilitate the PCP's efforts to effectively assess and resolve patients' experiences of acute pain. In this context, the BHS provides patients with information regarding the nature of both acute and chronic pain and emphasizes the importance of self-care and self-reliance to a speedy and full recovery. Basic education about the different forms of pain and associated sequelae has been demonstrated to be of benefit (Geneen et al., 2015), and instruction in self-care and self-reliance is considered one of the most basic and helpful interventions that can be provided to pain patients. It is also during the initial stages of pain assessment and management that the BHS can identify and problem-solve around pain coping behaviors (e.g., fear of reinjury, catastrophizing, and pain avoidance) that are among the best predictors of short- and long-term recovery.

Particularly important to the process of recovery from acute pain is the use of evidence-based management of patient expectations regarding the detrimental effects of pain, the course of pain and eventual recovery, and the interventions that are most beneficial to the recovery process. In a 2007 review of studies of whiplash associated disorders, McClune, Burton, and Waddell cited the following messages as having the most potential to reduce the risk of developing chronic pain: serious physical injury is rare; reassurance about good prognosis is important; over-medicalization is detrimental; recovery is improved by early return to normal (pre-pain) activities, self-exercise, and manual therapy; positive attitudes and beliefs are helpful in regaining activity levels; and collars, rest, and negative attitudes and beliefs delay recovery and contribute to chronicity. Such messages should be delivered by the PCP and can be reiterated by the BHS as part of an integrated approach to care delivery.

Evidence-Based Stepped Care and Brief Psychotherapeutic Approaches for Chronic Pain

In the face of the most judicious application of pain intervention strategies and the most articulate communication of recovery information and advice, some patients report continuing pain and impairment weeks after the initial PCP visit. This persistence of pain and impairment may point to the need for an individually tailored pain treatment plan in which specific functional limitations (e.g., difficulties standing, sitting, bending, lifting, etc.) and support needs (e.g., a limited number of phone contacts or visits with the BHS aimed at reinforcing recovery behaviors and managing barriers to such behaviors) are identified and managed. The BHS is perfectly positioned to perform a more detailed analysis of pain-related functional limitations and support needs and to put into effect a pain treatment plan that will result in more optimal outcomes for such patients.

Interventions that are used to managing pain may be placed on a continuum from least intensive/invasive to most intensive/invasive based on a variety of factors, including patient effort required, level of PCP contact required, and cost of the intervention. A stepped care model of healthcare delivery is one in which patients are first provided with less intensive/invasive interventions. More intensive/invasive interventions are employed only in the absence of an adequate treatment response to the least intensive/invasive interventions.

The mainstays of a stepped care model of chronic pain are reassurance, avoiding over-medicalization, and returning early as possible to usual daily activities. It is generally assumed that physician-delivered messages and instructions regarding patient health and health practices are of particular importance to patients and are more likely to be heeded than messages and instructions from others with less medical knowledge and authority. In the face of persisting reports of pain and suffering, the PCP should avoid unqualified statements that indicate that "nothing is physically wrong" with the pain patient. In the absence of positive diagnostic findings that would suggest physical compromise, the PCP might speak to the limitation of current diagnostic technology and reassure the patient that monitoring of symptoms will be continued. The PCP, in particular, also needs to be careful about messages around medication use, especially opioid medication use and overuse and combination of substance use and overuse (e.g., opioid and benzodiazepine). For some patients, the development of a substance abuse problem can become even more impactful than the basic pain condition. Finally, PCP messaging around returning to usual activities of daily functioning is valuable as it results in pain patients reporting pain of shorter duration and intensity, increased lumbar flexion, improved work function, and fewer days absent from work, while prescription for bed rest is associated with slower recovery (Malmivaara et al., 1995).

Different models of stepped care for management of chronic pain have been proposed (Dobscha et al., 2009; Otis, MacDonald, & Dobscha, 2006; Plagge, Lu, Lovejoy, Karl, & Dobscha, 2013). The most effective stepped care approaches to pain management share an emphasis on sequenced intervention that: (1) addresses patients' pain-related worries and concerns about pain, provides psychoeducation aimed at imparting accurate information about the patient's diagnosis, correcting misconceptions about the nature of pain, promoting a return to normal functioning, and discouraging activity avoidance; (2) provides structured support for self-management efforts such as physical exercise and activity engagement; and (3) provides more intensive psychological intervention aimed at addressing clinically significant emotional distress and lifestyle impairment.

Otis, MacDonald, and Dobscha (2006) have forwarded a three-step approach to pain management. In Step 1, intervention strategies are aimed at recognizing and addressing patient concerns about pain and enhancing patient readiness for self-care. Chronic pain patients who benefit most from Step 1 interventions are those who tend to experience less intense pain, rely less on medication, be more active across a variety of lifestyle domains, and experience less intense emotional distress. In Step 2, a more active approach to pain management is undertaken. At this step, the BHS reevaluates the treatment needs of the patient to determine which additional intervention strategies might serve best in maximizing treatment outcome. A variety of interventions are considered, including patient participation in a professional- or peer-led psychoeducational group and or brief individual therapy. Step 3 involves the use of more intensive psychological interventions aimed at managing psychological distress and addressing lifestyle impairments across occupational, interpersonal, and social domains of function. Otis and colleagues suggest that Step 3 is appropriate for patients who have not responded optimally to early interventions and who continue to report significant levels of pain, pain-related disability, and clinically significant emotional distress.

Although empirical examinations of the utility of stepped and integrated approaches to the management of chronic pain are few in number, several studies provide clear support for these approaches. Dobscha et al. (2009) conducted an empirical study of the effectiveness of integrated care for chronic pain patients. With Veterans Health Administration primary care facilities serving as recruitment sites for the study, these researchers randomly assigned 42 PCPs and 401 chronic pain patients served by these clinicians to either an assistance with pain treatment group or a treatment as usual group. The assistance with pain treatment group was structured (1) to provide clinicians with a two-session education program in which feedback and recommendations were provided and specialty care referrals facilitated by the integrated care team and (2) to provide patients with assessment as well as a variety of pain management strategies, all as part of a four-session workshop. The integrated care team was comprised of a full-time psychologist, a case manager, and an internist who was present and available 1 day per week. Clinicians and patients assigned to the treatment as usual group had regular access to the pain clinic and associated services. At 12-month follow-up, assistance with pain treatment group evidenced greater improvements in pain-related disability, pain intensity, and depression and reported greater impressions of positive change than the treatment as usual group. Although no significant group difference in the total number of ambulatory visits was revealed, the average number of physical therapy visits completed by patients in the assistance with pain treatment group was significantly greater than that for patients assigned to the treatment as usual group. These findings attest to the effectiveness of integrated care in improving clinical outcomes experienced by patients. Study findings also suggest that, when evaluating the impact of integrated care on healthcare utilization, a finer discrimination needs to be made between those healthcare visits that pertain to pain symptom management and those healthcare visits that serve to restore function and limit pain-related disability.

In a relatively recent, uncontrolled study of the effectiveness of integrated care in managing comorbid pain and post-traumatic stress disorder experienced by Iraqi and Afghanistan war veterans, Plagge, Lu, Lovejoy, Karl, and Dobscha (2013) determined that integrated care (defined as the provision of eight sessions of behavioral activation by a care team comprised of a primary care provider, psychologist, and physiatrist) was associated with improvement across a host of outcomes, including pain severity, pain interference, quality of life, post-traumatic stress symptoms, depression, and general emotional well-being. Overall, the empirical literature supports the role of the BHS and the effectiveness of collaborative and integrative, multidiscipline approaches to identifying and tailoring empirically supported healthcare services to the needs of patients with chronic conditions. Such approaches result in clinical benefits to patients and professional benefits to healthcare providers.

An integrated care team for chronic pain management embraces a biopsychosocial model of pain and, out of that model, works collaboratively across all phases of the patient's pain condition to manage pain, reduce functional limitations, and maximize outcome (Brown & Folen, 2005). The BHS would be considered essential to efforts aimed at reducing the number and complexity of treatment targets faced by the PCP. The recommendations made by the BHS to the care team are very much a function of the referral question and the assessment procedure required to effectively respond to that referral question. More often than not, assessment in the primary care setting will involve the use of brief screening instruments that confirm the intensity and impact of certain pain-relevant behaviors. Measures of pain intensity include a numeric, verbal, or visual rating scale that provides anchors (e.g., 0 = no pain and 5 = severe pain) to be used by patients in communicating the intensity of pain experienced. Measures of pain-relevant behavior usually assess pain-related changes in functional abilities, pain beliefs and expectations, pain coping styles and strategies, and pain-related changes in psychological distress. Relatively brief and standardized measures of these pain-relevant constructs include the West Haven-Yale Multidimensional Pain Inventory (MPI; Kerns et al., 1985), Medical Outcomes Study Short Form (SF-36; Ware et al., 1993), Pain Disability Index (PDI), Beck Depression Inventory-II (BDI-II; Beck et al., 1996), Beck Anxiety Inventory (BAI; Beck & Steer, 1993), and Coping Strategies Questionnaire (CSQ; Keefe et al., 1990). For a comprehensive and accessible review of both brief and more extensive measures of pain and pain-relevant behaviors, the authors recommend Dansie and Turk's (2013) review of chronic pain assessment processes and instruments.

On occasion, the patient's clinical presentation will require the BHS perform a comprehensive pain assessment, one that relies on both semi-structured interviewing and extensive psychological testing (see Duckworth, Iezzi, & Sewell, 2009 and Iezzi, 2008, for details). Psychological tests document changes in psychological functioning, quality of life, and coping. The aim of the interview and testing is to provide both an ideographic (i.e., within the individual) and nomothetic (i.e., the individual compared to other pain patients) perspective on the chronic pain patient. The information provided by the BHS allows the PCP to more fully appreciate and develop better management strategies that are tailored to the needs of the specific chronic pain patient. In addition, this information may be helpful in making a referral to a psychiatrist for an assessment of more disturbed thinking and need for more aggressive pharmacotherapy (Brown & Folen, 2005). The behavioral specialist also brings to the integrated care setting a sophisticated knowledge of the various demographic, psychological, and social factors to have been found to best predict the persistence of pain and disability. In consort with the PCP efforts, the behavioral healthcare specialist can assist in forecasting the probable course of the chronic pain problem. The ability of the PCP and the BHS to determine the prognosis of a chronic pain patient will assist in determining the patient's future care needs.

When tasked with providing brief, one- to five-session psychological intervention, the BHS has an extensive range of skills with which to treat chronic pain patients. At the most basic level, the BHS can provide reassurance about a number of issues. Perhaps the most common reassurances required by pain patients are those related to pain not being "in the head," which is often a primary concern for pain patients when pain continues for a protracted period. Statements that "normalize" pain patients' emotional reactions to pain and associated sequelae represent another powerful intervention. Early in the course of their recovery, pain patients are often consumed with concerns related to their pain condition and the benefit that can be expected from the healthcare services that are being provided. These concerns can reduce patients' willingness to participate in other pain interventions (e.g., physiotherapy).

In addition to normalizing a patient's pain experience, the BHS must identify and correct patients' maladaptive pain beliefs and expectations and enhance self-efficacy in pain patients, as these can have significant impacts on pain outcome (Jackson, Wang, & Fan, 2014; Jia & Jackson, 2016). This is often accomplished through psychoeducation. It is not uncommon for patients who present to primary care settings to possess misconceptions about their pain and the way in which it should be treated. Providing patients with accurate information about their condition as well as the data supporting or challenging certain pain interventions is a critical component in the treatment of chronic pain. Providing psychoeducation to chronic pain patients has been shown to improve pain symptoms, physical functioning, life satisfaction, and self-efficacy regarding pain management (LeFort, Gray-Donald, Rowat, & Jeans, 1998; McGillion et al., 2008). Patients should be oriented to the distinction between acute and chronic pain as well as the cause of their pain (i.e., tissue damage or nerve damage) and the variety of other factors that can contribute to pain including genetic factors, chronic medical conditions, psychological distress, social isolation, and lifestyle choices (Pozek, Beausang, Baratta, & Viscusi, 2016). By providing patients with information about factors that exacerbate pain, healthcare providers can help patients to implement behavioral changes and increase patients' sense of self-efficacy regardless of what is causing the patient to experience pain.

Helping patients move from using passive coping strategies (e.g., resting in bed for days or catastrophizing) to more active coping strategies (e.g., exercising or increasing the use of coping self-statements) can also be beneficial. The BHS can play an important role in moving the pain patient from a *pain relief* model of treatment to a *pain coping* model. A pain coping model emphasizes pain acceptance. McCracken (1998) defines acceptance of pain as involving responses to pain-related experiences that do not include attempts at pain control or pain avoidance as well as engagement in valued actions and pursuit of personal goals regardless of these experiences. In moving a pain patient away from pain relief and toward pain acceptance, the BHS encourages the patient to reflect on the less than satisfactory outcomes of past pain relief attempts, to assess the loss in quality of life that has been experienced as a function of pain avoidance and the pursuit of pain relief, to entertain the possibility of a life that is lived in the presence of pain, to identify valued actions and roles that define one's life, and to identify those functional and lifestyle adjustments that would be required to live as normal and satisfying a life as possible in the presence of pain. Research suggests that functional outcomes achieved by pain patients who participate in interventions that emphasize valued actions and goal-setting are equal to those achieved in the context of other cognitive-behavioral interventions for pain (Veehof, Oskam, Schreurs, & Bohlmeijer, 2011).

In terms of orienting patients to empirically supported behavioral interventions, healthcare providers can direct chronic pain patients to a variety of resources within a stepped care framework including bibliotherapy, eHealth options, and group interventions. The following sections will describe these triage alternatives for chronic pain patients.

Bibliotherapy for Chronic Pain Patients

Bibliotherapy can be a convenient resource for chronic pain patients, particularly if pain impacts a patient's physical functioning and mobility. Patients can access treatment within their home and complete treatment at a pace that corresponds to their individual level of strength and stamina. In addition to reducing multiple barriers to treatment for chronic pain patients, bibliotherapy has also been shown to be an effective intervention modality for patients suffering from chronic pain. Self-help interventions that adhere to acceptance and commitment therapy (ACT) have been shown to significantly improve quality of life, satisfaction, acceptance, functioning, and decrease pain ratings (Johnston, Foster, Shennan, Starkey, & Johnson, 2010; Thorsell et al., 2011). Other evidenced-based treatment and practices for the management of chronic pain include cognitive behavioral therapy (CBT) and mindfulness-based stress reduction (MBSR; see Sturgeon (2014) for a review of the distinctions between ACT, CBT, and MBSR). Similar to ACT self-help resources, CBT and MBRS protocols had been adapted to book and workbook formats as easily disseminable treatment options for chronic pain patients. Within an integrated care setting, healthcare providers should consider creating a brief summary of each evidence-based treatment approach as well as a list of self-help books corresponding to each approach to distribute to patients. It is important to encourage patients to pursue evidence-based self-help interventions while simultaneously empowering each individual to select the approach that specifically appeals to him/her.

eHealth Options for Chronic Pain Patients

In addition to bibliotherapy, there are a growing number of eHealth options that can address the common barriers to treatment (i.e., limited mobility, strength, and stamina) that self-help books historically addressed for chronic pain patients. eHealth resources can serve to educate patients or take the form of web-based or app-based interventions. Healthcare providers should encourage participants to learn about their condition by visiting research-based websites such as the Centers for Disease Control and Prevention, National Institutes of Health, and Mayo Clinic. Healthcare providers should orient patients to scientifically valid web-based resources to prevent the likelihood of patients obtaining inaccurate or harmful information from non-scientific web-based resources.

Web-based and app-based intervention for chronic pain patients have consisted of both adapted evidenced-based treatments for chronic pain as well as interventions aimed at self-management (Macea, Gajos, Calil, & Fregni, 2010; Ruehlman, Karoly, & Enders, 2012). Self-management interventions aim to provide pain patients with knowledge about their condition as well as strategies they can implement to optimize their physical and psychological functioning in the presence of their chronic pain and the lifestyle changes that have occurred consequent of their pain. Health behavior strategies may include changes to diet, exercise, or sleep, all of which can be tracked with specific mobile apps, allowing patients to set behavior change goals. Lalloo, Jibb, Rivera, Agarwal, and Stinson (2015) conducted a review of self-management apps for pain, identifying hundreds of apps that address pain management in some form. These authors identified CatchMyPain as the only app to have undergone empirical investigation. In attempting to select among the many untested pain management apps, patients should aim to identify those apps that contain intervention components that have proven beneficial in the larger pain intervention context. Lalloo et al. (2015) identified five specific components in pain self-management apps: self-care skills training, education, self-monitoring, social support, and goal setting. Healthcare providers should consider these components when recommending eHealth options to chronic pain patients.

Brief Psychotherapies

In addition to the cognitive-behavioral strategies described above as part of the BHS repertoire of behavior change strategies that can be employed in the management of both acute and chronic pain, other brief psychological interventions have been created and proved effective for the management of chronic pain. Included among the brief psychotherapies that are particularly amenable to pain management in the integrated care context are mindfulness-based interventions and motivational interviewing. Mindfulness-based interventions are being used more frequently for chronic pain (Chiesa & Serretti, 2011). Mindfulness-based interventions have significant nonspecific effects on pain reduction and improvement of emotional distress (Chiesa & Serretti, 2011). Although the standard program formally requires that patients attend weekly, 2-h sessions over a period of 8 weeks, mindfulness-based interventions can be customized to meet the care of patients treated in integrated care settings. In such settings, the BHS will assume the role of a mindfulness coach, with the bulk of mindfulness-based practice being self-guided and occurring outside of the treatment setting.

Motivational interviewing is also being used more extensively in treating chronic pain patients (Alperstein & Sharpe, 2016; Romano & Peters, 2015). Motivational interviewing is a person-centered approach that resolves ambivalence about behavior change by strengthening motivation and commitment to change. It is an ideal intervention for the BHS because of its brevity and cost-effectiveness. It can be administered over the phone or in person. This intervention is best suiting for addressing adherence issues in the management of chronic pain; for example, motivational interviewing can be used to address compliance with physiotherapy, return to work program, behavioral activation program, or medication schedule.

Group Interventions

In addition to the brief individual interventions that have been described, group interventions for chronic pain are available and can prove a cost-saving option for managing the needs of the large number of patients who present for management of pain. The initial aim of a group intervention should be orienting group members to the expectations of the group including: the number of scheduled sessions, the duration of each session, participation during group sessions, completion of homework assignments between sessions, and commitment to maintaining the confidentiality of other group members. The second aim of the group should be to orient patients to the impact of pain on multiple domains of functioning, including physical, occupational, social, and psychological, and the many interactions among these domains of functioning. Understanding these relations is critical to the success of chronic pain patient outcomes (Gatchel, Peng, Peters, Fuchs, & Turk, 2007). Following group orientation and education, consistent with other self-management interventions, group leaders should ask group members to identify treatment goals pertaining to each of the previously described domains of functioning.

Following the establishment of individual goals, group sessions will aim to address the physical variables including pain and physiological arousal, cognitive variables including unhelpful thinking strategies, and affective variables including mood and post-traumatic distress, all of which are associated with chronic pain (Kamper et al., 2012; Valentine, Gerber, Nobles, Shtasel, & Marques, 2016). To address these physiological, cognitive, and affective factors, group sessions should be characterized by the following four intervention modules: activity pacing, pain acceptance, interpersonal skill training, and relaxation techniques. Activity pacing refers to increasing behavior from a very low baseline rate, close to inactivity for some patients, to a consistent, manageable rate. Patients do not engage in excessive rest or excessively strenuous activities each day (Andrews, Strong, & Meredith, 2012). In the context of chronic pain, acceptance refers to "a behavior pattern that occurs with awareness of pain but is not directed at changing pain or otherwise influenced by pain" (p. 91; McCracken, & Vowles, 2006). Through acceptance, patients can focus on developing new coping skills instead of trying to avoid the experience of pain. Due to both the social consequences that often accompany chronic pain and the ongoing need for patients to act as their own healthcare advocates, group leaders should orient group members to assertiveness and communication skills (Cegala, McClure, Marinelli, & Post, 2000). Improved interpersonal functioning can decrease the likelihood of social isolation and conflict. Lastly, due to the physiological arousal associated with pain as well as pain-related psychological, occupational, and social stressors, relaxation training should be an integral part of chronic pain self-management groups. There is a large body of literature which demonstrates the effectiveness of relaxation techniques, including mindfulness and meditation practices, at improving quality of life among chronic pain patients (Chiesa & Serretti, 2011). In summary, an effective self-management group intervention for chronic pain patients must acknowledge and address the multiple domains of functioning that are impacted by the experience of chronic pain.

What Does Not Work

There are a number of patient beliefs, expectations, and coping behaviors and provider beliefs, messages, and recommendations that are considered to exacerbate pain behaviors, delay recovery from acute pain, and possibly contribute to the functional impairment, psychological distress, and disability that so often accompany chronic pain. Included among these less than beneficial patient and provider beliefs and behaviors are the following:

- Patient's unwavering focus on immediate and complete pain relief rather than on some balance between manageable pain and improved function
- Patient's primary use of catastrophizing and other passive pain coping strategies rather than active pain coping strategies
- Patient's overreliance on supportive others to assist with or complete activities that have been made difficult, but not impossible, to achieve in the presence of pain
- Patient's resistance to *paced* engagement in activities and a gradual return to pre-pain or optimal post-pain functioning
- Provider messages suggesting that, in the absence of identifiable pathophysiology, the patient's pain experience is psychological in origin
- Provider commitment to a pain relief model rather than a pain coping model
- Provider messages suggesting that complete pain relief is possible in the presence of certain interventions
- Provider messages that suggest that a return to normal function is best accomplished through rest and activity avoidance
- Provider stance toward the use of pain medications that results in the patient being either over-medicated or under-medicate.
- Provider reluctance to assess and address the impact of pain on major, nonphysical domains of life function, including intrapersonal, interpersonal, occupational, and social-recreational domains of function

Determining When a Referral to External Specialty Mental Health Is Necessary

It is also possible that a patient's report of continuing pain and impairment reflects an entire array of interacting physical, psychological, and social influences. These influences are usually first made evident to the PCP through the patient's report of increasing pain, suffering, disability, *and* emotional distress. Chronic pain is frequently accompanied by distress reactions, including symptoms of anxiety and depression. Again, the BHS is perfectly positioned to assist the PCP in determining the clinical significance of these distress reactions and in facilitating an appropriate referral should psychological symptoms warrant more aggressive pharmacotherapy and/or longer-term, specialized psychological management.

There are certain symptoms and behaviors that would indicate to the PCP that consultation and assistance is in order. In making a determination regarding the clinical import of emotional distress reactions and the need to enlist the assistance of behavioral/mental health specialists, Duckworth, Iezzi, and Sewell (2009) recommend that the following symptoms and behaviors be considered significant and to require psychological consultation: severe physical injury; significant pain or illness behaviors; increasing widespread pain; lack of acceptance of the chronicity of pain; kinesiophobia and fear of reinjury; excessive resistance or lack of compliance with return to work plan; simultaneous use of multiple, uncoordinated treatments; high levels of somatization; excessive medication-seeking behavior and repeated misuse of prescribed medications; passive coping and pain catastrophizing; increase in alcohol and/or illicit substance use/abuse; prominent marital discord; repeated episodes of property destruction and/or physical assault; prominent and multiple systems issue; little or no social support; and increase in severity of depression and suicidal ideations.

The importance of the relationship between pain and psychological variables was made most salient in a seminal literature review conducted by Linton (2000). He identified 37 prospective studies out of a larger group of 913 studies that examined psychological risk factors in back and neck pain. Based on Level A studies (support from two or more good-quality prospective studies), Linton concluded the following (p. 1153):

1. Psychosocial variables are clearly linked to the transition from acute to chronic pain disability.
2. Psychological factors are associated with reported onset of back and neck pain.
3. Psychosocial variables generally have more impact than biomedical or biomechanical factors on back pain disability.
4. Cognitive factors (attitudes, cognitive style, fear avoidance beliefs) are related to the development of pain and disability.
   (a) Passive coping is related to pain and disability.
   (b) Pain cognitions (e.g., catastrophizing) are related to pain and disability.
   (c) Fear-avoidance beliefs are related to pain and disability.
5. Depression, anxiety, distress, and related emotions are related to pain and disability.
6. Self-perceived poor health is related to chronic pain and disability.
7. Psychosocial factors may be used as predictors of the risk for developing long-term pain and disability.

In sum, the relation between pain and psychological variables is incontrovertible. Pain and psychological variables are associated with a cascade of pain-related lifestyle disruptions that move from lost work days to increased financial burden to increased interpersonal and intrapersonal distress. Research suggests that these pain-related lifestyle disruptions are predictive of the long-term recovery and well-being for patients with chronic pain (Duckworth & Iezzi, 2010; Duckworth, Iezzi, & Lewandowski, 2008; Duckworth, Iezzi, & Shearer, 2011).

The Role of the Primary Care Provider and Other Members of the Integrated Care Team in Managing Chronic Pain

In the context of chronic pain management, the PCP is tasked with monitoring, determining the significance of, and when warranted, medically treating any changes in the patient's experience of chronic pain and/or function. The PCP should examine any changes in a patient's experience of pain including intensity, location, and metrics of physical functioning (e.g., range of motion, strength, and stamina). The PCP should inquire about these symptom domains during each healthcare visit, prompting patients to provide a self-report of their experiences and any changes across these various domains. The PCP should meet with chronic pain patients across regular intervals of time, helping patients to appreciate the importance of consistent pain and lifestyle management. When healthcare visits are limited to periods characterized by high pain intensity and distress, patients may begin to conceptualize healthcare visits as a solution to increase pain intensity rather than a care regimen to improve their overall functioning. In the chronic pain context, the PCP is called upon to be particularly sophisticated in ensuring that pain medications are not being underprescribed or overprescribed but are being prescribed in an amount that facilitates functioning (for a full review of opioid prescribing practices, see Manchikanti et al., 2012).

The PCP is also responsible for coordinating the efforts of the other healthcare providers who are part of the patient's integrated care team. Nurses, physiotherapists, occupational therapists, chiropractors, and massage therapists are examples of other healthcare providers (HCPs) who are often part of the integrated care team and who actively contribute to the care of chronic pain patients. In addition to emphasizing the integration of the different treatments available through these HCPs, it is essential that there be routine evaluation of the usefulness of these treatments in reducing pain intensity and interference and improving physical function across those life domains that are most relevant to the patient's quality of life. As a member of the integrated healthcare team, the BHS can facilitate the patient experience of gains across all these functional domains. The BHS is uniquely skilled in identifying and managing barriers to treatment adherence as they occur at the level of the patient (e.g., motivation for treatment, knowledge of and expectations related to possible benefits and harms associated with treatment, presence of other physical or mental health problems) and at the level of the care environment (e.g., PCP knowledge and expertise in managing chronic pain, office scheduling, travel requirements to access care services, and cost of treatment and reimbursement issues; Glajchen, 2001).

Assessing the Impact of Care and Ensuring Quality Improvement

In order to reliably evaluate the effectiveness of care provided to chronic pain patients, assessment must be conducted in a systematic manner, with assessment occurring during the initial contact with the patient, in specific intervals of time during the course of treatment (i.e., 1-month to 6-week intervals, and during the final contact with the patient). This allows the PCP or BHS to observe changes in patient presentation over the course of treatment. Pain parameter assessment should consist of patient self-report as well as physical examination. In addition to pain parameters, systematic assessment should be conducted around the previously discussed factors that seem to be associated with changes in pain intensity and/or quality (i.e., activity level, level of fatigue, medication, and emotional distress). Through a comprehensive and systematic assessment approach, PCPs and BHSs can observe patients' progress and the degree to which these multiple presenting problems interact over the course of treatment.

Another mechanism for examining the impact of care involves the evaluation of healthcare utilization. In this context, it is typically the case that healthcare visits and healthcare costs are used as indices of improved patient outcomes. We would suggest that a finer analysis of healthcare utilization be performed, one that evaluates the exact services that are being sought and one that compares visits that are about pain symptom management (e.g., medication assessment) to those that reflect patients' efforts to improve function (e.g., physical therapy rehabilitation and behavioral health services). Additionally, consistent with the systematic assessment of pain parameters and related factors, an equally important strategy to improve the quality of care is the systematic assessment of patient satisfaction. Patient satisfaction assessment should aim to gather information about treatment strategies that patients found to be helpful as well as the treatment strategies patients found to be unhelpful, with members of the integrated healthcare team analyzing patient satisfaction data and making changes based on their feedback.

While it is important to consider patient feedback, it is also important to assess the PCPs' level of satisfaction with the approach to treating chronic pain implemented within the integrated care setting. PCP satisfaction assessment should aim to gather information about the following: knowledge, skills, and perceptions of the BHS, specifically the BHS's ability to provide direct patient care and the manner in which treatment is being implemented. Consistent with patient satisfaction data, PCP satisfaction data should be analyzed, shared with members of the integrated healthcare team, and changes should be implemented based on this feedback. It is important to note that data from one quality care improvement strategy should not be examined in isolation nor should changes be implemented without considering the data from other quality care improvement strategies. In summary, to effectively improve the quality of care for chronic pain patients in an integrated care setting, we recommend that all of the following information be considered: patient treatment outcomes, patient healthcare utilization, patient satisfaction, and provider satisfaction.

Conclusions

An integrated care effort between the PCP and BHS is absolutely essential to the process of ensuring the optimal management of patients with chronic pain. In trying to reduce the likelihood that injured persons will develop chronic pain, the PCP, in conjunction with the behavioral health specialist, presents an optimistic picture of recovery, encourages the pursuit of normal activities, discourages rest and activity avoidance, and normalizes the injured person's fears and other emotional reactions regarding reinjury and continuing functional compromise. In an effort to manage patients for whom pain persists and is associated with functional impairment and/or psychological distress, the behavioral health specialist, in conjunction with the PCP, assists the patient with pain acceptance, moves the patient away from pain relief efforts and toward pain coping strategies that reflect those actions and goals that the patient values most. Given the prevalence and diversity of pain problems that require management, the stepped care approach to pain management can be considered one of the most flexible and cost-effective approaches and an approach that is particularly well-suited to pain management in integrated care settings.

References

Alperstein, D., & Sharpe, L. (2016). The efficacy of motivational interviewing in adults with chronic pain: A meta-analysis and systematic review. *Journal of Pain, 17*, 393–403.

Andrews, N. E., Strong, J., & Meredith, P. J. (2012). Activity pacing, avoidance, endurance, and associations with patient functioning in chronic pain: A systematic review and meta-analysis. *Archives of Physical Medicine and Rehabilitation, 93*(11), 2109–2121.

Beck, A. T., & Steer, R. A. (1993). *Beck anxiety inventory manual*. San Antonio, TX: The Psychological Corporation.

Beck, A. T., Steer, R. A., & Brown, G. K. (1996). *The Beck depression inventory-II*. San Antonio, TX: Psychological Corporation.

Broderick, J. E., Keefe, F. J., Schneider, S., Junghaenel, D. U., Bruckental, P., Schwartz, J. E., … Gould, E. (2016). Cognitive behavioral therapy for chronic pain is effective, but for whom? *Pain, 157*, 2115–2123.

Brown, K. S., & Folen, R. A. (2005). Psychologists as leaders of multidisciplinary chronic pain management teams: A model for health care delivery. *Professional Psychology: Research and Practice, 36*, 587–594.

Cegala, D. J., McClure, L., Marinelli, T. M., & Post, D. M. (2000). The effects of communication skills training on patients' participation during medical interviews. *Patient Education and Counseling, 41*(2), 209–222.

Chiesa, A., & Serretti, A. (2011). Mindfulness-based interventions for chronic pain: A systematic review of the evidence. *Journal of Alternative and Complementary Medicine, 17*, 83–93.

Dansie, E. J., & Turk, D. C. (2013). Assessment of patients with chronic pain. British Journal of Anaesthesia, 111, 19–25.

Dobscha, S. K., Corson, K., Perrin, N. A., Hanson, G. C., Leibowitz, R. Q., Doak, M. N., … Gerrity, M. S. (2009). Collaborative care for chronic pain in primary care. *Journal of the American Medical Association, 301*, 1242–1252.

Duckworth, M. P., & Iezzi, T. (2010). Physical injuries, pain, and psychological trauma: Pathways to disability. *Psychological Injury and Law, 3*, 241–253.

Duckworth, M. P., Iezzi, T., & Lewandowski, M. (2008). Managing MVC-related sequelae in the primary care setting: Normalizing experiences of emotional distress. In M. P. Duckworth, T. Iezzi, & W. T.

O'Donohue (Eds.), *Motor vehicle collisions: Medical, psychosocial, and legal consequences* (pp. 167–180). New York: Academic Press.

Duckworth, M. P., Iezzi, T., & Sewell, T. (2009). Assessing and managing chronic pain in the primary care setting. In L. James & W. T. O'Donohue (Eds.), *The primary care consultant toolkit: Tools for behavioral medicine* (pp. 183–197). New York, NY: Springer.

Duckworth, M. P., Iezzi, T., & Shearer, E. (2011). Retraumatization associated with disabling physical injuries. In M. P. Duckworth & V. Follette (Eds.), *Retraumatization: Assessment, treatment, and prevention* (pp. 377–421). New York, NY: Routledge Press.

Gaskin, D. J., & Richard, P. (2012). The economic cost of pain in the United States. *Journal of Pain, 13*, 715–724.

Gatchel, R. J., & Okifuji, A. (2006). Evidence-based scientific data documenting the treatment and the cost-effectiveness of comprehensive pain programs for chronic nonmalignant pain. *Journal of Pain, 7*, 779–793.

Gatchel, R. J., Peng, Y. B., Peters, M. L., Fuchs, P. N., & Turk, D. C. (2007). The biopsychosocial approach to chronic pain: Scientific advances and future directions. *Psychological Bulletin, 133*(4), 581–624.

Geneen, L. J., Martin, D. J., Adams, N., Clarke, C., Dunbar, M., Jones, D., ... Smith, B. H. (2015). Effects of education to facilitate knowledge about chronic pain for adults: A systematic review with meta-analysis. *Systematic Reviews, 4*, 1–21.

Glajchen, M. (2001). Chronic pain: Treatment barriers and strategies for clinical practice. *The Journal of the American Board of Family Practice, 14*(3), 211–218.

Gureje, O., Simon, G. E., & Von Korff, M. (2001). A cross-national study of the course of persistent pain in primary care. *Pain, 92*, 195–200.

Iezzi, T. (2008). Medicolegal issues associated with motor vehicle collisions: A psychological perspective. In M. P. Duckworth, T. Iezzi, & W. T. O'Donohue (Eds.), *Motor vehicle collisions: Medical, psychosocial, and legal consequences* (pp. 503–539). New York: Elsevier.

Jackson, T., Wang, Y., & Fan, H. (2014). Self-efficacy and chronic pain outcomes: A meta-analytic review. *Journal of Pain, 15*, 800–814.

Jia, X., & Jackson, T. (2016). Pain beliefs and problems in functioning among people with arthritis: A meta-analytic review. *Journal of Behavioral Medicine., 39*, 735. https://doi.org/10.1007/s10865-016-9777-z

Johnston, M., Foster, M., Shennan, J., Starkey, N. J., & Johnson, A. (2010). The effectiveness of an acceptance and commitment therapy self-help intervention for chronic pain. *The Clinical Journal of Pain, 26*(5), 393–402.

Kamper, S. J., Maher, C. G., Costa, L. D. C. M., McAuley, J. H., Hush, J. M., & Sterling, M. (2012). Does fear of movement mediate the relationship between pain intensity and disability in patients following whiplash injury? A prospective longitudinal study. *Pain, 153*(1), 113–119.

Keefe, F. J., Crisson, J., Urban, B. J., & Williams, D. (1990). Analyzing chronic low back pain: The relative contribution of pain coping strategies. Pain, 40, 293–301.

Kerns, R. D., Turk, D. C., & Rudy, T. E. (1985). The West Haven-Yale multidimensional pain inventory. *Pain, 23*, 345–356.

Lalloo, C., Jibb, L. A., Rivera, J., Agarwal, A., & Stinson, J. N. (2015). "There's a pain App for that:" review of patient-targeted smartphone applications for pain management. *The Clinical Journal of Pain, 31*(6), 557–563.

LeFort, S. M., Gray-Donald, K., Rowat, K. M., & Jeans, M. E. (1998). Randomized controlled trial of a community-based psychoeducation program for the self-management of chronic pain. *Pain, 74*(2), 297–306.

Linton, S. J. (2000). A review of psychological risk factors in back and neck pain. *Spine, 25*, 1148–1156.

Macea, D. D., Gajos, K., Calil, Y. A. D., & Fregni, F. (2010). The efficacy of web-based cognitive behavioral interventions for chronic pain: A systematic review and meta-analysis. *The Journal of Pain, 11*(10), 917–929.

Malmivaara, A., Kakkinen, U., Aro, T., Heinrichs, M. L., Koskenniemi, L., Kuosma, E., ... Vaaranen, V. (1995). The treatment of acute low back pain—Bed rest, exercises, or ordinary activity? *New England Journal of Medicine, 332*, 351–355.

Manchikanti, L., Abdi, S., Atluri, S., Balog, C. C., Benyamin, R. M., Boswell, M. V., ... Burton, A. W. (2012). American Society of Interventional Pain Physicians (ASIPP) guidelines for responsible opioid prescribing in chronic non-cancer pain: Part I—Evidence assessment. *Pain Physician, 15*(3 Suppl), S1–65.

McClune, T., Burton, A. K., & Waddell, G. (2007). Whiplash associated disorders: A review of the literature to guide patient information and advice. *Emergency Medicine Journal, 19*, 499–506.

McCracken, L. M. (1998). Learning to live with pain: Acceptance of pain predicts adjustment in persons with chronic pain. *Pain, 74*, 21–27.

McCracken, L. M., & Vowles, K. E. (2006). Acceptance of chronic pain. *Current Pain and Headache Reports, 10*(2), 90–94.

McGillion, M. H., Watt-Watson, J., Stevens, B., LeFort, S. M., Coyte, P., & Graham, A. (2008). Randomized controlled trial of a psychoeducation program for the self-management of chronic cardiac pain. *Journal of Pain and Symptom Management, 36*(2), 126–140.

Merskey, H., & Bogduk, N. (1994). *Classification of chronic pain: Descriptions of chronic pain syndromes and definitions of pain terms*. Seattle, WA: IASP Press.

Nahin, R. L. (2015). Estimates of pain prevalence and severity in adults: United States, 2012. *Journal of Pain, 16*, 769–780.

Otis, J. D., MacDonald, A., & Dobscha, S. K. (2006). Integration and coordination of pain management in primary care. *Journal of Clinical Psychology*, *62*, 1333–1343.

Plagge, J. M., Lu, M. W., Lovejoy, T. I., Karl, A. I., & Dobscha, S. K. (2013). Treatment of comorbid pain and PTSD in returning veterans: A collaborative approach utilizing behavioral activation. *Pain Medicine*, *14*, 1164–1172.

Pozek, J. P. J., Beausang, D., Baratta, J. L., & Viscusi, E. R. (2016). The acute to chronic pain transition: Can chronic pain be prevented? *Medical Clinics of North America*, *100*(1), 17–30.

Romano, M., & Peters, L. (2015). Evaluating the mechanisms of change in motivational interviewing in the treatment of mental health problems: A review and meta-analysis. *Clinical Psychology Review*, *38*, 1–12.

Ruehlman, L. S., Karoly, P., & Enders, C. (2012). A randomized controlled evaluation of an online chronic pain self management program. *Pain*, *153*(2), 319–330.

Sturgeon, J. A. (2014). Psychological therapies for the management of chronic pain. *Psychology Research and Behavior Management*, *7*, 115–124.

Thorn, B. E., Cross, T. H., & Walker, B. B. (2007). Meta-analyses and systematic reviews of psychological treatments for chronic pain: Relevance to an evidence-based practice. *Health Psychology*, *26*, 10–12.

Thorsell, J., Finnes, A., Dahl, J., Lundgren, T., Gybrant, M., Gordh, T., & Buhrman, M. (2011). A comparative study of 2 manual-based self-help interventions, acceptance and commitment therapy and applied relaxation, for persons with chronic pain. *The Clinical Journal of Pain*, *27*(8), 716–723.

Valentine, S. E., Gerber, M. W., Nobles, C. J., Shtasel, D. L., & Marques, L. (2016). Longitudinal study of mental health and pain-related functioning following a motor vehicle collision. *Health Psychology*, *35*(7), 742–750. https://doi.org/10.1037/hea0000329

Veehof, M. M., Oskam, M. J., Schreurs, K. M. G., & Bohlmeijer, E. T. (2011). Acceptance-based interventions for the treatment of chronic pain: A systematic review and meta-analysis. *Pain*, *152*, 533–542.

Ware, J. E., Snow, K. K., Kosinski, M., & Gandek, B. (1993). *SF-36 health survey: Manual and interpretation guide*. Boston, MA: The Health Institute, New England Medical Center.

13 Conduct Disorder

Melissa Castle Heatly and Phyllis Lee

Definition and Etiology

Conduct disorder (CD) is a serious and persistent behavioral disorder that is characterized by hostile and sometimes physically violent behavior, callous disregard for others and societal norms, and persistent violation of rules and the rights, feelings, or personal space of other people (APA, 2013; Kazdin, 2007; Kimonis, Frick, & McMahon, 2014). Children and adolescents with CD may find aggression, coercion, deceit, and harming others gratifying and energizing and may even "get a rise" out of these behaviors. Signs that an older youth may have CD include picking fights, cheating and stealing, trespassing and vandalism, and abusive behavior including forced sex or using weapons to coerce others. For younger children, signs of CD are similarly coercive and may include intentional harm to peers or even animals, relentless bullying, and lying or stealing with little to gain aside from a power differential. These behaviors are differentiated from more typical "acting out" by their chronicity, persistence, severity, and appearance across a wide range of settings. Estimated prevalence rates range from 2 to 12% (Costello, Egger, & Angold, 2005), with higher prevalence in males than females (Nock, Kazdin, Hiripi, & Kessler, 2006).

Diagnostic criteria. The DSM-5 (APA, 2013) requires the presence of at least 3 out of 15 possible symptoms present within the past 12 months, including at least one symptom present within the past 6 months for diagnosis of CD. Symptoms are grouped into four categories: aggression to people and animals, destruction of property, deceitfulness or theft, and serious violations of rules. The DSM-5 diagnosis specifies the childhood-onset type for individuals displaying at least one symptom before age 10 and the adolescent-onset type for individuals without any symptoms before age 10. In addition, the DSM-5 specifies "with limited prosocial emotions" for individuals who demonstrate callous/unemotional (CU) traits such as limited empathy, remorse, guilt, emotionality, or responsiveness to discipline (Hawes & Dadds, 2005). Untreated CD can often precede the onset of antisocial personality disorder (Simonoff et al., 2004).

Etiology. The etiology and trajectories of CD are diverse and involve complex and interacting biological, psychological, and social factors (Bronfenbrenner, 1986; Kimonis et al., 2014). A systems level illustration of various factors and interactions is provided in Fig. 13.1. Notably, children who experienced abuse, parental rejection or neglect, and harsh or inconsistent

M.C. Heatly, Ph.D. (✉)
Pediatric Behavioral Health and Wellness, University of Rochester Medical Center, Rochester, NY, USA
e-mail: Melissa_heatly@URMC.rochester.edu

P. Lee, Ph.D.
University of Connecticut Health Center, Farmington, CT, USA
e-mail: phyllis124@gmail.com

A. Maragakis, W.T. O'Donohue (eds.), *Principle-Based Stepped Care and Brief Psychotherapy for Integrated Care Settings*, https://doi.org/10.1007/978-3-319-70539-2_13

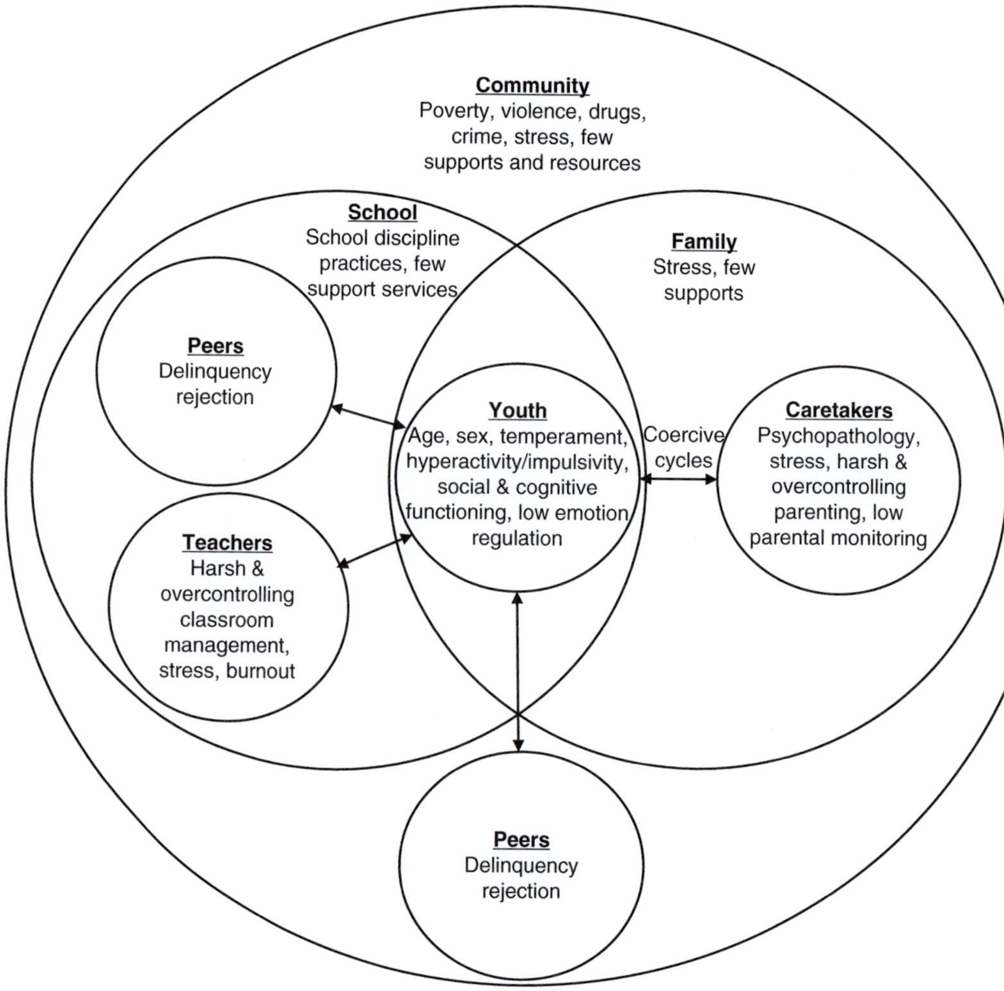

Fig. 13.1 A systemic perspective of conduct disorder

parenting are most at risk, as are those exposed to neighborhood violence, peer rejection, and peer delinquency.

Typically, youth with childhood-onset CD experience chronic and more severe conduct problems that persist into adulthood (Moffitt & Caspi, 2001). These children tend to display "undersocialized" behaviors in which they struggle with social interactions and engage in aggressive and other problem behaviors alone. In contrast, those with adolescent-onset CD are more likely to display "socialized delinquency," in which conduct problems are associated with peer delinquency and tend to remit after adolescence (Quay, 1987). There are also social and cognitive factors that contribute to conduct problems, including deficits in perception and interpretation of social cues (Dodge & Pettit, 2003). Specifically, youth with social cognitive deficits are more likely to make more hostile attributional biases and errors and also lack a repertoire of responses to social situations. CD is frequently comorbid with ADHD, academic difficulties and learning disorders, neurological impairments, substance use problems, and internalizing disorders. In turn, youth with CD and comorbid disorders are at risk for greater impairments (see McMahon & Frick, 2007 for review). For example, youth with ADHD and CD may have an increased likelihood of impulsively engaging in risky behaviors (Waschbusch, 2002), while those with depression and CD may be more likely to engage in suicidal behaviors (Vander Stoep et al., 2011).

Extensive research has also demonstrated the significance of parenting in the development of CD. Specifically, harsh and inconsistent discipline can trigger noncompliant behaviors, and parent-child interactions characterized by coercive cycles perpetuate conduct problems (Kazdin, 2007; Kimonis et al., 2014). For example, a parent may model aggressive ways of interacting by punishing a child for noncompliance and when the child argues back, the parent gets frustrated and gives up, thus reinforcing the child's noncompliant and argumentative behaviors. Low parental monitoring of youth activities is also related to CD as well as factors related to the parent or family may increase the risk of CD, including parental psychopathology and parent/family stressors (Frick et al., 1992). Children whose biological parents have a history of CD or ADHD or have substance use disorders, depression, bipolar disorder, or schizophrenia are also at risk.

In addition to the interactions that youth have with family members, interactions with deviant peers and dysfunctional communities may reinforce delinquency (Snyder et al., 2005). Especially in adolescence, association with delinquent peers increases the risk of CD. Youth with the social, cognitive, and self-regulatory deficits that place them at risk for CD may also experience peer rejection and also few opportunities to engage in positive social interactions (Miller-Johnson, Coie, Bierman, Maumary-Gremaud, & CPPRG, 2002). There are also community effects that may increase the likelihood of CD, and research has documented the negative effects of poverty, which is associated with increased exposure to crime, violence, stress, and compromised parenting practices (see Shaw & Shelleby, 2014 for review).

Assessment in Primary Care Settings

CD may present in a variety of ways within a primary care setting. Many youth with CD present with their parents regarding complaints of acting-out behavior at home, including non-compliance, aggression, argumentativeness, and disregard of rules. The youth likely also displays trouble at school or their community as well, with behaviors ranging from troubled teacher-child relationships, difficulty following classroom rules and expectations, targeted aggression toward peers, shoplifting, truancy, or frequent office disciplinary referrals or suspensions. The parent may have difficulty responding to these behaviors and may engage in coercive or overly harsh disciplinary strategies. Adolescents with CD will often verbalize remorse in order to avoid punishment or obtain favor, but may not experience any apparent guilt themselves (Searight, Rottnek, & Abby, 2001). Among children 10–14 years of age, cigarette smoking, sexual activity, and alcohol or drug use are also red flags for conduct disorder (Barry, Fleming, Manwell, & Copeland, 1997).

There are two main ways to assess for CD in primary care settings: behavior rating scales and interviews. Behavior rating scales are often the quickest and easiest ways to screen for a range of problem behaviors. Many pediatric offices offer generalized screeners for problem behavior, including the Pediatric Symptom Checklist-17 (PSC-17; Gardner et al., 1999). A high externalizing score on the PSC-17 provides an alert of possible oppositional or conduct problems, but further evaluation is necessary to distinguish the type of externalizing disorder. The Vanderbilt Rating Scale (Wolraich et al., 2003) is a longer questionnaire that includes ratings on specific symptoms of CD that could be helpful to distinguish CD from ODD or ADHD. Standardized broadband rating scales (e.g., CBCL; Achenbach & Rescorla, 2001, BASC-2; Reynolds & Kamphaus, 2004) are also useful to screen for a range of symptoms and disorders, assessing symptoms of CD as well as comorbid disorders and functioning (such as peer interactions and academic performance) that may inform case conceptualization. In using rating scales, it is often necessary to distinguish between CD and ODD. Generally, symptoms and behaviors of CD are more severe and include aggression toward others, destruction of property, and deceitfulness or theft (see DSM-5). CD is diagnosed if these behaviors are persistent (not occurring one time only) and are present within the past year.

How to further assess if a screen returns positive. If a potential diagnosis of CD is gleaned from the initial screening, more in-depth interviews from multiple sources are necessary to obtain comprehensive diagnostic information and to inform treatment. At a minimum, youth and parent/caretaker reports on standardized scales such as the BASC-2 or CBCL should be collected. In addition, reports from multiple parents/caretakers and teachers can provide different perspectives and information from different settings. Reports from different raters should also include structured or semi-structured clinical interviews (e.g., KSADS; Kaufman et al., 1997), which provide questions regarding specific symptoms or behaviors. It is also important to conduct an assessment of potential comorbidities such as ADHD or substance use disorders, with rating scales (e.g., Conners 3 for ADHD; Conners, Pitkanen, and Rzepa, 2011) or interviews (e.g., CRAFFT for substance use; Knight, Sherritt, Shrier, Harris, & Chang, 2002).

Once standardized and semi-structured reports are obtained, the physician should carefully assess details about noted patterns in symptoms and behaviors, including frequency, severity, age of onset, and functioning in multiple environments (at home with each parent/caretaker, with peers, at school). Information should also be gathered regarding risks and factors that may contribute to or maintain CD, including typical parent-child interactions related to conduct problem behaviors as well as antecedents and consequences of conduct problem behaviors. Assessment of parent psychopathology (e.g., antisocial personality traits, substance abuse, depression) and parent/family stressors (marital/partner conflict, stressful events) is also important, as families are essential in treatment and this information may inform treatment approaches.

For practitioners with limited time, the primary target of assessment should be differentiating between normal adolescent risk-taking behavior and more pathological and long-standing antisocial behaviors (Searight et al., 2001). Adolescence is often characterized by minor risk-taking behavior that is not indicative of a long-standing or significant problem. Isolated or short-term acting-out episodes may also be temporary reactions to external stressors such as recent parental separation, loss, school stress, or geographical moves. In order to determine the best treatment approach, it is necessary to gather more information about the frequency, severity, chronicity, and context of symptoms/behaviors. Physicians should inquire about such life changes or stressors and follow up with rating scales that include CD symptoms (e.g., Vanderbilt, CBCL, BASC-2). Examples of important interview questions to ask are provided in Table 13.1.

Table 13.1 Critical interview questions when assessing for conduct disorder

1. At what age did the child/adolescent start displaying conduct problems?
2. How often do conduct problems typically occur (how many times a day/week)?
3. How do the conduct problems impair functioning at home? At school? With peers?
4. In what situations are conduct problems most likely to occur?
5. What are the consequences for the youth's conduct problems?

Evidence-Based Stepped Care and Brief Psychotherapeutic Approaches

Primary care physicians are often the first professionals consulted by families of children with serious behavioral disorders like CD (Searight et al., 2001). Yet CD can be extremely difficult to treat due to its chronic nature and the diverse domains of associated dysfunction in child, family, and community systems. As a consequence, many youth with CD would benefit from specialty mental health treatment. Thus, a priority of primary care settings is to (1) focus on psychoeducation and then (2) motivate engagement with more intensive services (Ingoldsby, 2010).

Psychoeducation for conduct disorder. Psychoeducation is necessary to provide families with information of how CD develops and is maintained in order to effectively target the interactions and behaviors fueling CD. When CD is suspected, physicians should share their concerns, emphasize the seriousness of the child's behavior, and provide information about both the etiology and long-term prognosis of CD especially without significant parental interventions. Providing psychoeducation can help families identify processes and factors related to the youth's CD and empower both youth and caretakers in their roles in maintaining or changing behaviors. Practitioners should also discuss caretaker and youth expectations about treatment. For example, having a discussion with caretakers that working only with the youth is not effective for treating CD can decrease resistance when providing parent management training.

Motivating engagement with treatment. Supporting motivation for change is necessary for families to invest in treatment for CD (Emmons & Rollnick, 2001). Practitioners can particularly help empower caretakers in their role as caring adults and essential agents of change and can draw from engagement practices such as motivational interviewing. Building rapport and empathy is an essential first step. Begin discussing concerning behavior and invite parents or youth to describe the struggles they face with family members, peers, school, juvenile justice, and others. Open-ended questions, affirming responses, reflective listening statements, and summary statements are vital to this stage. Next, explore the youth or family's perspective on the pros and cons of their behaviors (e.g., "What are some of the good things about skipping school? What are some of the not so good things?"), and use summary statements to clarify and confirm what's been said. Then provide personalized feedback about the potential short-term and long-term risks and outcomes of untreated behaviors, and elicit initial reactions. Always reinforce the positives or readiness to change. Create an action plan outlining small options or steps that may work, and identify sources of support and strength that they can draw upon to help make changes. Finally, create a prescription for change by summarizing and writing down the plan and providing referrals to outpatient, family, or multi-systemic therapies, as appropriate.

Practical and Brief Interventions for Treating Conduct Disorder in Primary Care Settings

Though more serious cases of CD will need intensive treatment, subclinical conduct disorder symptoms or those with recent onset may be amenable to brief treatment approaches in primary care settings (Searight et al., 2001). In such cases, a broad array of effective tools have been distilled from common elements of the most effective evidence-based intervention programs tested and developed over the past 30 years (Rotheram-Borus, Swendeman, & Chorpita, 2012).

Teach calming and relaxation skills. Calming and relaxation skills teach youth how to change how one feels and to get a better grasp on anger and self-control (Chorpita & Weisz, 2009). Quick calming is best for when time is short, when caught off guard, or when in a public place. To quickly calm, teach youth relaxation and calming strategies. First relax their muscles, especially those that feel most tense. Second, discuss how to do slow breathing with deep breaths and slow exhalations. Third, encourage them to think of a peaceful place and imagine themselves relaxing there. After teaching these steps, practice using the steps with the youth in session. After this exercise, have the youth rate their mood again and debrief with the youth about their experience. During debriefing, discuss the difference between a relaxed body and a tense one and describe how quick calming strategies can help one cope with angry or upset feelings. Encourage the youth to identify at least one stressful situation in which they can practice quick calming exercises over the next week. A number of relaxing audio recordings, scripts, and even evidence-informed apps can also be found online to facilitate ongoing practice (Monshat, Vella-Brodrick, Burns, & Herrman, 2012). A list of commonly used apps and websites can be found in Appendix.

Teach and practice problem-solving. Youth with budding conduct disorder often have difficulty applying problem-solving skills to resolve challenges (Kazdin, 2007). In problem-solving skills training, youth are taught five problem-solving steps to both think and act differently when faced with obstacles. First, encourage the child to say what the problem is as specifically as possible (e.g., "The problem is that she nags me to do my math homework right away when I get home at night, and I never have time to relax!"). Next, encourage the youth to brainstorm at least three solutions—without judging their feasibility or their quality. Identify pros and cons of each one, and choose *one* to try out. Finally, discuss whether it worked or not—and if it did not, identify another solution to try. Present the child with a fun problem to solve in the session together, and then help the child identify a problem from his or her own life that can be worked on using the problem-solving procedure. At the end of the meeting, encourage the youth to use this in at least one situation that week.

Parental monitoring. Parental monitoring includes both structuring the child's environments and tracking the child's behavior (See Dishion & McMahon, 1998, for review) and is critical for both preventing and intervening with CD. While the specific methods and foci will change as children age, monitoring remains important from infancy through adolescence and perhaps even into young adulthood. Parents of school-age children should monitor the child's attendance at school, behavior (in the classroom, on the playground, with peers, etc.), academic progress, and homework. Neighborhood activity and peers are particularly relevant as children age, as selection of antisocial friends from the neighborhood is a characteristic of youth with conduct disorder. Parents should feel comfortable both in monitoring and setting limits on their children's whereabouts and asking youth to check in regularly. Compliance with an evening curfew is critical, as is ensuring the youth is in an appropriate setting during nonschool hours. For parents who work, engaging extended family members, family friends, or other trusted community members (pastors, youth group leaders, teachers, etc.) to help with monitoring may be particularly useful. Primary care providers can facilitate monitoring by offering lists or suggestions for structured opportunities for such youth to engage in such as sports, recreational programs, youth clubs, camps, scouting, and other activities, as well as connecting children/adolescents with mentors in the community. Older adolescents may benefit from employment or volunteer work within the community, and parents should be encouraged to track and encourage such involvement. Engaging and tracking youth in structured community activities are especially important during the summer months and other school breaks, when youth may otherwise have long periods of unstructured or unsupervised time.

Clear communication. Communication strategies and basic listening are also critical skills that are reasonably taught within a primary care setting (Searight et al., 2001). When asking children to perform desired tasks, parents should be coached to use calm, clear, direct, and specific behavioral requests (e.g., "Please take a seat at the dining room table and start your math homework"). After 30 s parents should give a verbal reminder; when the request is made for the third time, a clear, reasonable, and enforceable consequence should be added (e.g., "If you haven't started your math homework in the next 5 min, you will lose 15 min of computer time tonight"). Parents should be coached to avoid coercive, qualified, or negative statements (e.g., "If you'd spend as much time thinking about school as you do those video games you'd get straight A's! If you think you can ignore your math homework that needs to get done and still get to play games all day, you're dumber than I thought!"). These types of statements can lead to the "flight to peer" phenomenon, a process in which family conflict leads to the child spending more time with peers and away from home (Kazdin, 2007).

Positive reinforcement. When communicating, parents of youth with conduct disorder often rely on harsh, inconsistent, coercive, or negative exchanges rather than positive reinforcement (Patterson, 1982). Positive reinforcement of appropriate behaviors both decrease parents' reliance on punishment or coercion while also increasing the frequency of the child's desirable or prosocial behaviors (Chorpita & Weisz, 2009). Positive reinforcement can come in multiple forms, including praise (e.g., "Thanks for helping me load the dishwasher"), positive contingencies (e.g., "You can get the wi-fi password once you've finished your work"), or rewards including tokens, movies, or cellphone privileges. Importantly, reinforcement must be consistently applied, concrete, specific, and always provided immediately after the child demonstrates positive or expected behaviors.

An additional strategy for increasing positive interactions is encouraging parents to establish 10–15 min of one-on-one time with the youth each day (Chorpita & Weisz, 2009). One-on-one time helps build more positive feelings and exchanges between youth and parents, which can disrupt negative and coercive cycles, teach pro-social skills, and increase the likelihood of positive behaviors. This time should be spent doing an interactive activity of the child or adolescent's choosing. Parents should be encouraged to meet their child where they are at and engage and bond over children's preferred activities. Parents should be guided to comment positively and describe what the child is doing ("That was a creative move"), to say nice things ("I like how you…"), and to show interest. It is just about being together; this is not a time for parents to ask questions, teach, correct, or review daily problems.

Consistent discipline. All discipline strategies should be used after first working to develop a foundation of consistently positive and loving relationships and in concordance with positive reinforcement to increase appropriate behaviors. Once these are in place, discipline can be used to decrease or eliminate undesired behaviors (AACP, 1998). Encourage parents to use short time-outs for young children or temporary removal of privileges such as video games or television for older youth. Parents should be coached to avoid vague and unenforceable consequences as well as consequences that are extreme, far in the future, or difficult to follow through with (e.g., "You're never going to see your friends again! Forget going to summer camp next July!"). A major obstacle to effective discipline is inconsistency, which can come from disagreement about child-rearing strategies, cultural differences between parents, as well as parents' own psychopathology. Physicians should be mindful of these difficulties and offer guidance for how to resolve differences and challenges.

Medication management. Though there is no formally approved medication for conduct disorder, adjunct pharmacotherapy may be utilized to treat specific symptoms (Searight et al., 2001). Medication can be utilized to address symptoms of impulsivity, hyperactivity, and inattention, to increase inhibitory control, and to decrease reactivity. In turn, improvement in these symptoms may improve children's ability to benefit from other psychosocial interventions. Though a review of psychopharmacological treatments is beyond the scope of this chapter, stimulants, antidepressants, lithium, anticonvulsants, and clonidine have all been used to treat symptoms associated with conduct disorder (Campbell, Gonzalez, & Silva, 1992).

Ineffective Strategies

Given the extensive research demonstrating multi-systemic contributors to CD, interventions that only address one part of the system (such as only individual therapy with the child/adolescent) are unlikely to change behaviors. Furthermore, interventions that involve significant punishment, harsh relations, yelling, and overcontrol are ineffective and are likely to exacerbate symptoms. Physicians should especially discourage the use of spanking or other physical and overtly harsh discipline strategies, as large literature illustrates that such forms of punishment teaches aggressive behavior and feeds into the coercive family communication cycles often seen in conduct disorder (Paolucci & Violato, 2004).

Emerging data also indicates that several treatments may actually produce harm for youth with CD (see Lilienfeld, 2007, for review). Scared Straight programs were popularized in the 1970s for attempting to frighten at-risk adolescents away from criminal behavior by exposing them to prison life. However, evidence suggests that these interventions actually increase conduct problems and nearly double the odds of offending. Similarly, military-style boot camps that emphasize discipline and obedience to authority have revealed no significant effects on antisocial behavior and have been associated with several deaths and physical harm. Attachment therapy techniques such as rebirthing and holding therapy can also be harmful, intrusive, and aggressive. Such approaches can include verbal abuse and physical restraint and have not yielded any positive effects for childhood behavior problems.

Referring to External Specialty Mental Health

Because of the multi-systemic nature of CD, most youth who meet criteria for the disorder will need to be stepped into more intensive treatment. Given that families often have difficulty following through with referrals for mental health, practices should map the behavioral health resources communities have to offer, develop relationships and referral partnerships with local agencies who can offer comprehensive behavioral health treatment, and follow up with families after the referral is made. Some of these more intensive therapies are described below.

Parent and family interventions. Youth with CD almost always have major family issues and dysfunctions that contribute to conduct problems. Therefore, family-centered interventions are often the front-line treatment of choice, and modalities that involve parents and families in treatment can significantly improve outcomes (Kazdin, 1997, 2007). Treatments for younger children often focus more substantially on parent training and management strategies. In contrast, interventions for older children and adolescents often rely on family therapy, multi-systemic interventions, and individual cognitive-behavioral interventions.

Parent Management Training (PMT) trains parents in strategies, behaviors, and procedures to change children's behavior (Kazdin, 1997, 2007). This training is based on the general view that conduct problems are inadvertently developed and sustained by maladaptive parent-child interactions. Treatment sessions train parents in understanding and observing problem-behavior in new ways, delivering effective commands and prompts, applying positive reinforcement, as well as implementing mild punishments, negotiation, and contingency contracting (e.g., "If-then" statements). Sessions also provide opportunities for parents to observe how techniques are implemented, to practice using techniques, and to discuss implementation in the home.

Both Functional Family Therapy (FFT) and Brief Strategic Family Therapy (BSFT) are multi-systemic interventions focusing on multiple domains both within and outside of the family (Sexton & Alexander, 2003; Szapocznik & Williams, 2000). Both approaches focus on understanding how behavioral problems function within family relationship systems and promote family functioning from within. BSFT service providers specifically attend to problematic familial exchanges and determine maladaptive interactions that, if altered, are most likely to lead to desired outcomes (Szapocznik & Williams, 2000). FFT also emphasizes parental supervision and involvement as a mechanism for change within the family (Sexton & Alexander, 2000) and incorporates positive community and social systems within the family's natural environment. Average duration of service ranges from 8 to 15 sessions per family over a 3-month period and may include family therapy sessions, meetings with community resources, and phone calls.

Multi-systemic therapy (MST) is an effective home-based approach that provides integrative, multi-systemic, and family-based therapy for youth at risk of out-of-home placement (e.g., Henggeler, Clingempeel, Brondino, & Pickrel, 2002). MST may draw upon parent-management training to enhance positive interactions at home, school consultation and behavioral intervention plans to promote prosocial behavior at school, and problem-solving therapy or psychopharmacology to address the response repertoire of the child. MST can also include social supports to promote prosocial peer engagement, and employment or housing assistance as needed. Because of its interdisciplinary nature, MST often relies upon a team approach including a psychiatrist or psychiatric case manager, psychologists, social workers, and other specialists. Treatment duration typically ranges from 3 to 5 months, and therapists rotate an on-call schedule to respond to crises around the clock.

Multidimensional Treatment Foster Care (MTFC) is recommended when adult caregivers are unavailable or unable to provide the degree of structure and supervision required; temporary foster care or residential treatment may be necessary (Fisher & Gilliam, 2012). In MTFC, children are placed in a therapeutic family-based foster care for 6–9 months. The foster placement establishes a positive and predictable environment through a structured and individualized behavior management system that relies on frequent reinforcement of positive behavior in the home paired with consistent follow-through on consequences. Skill-building is offered for academic and social activities and is supplemented by additional services (e.g., therapeutic school or individual therapy) for the youth.

Individual interventions. Individual interventions can be powerful supplements to family and systemic treatment of CD—especially for adolescents. Cognitive behavioral therapy (CBT) is a short-term goal-oriented therapy geared toward helping youth better understand and alter the relationship between their thoughts, feelings, and actions (Kazdin, 1997, 2007). CBT for conduct disorder focuses on social cognitions and cognitive problem-solving skills training. Social cognitions and responses may be altered by generating alternative attributions to others' behaviors, learning alternative ways to perceive how another person may feel, and learning to more accurately evaluate the effects of one's own actions upon others. Problem-solving skills training (PSST) involves generating alternative perspectives and solutions to interpersonal problems, identifying alternative ways to achieve goals, or helping the youth think through the consequences of their actions. Anger management training, which generally involves teaching youth to better manage frustration feelings by learning to recognize and defuse anger sensations with reframing and relaxation techniques such as muscle relaxation or deep breathing, may also be taught.

Treatment for comorbidities. Conduct disorder is often comorbid with other diagnoses including ADHD, ODD, and substance use or abuse. At present, research has not provided clear guidelines for how to best address comorbidity in conduct disorder (Kazdin, 1997, 2007). However, the extant evidence suggests that substance use issue should be treated first, as behavior change under intoxication is challenging at best (Searight et al., 2001). Dual diagnosis treatment centers may be appropriate for those with serious substance use or dependence. Comorbid ADHD or mood disorders can be addressed with behavioral or CBT treatments noted above, and specific symptoms may also be treated with medication if needed.

The Role of the Primary Care Provider/Medical Team in Treatment

Due to the complexity of conduct disorder, collaborative relationships between primary care physicians and advancement of healthcare providers and services are vital for long-term treatment (Auxier et al., 2012). Upon referral, physicians should always obtain a release of information to coordinate care. Two-way coordination is critical, and physicians should consider proactively reaching out to external providers both before and throughout treatment as necessary. Indeed, one of the most powerful predictors of positive clinical outcomes in collaborative care is systematic follow-up by physicians. This is especially true when symptoms are not responding to intervention, when multiple systems are involved and when encouraging medication adherence. In such cases, physicians and behavioral health providers should consider developing an agreement that allows for updates on treatment recommendations and patients' progress on a quarterly basis (or as indicated). It is also reasonable to request follow-up from the external behavioral health provider if the patient has been discharged or dropped from treatment. In such cases, primary care providers may once more find themselves at the front lines of assessment, brief intervention, and referral to further care.

How to assess impact on care and quality improvement. Ongoing data collection and benchmarking provides physicians with important information on patient progress and can help target areas for continued improvement or indicate need to step youth into more intensive services (Taylor et al., 2013). Thus, physicians should plan to readminister rating scales or interviews described above every 3–6 months and compare to baseline assessments of symptoms and behaviors. Especially for CD, it is also important to consistently inquire about dangerous or more severe antisocial behaviors, as well as instances of abuse or neglect. Though privacy laws differ state-by-state, physicians should always be aware of limitations that allow for protection of others from harm, abuse, or neglect (Henderson, 2015) and be prepared to contact the appropriate agencies or authorities as necessary. Practices that have a significant number of patients with CD or other significant behavioral health disorders may also request expert behavioral health consultation to provide specific evidence-based knowledge from clinicians or staff specializing in treating severe behavioral disorders. Shared learning or learning collaboratives can also provide practices with a community in which they can share challenges, lessons learned, and best practices in CD intervention and quality improvement.

Summary

Conduct disorder can be a persistent and costly problem, with youth engaging in violent and criminal acts. Since families often seek help in primary care settings, practitioners in these settings are well-situated to assess, treat, and connect families with appropriate, evidence-based services to reduce CD.

Appendix: Youth-Friendly Websites to Teach and Facilitate Calming and Relaxation Skills

Facilitating calming and relaxation skills	
Name and website	Description
DBT Diary Card and Skills Coach available on iTunes. apple.com	This app works as a daily mood and thought diary, with a coaching module that gives tips on challenging emotional situations, like how to successfully resolve conflict or ask for what you need. Users get positive reinforcement when they're consistent with their entries.
ACT Coach available on iTunes.apple.com	Teaches users how to tolerate negative thoughts and feelings by virtually guiding them through awareness exercises and skills. Developed by the US Department of Veteran affairs.
Stop, Breathe, Think! http://www.stopbreathethink.org	Encourages teens to stop what they're doing and check in with what they are thinking and feeling. Provides support to practice mindful breathing, mindfulness, and mood tracking.
Smiling Mind https://smilingmind.com.au	Builds build individual mental health and wellbeing through positive, pre-emptive tools based on mindfulness meditation.
Breathe2Relax http://t2health.dcoe.mil/apps/breathe2relax	Teaches and encourage diaphragmatic breathing. Can be used as a stand-alone stress reduction tool, or can be used in tandem with clinical care directed by a healthcare worker. Developed by the National Center for Telehealth & Technology.

Note: This is a small sample of many therapeutic apps and websites available online and is not intended to be a comprehensive list or endorsement of those listed over others. These apps are maintained by independent third parties and may or may not be available at any given time. Thus, it is highly suggested that practitioners self-pilot apps prior to recommending to specific clients.

References

Achenbach, T. M., & Rescorla, L. (2001). *Manual for the ASEBA school-age forms and profiles*. Burlington, VT: University of Vermont, Research Center for Children, Youth, & Families.

American Academy of Pediatrics. (1998). Guidance for effective discipline. *Pediatrics, 101*(4), 723–728.

Alexander, J. F., Robbins, M. S., & Sexton, T. L. (2000). Family-based interventions with older, at-risk youth: From promise to proof to practice. The Journal of Primary Prevention, *21*(2), 185–205.

American Psychiatric Association. (2013). *Diagnostic and statistical manual of mental disorders* (5th ed.). Washington, DC: American Psychiatric Association.

Auxier, A., Runyan, C., Mullin, D., Mendenhall, T., Young, J., & Kessler, R. (2012). Behavioral health referrals and treatment initiation rates in integrated primary care: A collaborative care research network study. *Translational Behavioral Medicine*, 2(3), 337–344.

Barry, K. L., Fleming, M. F., Manwell, L. B., & Copeland, L. A. (1997). Conduct disorder and antisocial personality in adult primary care patients. *Journal of Family Practice, 45*(2), 151–158.

Bronfenbrenner, U. (1986). Ecology of the family as a context for human development: Research perspectives. *Developmental Psychology, 22*(6), 723–742.

Campbell, M., Gonzalez, N. M., & Silva, R. R. (1992). The pharmacologic treatment of conduct disorders and rage outbursts. *Psychiatric Clinics of North America, 15*(1), 69–85.

Chorpita, B. F., & Weisz, J. R. (2009). *MATCH-ADTC: Modular approach to therapy for children with anxiety, depression, trauma, or conduct problems*. Satellite Beach, FL: PracticeWise.

Conners, C. K., Pitkanen, J., & Rzepa, S. R. (2011). *Conners 3rd Edition (Conners 3; Conners 2008)*. New York, NY: Springer.

Costello, E. J., Egger, H., & Angold, A. (2005). 10-year research update review: The epidemiology of child and adolescent psychiatric disorders: I. Methods and public health burden. *Journal of the American Academy of Child & Adolescent Psychiatry, 44*(10), 972–986.

Dishion, T. J., & McMahon, R. J. (1998). Parental monitoring and the prevention of child and adolescent problem behavior: A conceptual and empirical formulation. *Clinical Child and Family Psychology Review, 1*(1), 61–75.

Dodge, K. A., & Pettit, G. S. (2003). A biopsychosocial model of the development of chronic conduct problems in adolescence. *Developmental Psychology, 39*(2), 349–371.

Emmons, K. M., & Rollnick, S. (2001). Motivational interviewing in health care settings: Opportunities and limitations. *American Journal of Preventive Medicine, 20*(1), 68–74.

Fisher, P. A., & Gilliam, K. S. (2012). Multidimensional treatment foster care: An alternative to residential treatment for high risk children and adolescents. *Psychosocial Intervention, 21*(2), 195–203.

Frick, P. J., Lahey, B. B., Loeber, R., Stouthamer-Loeber, M., Christ, M. A. G., & Hanson, K. (1992). Familial risk factors to oppositional defiant disorder and conduct disorder: Parental psychopathology and maternal parenting. *Journal of Consulting and Clinical Psychology, 60*(1), 49–55.

Gardner, W., Murphy, M., Childs, G., Kelleher, K., Pagano, M. E., Jellinek, M., … Sturner, R. (1999). The PSC-17. *Ambulatory Child Health, 5*(3), 225–236.

Hawes, D. J., & Dadds, M. R. (2005). The treatment of conduct problems in children with callous-unemotional traits. *Journal of Consulting and Clinical Psychology, 73*(4), 737–741.

Henderson, E. (2015). Potentially dangerous patients: A review of the duty to warn. *Journal of Emergency Nursing, 41*(3), 193–200.

Henggeler, S. W., Clingempeel, W. G., Brondino, M. J., & Pickrel, S. G. (2002). Four-year follow-up of multisystemic therapy with substance-abusing and substance-dependent juvenile offenders. *Journal of the American Academy of Child & Adolescent Psychiatry, 41*(7), 868–874.

Ingoldsby, E. M. (2010). Review of interventions to improve family engagement and retention in parent and child mental health programs. *Journal of Child and Family Studies, 19*(5), 629–645.

Kaufman, J., Birmaher, B., Brent, D., Rao, U., Flynn, C., Moreci, P., … Ryan, N. (1997). Schedule for affective disorders and schizophrenia for school-age children—Present and lifetime version (KSADS-PL): Initial reliability and validity data. *Journal of the American Academy of Child and Adolescent Psychiatry, 36*, 980–988.

Kazdin, A. E. (1997). Practitioner review: Psychosocial treatments for conduct disorder in children. *Journal of Child Psychology and Psychiatry, 38*(2), 161–178.

Kazdin, A. E. (2007). Psychosocial treatments for conduct disorder in children and adolescents. In P. E. Nathan & J. M. Gorman (Eds.), *A guide to treatments that work* (3rd ed., pp. 71–104). New York: Oxford University Press.

Kimonis, E., Frick, P. J., & McMahon, R. J. (2014). Conduct and oppositional defiant disorders. In E. J. Mash & R. A. Barkley (Eds.), *Child psychopathology* (pp. 145–179). New York, NY: Guilford Press.

Knight, J. R., Sherritt, L., Shrier, L. A., Harris, S. K., & Chang, G. (2002). Validity of the CRAFFT substance abuse screening test among adolescent clinic patients. *Archives of Pediatrics & Adolescent Medicine, 156*(6), 607–614.

Lilienfeld, S. O. (2007). Psychological treatments that cause harm. *Perspectives on Psychological Science, 2*(1), 53–70.

McMahon, R. J., & Frick, P. J. (2007). Conduct and oppositional disorders. In E. J. Mash & R. A. Barkley (Eds.),

Assessment of childhood disorders (pp. 132–183). New York, NY: Guilford Press.

Miller-Johnson, S., Coie, J. D., Bierman, K., Maumary-Gremaud, A., & CPPRG. (2002). Peer rejection and aggression and early starter models of conduct disorder. *Journal of Abnormal Child Psychology, 30*, 217–230.

Moffitt, T. E., & Caspi, A. (2001). Childhood predictors differentiate life-course persistent and adolescence-limited antisocial pathways among males and females. *Development and Psychopathology, 13*(2), 355–375.

Monshat, K., Vella-Brodrick, D., Burns, J., & Herrman, H. (2012). Mental health promotion in the internet age: A consultation with Australian young people to inform the design of an online mindfulness training programme. *Health Promotion International, 27*(2), 177–186.

Nock, M. K., Kazdin, A. E., Hiripi, E., & Kessler, R. C. (2006). Prevalence, subtypes, and correlates of DSM-IV conduct disorder in the National Comorbidity Survey Replication. *Psychological Medicine, 36*(5), 699–710.

Patterson, G. R. (1982). Coercive family process. Eugene, OR: Castalia.

Paolucci, E. O., & Violato, C. (2004). A meta-analysis of the published research on the affective, cognitive, and behavioral effects of corporal punishment. *The Journal of psychology, 138*(3), 197–222.

Quay, H. C. (1987). Patterns of delinquent behavior. In H. C. Quay & J. S. Werry (Eds.), *Handbook of juvenile delinquency* (pp. 118–138). New York, NY: Wiley & Sons.

Reynolds, C. R., & Kamphaus, R. W. (2004). *BASC-2: Behavior assessment system for children*. Pearson: Bloomington, MN.

Rotheram-Borus, M. J., Swendeman, D., & Chorpita, B. F. (2012). Disruptive innovations for designing and diffusing evidence-based interventions. *American Psychologist, 67*(6), 463–476.

Searight, H. R., Rottnek, F., & Abby, S. L. (2001). Conduct disorder: Diagnosis and treatment in primary care. *American Family Physician, 63*(8), 1579–1588.

Sexton, T. L., & Alexander, J. F. (2003). Functional family therapy: A mature clinical model for working with at-risk adolescents and their families. In T. L. Sexton, G. R. Weeks, & M. S. Robbins (Eds.), *Handbook of family therapy: The science and practice of working with families and couples* (pp. 323–348). New York, NY: Brunner-Routledge..

Shaw, D. S., & Shelleby, E. C. (2014). Early-onset conduct problems: Intersection of conduct problems and poverty. *Annual Review of Clinical Psychology, 10*, 503–528.

Simonoff, E., Elander, J., Holmshaw, J., Pickles, A., Murray, R., & Rutter, M. (2004). Predictors of antisocial personality. Continuities from childhood to adult life. *The British Journal of Psychiatry, 184*, 118–127.

Snyder, J., Schrepferman, L., Oeser, J., Patterson, G., Stoolmiller, M., Johnson, K., & Snyder, A. (2005). Deviancy training and association with deviant peers in young children: Occurrence and contribution to early-onset conduct problems. *Development and Psychopathology, 17*(2), 397–413.

Szapocznik, J., & Williams, R. A. (2000). Brief strategic family therapy: Twenty-five years of interplay among theory, research and practice in adolescent behavior problems and drug abuse. *Clinical Child and Family Psychology Review, 3*(2), 117–134.

Taylor, E. F., Genevro, J., Peikes, D., Geonnotti, K., Wang, W., & Meyers, D. (2013, April). *Building quality improvement capacity in primary care: Supports and resources*. Rockville, MD: Agency for Healthcare Research and Quality. Retrieved from http://www.ahrq.gov/professionals/prevention-chronic-care/improve/capacitybuilding/pcmhqi2.html

Vander Stoep, A., Adrian, M., Mc Cauley, E., Crowell, S. E., Stone, A., & Flynn, C. (2011). Risk for suicidal ideation and suicide attempts associated with co-occurring depression and conduct problems in early adolescence. *Suicide and Life-threatening Behavior, 41*(3), 316–329.

Waschbusch, D. A. (2002). A meta-analytic examination of comorbid hyperactive-impulsive attention problems and conduct problems. *Psychological Bulletin, 128*(1), 118–150.

Wolraich, M. L., Lambert, W., Doffing, M. A., Bickman, L., Simmons, T., & Worley, K. (2003). Psychometric properties of the Vanderbilt ADHD diagnostic parent rating scale in a referred population. *Journal of Pediatric Psychology, 28*(8), 559–568.

Depression

14

Cindy W. Mikeal and J. Arthur Gillaspy Jr.

A Brief Description of Depression

Depression is considered one of the most prevalent chronic illnesses in the USA (Community Care Network of Virginia, 2012). About 29.4% of individuals will have a depressive disorder in their lifetime, with 4.6% having chronic depression (Centers for Disease Control, 2016). To put this into context, approximately eight million patients with major depressive disorder annually seek services at primary care clinics, hospitals, or emergency departments. In addition, 10–30% of all individuals presenting in primary care clinics present with significant depressive symptoms (Hunter, Goodie, Oordt, & Dobmeyer, 2009). For individuals with another chronic illness (i.e., diabetes, cardiovascular disease, chronic pain) or stressful psychosocial factors, these rates are even higher (CDC, 2016; UMHS, 2011).

The good news is that depression is very treatable, but many individuals with depression never tell their primary care providers about their symptoms (Trangle et al., 2016). Considering the seriousness of depression and possible influences on overall health, the role of the behavioral health provider (BHP) in a primary care team setting is to conduct valid and reliable screening and assessment of symptoms and risk factors and to provide brief evidence-based psychological treatments for depression. This chapter will present an overview guide for BHPs for the assessment and care of patients with depressive disorders in an integrated care setting.

Effective Ways to Screen for Depression in the Primary Care Setting

The routine screening of patients for depressive symptoms is an important practice for medical and behavioral health providers. This is particularly important since primary care providers (PCPs) typically only recognize depression symptoms in about one-third to one-half of patients with major depression (Schonfeld et al., 1997; Williams, Noel, Cordes, Ramirez, & Pignone, 2002). This section will review several depression screening tools that are appropriate or routine use in integrated care and discuss how depression screening may promote better identification and tracking of patient progress.

There are multiple tools for screening for depression in primary care [e.g., Centers for Epidemiologic Studies Depression Scale-Revised (CESD-R; Eaton, Smith, Ybarra, Muntaner, & Tien, 2004) and the Geriatric Depression Scale-

C.W. Mikeal, Ph.D. (✉)
Psychology, CHI St. Vincent, Little Rock, AR, USA
e-mail: Cmikeal@stvincenthealth.com

J.A. Gillaspy Jr., Ph.D.
Psychology and Counseling, University of Central Arkansas, Conway, AR, USA
e-mail: artg@uca.edu

A. Maragakis, W.T. O'Donohue (eds.), *Principle-Based Stepped Care and Brief Psychotherapy for Integrated Care Settings*, https://doi.org/10.1007/978-3-319-70539-2_14

Short (GDS-S; Sheikh & Yesavage, 1986)]. The Patient Health Questionnaire-2 (PHQ-2; Kroenke, Spitzer, & Williams, 2003) is one of the most widely used (Ebell, 2008) and effective tools for identifying depressive symptoms for adult and geriatric patients (CCNV, 2012; Li, Friedman, Conwell, & Fiscella, 2007; Löwe, Kroenke, & Gräfe, 2005). The PHQ-2 is a quick screener that consists of the first two questions of the Patient Health Questionnaire-9 (PHQ-9; Kroenke, Spitzer, & Williams, 2001). These items ask the degree to which patients have experienced "little interest or pleasure in doing things" and "feeling down, depressed, or hopeless" within the last 2 weeks. Items are rated on a 3-point Likert scale with "0" indicating not at all and "3" representing "nearly every day." Scores totaling 3 or higher are considered a positive screen for depression and should be given the complete PHQ-9 to screen for additional depression symptoms such as sleep and appetite changes, problems with concentration, and suicidal thoughts. The entire PHQ-9 is free to use for patient care and monitoring outcomes. It can be found at the following website: http://www.psychcongress.com/saundras-corner/scales-screeners/depression. For primary care clinics that provide services to adolescents (12–17), the PHQ-A (Johnson, Harris, Spitzer, & Williams, 2002) is recommended.

Typically, the PHQ-2 is used as a global screener for identifying and tracking depressive symptoms for all individuals at each visit. While your primary care clinic may not choose to give the PHQ-2 to every patient, it is recommended to screen patients with any of the following (Intermountain Healthcare, 2015):

- Chronic diseases such as diabetes or cardiovascular disease
- Multiple somatic complaints that remain "unresolved"
- High utilizers (more than six visits per year)
- Postpartum status
- History of depression—personal or family
- Known and active substance abuse

For additional guidelines for providing best care practices and screening with special populations or those with comorbid chronic illness, see Trangle et al. (2016).

How to Further Assess if a Screen Returns Positive

Screening all patients can help providers more readily identify those with depressive symptoms, but further assessment may be necessary to better understand the nature of those symptoms and to inform treatment decisions. It is important that primary care clinics have a protocol in place for depression care if a patient screens positive.

A straightforward approach to this is that a positive screen would trigger a same-day follow-up assessment using the PHQ-9 or some other depression assessment measure. The PHQ-9 (Kroenke et al., 2001) is a nine-item measure assessing the most common symptoms (e.g., changes in appetite, poor sleep, ability to concentrate well, and suicidal ideations) associated with depression and include the two items from the PHQ-2. This measure is considered an effective tool for detecting depression in the primary care setting. Additionally, the PHQ-9 may be used as the initial screening instrument if desired since evidence exists that PCPs are not likely to follow-up a positive PHQ-2 screening with the PHQ-9 and are more likely to rely on their own knowledge about the patient as well as clinical judgment (Fuchs et al., 2015). This follow-up can be completed by a nurse or PCP; however, in many integrated care settings, BHPs are referred directly to the patient through a "warm handoff" where the BHP is introduced to the patient by the PCP and briefly assesses the severity of depression, impact of symptoms on daily functioning, and suicidal ideation. This is an appropriate time to administer a more thorough assessment of depression, such as the PHQ-9, to determine how severe patients view their symptoms.

A brief clinical interview is also recommended to better understand the nature of symptom severity, effects on daily functioning, and current coping strategies that the patient may be using (CCNV, 2012). With pediatric, geriatric, or pregnant/postpartum patients, additional self-report tools may be useful to further assess problematic symptoms or poor coping. For example, the Edinburgh Postnatal Depression Scale (EPDS; Cox, Holden, & Sagovsky, 1987) assesses current level of coping for postpartum patients, while the Geriatric Depression Scale – Short (GDS-S; Sheikh & Yesavage, 1986) contains specific questions about memory concerns. To rule out more serious mood concerns such as bipolar disorder, the Bipolar Spectrum Diagnostic Scale (BSDS; Nassir et al., 2005) or the Mood Disorder Questionnaire (MDQ; Hirschfield, 2002) is recommended. Table 14.1 includes a brief summary of common depression assessment tools.

Another brief measure that may be helpful for assessing distress experienced by patients with depression is the Outcome Rating Scale (ORS; Miller, Duncan, Brown, Sparks, & Claud, 2003). The ORS is a four-item measure of subjective distress that has been shown to be sensitive to patient change in traditional psychotherapy (Duncan & Reese, 2015; Gillaspy & Murphy, 2011). This scale may be useful for primary care by allowing BHPs and patients to monitor progress over time in addition to symptom change. In an exploratory study in a primary care setting, DeSantis, Jackson, Duncan, and Reese (2016) found that ORS scores were moderately correlated with the PHQ-9 and PHQ-2 for patients with depressive symptoms. Determining impact on work and home is important for persons with severe depression. Difficulty in any of these set-

Table 14.1 Depression screening scales

Scale	Website found	Description	Pros	Cons
Centers for epidemiologic studies depression scale-Revised	http://cesd-r.com/ or http://www.brandeis.edu/roybal/docs/CESD-10_website_PDF.pdf	20-item Self-report Asks about a range of behaviors associated with depression	Includes some symptoms associated with anxiety	The 20 items may make use for screening less desirable
Edinburgh postnatal depression scale	http://www2.aap.org/sections/scan/practicingsafety/Toolkit_Resources/Module2/EPDS.pdf	10-item Self-report Asks about symptoms associated with depression and anxiety as well as overall sense of level of coping	Addresses level of coping Is short enough to use as screener	Has been normed for a specific population
Geriatric depression scale-Short form	http://geriatrictoolkit.missouri.edu/cog/GDS_SHORT_FORM.PDF	15-item Self-report Asks about satisfaction with life, feelings of worthlessness, and general depression symptoms	Specifically asks about memory concerns	Does not include a question related to SI
Bipolar Spectrum diagnostic form	http://imaging.ubmmedica.com/all/editorial/psychiatrictimes/pdfs/clinical-scales-bipolar-spectrum-diagnostic-form.pdf	19-item Self-report Items are related to symptoms of mania and depression including asking about "noticeable shifts"	Screens for manic and depressive symptoms	Length makes it more appropriate for an intake measure if bipolar is suspected
Mood disorder questionnaire	http://www.integration.samhsa.gov/images/res/MDQ.pdf	17-item Self-report Asks about symptoms typically associated with mania	Screens for mania	May result in false positives suggesting the presence of bipolar disorder Does not screen for depression

tings is related to increase in symptom severity (Pratt & Brody, 2014). Monitoring distress in these areas may also help BHPs collaborate with patients and develop a working alliance.

Suicide assessment is also an important part of initial patient screening. Research suggests that 45–76% of those who commit suicide had contact with a PCP in the month prior (Luoma, Martin, & Pearson, 2002). Thus, any clinical interview should address suicidal ideation. The following steps should be taken in assessing patients with suicidal ideations (SI):

- Explore content of suicidal thoughts. It is not uncommon for patients with SI to have non-morbid thoughts of dying such as "I would be better off dead" or "If I did not wake up in the morning, I would be ok with that." If these thoughts exist, acknowledge that these are distressing but "normal" for many individuals with depression.
- Directly discuss the need to call or schedule a follow-up appointment if SIs become more frequent or more severe.
- Explore the severity of any plan and intent to commit suicide.
- Assess for previous suicidal behaviors, such as past or aborted attempts.
- Assess access to lethal means to carry out an attempt.
- Determine whether patient is at high, moderate, or low risk for suicide attempt. (Fig. 14.1 has been provided to give further details about how to approach care for each level of risk.)
- Assess for alcohol/substance use or misuse using the AUDIT-C (Bush, Kivlahan,

<table>
<tr><th>High Risk</th><th>Moderate Risk</th><th>Low Risk</th></tr>
<tr><td>Patient has frequent and intense SI and has started planning; multiple risk factors exist; few protective factor (e.g., poor social support).</td><td>Patient has SI with a limited plan and lower intent than found in high risk patients; may have a previous attempt, but with good self-control and limited emotional distress. Patient will also have multiple protective factors.</td><td>Patient has non-morbid SI with no plan or intent for self-harm; good social support and few risk factors.</td></tr>
<tr><td>If severe psychiatric symptoms, access to lethal means, poor social support, and impaired judgment exist; then arrange for hospitalization or call 911 immediately. Note: If patient refuses to voluntarily go for inpatient crisis care, then consider voluntary admission in accordance with your state rules and guidelines.

If patient has no access to lethal means, good social support, intact judgment, and stabilized psychiatric symptoms; then take immediate action to prevent a future crisis such as making a Crisis Response Plan (see figure 2).</td><td colspan="2">Evaluate for any additional psychiatric disorders, social stressors, and additional risk factors such as previous suicide attempts.

You may also do the following:

1) Create a Crisis Response Plan with the patient.
2) Refer (locally or via telemedicine) for medication management.
3) Refer for individual or family therapy.</td></tr>
<tr><td colspan="3">Encourage social support for patient – include any family, close friends and community members as appropriate. If patient currently has a therapist, obtain permission to call in the presence of the patient.</td></tr>
<tr><td colspan="3">Document risk assessment, rationale for what was done and the treatment plan. Continue to monitor and track patient's progress through follow-up interview/contacts. Provide a list of community resources as needed. Document all contact with the patient.</td></tr>
</table>

Fig. 14.1 Suicide risk assessment and care strategies

McDonnel, Fihn, & Bradley, 1998) or the CAGE-AID (Brown & Rounds, 1995). If positive for substance use, provide psychoeducation of how the use of substances lowers inhibition and increases the likelihood of suicide attempt.

- Assess for comorbid anxiety or high energy level or mania that may promote attempt to suicide. Studies have shown that patients with comorbid anxiety are more likely to attempt suicide (Davidson, LaRicka, Grant, Judah, & Mills, 2011; Nepon, Belik, Bolton, & Sareen, 2010; Pompili et al., 2012).
- Develop a crisis response plan (see Fig. 14.2). These plans work best when created in a collaborative manner taking into account patient preferences and available social support. Provide the patient with a copy of this plan or complete the plan on a 3 × 5 index card for the patient to take at the end of the session.
- Review limits of confidentiality in regard to the duty to protect. If patient is an adult, ask permission to bring a safe family member or friend into the session (if patient is under 18, have parent/guardian join the session).
- Explain options for inpatient psychiatric care. Always explain difference between voluntary and involuntary admission based on your state as well as federal guidelines. For example, in some states it is unlawful for individuals to sell firearms to patients that have been committed to a mental facility (NCSL, 2013). Patients need enough information to make the best decision possible for them and their families. Once a decision for care has been made, work with the patient and family to ensure that the patient has access to appropriate level of care.
- Document! Document! Document! Things to include the presence of suicidal ideation, severity of symptoms, creation of a crisis response plan, presence of access to lethal means, current substance use, breaking of confidentiality related to duty to protect, and plan for hospitalization. Complete documentation related to suicidal thoughts is important for continuing care of the patient. Remember, if you do not document it, it did not happen.

For additional tools and more information for suicide risk assessment, go to the website of the Suicide Prevention Resource Center (www.sprc.org).

Finally, when assessing depression in primary care, it is important to screen for other comorbid factors such as psychosis, trauma, and substance abuse. The presence of psychotic features may indicate the need for immediate inpatient care. Trauma and substance use disorders may indicate that longer-term treatment is necessary.

When thoughts of self-harm or of attempting suicide increase...
1. I will watch a funny T.V. show.
2. I will call my best friend.
3. I will go outside and take a walk.
4. Repeat # 1-3
If steps 1 – 4 do not help...
5. Call the clinic to speak to my BHP (provide phone contact) or call the National Suicide Prevention Lifeline at 1.800.273.8255
6. Go to the nearest Emergency Department

Fig. 14.2 Sample Crisis Response Plan

Evidence-Based Stepped Care and Brief Interventions

Treatment for depression in a primary care setting typically uses a stepped-care approach where brief interventions are used to help patients improve before more intensive services are implemented. Figure 14.3 provides details of a basic stepped-care approach to depression care (https://www.nice.org.uk/guidance/cg90/chapter/1-Guidance#stepped-care, p. 16).

Step 1 Care

For patients with subclinical depression, it is important to provide brief psychoeducation (15 min) about the possible course of depression, what to do if symptoms become worse or if suicidal thoughts are present, and simple ways to improve coping. If possible, include family members in these conversations to help prevent the further progression of depressive symptoms. There are many websites that provide free handouts for use by clinicians to explain the symptoms of depression and how early diagnosis may help (http://www.psnpaloalto.com/wp/wp-content/uploads/2010/12/Understanding-Depression-Handout-without-PAMF-logo.pdf, http://wellnessproposals.com/wellness-library/mental-health/anxiety-and-depression-handouts/, https://patienteducation.osumc.edu/Documents/depression.pdf, http://www.fammed.wisc.edu/integrative/resources/modules/, and http://www.champ-program.org/static/Patient%20Education%20booklet%20121010.pdf). Additionally, patients that have started to limit social activity because of depression symptoms may benefit from a referral to a local support group.

Step 2 Care

Patients with persistent subclinical depressive symptoms and mild to moderate depression may benefit from brief interventions such as the following:

Psychoeducation

- Provide information about the course of depression.
- If sleep has been affected, provide information about how the use of healthy sleep hygiene promotes a reduction in depression symptoms.
- Discuss the benefits of physical activity to improving depression symptoms.

Focus of the intervention	Types of the intervention
STEP 4: Severe depression or depression that includes risk to life and self-neglect	May include multiple professionals, intense psychological interventions, medication therapy, electroconvulsive therapy, crisis service, combined treatments, and possibly inpatient care
STEP 3: Treatment resistant mild to moderate depression or Persistent subthreshold depressive symptoms; moderate and severe depression	Use Medication, high-intensity psychological interventions, combined treatments, collaborative care with the PCP or an attending psychiatrist and referral for further assessment and interventions as appropriate.
STEP 2: Persistent subthreshold depressive symptoms; mild to moderate depression	Low-intensity psychosocial and psychological interventions, medication as appropriate and referral for further assessment and interventions
STEP 1: All known and suspected presentations of depression	Assessment, support, psychoeducation, active monitoring for poor response to interventions and need for more intensive services.

Fig. 14.3 The stepped-care model for depression

Brief Behavioral Interventions

- Make use of behavioral activation to help the patient make and track changes in sleep and other activities that promote improved well-being and symptom reduction.
- Use solution-focused brief therapy to help patient address presenting social stressors.
- Some websites provide free CBT handouts and worksheets that may be used for homework and timely implementation of brief depression therapy (www.psychology.tool/cbt.html, www.therapistaid.com/therapy-worksheets/depression/none and www.specialtybehavioralhealth.com/pdfs-cognitive-behavioral-therapy/).
- Make use of self-help/CBT via a book or a computerized CBT program (i.e., behavioral activation, problem solving, etc.); these should be guided and supported by a trained practitioner with six brief (15 min) in-person or telephone contacts over a 9-week period; two online programs that have been shown to be effective are Beating the Blues (www.beatingthebluesus.com) and MoodGYM (https://moodgym.anu.edu.au/welcome).

It is important to note here the research related to web- or computer-based interventions for depression. Studies have suggested that web- or computer-based interventions may promote a reduction of depression symptoms (Christensen, Griffiths, & Jorm, 2004; Clarke et al., 2014; Griffiths, Christensen, Jorm, Evans, & Groves, 2004; Mackinnon, Griffiths, & Christensen, 2008; Morris, Schueller, & Picard, 2015; Powell et al., 2013; Warmerdam, van Straten, Twisk, Riper, & Cuijpers, 2008). A recent meta-analysis (Cowpertwait & Clarke, 2013) found that web-based interventions had a medium effect compared to controls. Individuals in the treatment conditions showed significantly reduced depression symptoms particularly when they involved support or reminders to complete intervention components. Based on this evidence, we recommend that web-based interventions be used but with support and contact with the BHP.

Group Interventions

For some patients and in some settings, the use of brief group therapy may be helpful. The above brief interventions can also be used in a group setting and have the benefit of added social support from peers. Use of a structured group approach that includes topics or lessons address common problems for people with depression (e.g., improving sleep, understanding thoughts, feelings and behaviors, and improving interpersonal skills) can foster hope, lessen feelings of isolation and improve outcomes.

Step 3 Care

If the brief interventions mentioned above fail to address patient's symptoms and improve coping or initial assessment indicates moderately severe to severe depression, a more intensive outpatient therapy is required. BHPs will determine the next level of care required. For individuals presenting with severe depression, immediate referral to a specialty outpatient clinic and to their PCP or psychiatrist for medication management is indicated. As the BHP you will discuss these options and work with patients to make decisions about care that fits culture and needs. Individuals with subclinical depression or mild to moderate depression may benefit from continued services in the primary care setting. Rather than brief check-ins via an in-person office visit or phone call, the BHP will implement approximately six, 30 min sessions over an 8-week period. These brief interventions may resemble more traditional therapy and make use of more intense CBTs, interpersonal therapy, or behavioral activation depending on other presenting concerns. At this point, the BHP may decide to refer to longer-term therapy options if patients do not exhibit strong motivation to make changes and a willingness to commit to the short-term therapy over 8 weeks and have an overabundance of social stressors that impede brief work and low cognitive ability or education level (Cully & Teten, 2008).

CBTs—Cognitive-behavioral therapies are varied, and many have been found to be useful for improving depression symptoms especially those associated with dysfunctional thoughts about self and when behaviors as a result of these thoughts become problematic. To address these problems, therapist may:

- Provide additional psychoeducation about the way thoughts, feelings, and behaviors are connected, addressing that some thought-provoked behaviors have detrimental consequences for emotional states as well as in relationships.
- Use behavioral activation to promote small actions to promote movement and increase of previously pleasurable activities.
- Use solution-focused brief therapy to promote big changes over time by making small changes. The techniques of this therapy help patients focus on finding solutions rather than on past problems and to increase the use of behaviors that have been helpful in coping.
- Use acceptance and commitment therapy (ACT) to help patients better understand how avoidance of painful thoughts leads to more suffering and poor emotional regulation. Additionally, ACT focuses patients on making behavioral choices that are in accordance with defined values.

Interpersonal Therapy—Use of interpersonal therapy for depression places more focus on how the patient's relationships may be contributing to the maintenance of depression and how attention to the relationship may promote overall change for the patient (Robertson, Rushton, & Wurm, 2008). Some interventions that may be beneficial in addressing interpersonal disputes and role transitions relationships of persons with depression are listed below.

- Build a strong therapeutic alliance. This alliance is vital to helping the patient create a space to express emotions more freely without judgment. From this relationship the other techniques will be more impactful for patient change.
- Model and role play the use of active listening skills so that the patient (and supportive others) are better able to distinguish immediate beliefs about what a friend or family member is saying from what is truly being stated.
- Encourage emotional expression, and work with the patient to find different ways to express these emotions safely in family or work relationships. For example, teach patients to make use of "I statements."
- Johari window—This exercise promotes self-awareness and information processing about others, self, and relationships. A further explanation about this technique can be found at https://www.usc.edu/hsc/ebnet/Cc/awareness/Johari%20windowexplain.pdf.

While several of these strategies have been associated with more intensive, long-term therapy, it is possible to modify them for brief therapy by allowing yourself to be flexible in the moment. This flexibility calls on active listening skills to quickly hone in on the main one or two problems that are being identified by the patient and using clinical judgment to choose the intervention that may work best for the patient.

Step 4 Care

Patients in need of inpatient services or with severe or complex depression may begin treatment with more intensive interventions. These interventions may require a more immediate referral for specialty services such as inpatient crisis stabilization due to high risk for suicide attempt. However, there are services the BHP can provide until the patient is able to be seen by a specialty provider. First, the BHP can provide weekly follow-up sessions to monitor for deterioration in SI or psychosis that places the patient at higher risk. This weekly follow-up may also rely on a higher level of communication between the BHP and PCP and also may require a consult with a psychiatrist. For patients with a history of serious mental illness or in immediate danger from an abusive relationship, it may be important to help the patients make contacts into the community that will help them gain a safe place to be and help with the ongoing case management. For example, patients that are experiencing ongoing partner violence will benefit from information about local domestic violence shelters and planning for safety and leaving with the number to the National Domestic Violence Hotline—1.800.799.SAFE (7233).

What Does Not Work

Increasing access to care is a major reason why integrated care works. But are there things that we can do or fail to do that may result in harm to our patients? A few examples are listed below.

- Implement a depression care protocol without training everyone involved about the role that each individual plays as well as what to do when the BHP is absent from the clinic.
- Fail to conduct a risk assessment if a patient indicates SI. It is our duty to protect.
- Hesitate to refer immediately when the patient has severe depression, particularly when psychosis, substance use, chronic PTSD, or serious personality disorder is present. Other chapters in this book address these specific concerns more fully and will offer interventions that are appropriate to take.
- *Note: Some rural integrated care practices do not have extensive referral options. It is likely that these clinics will provide a wider range of services that also involve long-term more intensive psychotherapy due to a limitation in alternate care available. If a BHP is providing services in one of these types of clinics, work with the entire staff to increase training related to serious mental illness and how it can impact physical health as well as associated social risk factors.*

When to Refer to Specialty Mental Health

While many patients with depression can benefit from treatment in the primary care setting, sometimes it is in the best practice to refer the patient for more specialty care. It is important to help patients understand the nature or scope of the integrated model of your clinic. While some clinics, particularly in rural areas, provide a wide range of behavioral health services, most integrated care sites only provide brief interventions. Thus, it is important to discuss the options for care within your primary care settings and set expectations regarding number of sessions and continuity of care.

With this in mind, the following are general guidelines for referral to specialty care or co-management of therapy with another BHP (Trangle et al., 2016):

- Refer when there are emergency cases (e.g., high risk of death by suicide, presence of psychosis, etc.).
- Refer if the patient has comorbid substance use or PTSD that is seriously impacting daily functioning.
- Refer when the patient has complex psychosocial concerns or intellectual disability.
- Refer when patients also have a diagnosis of a personality disorder that is particularly severe and requires more intensive approaches such as dialectical behavioral therapy.

Role of the Primary Care Team in Depression Care

The above sections have addressed interventions for depression in primary care settings. It is important to know who may play a role in the depression care team. We recommend that a collaborative care (CC) approach be implemented. Practically, implementing CC requires monitoring and tracking changes with a clinical rating scale such as the PHQ-9 (Kroenke et al., 2001) and adjusting treatment as needed (Unützer, Harbin, Schoenbaum, & Druss, 2013).

The first and most important member of this team is the patient. The patient is the center of care and collaborates with the care team related to their concerns about medication and interventions that may be a best fit. While the patient is the most important member of the team, others in the primary care setting play major roles in supporting the patient in recovery. These members include the PCP, the care management staff (LPN or RN), a BHP (a doctoral level trained clinician is preferred; however, masters level trained clinicians may work in many settings), and, if available, a psychiatric consultant (Corso, 2016; Unützer et al., 2013). The role that each plays varies but should complement the other for best patient outcomes.

During an appointment the care management staff are the first trained staff to interact with the patient in regard to health concerns. During triage it is common for a nurse or medical assistant (MA) to ask about depression using the PHQ-2 or PHQ-9. Beyond screening, the nurse or MA may be the team member that alerts the PCP to patient concerns and symptoms related to depression so that this can be addressed during the visit. Care management staff may also be the facilitator between the PCP and psychiatric consultant as well as following up with patients in regard to adherence to medication therapy (Korso, Hunter, Dahl, Kallenberg, & Manson,, 2016; Unützer et al., 2013).

The PCP may be considered the head of the team promoting patient care related to depression. The PCP will be the provider who initially discusses depression symptoms with the patient and helps initiate a plan of action. The PCP can use the PHQ-9 to determine the patient's symptom severity and provide brief information about overall medication efficacy for the patient's current symptom severity. For example, research indicates that individuals with mild to moderate depression will find benefit in brief cognitive-behavioral therapies (CBTs) without the assistance of medication, while those with severe depression will likely need a combination of medication and more intensive therapy services (Davidson, 2010; DeRubeis et al., 2005). Once a decision has been made about approach, the PCP acts as a liaison between the patient and the BHP by introducing the BHP to the patient on a warm handoff.

BHPs can help fulfill several roles on the depression care team. Their primary role is to support the PCP in helping the patient manage or resolve depression symptoms. This will be done by providing brief therapy for depression (e.g., behavioral activation, solution-focused brief therapy), making referrals for specialty mental health as needed, and helping to monitor changes in depression symptoms as a result of interventions. Another major role for BHPs in primary care involves the screening of risks associated with suicidal ideation and helping high-risk patients acquire emergency services. As a part of helping adequately screen for suicidal ideation, they also may act as educators for the medical staff about additional warning signs and risk factors of suicidal ideations in patients with depression. These risks include substance use disorders, PTSD or other anxiety disorders, chronic pain, and serious physical illness (particularly those with traumatic brain injury or other central nervous system disorders). BHPs may also be called upon to help set standards for depression care that includes a schedule for screening all patients for depression along with protocols for care when a screening in positive. Lastly, BHPs may also be responsible in their settings for assessing clinic process and outcomes related to depression care. This topic will be addressed in the following section.

Finally, some collaborative care teams include a psychiatric consultant (psychiatrists and psychiatric nurse practitioners) who act as an advisor to the depression care team for patients that are not demonstrating improvements or may have treatment-resistant depression. Some locations may have a psychiatric consultant on staff that acts as the primary medication manager for patients with severe symptoms when the PCP views this as a necessity for best care.

Quality Improvement

Assessing the impact of care for depression care involves monitoring outcomes for individual patients and the overall success of the entire team. Depressive symptoms, as well as other health symptoms, should to be monitored with the PHQ-9 or other outcome measures throughout treatment. Monitoring patients change visit to visit also allows the team to more easily adjust interventions as needed to improve outcome. Additionally, it is important to measure how well the team's efforts to improve patients' health clinic-wide (fidelity to routinely screen all patients with the PHQ-2, to consistently provide diabetes education, and to follow up calls to ED visits) have impacted the overall patient health. Below are several suggestions for what to monitor to determine if interventions have been successful.

- Access to care—a standard assessment of access in healthcare is time to the third next available appointment (Institute for Healthcare Improvement, 2016). If this appointment is in 2 weeks, then the BHP will need to increase referral to outside specialty care or reduce the number of visits for less serious patient concerns (IHI, 2016).
- Along with access to care, measuring acceptance or refusal of recommended behavioral health services may help BHPs. This information may help the clinic change education practices about the mind-body connection.
- Response to treatment interventions—track overall change on the PHQ-9 across all patients.
- Impact of depression care on other healthcare (i.e. A1Cs, blood pressure, ED visits, etc.).

Much of this data can be obtained from the electronic health records (EHR). The ease of this data retrieval will mostly be a function of the type of EHR your clinic uses as well as how the related information is placed in the system. Information that is input via a free text method will be more difficult to remove from records. Data placed in the system through selection or check boxes are easier to collect. We advise working with your IT department to design templates that allows for easier extraction of data related to depression.

Depression care in the integrated care setting has been shown to reduce depression symptoms, improve access to care, and increase adherence to treatment and improve outcomes for those with comorbid diabetes (Katon et al., 2010; Lamers, Jonkers, Bosma, Knottnerus, & Van Eijk, 2011; Lang, 2003). However, effective outcomes start with a systematic and routine method of screening patients for depression symptoms, having a structured protocol for how patients that screen positive for depression will be further assessed, and making sure you have plenty of tools in your depression care toolbox which are important for improved patient outcomes. This chapter provides the reader with a basic structure to begin to care for patients with depression in the primary care setting.

References

Beating the Blues. (2016). Retrieved from https://www.beatingthebluesus.com/

Beekman, A. T. F., Deeg, D. J. H., Van Limbeek, J., Braam, A. W., De Vries, M. Z., & Van Tilburg, W. (1997). Criterion validity of the Center for Epidemiologic Studies Depression scale (CES-D): Results from a community-based sample of older subjects in the Netherlands. *Psychological Medicine, 27*, 231–235. Retrieved from https://www.researchgate.net/publication/14096630_Criterion_validity_of_the_Center_for_Epidemiologic_Studies_Depression_scale_CES-D_Results_from_a_community-based_sample_of_older_subjects_in_The_Netherlands

Bower, P., & Gilbody, S. (2005). Stepped care in psychological therapies: Access, effectiveness and efficiency. *The British Journal of Psychiatry, 186*, 11–17. https://doi.org/10.1192/bjp.186.1.11

Brown, R. L., & Rounds, L. A. (1995). Conjoint screening questionnaires for alcohol and drug abuse. *Wisconsin Medical Journal, 94*, 135–140. Retrieved from https://www.ncbi.nlm.nih.gov/pubmed/7778330

Bush, K., Kivlahan, D. R., McDonnel, M. B., Fihn, S. D., & Bradley, K. A. (1998). The AUDIT alcohol consumption questions (AUDIT-C): An effective brief screening test for problem drinking. *Archives of Internal Medicine, 158*, 1789–1795. https://doi.org/10.1001/archinte.158.16.1789

Centers for Disease Control and Prevention. (2016, September). Depression. Retrieved from http://www.cdc.gov/mentalhealth/basics/mental-illness/depression.htm

Christensen, H., Griffiths, K. M., & Jorm, A. F. (2004). Delivering interventions for depression by using the internet: Randomised controlled trial. *British Medical Journal, 328*, 265–270. https://doi.org/10.1192/bjp.185.4.342

Clarke, J., Proudfoot, J., Birch, M. R., Whitton, A. E., Parker, G., Manicavasgar, V., … Hadzi-Pavlovic, D. (2014). Effects of mental health self-efficacy on outcomes of a mobile phone and web intervention for mild-to-moderate depression, anxiety and stress: Secondary analysis of a randomized controlled trial. *BMC Psychiatry, 14*, 272. https://doi.org/10.1186/s12888-014-0272-1

Community Care Network of Virginia. (2012). Depression clinical care guideline.

Cox, J. L., Holden, J. M., & Sagovsky, R. (1987). The Edinburg postnatal depression scale. *British Journal of Psychiatry*, *150*, 782–786. https://doi.org/10.1192/bjp.150.6.782

Cowperwait, L., & Clarke, D. (2013). Effectiveness of web-based psychological interventions for depression. *International Journal of Mental Health and Addiction*, *11*,247-260. https://doi.org/10.1007/s11469-012-9416-z

Cully, J. A., & Teten, A. L. (2008). *A therapist's guide to brief cognitive behavioral therapy*. Houston: Department of Veteran's Affairs South Central MIRECC. Retrieved from http://www.mirecc.va.gov/visn16/docs/Therapists_Guide_to_Brief_CBTManual.pdf

Davidson, J. R. T. (2010). Major depressive disorder treatment guidelines in America and Europe. *Journal of Clinical Psychiatry*, *71*, e04. https://doi.org/10.4088/JCP.9058selc.04gry

Davidson, C. L., LaRicka, R., Grant, D. M., Judah, M. R., & Mills, A. C. (2011). Interpersonal suicide risk and ideation: The influence of depression and social anxiety. *Journal of Social and Clinical Psychology*, *30*, 842–855. https://doi.org/10.1521/jscp.2011.30.8.842

Depression in adults: recognition and management. (2016). Clinical guideline [CG90], p.16. Retrieved from https://www.nice.org.uk/guidance/cg90/chapter/1-Guidance#stepped-care

DeRubeis, R. J., Hollon, S. D., Amsterdam, J. D., Shelton, R. C., Young, P. R., Salomon, R. M., … Gallop, R. (2005). Cognitive therapy vs medications in the treatment of moderate to severe depression. *Archives of General Psychiatry*, *62*, 409–416. https://doi.org/10.1001/archpsyc.62.4.409

DeSantis, B., Jackson, M. J., Duncan, B. L., & Reese, R. J. (2016). Casting a wider net in behavioral health screening in primary care: A preliminary study of the outcome rating scale. *Primary Health Care Research & Development*, *18*, 1–6. https://doi.org/10.1017/S1463423616000311

Duncan, B. L., & Reese, R. J. (2015). The Partners for Change Outcome Management System (PCOMS): Revisiting the client's frame of reference. *Psychotherapy*, *52*, 391–401. https://doi.org/10.1037/pst0000026

Eaton, W. W., Smith, C., Ybarra, M., Muntaner, C., & Tien, A. (2004). Center for Epidemiologic Studies Depression Scale: Review and revision (CESD and CESD-R). In M. E. Maruish (Ed.), *The use of psychological testing for treatment planning and outcomes assessment: Instruments for adults* (Vol. 3, 3rd ed., pp. 363–377). Mahwah, NJ: Lawrence Erlbaum.

Ebell, M. H. (2008). Screening instruments for depression. *American Family Physician*, *78*, 244–246. Retrieved from http://www.aafp.org/afp/2008/0715/p244.html

Fuchs, C. H., Haradhvala, N., Hubley, S., Nash, J. M., Keller, M. B., Ashley, D., … Uebelacker, L. A. (2015). Physician actions following a positive PHQ-2: Implications for the implementation of depression screening in family practice. *Family Systems Health*, *33*, 18–27. https://doi.org/10.1037/fsh0000089

Gillaspy, J. A., & Murphy, J. J. (2011). Incorporating outcome and session rating scales in solution-focused brief therapy. In C. Franklin, T. Trepper, W. Gingerich, & E. McCollum (Eds.), *Solution-focused brief therapy*. New York: Oxford University Press.

Griffiths, K. M., Christensen, H., Jorm, A. F., Evans, K., & Groves, C. (2004). Effect of web-based depression literacy and cognitive-behavioural therapy interventions on stigmatizing attitudes to depression: Randomized controlled trial. *British Journal of Psychiatry*, *185*, 342–349. https://doi.org/10.1192/bjp.185.4.342

Hirschfield, R. M. A. (2002). The mood disorder questionnaire: A simple screening instrument for bipolar disorder. *Primary Care Companion, Journal of Clinical Psychology*, *4*, 9–11.

Hunter, C. L., Goodie, J. L., Oordt, M. S., & Dobmeyer, A. C. (2009). *Integrated behavioral health in primary care: Step-by-step guidance for assessment and intervention*. Washington, DC: American Psychological Association.

Institute for Healthcare Improvement. (2016). Third next available appointment. Retrieved from http://www.ihi.org/resources/Pages/Measures/ThirdNextAvailableAppointment.aspx

Intermountain Healthcare. (2015, February). *Management of Depression*. Retrieved from https://intermountainhealthcare.org/ext/Dcmnt?ncid=51061767

Johnson, J., Harris, E. S., Spitzer, R. L., & Williams, J. B. (2002). The patient health questionnaire for adolescents: Validation of an instrument for the assessment of mental disorders among adolescent primary care patients. *Journal of Adolescent Health*, *30*, 196–204.

Katon, W. J., Lin, E. H., Von Korff, M., Ciechanowski, P., Ludman, E. J., Young, B., … McCulloch, D. (2010). Collaborative care for patients with depression and chronic illnesses. *New England Journal of Medicine*, *363*, 2611–2620. https://doi.org/10.1056/NEJMoa1003955

Korso, K. A., Hunter, C. L., Dahl, O., Kallenberg, G. A., & Manson, L. (2016) Integrating behavioral health into the medical home: A rapid implementation guide. Phoenix, MD:Greenbranch Publishing.

Kroenke, K., Spitzer, R. L., & Williams, J. B. W. (2001). The PHQ-9: Validity of a brief depression severity measure. *Journal of General Internal Medicine*, *16*, 606–661. https://doi.org/10.1046/j.1525-1497.2001.016009606.x

Kroenke, K., Spitzer, R. L., & Williams, J. B. (2003). The patient health Questionnaire-2: Validity of a two-item depression screener. *Medical Care*, *41*, 1284–1292. https://doi.org/10.1097/01.MLR.0000093487.78664.3C

Lamers, F., Jonkers, C. C., Bosma, H., Knottnerus, J. A., & van Eijk, J. T. (2011). Treating depression in diabetes patients: Does a nurse-administered minimal psychological intervention affect diabetes-specific quality of life and glycemic control. *Journal of Advanced Nursing*, *67*, 788–799. https://doi.org/10.1111/j.1365-2648.2010.05540.x

Lang, A. J. (2003). Brief intervention for co-occurring anxiety and depression in primary care: A pilot study. *International Journal of Psychiatry in Medicine, 33*, 141–154. Retrieved from http://journals.sagepub.com/doi/pdf/10.2190/4FM9-T915-L7E3-EFMX

Li, C., Friedman, B., Conwell, Y., & Fiscella, K. (2007). Validity of the patient health questionnaire 2 (PHQ-2) in identifying major depression in older people. *Journal of the American Geriatrics Society, 55*, 596–602. https://doi.org/10.1111/j.1532-5415.2007.01103.x

Löwe, B., Kroenke, K., & Gräfe, K. (2005). Detecting and monitoring depression with a two-item questionnaire (PHQ-2). *Journal of Psychosomatic Research, 58*, 163–171. https://doi.org/10.1016/j.jpsychores.2004.09.006

Luoma, J. B., Martin, C. E., & Pearson, J. L. (2002). Contact with mental health and primary care providers before suicide: A review of the evidence. *American Journal of Psychiatry, 159*, 909–916. https://doi.org/10.1176/appi.aip.159.6.909

Mackinnon, A., Griffiths, K. M., & Christensen, H. (2008). Comparative randomized trial of online cognitive-behavioural therapy and an information website for depression: 12-month outcomes. *British Journal of Psychiatry, 192*, 130–134. https://doi.org/10.1192/bjp.bp.106.032078

Miller, S. D., Duncan, B. L., Brown, J., Sparks, J. A., & Claud, D. A. (2003). The outcome rating scale: A preliminary study of the reliability, validity, and feasibility of a brief visual analog measure. *Journal of Brief Therapy, 2*, 91–100. Retrieved from http://www.researchgate.net/profile/Scott_Miller12/publication/242159752_The_Outcome_Rating_Scale_A_Preliminary_Study_of_the_Reliability_Validity_and_Feasibility_of_a_Brief_Visual_Analog_Measure/links/02e7e52e7b2daab9a1000000.pdf

MoodGYM. (2016). Retrieved from https://moodgym.anu.edu.au/welcome

Morris, R. R., Schueller, S. M., & Picard, R. W. (2015). Efficacy of a web-based, crowdsourced peer-to-peer cognitive reappraisal platform for depression: Randomized controlled trial. *Journal of Medical Internet Research, 17*, e72. https://doi.org/10.2196/jmir.4167

Nassir, G. S., Miller, C. J., Berv, D. A., Klugman, J., Rosenquist, K. J., & Pies, R. W. (2005). Sensitivity and specificity of a new bipolar spectrum diagnostic scale. *Journal of Affective Disorders, 84*, 273–277. https://doi.org/10.1016/S0165-0327(03)00196-4

National Council of State Legislature. (2013, January). *Possession of firearms by people with mental illness*. Retrieved from http://www.ncsl.org/research/civil-and-criminal-justice/possession-of-a-firearm-by-the-mentally-ill.aspx

Nepon, J., Belik, S., Bolton, J., & Sareen, J. (2010). The relationship between anxiety disorders and suicide attempts: Findings from the national epidemiologic survey on alcohol and related condition. *Depression and Anxiety, 27*, 791–798. https://doi.org/10.1002/da.20674.

Pompili, M., Innamoratia, M., Rihmerc, Z., Gondac, X., Serafinia, G., Akiskald, H., … Girardia, P. (2012). Cyclothymic–depressive–anxious temperament pattern is related to suicide risk in 346 patients with major mood disorders. *Journal of Affective Disorders, 136*, 405–411.

Powell, J., Hamborg, T., Stallard, N., Burls, A., McSorley, J., Bennett, K., … Christensen, H. (2013). Effectiveness of a web-based cognitive-behavioral tool to improve mental well-being in the general population: Randomized controlled trial. *Journal of Medical Internet Research, 15*, e2. https://doi.org/10.2196/jmir.2240

Pratt, L. A., & Brody, D. J. (2014). *Depression in the U.S. household population, 2009-2012* (National Center for Health Statistics: Data Brief No. 172). Retrieved from http://www.cdc.gov/nchs/data/databriefs/db172.htm

Robertson, M., Rushton, P., & Wurm, C. (2008). Interpersonal psychotherapy: An overview. *Psychotherapy in Australia, 14*, 46–54. Retrieved from http://www.psychotherapy.com.au/fileadmin/site_files/pdfs/InterpersonalPsychotherapy.pdf

Rush, A. J., Trivedi, M. H., Ibrahim, H. M., Carmody, T. J., Arnow, B., Klein, D. N., … Keller, M. B. (2003). The 16-item quick inventory of depressive symptomatology (QIDS), clinician rating (QIDS-C), and self-report (QIDS-SR): A psychometric evaluation in patients with chronic major depression. *Biological Psychiatry, 54*, 573–583. https://doi.org/10.1016/S0006-3223(02)01866-8

Schonfeld, W. H., Verboncoeur, C. J., Fifer, S. K., Lipschutz, R. C., Lubeck, D. P., & Buesching, D. P. (1997). The functioning and well-being of patients with unrecognized anxiety disorders and major depressive disorder. *Journal of Affective Disorder, 43*, 105–119.

Sheikh, J. I., & Yesavage, J. A. (1986). Geriatric depression scale (GDS): Recent evidence and development of a shorter version. *Clinical Gerontology, 5*, 165–173.

Suicide. (2016, September). World Health Organization. Retrieved from http://www.who.int/mediacentre/factsheets/fs398/en/

Trangle, M., Gursky, J., Haight, R., Hardwig, J., Hinnenkamp, T., Kessler, D. … Myszkowski, M. (2016). Adult depression in primary care, 17th edition. *Institute for Clinical Systems Improvement*. Retrieved September 21, 2016, from http://icsi.org/assest/fnhdm3/Depr.pdf

University of Michigan Health System (UMHS). Depression. Ann Arbor (MI): Augest 2011.

Unützer, J., Harbin, H., Schoenbaum, M., & Druss, B. (2013). The collaborative care model: An approach for integrating physical and mental health care in Medicaid health homes. *Centers for Health Care Strategies*. Retrieved from https://www.medicaid.gov/state-resource-center/medicaid-state-technical-assistance/health-homes-technical-assistance/downloads/hh-irc-collaborative-5-13.pdf

Warmerdam, L., van Straten, A., Twisk, J., Riper, H., & Cuijpers, P. (2008). Internet-based treatment for adults with depressive symptoms: Randomized controlled trial. *Journal of Medical Internet Research, 10*, e43. https://doi.org/10.2196/jmir.1094

Weissman, M. M., Orvaschel, H., & Padian, N. (1980). Children's symptom and social functioning self-report scales: Comparison of mothers' and children's reports. *Journal of Nervous and Mental Disorders, 168*, 736–740.

Williams, J. W., Jr., Noel, P. H., Cordes, J. A., Ramirez, G., & Pignone, M. (2002). Is this patient clinically depressed. *Journal of the American Medical Association, 287*, 1160–1170. https://doi.org/10.1001/jama.287.9.1160

Yesavage, J. A., Brink, T. L., Rose, T. L., Lum, O., Huang, V., Adey, M., & Leirer, V. O. (1983). Development and validation of a geriatric depression screening scale: A preliminary report. *Journal of Psychiatry Research, 17*, 37–49.

Diabetes Management 15

David E. Bauman, Bridget R. Beachy, and Stacy A. Ogbeide

Never in human history has there been as many medications and technologies available to help people manage their diabetes, yet the sequelae of poorly managed diabetes continue to wreak havoc on patients and health-care systems alike. While estimates of the prevalence rates of diabetes mellitus (DM) in the United States range from 6 to 13% (Centers for Disease Control [CDC], 2011; Li et al., 2011), upward to 14% of *all* health-care expenditures can be traced back to poor DM management (Mokdad et al., 2003). Diabetes management, especially for type 2 DM, is largely contingent upon behavioral factors related to ones' eating, physical activity, and medication treatment adherence habits. Viewing DM management through the lens of the Quadruple Aim (i.e., improved outcomes, decreased cost, improved patient experience, and increased support for medical providers), health-care systems and agencies are in dire need of implementing evidence-informed/evidence-based treatments in a cost-effective, stepped-care, and team-based manner. The authors of this chapter aim to organize ideas for accomplishing this all while honoring the humanity of patients. To this end, we will provide a brief overview of DM, screening and diagnostic procedures, and the research on tried and true behavioral interventions. We will also address the barriers and obstacles to DM management and the specific roles and strategies the interdisciplinary teams can utilize to help patients manage DM, starting from the least to the most intensive.

Before we "jump into the deep," we want to take a moment to expand upon what we mean by providing care while honoring the humanity of patients. Currently, there is a subtle but radical and powerful philosophical shift that is happening in health care. "Good" health is no longer achieved by merely producing a reduction in symptoms; rather we want to help patients in the pursuit of living a meaningful life. This means we may say to patients, "we don't just want to help you lower your A1C, we want to help you live with purpose and meaning." This is a powerful message. It is a message of humanity. Ponder the difference between saying, "we are here to treat your diabetes," versus "we are interested in helping you live life to its fullest while living with diabetes." Not tying data outcomes to what matters to people in real life may be one missing ingredient that has contributed to limited gains in

D.E. Bauman, Psy.D. (✉)
Family Medicine, Central Washington Family Medicine Residency, Yakima, WA, USA
e-mail: Davidbauman4@gmail.com

B.R. Beachy, Psy.D.
Behavioral Health, Community Health of Central Washington, Yakima, WA, USA
e-mail: bridgetbeachy@gmail.com

S.A. Ogbeide, Psy.D.
Departments of Family and Community Medicine and Psychiatry, UT Health San Antonio, San Antonio, TX, USA
e-mail: stacy.ogbeide@gmail.com

A. Maragakis, W.T. O'Donohue (eds.), *Principle-Based Stepped Care and Brief Psychotherapy for Integrated Care Settings*, https://doi.org/10.1007/978-3-319-70539-2_15

DM management, despite advances in technology. Many refer to this as a shortcoming of the biomedical model and call for the implementation of the biopsychosocial perspective to help infuse "whole person care."

Another missing ingredient that may be contributing to the paradox of advanced technologies without the leaps and bounds we were hoping to gain is the notion that we may be focusing on symptoms rather than the real problem. Meaning, DM and its associated risk factors may be symptoms of much deeper issues. As evidence regarding adverse childhood experiences (ACEs) continues to mount (for more information on ACEs, please see https://www.cdc.gov/violenceprevention/acestudy/), we must understand that behavior does not happen in a vacuum. People engage in certain behaviors for a reason, and that reason may lie in hardships experienced in peoples' lives. Ranging from enduring parental separation, parental mental illness, parental substance use, and family member imprisonment to incurring physical, sexual, and emotional abuse and neglect and living without sufficient resources, these ACEs often create conditions in which patients have a hard time valuing themselves. While we focus on stepped-care, behavioral approaches to DM management, we will do so with the overarching goal of encouraging providers of all disciplines to simultaneously work with patients on helping them value themselves while linking their DM management with what they find important in this life.

Overview of Diabetes

Diabetes mellitus can be broken into two distinct conditions or types (i.e., type 1 and type 2), with each having a different prevalence rate, etiology, management/treatment strategy, and presentation of symptoms. Specifically, type 1, which accounts for less than 10% of all DM cases, is largely based on genetic predispositions. Individuals with no family history of type 1 DM have less than half a percent chance of being diagnosed (Tillil & Köbberling, 1987); however, for monozygotic twins, there is a 65% concordance rate by the age of 60 (Redondo, Jeffrey, Fain, Eisenbarth, & Orban, 2008). Forty-five percent of all type 1 cases are diagnosed before the age of 10; however, 25% are diagnosed in adulthood (Duncan, 2006; Fagot-Campoagna et al., 2000; Lipton et al., 2005). Furthermore, there appears to be a distinct bimodal distribution of age of diagnosis, with a peak being seen at the age of 4–6 years old and another at the age of 10–14 years old (Elamin, Omer, Zein, & Tuvemo, 1992; Felner et al., 2005). Due to type 1 being caused by the body's inability to produce insulin, symptoms range from increased thirst and frequent urination, bedwetting in children, extreme hunger, unintended weight loss, irritability and other mood changes, as well as fatigue and weakness (Mayo Clinic, 2014). Due to these symptoms overlapping greatly with common mental and behavioral health disorders seen in adolescents, it is paramount that medical and behavioral health providers are cognizant of these symptoms.

Type 2 accounts for over 90% of all DM cases (Mokdad et al., 2003) and is typically diagnosed after puberty; however, rates in children are increasing at an alarming pace (Mokdad et al., 2003). As we mentioned, type 1 is largely dependent on genetic factors, and while type 2 appears to have an association with genetic predispositions, it is more related to lifestyle factors (Meigs, Cupples, & Wilson, 2000). Type 2 DM is due to the body's resistance to insulin and being unable to produce impactful levels of insulin (Mayo Clinic, 2016). Symptoms of type 2 include increased thirst and frequent urination, increased hunger, weight loss, fatigue, blurred vision, slow-healing sores or frequent infections, and areas of darkened skin (Mayo Clinic, 2016). Due to the symptoms of type 2 DM overlapping with other common medical and behavioral concerns, vigilance and proper assessment are needed to ensure accurate diagnosis and intervention.

Risk factors to assess/screen. Risk factors have been identified for both type 1 and type 2 DM. Both type 1 and type 2 DM have links to genetic predispositions, with type 1 having significant genetic underpinnings. Additionally, researchers are beginning to identify potential risk factors associated with type 1, including viral infections, poor diet, and different levels of socioeconomic statuses (Levitsky & Misra, 2016).

There have been a number of risk factors associated with type 2 DM. Specifically, having a family history of DM increases (i.e., fivefold) the likelihood of an individual developing the condition (Meigs et al., 2000). Ethnicity also appears to be a risk factor, with Asians, Hispanics, and African-Americans having higher-risk levels (Shai et al., 2006). Being overweight or obese further increases one's risk for developing type 2 DM (Helmrich, Ragland, Leung, & Paffenbarger, 1991; Mokdad et al., 2003; Nguyen, Nguyen, Lane, & Wang, 2011). Lastly, lifestyle factors, including, lack of exercise, poor diet, smoking, sleep problems, and high alcohol consumption, have all been associated with increased risk of type 2 DM (Reis et al., 2011).

Effective Ways to Screen in the Primary Care Setting

While type 1 and 2 DM have distinctive differences, screening and diagnosing procedures are largely similar. Recommendation for screening all patients for DM has not been established; thus, having the health-care team educated on the appropriate indicators of DM will assure more appropriate diagnostic procedures are conducted. The United States Preventive Service Task Force (USPSTF) has assigned a "B" rating (i.e., high confidence that the net benefit is moderate or substantial and is highly recommend) to screening asymptomatic adults for type 2 DM who have a blood pressure greater than 135/80 mmHg and all overweight or obese adults aged 40–70 years old (Norris, Kansagara, Bougatsos, Nygren, & Fu, 2008; USPSTF, 2016).

Diabetes mellitus is diagnosed through assessing an individual's fasting glucose, or blood sugar, levels (McCulloch & Hayward, 2017). It is important to note that individuals may be asymptomatic; however, if risk factors of DM are present, screening the individual's glucose levels is appropriate. For both type 1 and 2, a fasting (i.e., no caloric intake in the past 8 h) glucose greater than 100 mg/dL is considered abnormal and could be grounds, if paired with simultaneous symptoms of DM, for initiating further testing. A fasting blood glucose level greater than 126 mg/dL, regardless of concurrent symptoms, is considered abnormal and should initiate further testing. If an abnormal fasting glucose level is identified, initiating a hemoglobin A1C (A1C), which is the most common DM measure, is recommended. The A1C is a 3-month average of an individual's blood sugar levels. Scores ranging from 5.7 to 6.4 identify individuals who are at risk for developing DM or who are considered to have prediabetes. When identified, individuals should be initiated into a preventative protocol, or pathway, which will be discussed in further sections.

While assessing one's A1C when diagnosing DM is paramount, we also suggest using functionality screeners to help provide additional perspective to the patient's situation. Two brief functionality measures that have been developed for primary care are the DUKE Health Profile (Parkerson, Broadhead, & Tse, 1990) and the World Health Organization Quality of Life Brief (WHOQOL-BREF; WHO, 1998). By using such screeners, providers are able to identify other potential barriers that may be impacting the patient's ability in managing their DM. Furthermore, by utilizing a functionality screener, the focus of subsequent treatment will not solely be on improving one's AlC; rather, focus will simultaneously be on improving the individual's quality of life. While we highly recommend using the DUKE or WHOQOL-BREF for individuals being assessed for DM, we also recommend all patients within medical centers have yearly assessments of their functionality or quality of life.

Other assessment measures that should be considered with DM are the Patient Health Questionnaire-9 item (PHQ-9; Kroenke, Spitzer, & Williams, 2001) and the 17-item Diabetes Distress Scale (DDS17; Polonsky et al., 2005). The PHQ-9 is a brief screener for depression that is routinely used in the primary care setting. Egede and Ellis (2010) found a significant link between DM and depression, as well as individuals who are depressed having significant difficulty with treatment adherence, poor A1C control, as well as higher rates of complications and health-care costs. Using the PHQ-9 routinely with patients with DM can be a useful way of quickly identifying and intervening with depressive symptoms, which may in turn improve DM management. Furthermore, the DDS17 is a brief measure that assesses the emotional distress of being diagnosed with DM. Fisher, Hessler, Polonsky, and Mullan (2012) found higher scores on the DDS17 are associated with poorer A1C control, lower self-efficacy, as well poorer diet and physical inactivity. Both the PHQ-9 and DDS17 are appropriate brief measures for primary care and should be considered when developing assessment measures for DM management.

How to Further Assess if a Screen Returns Positive

Individuals who have an A1C of 6.5 or greater are deemed to have DM, and behavioral and medical intervention should be considered and subsequently initiated. As we discussed earlier, once a positive A1C is identified, further assessments (e.g., quality of life, depression, distress, etc.) should be completed to help identify proper interventions, which will most likely include a combination of behavioral and pharmacology treatments. As we have and will continue to discuss throughout this chapter, the patient's context should be evaluated before any treatment plan is implemented. Research has shown that providers that understand the patient's perspective or context have a higher likelihood of establishing realistic goals, as well as having patients adhere to treatment recommendations (Martin, Williams, Haskard, & DiMateo, 2005). We suggest using the Contextual Interview (Fig. 15.1), which is an efficient and effective way of gathering this information and allows for accurate and intentional interventions that can promote the desired behavioral change. This interview has been adapted from Robinson, Gould, & Strosahl (2010) *Love, Work, Play, Health Behaviors.* Physicians and advanced practice clinicians (APCs) can also be taught to use this interview; however, we are aware of time constraints, especially if they are managing other aspects of care.

Contextual Interview
❖ **Love (Identify the patient's social relationships)** ➢ Living situation ➢ Relationship status ➢ Family ➢ Friends ➢ Spiritual life
❖ **Work (Identify the patient's work and financial situation)** ➢ Work ➢ Source of income
❖ **Play (Identify meaningful activities to patient)** ➢ Hobbies ➢ Fun activities
❖ **Health Risk & Behaviors** ➢ Tobacco use ➢ Alcohol use ➢ Marijuana use ➢ Street drugs use ➢ Caffeine use ➢ Diet/supplements ➢ Exercise ➢ Sleep ➢ Sexual activity

Fig. 15.1 Contextual Interview

Depending on the availability of a multidisciplinary team, different pathways can be established to help guide the intensity of treatment and the providers involved when working with patients who have DM. In robust medical systems that have integrated care teams, which include behavioral health providers (BHPs) and nutritionists, patients that are identified as prediabetic (i.e., A1C = 5.7–6.4) could be referred immediately to these providers in hopes of preventing the individual from developing DM. This same pathway could be made for all patients who have been newly diagnosed with DM. However, if availability of BHPs is limited, ensuring that highly uncontrolled DM (e.g., A1C > 9.0) and patients with DM who have significant contextual factors influencing their treatment adherence and care should be regularly referred to BHPs. Again, the correct pathway is dependent on the availability of these providers.

While developing pathways for patients that are identified as DM is important, we also believe it is important to be aware of and assess possible barriers to DM management. To us, these barriers are multifaceted and interconnected. As BHPs working in integrated care settings, we see the toll poor DM management takes on the patient, provider, and health-care system. We have witnessed firsthand what does not work on a daily basis, which does serve as fodder to figure out what can work better. Table 15.1 provides an

Table 15.1

Barriers for successful prevention and management of diabetes
• Patient factors: Patients who have…
– *Fear of judgment*: Due to fear of judgment and insecurity, patients often have a hard time being fully transparent with their medical team
– *Depression*: High levels of depression often make it hard for patients to connect with what they value; high comorbidity between depression and DM
– *Low health literacy*: Difficulty understanding medication regimen
– *Asymptomatic presentations*: Asking patients to take medications when they don't feel sick
– *Difficulty foreseeing long-term consequences*: Peoples' difficulty in seeing future problems with the same level of urgency as imminent problems
– *Adverse childhood experiences*: Patients often have deep-seated difficulties with self-esteem in which taking care of themselves is often put on the back burner
– *The tendency to put other family members' care above their own*: Parents who neglect their own health while taking care of kids or children taking care of aging parents
– *Stress*: It is hard for patients with ubiquitously high stress levels to make these lifestyle changes, as making changes is stressful in and of itself
– *Reduced opportunities for joy and pleasure in life*: Patients may over rely on eating behavior as a means of coping and gratification
– *Misconceptions about DM medications*: Patient who worry about "getting hooked" on insulin or the medication worsening the condition
– *Cultural belief systems that are leery of medication*: Apprehension about taking medication due to cultural norms
• Provider factors: Providers who…
– *Use "scared straight" strategies*: Although it may seem like common sense to "scare" patients about the severity of their condition, it can actually have the opposite of intended effect
– *Experience demoralization*: Physicians may feel demoralized, especially if they feel they are being held accountable for so many factors that are seemingly outside their reach
– *Lecture patients*: This only works to increase patients' fear and judgment
– *Are overworked and underpaid in primary care*: Long hours take their toll on primary care providers, who often are the least paid
– *Experience time constraints*: It is hard to address issues in depth in 15–20 min appointments
– *Manage complex comorbidities*
– *Lack training in teaching patients behavioral management strategies*
– *Lack of training in patient-centered communication skills*: It is crucial for providers to be able to elicit the patients' perspectives, engage in shared decisionmaking, and/or use the teach-back method (i.e., patients teach the treatment plan back to the provider)

(continued)

Table 15.1 (continued)

Barriers for successful prevention and management of diabetes
• *Societal factors include*: – *Overemphasis on medications*: Seeing medications as the sole key to managing one's health problems – *Stigma*: Conditions being associated with lifestyle factors may lead to patients feeling "blamed" and ashamed of their health problems – *Financial barriers*: Cost of medication, lack of appropriate health care, lack of transportation, etc.
• *System factors include*: – *Inefficient electronic health records*: Arduous process to charting and inefficient electronic health records that stymy health-care systems in providing appropriate care – *Siloed approach to health care*: This makes communication difficult between primary care providers, the specialty mental and behavioral health systems, and the medical specialists

overview of some of the notable barriers for successful prevention and management of diabetes broken up into four major categories including patient, provider, societal, and systemic factors. These barriers should be considered and assessed when working on pathway protocols to help assess and intervene with patients who have DM.

Evidence-Based Stepped-Care and Brief Psychotherapeutic Approaches

It can be overwhelming looking at these obstacles; however, it is essential that these difficulties are addressed in order to achieve the desired outcome. If we begin to apply solutions to an equation that we have yet to fully understand, we will never be able to solve the equation accurately. One of the antidotes to the above obstacles is employing stepped-based care. It is important to note that stepped-care goes beyond interventions and does not only include an increase in intervention intensity but also providers and staff members involved. In integrated care models, particularly the Primary Care Behavioral Health (PCBH) model (Robinson & Reiter, 2016), BHPs do not only provide brief interventions but work with the staff, providers, and medical system to fortify primary care services. In the following section, we will discuss both aspects of stepped-care, ways of increasing the intensity of behavioral interventions, as well as the individuals involved in care.

Before we discuss stepped-based care that can be implemented (i.e., psychoeducation, bibliotherapy/e-health, group and brief individual interventions), we wanted to provide an overview of the evidence of behavioral interventions for DM management. Specifically, we will focus on the evidence regarding lifestyle changes, including diet and physical activity when managing DM.

Table 15.2 Diabetes self-management education content areas

1. Diabetes disease process and treatment options
2. Nutritional management
3. Physical activity
4. Using medications safely and for maximal therapeutic effectiveness
5. Monitoring blood glucose
6. Preventing, detecting, and treating acute complications
7. Preventing, detecting, and treating chronic complications
8. Personal strategies to address psychosocial issues and concerns
9. Personal strategies to promote health and behavior change

What works behaviorally? For any provider who works in primary care, it is a common place to recommend lifestyle changes for individuals who have been identified as having prediabetes or DM. These lifestyle changes are usually in the form of improved diet and exercise. The American Diabetes Association (ADA) recommends that individuals receive information regarding the standards for diabetes self-management education (DSME; Haas et al., 2012). These standards can be found in Table 15.2.

These standards are commonly disseminated in formal diabetic education classes. With appropriate DSME, there appears to be a moderate improvement of A1C control (Cavanaugh et al., 2008). Increasing, fortifying, and fostering the patients' social support have been deemed to be a significant factor in the delivery and implementation of DSME (Hassan & Heptulla, 2010). Having interventions that are tailored to individuals and their families, as well as avoiding scare tactics, is also associated with improved effectiveness of DSME (Anderson, Funnell, Burkhart, Gillard, & Nwankwo, 2003).

Although DSME can be effective in assisting patients to initiate lifestyle changes and subsequently lowering their A1Cs, at times upward to a full percentage point in children (Haas et al., 2012; Norris, Lau, Smith, Schmid, & Engelgau, 2002), it can take significant time to implement. Specifically, UpToDate (Schreiner & Ponder, 2016) recommends 4–6 h for initial DSME implementation, as well as routine follow-up when working with children who have DM. The feasibility of such interventions for both primary care and patients is dubious.

Further, long-term research is lacking regarding patients' ability to maintain behavioral changes made through DSME interventions. While there is a small but significant improvement in A1Cs for individuals who attend diabetic education classes, there appears to be no significant difference in quality of life measures (Liang et al., 2011; Pal et al., 2013; Saffari, Ghanizadeh, & Koenig, 2014). Which begs the question, if a person is not able to improve their quality of life, how meaningful is the intervention? Further looking into research regarding diet-only interventions for DM management, there is a clear relationship between improved diet and lowered A1C (Henry, Scheaffer, & Olefsky, 1985; Niskanen, Uusitupa, Sarlund, Siitonen, & Pyörälä, 1990; Norris et al., 2004). However, there is actually very little evidence that patients with DM will maintain dietary improvements long term (Niskanen et al., 1990; Norris et al., 2004), which is a common shortcoming seen across the board for chronic conditions (e.g., obesity, hypertension, etc.). Thus, while education regarding appropriate diet for DM is suggested and should be provided, the evidence suggests there is more needed to sufficiently manage one's DM.

Exercise and increased physical activity appears to be beneficial in DM management. Specifically, after controlling for weight loss, exercise alone has been shown to lower patients' A1C levels (Jeon, Lokken, Hu, & van Dam, 2007; Umpierre et al., 2011). Recommendations for exercise mirror standard recommendations for adults, which is 30–60 min per day, totaling 150 min per week that combines cardio with resistance activities. Unfortunately similar to diet interventions, it is estimated that 50% of individuals are unable to maintain the recommended physical activity long term (Jeon et al., 2007; Umpierre et al., 2011).

Psychoeducation. At the most basic level, BHPs can meet directly with patients with DM and implement psychoeducation regarding DSME. BHPs should focus on interventions that educate patients on the condition itself, ways of identifying acute and chronic concerns, and improving diet and physical activity. The most basic stepped-care approach in managing diabetes is providing information and psychoeducation through reading materials. We recommend utilizing handouts from the American Diabetes Association (ADA; http://www.diabetes.org/research-and-practice/we-support-your-doctor/patient-education-materials.html), as well as the website Learning About Diabetes, which provides all handouts in English and Spanish (www.learningaboutdiabetes.org). It is paramount that any reading materials provided, whether from an aforementioned website or preexisting electronic health record, to be screened for reading and literacy levels. We also recommend to not overload the patient with reading materials. A great way of ensuring this is to identify one or two handouts that are relevant to the patient's situation and provide hard copies of these handouts for the patient to take home while also providing information to them regarding how they can obtain additional handouts/information.

Bibliotherapy and e-health resources. Bibliotherapy and e-health resources are another minimal intensity stepped-care approach that can have profound impacts on DM management and patients' understanding of DM. Regarding DM self-help books, we again recommend utilizing the ADA in identifying potential diabetes self-help books and other reading materials (http://www.diabetes.org/living-with-diabetes/). We also recommend Gregg, Callaghan, and Hayes (2007) self-help book that provides readers a contextual approach to managing DM. Regarding websites or e-health resources, we recommend utilizing the same websites (i.e., ADA and Learning About Diabetes) mentioned earlier. While having lists of these resources readily available for patients is useful, we also recommend medical centers to keep these reading materials on-site and offer them to patients who are interested. Particularly in low SES settings, having these materials free and available may prove to be beneficial. As was the case with psychoeducation, reading levels must be assessed before providing to patients to ensure patient comprehension.

Group classes. Group classes are another way to amplify the intensity and population served by the medical team. We recommend having group diabetic classes include a number of team members. If possible, having a dietician/nutritionist, medical provider, and BHP is ideal. We have completed such groups with these team members and found great success. Groups should be open, stand-alone classes that focus on providing basic DSME, as well as experiential exercises that promote wellness, self-compassion, and valued engagement (Strosahl, Robinson, & Gustavsson, 2012). Families of patients should be welcomed to attend, as familial factors can interfere with treatment success.

Individual interventions. BHPs can also meet with patients individually to set SMART goals that include the DSME recommendations. We again want to emphasize the importance of gathering the patient's contextual information before any goals are established. Without this information, treatment plans and interventions will often fall short due to major factors impacting treatment adherence not being addressed or identified.

Once patients are provided information regarding DM and subsequent management, as well as patient contextual information is gathered, we recommend working with patients on self-management goals. However, before doing so we must first establish the reasons it is important for patients to manage their DM. This is a technique taken from Motivational Interviewing, as well as Acceptance and Commitment Therapy. Asking the question, "what makes it important for you to manage your diabetes?" is a great way of ascertaining this information. If the patient replies, "it is important for my health," we recommend following up with, "If you had improved health, what types of activities would you be doing? What could you do more of in your life?" The purpose of this clarification is to identify what is driving the patient to take care of themselves. As we said at the beginning of this chapter, patients will struggle to care for themselves if they do not view themselves as being worthy of care. If the patient is able to identify a specific reason or value related to managing their health, such as being able to spend more time with family or interact with their children, the likelihood of their self-management goal increases significantly. If the patient is unable to identify what makes taking care of their DM important to them, it may be a futile endeavor to set a self-management goal.

Higher levels of individual intervention intensity may include motivational interviewing, solution-focused, behavioral, cognitive behavioral, third-wave cognitive behavioral (e.g., Acceptance and Commitment Therapy [ACT], Focused Acceptance and Commitment Therapy [FACT], mindfulness based, etc.), and other problem-solving techniques.

When to Refer to External Specialty Care

Poorly managed psychiatric conditions lead to poor management of self-care behaviors (e.g., diet and exercise), poor metabolic control, and a decrease in overall functioning (Groot, Golden, & Wagner, 2016). Patients with severe mental illness (e.g., bipolar disorder, schizophrenia) are twice as likely to develop type 2 DM and experience premature mortality compared to the general population due to complications (Groot et al., 2016). Thus, primary care teams should recognize and treat comorbid conditions in addition to diabetes-related distress. Rubin and Peyrot (2001) suggest the following step-by-step for clinical care of comorbid psychiatric conditions:

1. Identify patients with diabetes-related distress.
2. Apply evidence-based behavioral treatments to treat diabetes-related distress.
3. Identify patients with psychiatric disorders (e.g., routine screening of depression with the PHQ-9).
4. Treat psychiatric conditions or refer patients to specialty mental health services when appropriate.

Primary care teams are encouraged to begin with behavioral interventions that can be implemented during clinic visits prior to using more intensive behavioral interventions. If psychiatric symptoms are identified and severe, and the BHP is appropriately trained, psychiatric symptoms should be treated first. If the BHP is unable to treat the psychiatric condition within the clinic, the patient should be referred to specialty mental health services. Once the current episode of the psychiatric condition is treated, the DM care team should closely monitor patients' symptoms in the instance of a return of symptoms. Of note, we encourage primary care teams that have established and robust integrated models of care to first treat these concerns in primary care. This again, is the essence of the stepped-care approach, and when the initial intensity levels of treatment are not providing desired outcomes, a referral to specialty services should be considered. However, it is paramount to not skip the first step, which is to apply the first level of stepped-care, which usually occurs in primary care.

The Role of the Medical Team

We want our clinical team to help neutralize the barriers every step of the way. Many clinical teams may consist of medical assistants, nurses, advanced practice clinicians (i.e., nurse practitioners and physician assistants), and physicians. Depending on resources, pharmacists, case managers or social workers, dieticians, care managers, or behavioral health providers may round out the interdisciplinary clinical team. These interprofessional teams have shown success in improving outcomes for patients with DM (Willens, Cripps, Wilson, Wolff, & Rothman, 2011). Having the overall organization committed to providing excellent service is also important; thus clinic managers and front desk staff can also have a role to play. We also suggest your clinic look to make connections with specialty services, both medical and behavioral health. Of course, having as many resources in-house will reduce barriers; however, we know this may not always be feasible, particularly for rural and underserved areas.

Front desk staff. One often overlooked aspect is the role clinic managers and front desk staff can play. Having reading material available and accessible in the waiting rooms is a good way to help educate patients about preventive lifestyle strategies. Make sure these materials are written at approximately a sixth grade reading or less to increase the likelihood of knowledge acquisition and retention. Having warm and empathic front desk staff as the first people the patients interact with sets the stage for putting patients at the center of care. It gives them the message that they are respected and cared for.

Front desk staff can also be one of the "gatekeepers" in getting patients on board with additional services that will assist with their DM management (e.g., behavioral health, nutrition, etc.). Training front desk staff on how to introduce these services and answer questions will present a united front, as well as demonstrate to patients that the additional resources are part of usual care.

Nurses and medical assistants. The medical assistants and nurses should be well versed in how exercise and diet changes can impact diabetes. They should readily have on hand diabetes blood sugar logs, exercise and diet logs, and other handouts with sample meal plans in English and other common languages served at the clinic. They may have an up-to-date list of the most helpful free apps that can be downloaded on smartphones to help increase adhering to dietary recommendations and increasing physical activity. Having training in techniques such as motivational interviewing is also a sound strategy for helping to improve the chances the information will be processed. Also, training nurses and medical assistants to alert providers regarding patients who may have health literacy concerns would be beneficial. Additionally, the research on helping patients with DM calls for frequent contact and follow-ups by the medical team; thus, having nurses make phone calls to check in on patients is another strategy that can be utilized. Specifically, having the nursing team contact patients to check on their dietary and exercise goals, as well as ask if they have any questions or concerns regarding medications are a minimal intensity intervention that may prove to be quite robust. Research has shown that social media and/or text messaging can be beneficial in assisting patients manage their diabetes, particularly in adolescents (Harvey, 2015). Lastly, having the nursing team assess the patient's understanding of their medication regimen could be a vital part of the patient's ability to adhere to treatment. Asking inquisitive questions such as, "can you remind me how you are supposed to take your medication?" is a teach-back method to ensure patients' understanding.

Pharmacists. Another way of dispersing psychoeducation on how to properly take medication is by having on-site pharmacists work with patients. They, too, can give tips as well as check in on patients' understanding of their medication regimen. Whether this is directly meeting with patients regarding their medication management or solely providing education when patients request refills, pharmacists are often a very underutilized resource in primary care.

Social work/case management. As anyone who works in a primary care organization can attest, and as we have discussed already in this chapter, patients' adherence to treatment is largely dependent on their psychosocial context. Patients who are homeless or do not have access to consistent food sources are going to have significant problems in adhering to treatment recommendations. Having social workers and case managers on the team can be a game changer. Ensuring means to transportation, housing, and other basic resources makes a world of difference for some patients.

Dieticians. If organizations have enough resources, a dietician can not only provide psychoeducation to patients, but they can help provide all ancillary staff with useful materials. They can start setting the stage for self-management goals. We have found dieticians to be as beneficial to providers as they are to patients. This additional team member can greatly strengthen the entire care team with accurate nutritional information and handouts.

Care managers. One of the higher intensity interventions and staff members are care managers. Care managers can be useful in identifying, tracking, and assisting those with highly uncontrolled DM, as well as individuals who regularly no-show for appointments. Care managers can develop a registry of all patients who have DM and follow-up with high-risk patients regularly. The care manager can also communicate and coordinate with the team to ensure the patient is receiving adequate and appropriate care. For more information on the use of care managers within the collaborative care model, please see the following resources (https://aims.uw.edu/collaborative-care).

Advanced practice clinicians and physicians. In addition to the staff, the APCs and physician themselves can also use motivational interviewing strategies, basic counseling skills, and behavioral principles to help encourage health behavior change. For example, physicians can learn to use open-ended questions and reflective listening and adopt a nonjudgmental stance with patients. They can help patients to set specific, measurable, attainable/achievable, relevant, and time oriented (SMART) goals. When faced with barriers, they can use an open, nonjudgmental stance to elicit the patient's perspective about their current state. They can employ the teach-back method when implementing a treatment plan. For more information on patient-centered communication skills and basic behavioral principles, please see Hunter, Goodie, Oordt, & Dobmeyer (2016), Mauksch, Dugdale, Dodson, & Epstein (2008), Robinson et al. (2010).

It is important to note that all the team members above will most likely need training to implement these stepped-care approaches. BHPs are uniquely trained to not only provide interventions to patients but teach and train team members on how to communicate effectively. BHPs are also able to assist in developing protocols, procedures, registries, etc. that standardizes the way patients with DM are treated. This grows the behavioral health provider's reach exponentially and is the ultimate depiction of stepped-care; while the behavioral health provider may never directly meet with every patient, they may indirectly improve the care of countless patients.

Quality Improvement

It is important to discuss how to assess the impact of the interventions instituted by the medical agency. Clearly, tracking patients' A1Cs is paramount and a part of meaningful use. BHPs should partner with medical providers and receive information regarding the patients they have seen and their subsequent A1C scores. We have routinely been part of provider meetings where A1C scores are reported, and we then work with the providers who are having the most difficult time improving their panel's scores. This makes our intervention intentional and allows us to target the patients who have the highest need.

In addition to tracking A1C scores, medical systems should also track quality of life or overall functioning scores. As we have discussed, there is a growing movement to discard the "symptom reduction" approach to evaluating success; rather, pairing the symptom reduction outcome with a quality of life measure provides a better picture of success for the patient. We again recommend using brief functionality measures, such as the DUKE Health Profile (Parkerson et al., 1990) or the World Health Organization Quality of Life Brief (WHOQOL-BREF; WHO, 1998).

Lastly, tracking patient satisfaction, as well as provider satisfaction, is an important outcome measure for BHPs, as well as pathways and stepped-care approaches.

Conclusion

Diabetes mellitus is a chronic condition that, despite continued medical advances, continues to wreak havoc on medical systems, patients, and providers. We have discussed a number of stepped-care approaches, including increasing the intensity of both interventions and team members' involvement. We also need to continue to connect DM management to the humanity of our patients. We need to understand that behavior does not happen in a vacuum, and if we can understand a patients' context, this may be a more effective way of helping patients to engage in and maintain meaningful health behavior change.

References

Anderson, R., Funnell, M., Burkhart, N., Gillard, M. L., & Nwankwo, R. (2003). *101 tips for behavior change in diabetes education*. Alexandria, VA: American Diabetes Association.

Cavanaugh, K., Huizinga, M. M., Wallston, K. A., Gebretsadik, T., Shintani, A., Davis, D., … Rothman, R. L. (2008). Association of numeracy and diabetes control. *Annals of Internal Medicine*, *148*(10), 737–746.

Centers for Disease Control and Prevention. (2011). National diabetes fact sheet: National estimates and general information on diabetes and prediabetes in the United States. *US Department of Health and Human Services,* Centers for disease control and prevention. Retrieved February 11, 2017, from https://www-cdc-gov.offcampus.lib.washington.edu/diabetes/pubs/pdf/ndfs_2011.pdf

Duncan, G. E. (2006). Prevalence of diabetes and impaired fasting glucose levels among US adolescents: National Health and nutrition examination survey, 1999-2002. *Archives of Pediatrics & Adolescent Medicine*, *160*(5), 523–528.

Egede, L. E., & Ellis, C. (2010). Diabetes and depression: Global perspectives. *Diabetes Research and Clinical Practice*, *87*, 302–312.

Elamin, A., Omer, M. I., Zein, K., & Tuvemo, T. (1992). Epidemiology of childhood type I diabetes in Sudan, 1987-1990. *Diabetes Care*, *15*(11), 1556–1559.

Fagot-Campoagna, A., Pettitt, D. J., Engelgau, M. M., Burrows, N. R., Geiss, L. S., Valdez, R., … Narayan, K. M. (2000). Type 2 diabetes among north American children and adolescents: An epidemiologic review and a public health perspective. *The Journal of Pediatrics*, *136*(5), 664–672.

Felner, E. I., Kiltz, W., Ham, M., Lazaro, A. M., Stastny, P., Dupont, B., & White, P. C. (2005). Genetic interaction among three genomic regions creates distinct contributions to early- and late-onset type 1 diabetes mellitus. *Pediatric Diabetes*, *6*(4), 213–220.

Fisher, L., Hessler, D. M., Polonsky, W. H., & Mullan, J. (2012). When is diabetes distress clinically meaningful? Establishing cut points for diabetes distress scale. *Diabetes Care*, *35*(2), 259–264. https://doi.org/10.2337/dc11-1572

Gregg, J., Callaghan, G., & Hayes, S. C. (2007). *The diabetes lifestyle book: Facing your fears and making changes for a long and healthy life*. Oakland, CA: New Harbinger.

Groot, M., Golden, S. H., & Wagner, J. (2016). Psychological conditions in adults with diabetes. *American Psychologist*, *71*(7), 552–562. https://doi.org/10.1037/a0040408.

Haas, L., Maryniuk, M., Beck, J., Cox, C. E., Duker, P., Edwards, L., … Youssef, G. (2012). National standards for diabetes self-management education and support. *Diabetes Care*, *35*(11), 2392–2401. https://doi.org/10.2337/dc12-1707.

Harvey, J. N. (2015). Psychosocial interventions for the diabetic patient. *Diabetes, Metabolic Syndrome and Obesity: Targets and Therapy*, *8*, 29–43. https://doi.org/10.2147/DMSO.S44352

Hassan, K., & Heptulla, R. A. (2010). Glycemic control in pediatric type 1 diabetes: Role of caregiver literacy. *Pediatrics*, *125*(5), 1104–1108. https://doi.org/10.1542/peds.2009-1486.

Helmrich, S. P., Ragland, D. R., Leung, R. W., & Paffenbarger, R. S., Jr. (1991). Physical activity and reduced occurrence of non-insulin-dependent diabetes mellitus. *The New England Journal of Medicine*, *325*(3), 147–152.

Henry, R. R., Scheaffer, l., & Olefsky, J. M. (1985). Glycemic effects of intensive caloric restriction and isocaloric refeeding in noninsulin-dependent diabetes mellitus. *The Journal of Clinical Endocrinology and Metabolism*, *61*(5), 917–925.

Hunter, C. L., Goodie, J. L., Oordt, M. S., & Dobmeyer, A. C. (2016). *Integrated behavioral health in primary care* (2nd ed.). Washington, DC: American Psychological Association.

Jeon, C. Y., Lokken, R. P., Hu, F. B., & van Dam, R. M. (2007). Physical activity of moderate intensity and risk of type 2 diabetes: A systematic review. *Diabetes Care*, *30*(3), 744–752.

Kroenke, K., Spitzer, R. L., & Williams, J. B. (2001). The PHQ-9: Validity of a brief depression severity measure. *Journal of General Internal Medicine*, *16*(9), 606–613. https://doi.org/10.1046/j.1525-1497.2001.016009606.x

Levitsky, L. L., & Misra, M. (2016). Epidemiology, presentation, and diagnosis of type 1 diabetes mellitus in children and adolescents. *UpToDate*. Retrieved February 11, 2017.

Li, C., Balluz, L. S., Okoro, C. A., Strine, T. W., Lin, J. M., Town, M., … Valluru, B. (2011). Surveillance of certain health behaviors and conditions among states and selected local areas—Behavioral risk factor surveillance system, United States, 2009. *Morbidity and Mortality Weekly Report. Surveillance Summaries*, *60*(9), 1–250.

Liang, X., Wang, Q., Yang, X., Cao, J., Chen, J., Mo, X., … Gu, D. (2011). Effect of mobile phone intervention for diabetes on glycaemic control: A meta-analysis. *Diabetes medicine*, *28*(4), 455–463. https://doi.org/10.1111/j.1464-5491.2010.03180.x

Lipton, R. B., Drum, M., Burnet, D., Rich, B., Copper, A., Baumann, E., & Hagopian, W. (2005). Obesity at the onset of diabetes in an ethnically diverse population of children: What does it mean for epidemiologists and clinicians? *Pediatrics*, *115*(5), 553–560.

Martin, L. R., Williams, S. L., Haskard, K. B., & DiMateo, M. R. (2005). The challenge of patient adherence. *Therapeutics and Clinical Risk Management*, *1*(3), 189–199.

Mauksch, L. B., Dugdale, D. C., Dodson, S., & Epstein, R. (2008). Relationship, communication, and efficiency in the medical encounter: Creating a clinical model from a literature review. *Archives of Internal Medicine*, *168*(13), 1387–1395. https://doi.org/10.1001/archinte.168.13.1387.

Mayo Clinic. (2014). Type 1 diabetes. *Diseases and Conditions*. Retrieved February 11, 2017, from http://www.mayoclinic.org/diseases-conditions/type-1-diabetes/basics/symptoms/con-20019573

Mayo Clinic. (2016). Type 2 diabetes. *Diseases and Conditions*. Retrieved February 11, 2017, from http://www.mayoclinic.org/diseases-conditions/type-2-diabetes/symptoms-causes/dxc-20169861

McCulloch, D., & Hayward, R. A. (2017). Screening for type 2 diabetes mellitus. *UpToDate*. Retrieved February 11, 2017.

Meigs, J. B., Cupples, L. A., & Wilson, P. W. (2000). Parental transmission of type 2 diabetes: The Framingham offspring study. *Diabetes*, *49*(12), 2201–2207.

Mokdad, A. H., Ford, E. S., Bowman, B. A., Dietz, W. H., Vinicor, F., Bales, V. S., & Marks, J. S. (2003). Prevalence of obesity, diabetes, and obesity-related health risk factors, 2001. *JAMA*, *289*(1), 76–79.

Nguyen, N. T., Nguyen, X. T., Lane, J., & Wang, P. (2011). Relationship between obesity and diabetes in a US adult population: Findings from the National Health and nutrition examination survey, 1999-2006. *Obesity Surgery*, *21*(3), 351–355. https://doi.org/10.1007/s11695-010-0335-4

Niskanen, L. K., Uusitupa, M. I., Sarlund, H., Siitonen, O., & Pyörälä, K. (1990). Five-year follow-up study on plasma insulin levels in newly diagnosed NIDDM patients and nondiabetic subjects. *Diabetes Care*, *13*(1), 41–48.

Norris, S. L., Kansagara, D., Bougatsos, C., Nygren, P., & Fu, R. (2008). Screening for type 2 diabetes mellitus: A review of the evidence for the U.S. Preventive Services Task Force. *Annals of Internal Medicine*, *148*(11), 855–868.

Norris, S. L., Lau, J., Smith, S. J., Schmid, C. H., & Engelgau, M. M. (2002). Self-management education for adults with type 2 diabetes: A meta-analysis of the effect on glycemic control. *Diabetes Care*, *25*(7), 1159–1171.

Norris, S. L., Zhang, X., Avenell, A., Gregg, E., Bowman, B., Serdula, M., … Lau, J. (2004). Long-term effectiveness of lifestyle and behavioral weight loss interventions in adults with type 2 diabetes: A meta-analysis. *The American Journal of Medicine, 117*(10), 762–774.

Pal, K., Eastwood, S. V., Michie, S., Farmer, A. J., Barnard, M. L., Peacock, R., … & Murry, E. (2013). Computer-based diabetes self-management interventions for adults with type 2 diabetes mellitus. *The Cochrane database of systematic reviews, 28*(3). doi:https://doi.org/10.1002/14651858.CD008776.pub2.

Parkerson, G. F., Jr., Broadhead, W. E., & Tse, C. K. (1990). The Duke Health Profile. A 17-item measure of health and dysfunction. *Medical Care, 28*(11), 1056–1072.

Polonsky, W. H., Fisher, L., Earles, J., Dudl, R. J., Lees, J., Mullan, J., & Jackson, R. A. (2005). Assessing psychosocial distress in diabetes: Development of the diabetes distress scale. *Diabetes Care, 28*(3), 626–631.

Redondo, M. J., Jeffrey, J., Fain, P. R., Eisenbarth, G. S., & Orban, T. (2008). Concordance for islet autoimmunity among monozygotic twins. *The New England Journal of Medicine, 359*(26), 2849–2850.

Reis, J. P., Loria, C. M., Sorlie, P. D., Park, Y., Hollenbeck, A., & Schatzkin, A. (2011). Lifestyle factors and risk for new-onset diabetes: A population-based cohort study. *Annals of Internal Medicine, 155*(5), 292–299. https://doi.org/10.7326/0003-4819-155-5-201109060-00006

Robinson, P. J., Gould, D. A., & Strosahl, K. D. (2010). *Real behavior change in primary care: Improving patient outcomes & increasing job satisfaction*. Oakland, CA: New Harbinger.

Robinson, P., & Reiter, J. (2016). *Behavioral consultation and primary care: A guide to integrating services* (2nd ed.). New York: Springer.

Rubin, R., & Peyrot, M. (2001). Psychological issues and treatments in people with diabetes. *Journal of Clinical Psychology, 57*, 457–478.

Saffari, M., Ghanizadeh, G., & Koenig, H. G. (2014). Health education via mobile text messaging for glycemic control in adults with type 2 diabetes: A systematic review and meta-analysis. *Primary Care Diabetes, 8*(4), 275–285. https://doi.org/10.1016/j.pcd.2014.03.004

Schreiner, B., & Ponder, S. (2016). Self-management for the child with diabetes mellitus. *UpToDate*. Retrieved February 11, 2017.

Shai, I., Jiang, R., Manson, J. E., Stampfer, M. J., Willett, W. C., Colditz, G. A., & Hu, B. F. (2006). Ethnicity, obesity, and risk of type 2 diabetes in women: A 20-year follow-up study. *Diabetes Care, 29*(7), 1585–1590.

Strosahl, K. D., Robinson, P. J., & Gustavsson, T. (2012). *Brief interventions for radical change: Principles and practice of focused acceptance and commitment therapy*. Oakland, CA: New Harbinger.

Tillil, H., & Köbberling, J. (1987). Age-corrected empirical genetic risk estimates for first-degree relatives of IDDM patients. *Diabetes, 36*(1), 98–99.

Umpierre, D., Ribeiro, P. A., Kramer, C. K., Leitão, C. B., Zucatti, A. T., Azevedo, M. J., & Gross, J. L. (2011). Physical activity advice only or structured exercise training and association with HbA1c levels in type 2 diabetes: A systematic review and meta-analysis. *JAMA, 305*(17), 1790–1799. https://doi.org/10.1001/jama.2011.576

USPSTF. (2016). Abnormal blood glucose and type 2 diabetes mellitus: Screening. *Final Recommendation Statement*. Retrieved February 11, 2017, from https://www.uspreventiveservicestaskforce.org/Page/Document/RecommendationStatementFinal/screening-for-abnormal-blood-glucose-and-type-2-diabetes

Willens, D., Cripps, R., Wilson, A., Wolff, K., & Rothman, R. (2011). Interdisciplinary team care for diabetic patients by primary care physicians, advanced practice nurses, and clinical pharmacists. *Clinical Diabetes, 29*(2), 60–68. https://doi.org/10.2337/diaclin.29.2.60

World Health Organization (WHO). (1998). *WHOQOL user manual*. Geneva, Switzerland: World Health Organization.

Eating Disorders

16

Sarah L. Russell, Carol B. Peterson, and Ann F. Haynos

Description of the Disorders

There are several eating disorders recognized by the Diagnostic and Statistical Manual of Mental Disorders (DSM-5; American Psychiatric Association, 2013). Anorexia nervosa (AN), bulimia nervosa (BN), and binge eating disorder (BED) are the most recognizable eating disorder diagnoses. AN is characterized by restriction of caloric intake relative to necessary energy requirements leading to significantly low body weight (often defined as <85% ideal body weight or IBW; American Psychiatric Association, 2006), accompanied by an intense fear of weight gain and distorted body image. Individuals with AN regularly engage in behaviors that impede weight gain (e.g., excessive dietary restriction, compulsive exercise, purging) regardless of their significantly low weight and may also engage in intermittent binge eating (i.e., eating a large amount of food in a short period of time while experiencing a sense that eating is out of control). BN is characterized by recurrent episodes of binge eating and inappropriate compensatory behaviors (e.g., self-induced vomiting, use of laxatives or other weight-loss medications, fasting, compulsive exercise) used to prevent weight gain from binge eating that do not result in the individual being underweight. Finally, BED is characterized by recurrent episodes of binge eating without accompanying compensatory behaviors. In addition, a substantial portion of individuals with eating disorders fall into the category of Other Specified Feeding or Eating Disorders (OSFED), which is characterized by disordered eating causing significant distress and/or clinical impairment that does not meet full criteria for AN, BN, or BED.

Eating disorders are relatively common. Lifetime population prevalence of DSM-5 eating disorders is approximately 1–4% for AN, 2% for BN, and 1–5% for BED (Smink, van Hoeken, & Hoek, 2013). Although few population estimates exist for OSFED, it is by far the most common eating disorder diagnosis and may affect more than 14% of the population over their lifetime (Smink et al., 2013). Psychological comorbidity, especially co-occurrence of depressive, anxiety, and substance disorders, use is extremely common among individuals with eating disorders (Braun, Sunday, & Halmi, 1994). There are also

S.L. Russell (✉)
Department of Social Work, St. Catherine University and the University of St. Thomas, St. Paul, MN, USA
e-mail: sarah.e.lemay@gmail.com

C.B. Peterson
Department of Psychiatry, University of Minnesota Medical Center, Minneapolis, MN, USA

The Emily Program, Minneapolis, MN, USA
e-mail: peter161@umn.edu

A.F. Haynos
Department of Psychiatry, University of Minnesota Medical Center, Minneapolis, MN, USA
e-mail: afhaynos@umn.edu

A. Maragakis, W.T. O'Donohue (eds.), *Principle-Based Stepped Care and Brief Psychotherapy for Integrated Care Settings*, https://doi.org/10.1007/978-3-319-70539-2_16

severe physical consequences associated with eating disorders, including complications of the gastrointestinal (e.g., gastric dilatation, liver dysfunction), cardiovascular (acrocyanosis, arrhythmia), skeletal (osteopenia/osteoporosis), and nutritional (e.g., sodium depletion, hypophosphatemia, hypomagnesemia) systems (Mitchell & Crow, 2006). Additionally, eating disorders have the highest mortality rate of any psychiatric illness, with death resulting from suicide or physical complications (Crow et al., 2009).

Effective Ways to Screen for Eating Disorders in Primary Care Settings

Given the relatively high lifetime rates of disordered eating (Smink et al., 2013), and the severity of consequences associated with eating disorder behaviors (Crow et al., 2009; Mitchell & Crow, 2006), routine eating disorder screening in primary care is encouraged. Screening is particularly encouraged for patients demonstrating physical and/or psychological symptoms consistent with an eating disorder, such as low BMI, sudden or dramatic weight change, electrolyte disturbance, menstrual irregularity, self-reported disordered eating (e.g., fasting, purging, diet pill use), or concerns about weight/shape (Sangvai, 2016).

Several eating disorder screening measures have been developed for the use in primary care settings. The Primary Care Evaluation of Mental Disorders (PRIME-MD; Spitzer et al., 1994) was designed to screen for a number of psychiatric disorders, including eating disorders, with the administration of a 26-item questionnaire that asks about the occurrence of specific symptoms over the past month (e.g., loss of control eating) and interview modules to further evaluate any symptoms endorsed on the questionnaire. The PRIME-MD takes less than 9 min to administer and has been shown to have good inter-rater agreement on diagnoses (Spitzer et al., 1994). The PRIME-MD has been adapted into a widely used questionnaire format, the Patient Health Questionnaire (PHQ), in order to reduce physician administration screening (Spitzer, Kroenke, & Williams, 1999). However, because this questionnaire only contains one item that asks about overeating or loss of appetite, it may be most useful for diagnosing binge eating and less helpful for identifying eating disorders characterized by other symptoms (e.g., purging, dietary restriction). Given the high rates of psychiatric comorbidity associated with eating disorders (Smink et al., 2013), the use of the full PRIME-MD or PHQ is encouraged. However, if time is limited, the eating disorder questions from these measures can be administered in a stand-alone fashion.

The SCOFF (Morgan, Reid, & Lacey, 1999) was originally developed as an interview and later adapted to a questionnaire format for the use to screen for eating disorder symptoms (Hills, Reid, Morgan, & Lacey, 2010). Developed in England, the SCOFF abbreviation refers to each of the five questions (e.g., S = "Do you make yourself *s*ick…?" C = "Do you worry that you have lost *c*ontrol over how much you eat?" O = "Have you recently lost more than *o*ne stone (14 lbs) in a 3-month period?" F = "Do you believe yourself to be *f*at when others say you are thin?" F = "Would you say that *f*ood dominates your life?"). Its brevity, translation into a number of languages, and inclusion of multiple aspects of eating disorders (e.g., purging, binge eating, weight loss, concerns about shape and eating) make it particularly useful as a screening instrument in primary care settings. Several studies have supported the reliability and validity of the SCOFF, including a recent meta-analysis (Botella, Sepulveda, Huang, & Gambara, 2013). However, this measure has been found to generate a high rate of false negatives in a multiethnic sample (Solmi, Hatch, Hotopf, Treasure, & Micali, 2015), which is a limitation that should be considered when using this measure.

Although less commonly used in primary care settings, several other questionnaires can be used to screen for eating disorders (see review by Tury, Gulec, & Kohls, 2010), including the Eating Attitudes Test (EAT-26; Garner, Olmsted, Bohr, & Garfinkel, 1982) and the Eating Disorder Examination-Questionnaire (EDE-Q; Fairburn & Beglin, 1994), which provide more comprehensive assessment information about eating disorder behaviors, including binge eating and purging, attitudes about weight and shape, and dietary restraint.

How to Further Assess If a Screen Returns Positive

Any indication of eating disorder symptoms in the screening process requires a more thorough diagnostic and physical evaluation. In primary care settings, the clinician can use an established diagnostic measure including the Eating Disorder Examination interview (EDE; Fairburn, 2008), which is available in the public domain (http://credo-oxford.com) and contains questions to assess concerns about eating, weight, and shape as well the frequency of binge eating, purging, and driven exercise. The EDE and, its questionnaire adaptation, the EDE-Q (Fairburn & Beglin, 1994) have extensive psychometric data to support their reliability and are widely used in research and clinical settings (Berg, Peterson, Frazier, & Crow, 2012; Fairburn, 2008). The primary care provider can also refer to the DSM-5 (APA, 2013) for a list of symptoms and descriptions of diagnostic markers. The provider can use this information to conduct a clinical interview to establish an eating disorder diagnosis.

Because patients with eating disorders are often hesitant to discuss their symptoms because of fear, shame, symptom minimization, or concerns about forced treatment, clinical rapport and emotional validation are crucial (Peterson, 2005). Asking for specific examples (e.g., types and amounts of food consumed during meals and binge eating episodes) can be especially useful in evaluating diagnostic criteria. In addition, body mass index (BMI) should be measured for accuracy rather than relying on self-report. Offering for the patient to be weighed without having to see their weight can help them feel more comfortable with the procedure. Risk assessment is extremely important with all types of eating disorders, regardless of weight status. Given the high rate of psychiatric comorbidity and suicide risk (Braun et al., 1994; Crow et al., 2009; Mitchell & Crow, 2006), the primary care clinician should be certain to assess for suicidal ideation, intent, and recent attempts. In addition, a thorough medical examination by medical provider (as described below) is indicated.

Evidence-Based Stepped Care and Brief Psychotherapeutic Approaches

Stepped care for eating disorders allows the care to provider to administer treatments that are sequenced in intensity according to the need and response of the client (Wilson, Vitousek, & Loeb, 2000). There is a growing literature to support stepped care in the treatment of eating disorders, especially BN and BED (Mitchell et al., 2011; Sysko & Walsh, 2008), but also OSFED (Traviss, Heywood-Everett, & Hill, 2011). A stepped care approach has been shown to reduce cost and time of treatment compared to specialized care (Haaga, 2000).

The stepped care model for treating BN, BED, or OSFED begins with utilizing self-help cognitive behavioral therapy (CBT) (Grilo et al., 2014; Mitchell et al., 2011). The self-help book, *Overcoming Binge Eating* (Fairburn, 2013), is the most commonly used in this stepped care model (Grilo et al., 2014; Hilbert, Hildebrandt, Agras, Wilfley, & Wilson, 2015; Mitchell et al., 2011); however, several other self-help books are available (see APA, 2006). *Overcoming Binge Eating* follows the standard model of CBT for eating disorders and has three stages (Fairburn, 2013). In the first stage, the CBT model is described, and methods for self-monitoring and normalizing eating behaviors are explained. The second stage asks individuals to maintain normalized eating patterns and self-monitoring, integrate cognitive procedures, and learn skills for coping with triggers of disordered eating. The third stage encourages individuals to maintain progress and learn relapse prevention techniques.

Studies have shown that self-help CBT provides more support than remaining on a waitlist for specialized care (Sysko & Walsh, 2008). Evidence suggests access to 30-min sessions with an eating disorder specialist in order to go over homework, address possible difficulties, and provide additional support and encouragement that can enhance symptom improvement from CBT self-help (Vaz, Conceição & Machado, 2013). Therefore, circumscribed clinician support in addition to self-help is recommended. There is some evidence that the addition of psychotropic medication, such as fluoxetine, may also enhance therapist-assisted self-help for eating disorders (Mitchell et al., 2011).

Researchers are also beginning to explore the use of technology to support individuals in eating disorder treatment, including online and mobile self-help programs (Keyes & Schmidt, 2016; Nitsch et al., 2016; Tregarthen, Lock, & Darcy, 2015). The most popular of these methods is a widely available mobile phone application, *Recovery Record* (https://www.recoveryrecord.com/), which follows CBT principles to guide users through behavioral self-monitoring and the use of coping strategies (Tregarthen et al., 2015). This application includes an online forum, allowing users to interface with others working toward recovery in order to provide peer support. Users are also able to send clinical information to treatment providers through this application. While early studies have shown that internet-based CBT is popular and can be effective, there is often low adherence to treatment (Keyes & Schmidt, 2016; Tregarthen et al., 2015). Therefore, while online and mobile applications can be used as tools to support recovery in an integrated care setting, they are not yet recommended as stand-alone treatments.

If self-help treatment is not successful, or otherwise not appropriate as a first line of care, a brief course of clinician-led CBT for eating disorders would be an appropriate next approach for treatment of BN, BED, or OSFED. The recommended length of CBT for eating disorders is 20 sessions (Fairburn, 2008). However, studies have shown that significant portion of individuals demonstrate a rapid response (e.g., a significant reduction ≥65–70% in binge eating) by the fourth week of treatment and that rapid response is an excellent predictor of good clinical outcomes (Grilo, White, Masheb & Gueorguieva, 2015; Hilbert et al., 2015). Therefore, a clinician in an integrated care setting may initiate a brief course (e.g., 4 weeks) of CBT. If a patient demonstrates a rapid clinical response in this period of time, the provider and patient can discuss whether to maintain these gains through continued therapy sessions or to transition to a lower level of care (e.g., guided self-help). However, if the patient does not show symptom reduction in this period, this may be an indicator that the patient is more appropriate for treatment in specialty care by a therapy specifically trained to treat eating disorders.

There is no established research supporting nonspecialized care for individuals with AN. Therefore, the current recommendation is to refer these individuals to specialized care immediately upon establishing a diagnosis.

What Not to Do

There are some common pitfalls that providers in a primary care setting should take precautions to avoid. First, there is evidence that healthcare providers often have negative perceptions of eating disorders, viewing individuals with eating disorders as selfish, vain, weak, unlikeable, and/or blameworthy (Bannatyne & Stapleton, 2016; Fleming & Szmukler, 1992; Yu, Hildebrandt, & Lanzieri, 2015). These perceptions may result from the commonly held belief that eating disorders result from sociocultural pressures and lack of willpower (Bannatyne & Stapleton, 2016; Fleming & Szmukler, 1992). Such attitudes can be shaming to patients with eating disorders (Goss & Allan, 2009) and can lead to alienation from the healthcare system and treatment nonengagement (Swan & Andrews, 2003) or can indirectly perpetuate eating disorder symptoms (Berg et al., 2013; Haynos et al., 2017). In addition, misperceptions about the seriousness of eating disorders can cause providers to inappropriately minimize treatment (Rodgers et al., 2015) or to use unhelpful critical or confrontational approaches to eliciting change (Treasure, Crane, McKnight, Buchanan, & Wolfe, 2011).

Weight stigmatization is a related concern. Eating disorders and obesity frequently co-occur (Darby et al., 2009). Evidence suggests that overweight and obese individuals are often negatively perceived as lazy, weak, and unmotivated (Puhl & Suh, 2015), even by healthcare professionals (Puhl & Brownell, 2006). Weight stigma can excaerbate eating disorder symptoms (Nolan & Eshleman, 2016) and overeating (Schvey, Puhl, & Brownell, 2011) and can encourage individuals to avoid engaging with the healthcare system (Drury & Louis, 2002). Further, there is evidence that individuals who are overweight or obese receive poorer quality care as a result of these misperceptions (Phelan et al., 2015). Because overvaluation of weight and shape is a critical component of most eating disorders (APA, 2013), it is important to be sensitive in discussions of weight among individuals with disordered eating and to focus to a greater degree on symptom reduction, rather than weight loss. Providers are encouraged to monitor and intervene upon tendencies toward eating disorder and weight stigmatization.

There are other unhelpful patterns that are common for care providers (Treasure et al., 2011). On the opposite pole from trivializing eating disorders, providers can become overreactive and overprotective of individuals with eating disorders, demonstrating anxiety regarding eating disorder symptoms and recommending higher levels of care for longer periods of time than guidelines suggest. Alternatively, providers can accomodate an individual's eating disorder symptoms (e.g., relaxing weight standards, not targeting purging) out of fear of alienating the patient. These behaviors are iatrogenic and to be avoided.

When to Refer to External Specialty Mental Health

Because eating disorders have such serious consequences, it is important to know when the outpatient level of care is no longer sufficient, and an individual needs to be referred to specialty care. The following recommendations follow the practice guidelines for the treatment of patients with eating disorders (APA, 2006).

To be considered appropriate for outpatient care, patients must (1) be medically stable (e.g., heart rate >40 bpm, blood pressure >90/60 mmHg, glucose >60 mg/dL, potassium >3 mEq/L, temperature >97.0 °F, no evidence of electrolyte imbalance, dehydration, or hepatic, renal, or cardiovascular compromise), (2) have >85% of IBW, (3) be not experiencing suicidal ideation or significant comorbid concern requiring intensive or specialist care (e.g., substance abuse), (4) be motivated to recover, (5) be able to have insight into their illness, (6) be able to obtain the structure necessary to normalize eating and exercise and reduce or eliminate purging, (7) have a support system available, and (8) live within a reasonable distance of the treatment setting (APA, 2006). If a patient does not meet these outpatient guidelines at any point in evaluation or treatment, they should be recommended for more intensive specialty eating disorder care.

Role of Primary Care Provider

Current recommendations suggest that optimal treatment of eating disorders at all levels of care involves a comprehensive, multidisciplinary team, including a primary care physician (in addition to a psychotherapist, nutritionist, and psychiatrist as needed) that regularly communicates in order to coordinate care (APA, 2006; Halmi, 2009). The primary care physician is responsible for the initial physical assessment, as well as the monitoring and management of ongoing medical issues in the case of outpatient treatment. The initial physical assessment should involve vital signs, blood work (complete blood count with white blood cell differential, complete metabolic profile, and thyroid laboratory tests), an echocardiogram, and a bone density scan for individuals who have been amenorrheic for ≥6 months (APA, 2006; Halmi, 2009; Sangvai, 2016). Individuals engaging in vomiting as a compensatory behavior should be referred for a dental examination (APA, 2006). For a thorough description of common physicial symptoms of eating disorders, the primary care provider is referred to the APA (2006) treatment guidelines. Patients will often present with a normal physical examination despite severe eating disorder symptoms (Sangvai, 2016). It is important that a lack of physical manifestation will not be interpreted as evidence that the eating disorder is unconcerning. Rather, the primary care physician is encouraged to take symptoms seriously and to stress to the patient that physical abnormalities are not required for the diagnosis of an eating disorder.

Ongoing monitoring and treatment of physical concerns by the primary care provider is recommended for outpatient treatment (APA, 2006). The physician should determine whether any ongoing physical abnormalities are likely to be primary or secondary to the eating disorder (Sangvai, 2016), as many physical symptoms will resolve with cessation of eating disorder behavior. Additionally, new physical complaints may arise upon decreasing or ceasing eating disorder behavior (e.g., bloating or constipation from reduced gut motility) (APA, 2006). These physical concerns may be temporarily alleviated with medical intervention and are also likely to resolve over time with improvement of eating disorder symptoms.

Weight may also be monitored by the primary care physician, although the patient's individual therapist may assume this role. Restoration of weight to a healthy range is an essential goal for individuals who are underweight (APA, 2006; Halmi, 2009). The ideal weight range recommended is >90% IBW (roughly equivalent to BMI > 19.5 kg/m^2; APA, 2006); however, restoration to a higher BMI is associated with better clinical outcomes (El Ghoch, Calugi, Chignola, Bazzani, & Dalle Grave, 2016), and it is suggested that weight goals be adjusted higher if mecharche has not resumed at 90% IBW (Sangvai, 2016). The recommended rate of weight gain for underweight individuals with eating disorders is approximately 0.5–1 lb/week (APA, 2006). For eating disorder patients within a normal weight range, the goal is healthy weight maintenance (Sangvai, 2016). These individuals are monitored for dramatic weight decreases or increases that may indicate a concern (e.g., escalation of binge eating, purging, or dietary restriction). Although it is debated whether weight loss should be a treatment goal for overweight or obese individuals with eating disorders, there is evidence that overweight individuals with BED respond effectively to weight loss interventions (APA, 2006). Weight loss goals for the overweight or obese individual with an eating disorder should be determined collaboratively between patient and provider, with the understanding that weight loss efforts should not trump symptom cessation.

Medication management may also be assumed by the primary care physician, although this function could be managed by a psychiatrist. Currently, the only psychotropic medications approved by the Food and Drug Administration (FDA) for eating disorders are fluoxetine (60 mg/day) for BN and lisdexamfetamine for moderate to severe BED (30–70 mg/day) (Sangvai, 2016). Medications have not been found to be helpful for individuals with AN. Some medications are not appropriate for individuals with eating disorders. For instance, the FDA has issued a black box warning on the use of bupropion among individuals with eating disorders, due to an elevated seizure risk among this population (APA, 2006). Use of medications with addictive properties (e.g., benzodiazepines) and/or appetite suppressant properties (e.g., stimulant medications) should be considered cautiously among individuals with eating disorders, due to increased propensity for addictive behaviors and unhealthy weight loss (APA, 2006).

Quality Improvement

There is no evidence base to suggest how to implement quality improvement practices related to screening and treating eating disorders in an integrated care setting. In the absence of specific recommendations from the eating disorder field, it is suggested that any quality improvement process follows the standards outlined by the Institute of Medicine (2001) to assess the degree to which the system of care is (a) effective, (b) patient-centered, (c) safe, (d) timely, (e) efficient, and (f) equitable.

Providers can assess *effectiveness* outcomes by evaluating the degree to which patients' symptoms improve from the time the eating disorder is detected in primary care using the EDE, EDE-Q, or another standard eating disorder assessment. Ideally, a system would aim to have outcomes match benchmarks established in eating disorder treatment trials (Berkman et al., 2006). *Patient-centered* outcomes can be monitored using quality of life measures, such as the Eating Disorder Quality of Life (Engel et al., 2006) or the Clinical Impairment Assessment (Bohn et al., 2008) questionnaires, as well as visual analogue scales to rate treatment acceptability (e.g., Zainal et al., 2016). *Safety* can be monitored through routine review of electronic health records to determine whether integrated care for eating disorders is associated with a reduction in physical and psychological complaints. Assessment of the degree to which treatment is *timely* will involve examining the length of time between symptom initiation, detection in primary care, and treatment initiation. Early detection and timely treatment are associated with improved outcomes for individuals with eating disorders (Cadwallader, Godart, Chastang, Falissard, & Huas, 2016). However, evidence suggests that most eating disorder cases are not detected in a primary care setting (Cadwallader et al., 2016). Quality care practices should aim to improve upon the number of cases detected, as well as how quickly treatment is initiated. Monitoring whether a treatment is *efficient* requires examining the degree to which the length of treatment in the integrated care system matches standards for eating disorder treatment, which are generally 20 sessions of treatment for individuals without weight restoration goals and 40 sessions for those requiring weight restoration (APA, 2006). It is also important to assess the degree to which eating disorder screening and care is *equitable* across demographics. There is evidence that individuals who are male, overweight or obese, or belong to a minority group are less likely to receive an eating disorder diagnosis and be referred to treatment (Cachelin, Rebeck, Veisel, & Striegel-Moore, 2001; MacCaughelty, Wagner, & Rufino, 2016). Therefore, it is especially important to monitor if individuals from these groups are receiving comparable screening and treatment procedures. Quality improvement procedures can provide information regarding how effectively the integrated care system is addressing the significant and serious concern of eating disorders within the healthcare setting.

References

American Psychiatric Association. (2013). *Diagnostic and statistical manual of mental disorders* (5th ed.). Washington, DC: American Psychiatric Association.

American Psychiatric Association. (2006). Treatment of patients with eating disorders (3rd edition). *American Journal of Psychiatry*, *163*, 4–54.

Bannatyne, A. J., & Stapleton, P. B. (2016). Attitudes towards anorexia nervosa: Volitional stigma differences in a sample of pre-clinical medicine and psychology students. *Journal of Mental Health*, *29*, 1–7.

Berg, K. C., Crosby, R. D., Cao, L., Peterson, C. B., Engel, S. G., Mitchell, J. E., et al. (2013). Facets of negative affect prior to and following binge-only, purge-only, and binge/purge events in women with bulimia nervosa. *Journal of Abnormal Psychology*, *122*, 111–118.

Berg, K. C., Peterson, C. B., Frazier, P., & Crow, S. J. (2012). Psychometric evaluation of the Eating Disorder Examination and Eating Disorder Examination-Questionnaire: A systematic review of the literature. *International Journal of Eating Disorders*, *45*, 428–438.

Berkman, N. D., Bulik, C. M., Brownley, K. A., Lohr, K. N., Sedway, J. A., Rooks, A., et al. (2006). Management of eating disorders. *Evidence Report/Technology Assessment (Full Report)*, *135*, 1–166.

Bohn, K., Doll, H. A., Cooper, Z., O'Connor, M., Palmer, R. L., & Fairburn, C. G. (2008). The measurement of impairment due to eating disorder psychopathology. *Behavior Research and Therapy*, *46*, 1105–1110.

Botella, J., Sepulveda, A. R., Huang, H., & Gambara, H. (2013). A meta-analysis of the diagnostic accuracy of the SCOFF. *Spanish Journal of Psychology*, *16*, E92.

Braun, D. L., Sunday, S. R., & Halmi, K. A. (1994). Psychiatric comorbidity in patients with eating disorders. *Psychological Medicine*, *24*, 859–867.

Cachelin, F. M., Rebeck, R., Veisel, C., & Striegel-Moore, R. H. (2001). Barriers to treatment for eating disorders among ethnically diverse women. *International Journal of Eating Disorders*, *30*, 269–278.

Cadwallader, J. S., Godart, N., Chastang, J., Falissard, B., & Huas, C. (2016). Detecting eating disorder patients in a general practice setting: A systematic review of heterogeneous data on clinical outcomes and care trajectories. *Eating and Weight Disorders*, *21*(3), 365–381.

Crow, S. J., Peterson, C. B., Swanson, S. A., Raymond, N. C., Specker, S., Eckert, E. D., et al. (2009). Increased mortality in bulimia nervosa and other eating disorders. *American Journal of Psychiatry, 166*, 1342–1346.

Darby, A., Hay, P., Mond, J., Quirk, F., Buttner, P., & Kennedy, L. (2009). The rising prevalence of comorbid obesity and eating disorder behaviors from 1995 to 2005. *International Journal of Eating Disorders, 42*, 104–108.

Drury, C. A., & Louis, M. (2002). Exploring the association between body weight, stigma of obesity, and health care avoidance. *Journal of the American Academy of Nurse Practitioners, 14*, 554–561.

El Ghoch, M., Calugi, S., Chignola, E., Bazzani, P. V., & Dalle Grave, R. (2016). Body mass index, body fat and risk factor of relapse in anorexia nervosa. *European Journal of Clinical Nutrition, 70*, 194–198.

Engel, S. G., Wittrock, D. A., Crosby, R. D., Wonderlich, S. A., Mitchell, J. E., & Kolotkin, R. L. (2006). Development and psychometric validation of an eating disorder-specific health-related quality of life instrument. *International Journal of Eating Disorders, 39*, 62–71.

Fairburn, C. G. (2008). *Cognitive-behavioral therapy and eating disorders*. New York: Guilford.

Fairburn, C. G. (2013). *Overcoming binge eating*. New York: Guilford.

Fairburn, C. G., & Beglin, S. J. (1994). Assessment of eating disorders: interview or self-report questionnaire? *International Journal of Eating Disorders, 16*, 363–370.

Fleming, J., & Szmukler, G. I. (1992). Attitudes of medical professionals towards patients with eating disorders. *The Australian and New Zealand Journal of Psychiatry, 26*, 436–443.

Garner, D. M., Olmsted, M. P., Bohr, Y., & Garfinkel, P. E. (1982). The Eating Attitudes Test: Psychometric features and clinical correlates. *Psychological Medicine, 12*, 871–878.

Goss, K., & Allan, S. (2009). Shame, pride and eating disorders. *Clinical Psychology & Psychotherapy, 16*, 303–316.

Grilo, C. M., Masheb, R. M., White, M. A., Gueorguieva, R., Barnes, R. D., Walsh, B. T., et al. (2014). Treatment of binge eating disorder in racially and ethnically diverse obese patients in primary care: Randomized placebo-controlled clinical trial of self-help and medication. *Behaviour Research and Therapy, 58*, 1–9.

Grilo, C. M., White, M. A., Masheb, R. M., & Gueorguieva, R. (2015). Predicting meaningful outcomes to medication and self-help treatments for binge-eating disorder in primary care: The significance of early rapid response. *Journal of Consulting and Clinical Psychology, 83*, 387–394.

Haaga, D. A. (2000). Introduction to the special section on stepped care models in psychotherapy. *Journal of Consulting and Clinical Psychology, 68*, 547–548.

Halmi, K. A. (2009). Salient components of a comprehensive service for eating disorders. *World Psychiatry, 8*, 150–155.

Haynos, A. F., Berg, K. C., Cao, L., Crosby, R. D., Lavender, J. M., Utzinger, L. M., et al. (2017). Trajectories of higher- and lower-order dimensions of negative and positive affect relative to restrictive eating in anorexia nervosa. *The Journal of Abnormal Psychology, 126*(5), 495–505.

Hilbert, A., Hildebrandt, T., Agras, W. S., Wilfley, D. E., & Wilson, G. T. (2015). Rapid response in psychological treatments for binge eating disorder. *Journal of Consulting and Clinical Psychology, 83*, 649–654.

Hills, L. S., Reid, F., Morgan, J. F., & Lacey, J. H. (2010). SCOFF, the development of an eating disorder screening questionnaire. *International Journal of Eating Disorders, 43*, 344–351.

Institute of Medicine. (2001). *Crossing the quality chasm: A new health system for the 21st century*. Washington, DC: National Academy Press.

Keyes, A., & Schmidt, U. (2016). ICBT for eating disorders. In N. Lindefors & G. Andersson (Eds.), *Guided internet-based treatments in psychiatry* (pp. 175–196). Switzerland: Springer.

MacCaughelty, C., Wagner, R., & Rufino, K. (2016). Does being overweight or male increase a patient's risk of not being referred for an eating disorder consult? *International Journal of Eating Disorders, 49*, 963–966.

Mitchell, J. E., & Crow, S. (2006). Medical complications of anorexia nervosa and bulimia nervosa. *Current Opinion in Psychiatry, 19*, 438–443.

Mitchell, J. E., Agras, S., Crow, S., Halmi, K., Fairburn, C. G., Bryson, S., & Kraemer, H. (2011). Stepped care and cognitive-behavioural therapy for bulimia nervosa: Randomised trial. *The British Journal of Psychiatry, 198*, 391–397.

Morgan, J. F., Reid, F., & Lacey, J. H. (1999). The SCOFF questionnaire: Assessment of a new screening tool for eating disorders. *British Medical Journal, 319*, 1467–1468.

Nitsch, M., Dimopoulos, C. N., Flaschberger, E., Saffran, K., Kruger, J. F., Garlock, L., et al. (2016). A guided online and mobile self-help program for individuals with eating disorders: An iterative engagement and usability study. *Journal of Medical Internet Research, 18*, e7.

Nolan, L. J., & Eshleman, A. (2016). Paved with good intentions: Paradoxical eating responses to weight stigma. *Appetite, 102*, 15–24.

Peterson, C. B. (2005). Conducting the diagnostic interview. In J. E. Mitchell & C. B. Peterson (Eds.), *Assessment of eating disorders* (pp. 32–58). New York: Guilford.

Phelan, S. M., Burgess, D. J., Burke, S. E., Przedworski, J. M., Dovidio, J. F., Hardeman, R., et al. (2015). Beliefs about the causes of obesity in a national sample of 4th year medical students. *Patient Education and Counseling, 98*, 1446–1449.

Puhl, R. M., & Brownell, K. D. (2006). Confronting and coping with weight stigma: An investigation of overweight and obese adults. *Obesity (Silver Spring), 14*, 1802–1815.

Puhl, R., & Suh, Y. (2015). Stigma and eating and weight disorders. *Current Psychiatry Reports, 17*, 552.

Rodgers, R. F., Paxton, S. J., McLean, S. A., Massey, R., Mond, J. M., Hay, P. J., et al. (2015). Stigmatizing attitudes and beliefs toward bulimia nervosa: The importance of knowledge and eating disorder symptoms. *Journal of Nervous and Mental Disease, 203*, 259–263.

Sangvai, D. (2016). Eating disorders in the primary care setting. *Primary Care, 43*, 301–312.

Schvey, N. A., Puhl, R. M., & Brownell, K. D. (2011). The impact of weight stigma on caloric consumption. *Obesity (Silver Spring), 19*, 1957–1962.

Smink, F. R., van Hoeken, D., & Hoek, H. W. (2013). Epidemiology, course, and outcome of eating disorders. *Current Opinion in Psychiatry, 26*, 543–548.

Solmi, F., Hatch, S. L., Hotopf, M., Treasure, J., & Micali, N. (2015). Validation of the SCOFF questionnaire for eating disorders in a multiethnic general population sample. *International Journal of Eating Disorders, 48*, 312–316.

Spitzer, R. L., Kroenke, K., & Williams, J. B. (1999). Validation and utility of a self-report version of the PRIME-MD: The PHQ primary care study. Primary Care Evaluation of Mental Disorders. Patient Health Questionnaire. *Journal of the American Medical Association, 282*, 1737–1744.

Spitzer, R. L., Williams, J. B., Kroenke, K., Linzer, M., DeGruy, F. V., III, Hahn, S. R., et al. (1994). Utility of a new procedures for diagnosing mental disorders in primary care. The PRIME-MD 1000 study. *Journal of the American Medical Association, 14*, 1749–1756.

Swan, S., & Andrews, B. (2003). The relationship between shame, eating disorders and disclosure in treatment. *British Journal of Clinical Psychology, 42*, 367–378.

Sysko, R., & Walsh, B. T. (2008). A critical evaluation of the efficacy of self-help interventions for the treatment of bulimia nervosa and binge-eating disorder. *International Journal of Eating Disorders, 41*, 97–112.

Traviss, G. D., Heywood-Everett, S., & Hill, A. J. (2011). Guided self-help for disordered eating: A randomised control trial. *Behaviour Research and Therapy, 49*, 25–31.

Tury, F., Gulec, H., & Kohls, E. (2010). Assessment methods for eating disorders and body image disorders. *Journal of Psychosomatic Research, 69*, 601–611.

Treasure, J., Crane, A., McKnight, R., Buchanan, E., & Wolfe, M. (2011). First do no harm: Iatrogenic maintaining factors in anorexia nervosa. *European Eating Disorders Review, 19*, 296–302.

Tregarthen, J. P., Lock, J., & Darcy, A. M. (2015). Development of a smartphone application for eating disorder self-monitoring. *International Journal of Eating Disorders, 48*, 972–982.

Vaz, A. R., Conceição, E., & Machado, P. P. (2013). Guided self-help CBT treatment for bulimic disorders: Effectiveness and clinically significant change. *Psychotherapy Research, 23*, 324–332.

Wilson, G. T., Vitousek, K. M., & Loeb, K. L. (2000). Stepped care treatment for eating disorders. *Journal of Consulting and Clinical Psychology, 68*, 564–572.

Yu, J., Hildebrandt, T., & Lanzieri, N. (2015). Healthcare professionals' stigmatization of men with anabolic androgenic steroid use and eating disorders. *Body Image, 15*, 49–53.

Zainal, K. A., Renwick, B., Keyes, A., Lose, A., Kenyon, M., DeJong, H., et al. (2016). Process evaluation of the MOSAIC trial: Treatment experience of two psychological therapies for out-patient treatment of Anorexia Nervosa. *Journal of Eating Disorders, 4*, 2.

Elimination Disorders

17

Stu Law, Mark Malady, Tom Buqo, and Larry Williams

Description of the Disorders

The Diagnostic and Statistical Manual of Mental Disorders (American Psychiatric Association, 2013) separates elimination disorders into enuresis and encopresis. Enuresis is defined as repeated urination into bed or clothing at least twice a week for a period of at least 3 months that is not due directly to a physiological condition or substance and occurs for an individual who is at least 5 years of age (American Psychiatric Association, 2013). Encopresis is defined as repeated bowel movements into bed or clothing at least one time per month for a period of at least 3 months, is not due directly to a physiological condition or substance, and occurs for an individual who is at least 4 years of age (American Psychiatric Association, 2013). Alternative diagnostic systems include the Rome-III criteria and the International Children's Continence Society's classification system (Nevéus et al., 2006; Rasquin et al., 2006). The three systems differ on the minimum age, the various subtypes, and the specific language of the descriptions (for a full review, see von Gontard, 2013). All three systems differentiate between urinary and bowel movement-based incontinence, and translation across the three systems does not exclude research based on one system versus the other. However, some offer more specification on the subtype of elimination disorders.

Most elimination disorders are diagnosed for children between the age of 7 and 12 years (Christophersen, Christophersen, & Friman, 2010). The most common elimination disorders are nocturnal enuresis, diurnal enuresis, constipation, and encopresis. Nocturnal enuresis is identified by urinating into garments during periods of sleep more than two times per week for at least 3 months for children over the age of 5. Diurnal enuresis is defined by urination into garments during waking hours for at least more than two times per week for at least 3 months for children over the age of 5. For the purposes of this chapter, enuresis and encopresis will serve as primary focal points.

With regard to encopresis, examination of co-occurring constipation should be conducted, as its presence or absence within encopresis appears to contribute to clinically important differences such as impacted bowels and severe discomfort (Beninga, Büller, Heymans, Tytgat, & Taminia, 1994). Two subtypes of encopresis can be considered: encopresis with constipation and encopresis without consti-

S. Law, M.A. (✉) • L. Williams, Ph.D., B.C.B.A.-D.
Department of Psychology, University of Nevada, Reno, NV, USA
e-mail: StuLaw34@gmail.com; LarryW@unr.edu

M. Malady, M.S., B.C.B.A.
Bx Plus, Reno, NV, USA
e-mail: Markmalady@yahoo.com

T. Buqo, B.A.
Department of Psychology, Hofstra University, Hempstead, NY, USA
e-mail: TomBuqo@gmail.com

A. Maragakis, W.T. O'Donohue (eds.), *Principle-Based Stepped Care and Brief Psychotherapy for Integrated Care Settings*, https://doi.org/10.1007/978-3-319-70539-2_17

pation. A more complete examination of these two disorders will be discussed, as well as the implications for treatment. While many cases of encopresis are the result of constipation, this is not true for all cases, and this distinction is valuable in informing clinical practice (Beninga et al., 1994).

The prevalence rates of both primary types of elimination disorders vary based on the demographic features of sampled populations such as age and geographical region. However, nighttime enuresis is typically 10% among 6-year-old children and around 5% among 10-year-old children (von Gontard, 2013). Prevalence rates for encopresis for children tend to be much lower with a range of 1.1–1.2% for 6-year-old children (Equit, Klein, Braun-Bither, et al., 2014; von Gontard & Equit, 2015). Enuresis for teenagers has been estimated at 1–3% (Feehan, McGee, Stanton, & Silva, 1990). However, even in adulthood there appears to be a prevalence of 2–3% (Yeung, Sreedhar, Sihoe, Sit, & Lau, 2006).

Comorbidity with other psychological disorders is found with 20–30% of children diagnosed with an elimination disorders (Nevéus et al., 2006). Comorbidity with being overweight, eating concerns, and self-image is further correlated at a higher degree with encopresis over enuresis according to Wagner, Equit, Niemczyk, and von Gontard (2015). Elimination disorders have been primarily associated with attention deficit hyperactivity disorder and oppositional defiant disorder, although mediational variables have not been addressed at this time.

Effective Ways to Screen for Elimination Disorders in Primary Care Settings

In primary care settings, screening for elimination disorders is conducted based upon the information provided by the parent or guardian of the person. Narrative descriptions typically initially identify elimination disorders. Once an elimination disorder is suspected, the physician should start a formal screening process. Part of the formal screening process should involve a brief screening to further assess if other psychological disorders might be present.

Several general psychological screening assessments for children have been developed for the use of primary care settings, such as the Pediatric Symptom Checklist (http://www.massgeneral.org/psychiatry/services/psc_forms.aspx) and the Early Childhood Screening Assessment (http://www.infantinstitute.org/measures-manuals/). For a more thorough review, please see American Academy of Pediatrics (2010). These general screens can then be used for entry level treatments or for referral as needed. Given the high prevalence rate of elimination disorders for children age 6–10, Van Herzeele, De Bruyne, De Bruyne, and Walle (2015) recommended utilization of a tiered style of screening in order to detect the largest possible number of cases and provide the appropriate level of empirically supported treatment.

How to Further Assess If a Screen Returns Positive

If a screen returns positive or if there is further concern that an elimination disorder is probable, then standard assessment procedures should be followed. Per von Gontard (2013), "The standard assessment consists of a thorough history, frequency/volume charts, specific questionnaires, a full physical examination, sonography and urinalysis" (p. s65). Follow-up assessment can be completed in primary care settings such as pediatric and child psychiatry settings. If organic causes cannot be identified, voiding journals or standardized questionnaires can be used to further assess the type of elimination disorder and first-pass treatment options.

Physical examinations should look for organic variables that have known influence on the incontinence type of interest, given the symptoms presented by the person. Both sonography and urinalysis should be considered in order to further rule out organic variables if deemed necessary, at which point intrusive procedures such as further medication or surgery may be required to provide adequate treatment. However, these assessments can be costly (roughly $300–$800), often require multiple visits and professionals, and can be unnecessary given low-risk situations. Positive results from these screens would exclude a formal diagnosis of an elimination disorder, as elimination disorder requires that voiding patterns are not accounted for by a physiological condition.

In the case of encopresis, additional physical examination should assess for the presence of bowel impaction, or constipation must occur to inform future treatment and determine the subtype of encopresis present (von Gontard, 2013). Sonography and rectal examination are, again, somewhat costly assessments that can provide options and concerns upon initial diagnosis. These diagnostic tools can assist in making this determination of the cause of the encopresis, as can other forms of physical examination which are crucial additional points of assessment in encopresis. In addition, examination of the spinal cord could occur in order to rule out possible organic causes (Loening-Baucke, 2002). If no bowel impaction or constipation is observed, assessment for additional emotional and behavioral problems may be warranted, though there is some disagreement over this (Loening-Baucke, 2002).

Frequency/volume charts can be used to identify the severity of the amount that is being voided through a standard procedure that can be completed in the natural environment. Nevéus et al. (2006) recommend that at least seven nights of a voiding journal are used to record the weight of the void and provide the information to the general practitioner to further select the best treatment interventions available.

The ICCL currently has distinguished two questionnaires as evidence based for elimination disorders. Although the ICCL uses a different diagnostic approach to elimination disorders than the DSM-5, there is compatibility across the two systems.

Evidence-Based Stepped Care and Brief Psychotherapeutic Approaches

Over the past 30 years, there has been a steady increase in evidence-based evaluations of treatments for several of the elimination disorders (Williams, Jackson, & Friman, 2007). However, it appears that elimination disorders have not been conceptualized in the framework of evidence-based stepped care. Currently, there is a lack of evidence-based stepped care, although several of the evidence-based approaches do hint at effective treatment elements that can be conceptualized in a stepped care framework. This section will aim to highlight the elements that have been evaluated in evidence-based fashion and will build a basic stepped care formulation.

Nocturnal enuresis has received a wide amount of empirical research including single-subject designs and randomized controlled trials comparing treatment approaches (von Gontard, 2013). Currently, the most supported intervention is the use of the bedtime alarm in combination with a voiding journal and brief education. Responsiveness to the use of the bedtime alarm procedure typically falls between 50 and 70%, with minimal relapse rates within a 6-month period (Glazener & Evans, 2004). Although the bedtime alarm has strong efficacy within the intervention, it also has a high level of resistance due to the complexity of the intervention, the intrusiveness, and social variables due to disruption of cultural features such as sleepovers (Christophersen et al., 2010). Most of the current research base, however, is composed of treatment packages that combine multiple treatment elements.

With regard to encopresis, the vast majority of primary care providers report treatment success rates in the range of 75–100% with little reason to refer to specialty care (Philichi & Yuwono, 2010). The case of referral for encopresis often relates to treatment resistance or a desire for additional assessment, rather than any difficulty in treatment. Treatment interventions in primary care settings typically utilize pharmacological or dietary intervention, though the types of dietary interventions vary (Philichi & Yuwono, 2010). For a list of options and manufacturers, see http://www.encopresis.com/bedwetting-device-manufacturers.

Evidence-Based Treatment: Enuresis

Key treatment elements that have empirical support include the use of a bladder diary, diet and exercise, the use of a reward system, relaxation training, biofeedback, nighttime awakening, and the use of desmopressin (von Gontard, 2013). Treatment elements should be incorporated into a treatment plan that fits the lifestyle of the child and the family. More intrusive elements should be used as non-responsiveness to less intrusive elements is observed.

Bladder diary is based on recording key information related to fluid intake, food intake, and urination into fabric (Nevéus et al., 2006). The bladder diary should be used for a minimum of 14 days; however, a minimum of seven nights of weighted volume of void should be recorded for nocturnal enuresis. The literature has referred to this approach by a number of different names, including charts, volume charts, frequency charts, voiding journal, or bladder diary (Nevéus et al., 2006; von Gontard, 2013). Bladder diary captures the total range of information that can be gathered depending on the type of information that is needed. The bladder diary is a flexible evidence-based practice that allows the practitioner to tailor the approach to the needs of each person.

Basic bladder advice, education, or counseling is typically used in order to explain the function of the bladder, to remove stigma related to elimination disorders, and to create buy-in for other treatment elements that typically can be resource intensive (von Gontard, 2013). General advice should focus on the importance of fluid intake, encouraging typical toilet usage of four to seven times per day, the common occurrence rates of enuresis, and the importance of support for parents/guardians (O'Flynn, 2011). Randomized controlled trials have been met with mixed results for basic bladder advice (Cederblad et al. 2015). But given the relative ease of the treatment component, and only initial formal criticism of the evidence behind its support, providing education and support to families in this manner is still generally recommended as a component of treatment (Vande Walle et al. 2017)

Reward systems should be used for toileting compliance, following fluid consumption recommendations, and follow-through with commitments related to treatment recommendations. Specific subtypes of enuresis such as nocturnal enuresis have specific recommendations such as not having rewards for dry nights but instead rewards for compliance with the treatment package (O'Flynn, 2011). Reward systems and basic bladder advice in combination with the use of a bladder diary has commonly been referred to as urotherapy and is typically the first line of treatment for daytime enuresis and is usually included with nocturnal enuresis treatment as well (Sinha & Raut, 2016). A basic package of education plus reward system and a waking procedure based on the baseline of nighttime voids has been found to be successful for a subgroup of individuals with nocturnal enuresis. However, longevity of results tends to be significantly less than the use of some medications or an enuresis alarm (Sinha & Raut, 2016). For a recent training manual based on current best practices, see Equit, Sambach, Niemczyk, and von Gontard (2015).

For nocturnal enuresis, an enuresis alarm is the next line of treatment following basic bladder diary, rewards, and bladder advice (von Gontard, 2013). Results of several studies have demonstrated that the enuresis alarm has the highest level of success for dry nights both during treatment and a relatively high rate of continued dryness post-intervention with 75% of responders having success following the removal of the intervention (Glazner, Evans, & Peto, 2003). As Sinha and Raut indicated in 2016:

> *[e]nuresis alarm should not be tried if: (1) The child wets the bed only once or twice per week; (2) The child or parents do not seem to be enthusiastic about the enuresis alarm; (3) Rapid or short-term improvement seems to be the goal for the parents; and (4) The parents seem to express negative feelings/blame their child for wetting the bed. (p. 334)*

The enuresis alarm has physically changed with the advancement of technologies, and currently the common enuresis alarms are small sensors placed in strategic area of the person's body. In order for the procedure to be most effective, it must have a high level of support from the care providers, and data should be recorded on the number of dry versus wet nights. Dry and wet nights should be included into the reward system, though it should not be the only element that earns rewards so that the reward system may be sensitive to small levels of change (O'Flynn, 2011; Sinha & Raut, 2016).

Evidence-Based Treatment: Encopresis

One of the primary differences between encopresis treatments when compared to enuresis is that effective treatment almost always involves the ingestion of specific foods such as high-fiber foods or substances that soften stool (Friman & Jones, 1998; Houts, 1991; Mellon & Houts, 1995; McGrath, Mellon, & Murphy, 2000). In addition, reduction or elimination of dairy is often recommended by a number of primary care providers (Philichi & Yuwono, 2010) and specialists (Loening-Baucke, 2002).

Bowel impaction may cause involuntary passage of large stools. Soft stool may also be evacuated around the obstruction as seepage. This seepage is often referred to as "paradoxical diarrhea" as severe constipation leads to the passage of only very soft stool which may appear to be diarrhea. As a result, unaware parents may administer medication to further slow bowel motility and further exacerbate the issue (Friman, Hofstadter, & Jones, 2006; Friman & Jones, 1998). Due to these issues it is important that encopresis be differentiated in its treatment and assessment as falling into two subtypes: with and without constipation (von Gontard, 2013).

In a biobehavioral approach, physical examination is, again, essential to the process. As noted by von Gontard (2013):

> *The perianal and perigenital areas should be inspected. Spine, reflex differences and asymmetries of buttocks should be noted. A rectal examination should be performed at least once. If sonography is available, this can replace the rectal exam if no organic form or fecal incontinence is suspected. If available, sonography of abdomen, kidneys, bladder and retrovesical region is helpful. (2012 p. 6)*

Following this examination, toilet training, laxatives, and functional behavioral treatments should be considered to address issues of impaction or other causes of encopresis that are determined. If constipation due to bowel impaction is the cause, treatment of the impaction should begin according to these methods in addition to dietary interventions and laxatives. After successful disimpaction, a long-term maintenance treatment over a minimum of 6 months to 2 years should follow to avoid re-accumulation of stool masses (Felt, Wise, Olsen, Kochhar, Marcus, & Coran, 1999).

In the case that constipation or impaction is not present, toilet training, dietary modification, and functional behavioral treatment are warranted. However, in such a case, the use of laxatives or bowel impaction treatment is not necessarily useful (Loening-Baucke, 2002). While some have argued that soiling in the absence of constipation is an expression of an additional behavioral or emotional problem, such a viewpoint remains a contention within the literature and the field (Loening-Baucke, 2002).

What Does Not Work

Early studies demonstrated an effect for hypnotherapy when compared to other available treatments such as imipramine. In a 1993 study, treatment utilizing hypnosis was reported to have lasting positive effects for roughly three-quarters of participants ($n = 25$) (Banejeree et al. 1993). However, more recently, the same hypnotherapy protocols were replicated and compared to alarm therapy. Subjects received an audiotape which they were to listen to nightly. While 55.3% of alarm-therapy participants achieved dryness, only 19.4% achieved this same outcome in the hypnotherapy condition ($n = 96$) (Seabrook, Gorodzinsky, & Freedman, 2005). This poor outcome should yield some skepticism among practitioners regarding hypnotherapy at this time, until further studies are conducted.

Some treatments, when delivered by trained practitioners, have been demonstrated to be effective but are designed to contain some treatment elements which can be aversive to the treatment recipient. For example, some behavioral approaches can include negative reinforcement or overcorrection elements which have been shown to be helpful pieces of some behavioral treatment packages (Crowley & Armstrong, 1977; Rolider & Van Houten, 1985). A commonly used book among behavior analytic practitioners and parents alike, *Toilet Training in Less Than a Day*, recommends overcorrection as part of its treatment package.

One overcorrection procedure suggested within this book is that children rapidly go to and from the bathroom numerous times if they void or urinate outside of the toilet (Azrin & Fox, 1974, p. 85). This treatment element is designed to address behavioral functions around the general response effort involved when a child is engaged in a potentially fun, relaxing, or otherwise reinforcing activity and must leave that activity to engage in high-effort responding away from all of the reinforcing stimulation. Balancing the scale of disproportional response effort and manipulating the reinforcing value of voiding successfully in the toilet against other competing activities are practices that have been shown to often be effective at quickly reducing or eliminating issues of enuresis and encopresis.

However, in many cases, it should be recommended that these procedures be done under the supervision and guidance of a practitioner who is trained in function-based approaches to behavior, particularly in cases where elimination disorders are comorbid with other conduct or developmental disorders and parent burnout is likely or parent follow-through is otherwise unlikely. Untrained and unsupervised parents or guardians should certainly avoid situations in which they are delivering aversive consequences such as social disapproval or other more extreme forms of punishment when the child does not use the bathroom to void. These procedures can be unnecessarily divisive and carry a risk of worsening behavioral issues, as parents may provide social disapproval and shaming, which could compound issues of guilt and anxiety around elimination. Many behavioral treatments include careful consideration of current behavioral targets to ensure shaping processes which are likely to emphasize success, reinforcement, and reward over punitive consequences.

In short, while potentially aversive procedures such as response cost, negative reinforcement, or overcorrection have demonstrated some efficacy, they should be utilized only when other options have been attempted, should likely be under the supervision of a trained professional such as a clinical psychologist or Board Certified Behavior Analyst, and should never be accompanied by social admonishment, shaming, or reprimand. More generally, behaviorally oriented treatments for encopresis and enuresis should always follow a thorough medical assessment as previously mentioned.

Related to behavioral treatments, which look at the contingencies surrounding voiding, are psychological and behavioral awareness treatments which seek to provide the child with training and practice in recognizing and controlling elimination processes. Bladder training exercises, which intend to increase maximum volume voided (MVV), have yet to demonstrate a clear positive effect in isolation (Starfield & Mellits, 1968; Harris & Purohit, 1977; Geffken, Johnson, & Walker, 1986). The idea behind this treatment is to have the child ingest large quantities of fluid and to subsequently hold urine in the bladder or practice stopping and starting urination. This method is meant to foster the bladder's ability to retain liquid through practice and muscle awareness and strengthening. Van Hoeck et al. (2008) found the MVV training component to be an inert part of a larger composite treatment for monosymptomatic nocturnal enuresis. In their study, alarm treatment alone served as a control for the use of oxybutynin and MVV training. The enuresis alarm alone resulted in the highest rate of full response and "lasting cure rate" of 50–67% 1 year after treatment. They note that "unfortunately, increasing MVV with pretreatment did not improve response or cure rate of subsequent alarm treatment (p. 1125)." This finding is coherent with another similar study which found minimal to no differences between these conditions (Van Hoeck et al., 2007).

When to Refer to External Specialty Mental Health

Elimination disorders are often conceived as simple problems but often necessitate a multidisciplinary approach including primary care providers, pediatric gastroenterologists, behavior analysts, and mental health practitioners. Given high rates of comorbidity and the relative success of behavioral and clinical approaches in the treatment of both elimination disorders and other psychological disorders, referral to external specialty mental health may be warranted. In particular, enuresis is frequently associated with developmental delays in domains such as speech, language, learning, and motor skills, as well as certain sleep-wake disorders (i.e., sleepwalking and sleep terror disorder) (American Psychiatric Association, 2013). Due to the high comorbidity rate, a child psychiatric assessment is recommended in child psychiatric settings (von Gontard, 2013). In other settings, screening with validated questionnaires (such as the Child Behavior Checklist; Achenbach, 1991) is recommended. If scores are in the clinical range, further assessment or child psychiatric referral is recommended (von Gontard, Baeyens, Van Hoecke, et al., 2011).

In addition, in the case of encopresis, if resistance to treatment is observed, referral to a mental health specialist may be warranted, as such issues may relate to problems in the areas of noncompliance or control (Loening-Baucke, 2002). If additional behavior problems are observed, or treatment adherence on the part of parent(s)/care provider(s) is low, referral to a mental health specialist for psychological intervention, family counseling, or, on occasion, hospitalization may be warranted. Treatment adherence might be challenging for some, as patterns of voiding can occur late at night, or while care providers are engaged with competing daily activities.

The Role of the Primary Care Provider/Medical Team

In general, most interventions can be provided in primary care settings, and most patients can be treated on an outpatient basis (von Gontard, 2013). However, primary care providers may wish to refer or work alongside integrated teams when treating cases where comorbid disorders and symptoms are present. In addition, treatment resistance and the desire for a second opinion are common reasons for referral requests in encopresis cases (Philichi & Yuwono, 2010). Primary care providers may follow steps from a treatment protocol which may include self-management, parent management, various approaches as mentioned in earlier sections, and even prescription and monitoring of medications (Borch, 2015).

How to Assess Impact on Care/ Quality Improvement Processes

Treatment success rates for the treatment of elimination disorders tend to be high, and success can be determined by the elimination of inappropriate voiding or the treatment of any co-occurring constipation in the case of encopresis. If inappropriate soiling continues and is resistant to treatment, improvement or referral to treat other potentially co-occurring issues is warranted.

In addition, parents provide an information source when examining the success or quality of care provided in the treatment process. When seeking referrals to an outside source, the primary reasons provided are the desire for a second opinion or treatment resistance (Philichi & Yuwono, 2010). As such, parental observations of behavior outside of the primary care setting or clinical context can provide a valuable source of data related to treatment improvement and quality of care provided. If parents seek outside referrals or additional information, an examination of the care provided by the practitioner and the communication of important health information to the consumer may be needed to address any barriers to successful service administration.

References

Achenbach, T. M. (1991). *Manual for the child behavior checklist/4-18 and 1991 profile*. Burlington: University of Vermont.

American Academy of Pediatrics. (2010). *Addressing mental health concerns in primary care: A clinician's toolkit*. Elk Grove Village, IL: American Academy of Pediatrics.

American Psychiatric Association. (2013). *Diagnostic and statistical manual of mental disorders* (5th ed.). Arlington, VA: American Psychiatric Publishing.

Azrin, & Fox. (1974). *Toilet training in less than a day*. New York, NY: Simon and Schuster.

Banerjee, S., Srivastav, A., & Palan, B. M. (1993). Hypnosis and self-hypnosis in the management of nocturnal enuresis: A comparative study with imipramine therapy. *The American Journal of Clinical Hypnosis*, *36*(2), 113.

Beninga, M. A., Büller, H. A., Heymans, H. S. A., Tytgat, G. N. J., & Taminia, J. A. J. M. (1994). Is encopresis always the result of constipation? *Archives of Disease in Childhood.*, *71*, 186–193.

Borch, L. (2015). Urinary and Fecal Incontinence. A Training Program for Children and Adolescents including CD-ROM with 109 pages of colour worksheets by Equit M, Sambach H, Niemczyk J, von Gontard A, 2014. Ashland, OH, USA.

Cederblad, M., Sarkadi, A., Engvall, G., & Nevéus, T. (2015). No effect of basic bladder advice in enuresis: A randomized controlled trial. *Journal of Pediatric Urology*, *11*(3), 153.e151–153.e155.

Christophersen, E. C., Christophersen, E. R., & Friman, P. C. (2010). *Elimination disorders in children and adolescents* (Vol. 16). Göttingen: Hogrefe Publishing.

Crowley, C. P., & Armstrong, P. M. (1977). Positive practice, overcorrection and behavior rehearsal in the treatment of three cases of encopresis. *Journal of Behavior Therapy and Experimental Psychiatry*, *8*(4), 411–416.

Equit, M., Klein, A., Braun-Bither, K., Gräber, S., & von Gontard, A. (2014). Elimination disorders and anxious-depressed symptoms in preschool children: A population-based study.European Child & Adolescent Psychiatry, *23*(6), 417–423. doi:10.1007/s00787-013-0468-9

Equit, M., Sambach, H., Niemczyk, J., & von Gontard, A. (2015). Urinary and fecal incontinence: A training program for children and adolescents.

Feehan, M., McGee, R., Stanton, W., & Silva, P. A. (1990). A 6 year follow-up of childhood enuresis: prevalence in adolescence and consequences for mental health. *Journal Paediatric Child Health.*, *26*, 75–79.

Felt, B., Wise, C. G., Olsen, A., Kochhar, P., Marcus, S., & Coran, A. (1999). Guideline for the management of pediatric idiopathic constipation and soiling. *Archives of Pediatric and. Adolescent Medicine*, *153*, 380–385.

Friman, P. C., & Jones, K. M. (1998). Elimination disorders in children. In S. Watson & F. Gresham (Eds.), *Handbook of child behavior therapy* (pp. 239–260). New York: Plenum.

Friman, P. C., Hofstadter, K. L., & Jones, K. M. (2006). A biobehavioral approach to the treatment of functional encopresis in children. *Journal of Early and Intensive Behavior Intervention, 3*(3), 263–272.

Geffken, G., Johnson, S. B., & Walker, D. (1986). Behavioral interventions for childhood nocturnal enuresis: the differential effect of bladder capacity on treatment progress and outcome. *Health and Psychology*, *5*, 261.

Glazener, C. M., Evans, J. H., & Peto, R. E. (2003). Alarm interventions for nocturnal enuresis in children. The Cochrane Database of Systematic Reviews, (2), CD002911.

Glazener, C. M., & Evans, J. H. (2004). Simple behavioural and physical interventions for nocturnal enuresis in children. *Cochrane Database Syst Rev*, (2), CD003637.

Harris, L. S., & Purohit, A. P. (1977). Bladder training and enuresis: A controlled trial. *Behavior Research and Therapy*, *15*, 485.

Houts, A. C. (1991). Nocturnal enuresis as a biobehavioral problem. *Behavior Therapy*, *22*, 133–151.

Loening-Baucke, V. (2002). Encopresis. *Current Opinion in Pediatrics.*, *14*, 570–575.

McGrath, M. L., Mellon, M. W., & Murphy, L. (2000). Empirically supported treatments in pediatric psychology: Constipation and encopresis. *Journal of Pediatric Psychology*, *25*(4), 225–254.

Mellon, M. W., & Houts, A. C. (1995). Elimination disorders. In R. T. Ammerman & M. Hersen (Eds.), Handbook of child behavior therapy in the psychiatric setting (pp. 341–366). New York: Wiley.

Nevéus, T., von Gontard, A., Hoebeke, P., Hjälmås, K., Yeung, C. K., Vande Walle, J., … Djurhuus, J. C. (2006). The standardization of terminology of lower urinary tract function in children and adolescents: Report from the Standardization Committee of the International Children's Continence Society (ICCS). *Journal of Urology*, *176*, 314–324.

O'Flynn, N. (2011). Nocturnal enuresis in children and young people: NICE clinical guideline. *The British Journal of General Practice*, *61*(586), 360–362.

Philichi, L., & Yuwono, M. (2010). Primary care: Constipation and encopresis treatment strategies and reasons to refer. *Gastroenterology Nursing.*, *33*(5), 363–366.

Rasquin, A., Di Lorenzo, C., Forbes, D., Guiraldes, E., Hyams, J. S., Staiano, A., & Walker, L. S. (2006). Childhood functional gastrointestinal disorders: child/adolescent. *Gastroenterology.*, *130*, 1527–1537.

Rolider, A., & Van Houten, R. (1985). Treatment of constipation-caused encopresis by negative reinforcement procedure. *Journal of Behavior Therapy and Experimental Psychiatry*, *16*, 67–70.

Seabrook, J. A., Gorodzinsky, F., & Freedman, S. (2005). Treatment of primary nocturnal enuresis: A randomized clinical trial comparing hypnotherapy and alarm therapy. *Paediatrics & Child Health*, *10*(10), 609–610.

Sinha, R., & Raut, S. (2016). Management of nocturnal enuresis – Myths and facts. *World Journal of Nephrology*, *5*(4), 328.

Starfield, B., & Mellits, D. M. (1968). Increase in functional bladder capacity and improvements in enuresis. *Journal of Pediatrics*, *72*, 483.

Van Herzeele, C., De Bruyne, P., De Bruyne, E., & Walle, J. V. (2015). Challenging factors for enuresis treatment: Psychological problems and non-adherence. *Journal of Pediatric Urology*, *11*(6), 308–313.

Van Hoeck, K., Bael, A., Lax, H., Hirche, H., Van Dessel, E., Van Renthegem, D., et al. (2007). Urine output rate and maximum volume voided in school-age children with and without nocturnal enuresis. *Journal of Pediatric Urology*, *151*, 575.

Van Hoeck, K. J., Bael, A., Lax, H., Hirche, H., Bernaerts, K., Vandermaelen, V., & van Gool, J. D. (2008).

Improving the cure rate of alarm treatment for monosymptomatic nocturnal enuresis by increasing bladder capacity—A randomized controlled trial in children. *The Journal of Urology*, *179*(3), 1222–1226.

Vande Walle, J., Rittig, S., Tekgül, S., Austin, P., Yang, S. S.-D., Lopez, P.-J., & Van Herzeele, C. (2017). Enuresis: practical guidelines for primary care. *The British Journal of General Practice, 67*(660), 328–329. http://doi.org/10.3399/bjgp17X691337.

von Gontard, A., Baeyens, D., Van Hoecke, E., Warzak, W. J., & Bachmann, C. (2011). Psychological and psychiatric issues in urinary and fecal incontinence. *Journal of Urology*, *185*, 1432–1437.

von Gontard, A. (2013). The impact of DSM-5 and guidelines for assessment and treatment of elimination disorders. *European Child & Adolescent Psychiatry*, *22*(S1), 61–67.

von Gontard, A., & Equit, M. (2015). Comorbidity of ADHD and incontinence in children. *European Child & Adolescent Psychiatry*, *24*(2), 127–140.

Wagner, C., Equit, M., Niemczyk, J., & von Gontard, A. (2015). Obesity, overweight, and eating problems in children with incontinence. *Journal of Pediatric Urology*, *11*(4), 202–207.

Williams, W. L., Jackson, M., & Friman, P. C. (2007). *Encopresis and enuresis-9* (pp. 171–190). Elsevier. https://doi.org/10.1016/B978-012372544-8/50010-0

Yeung, C. K., Sreedhar, B., Sihoe, J. D., Sit, F. K., & Lau, J. (2006). Differences in characteristics of nocturnal enuresis between children and adolescents: A critical appraisal from a large epidemiological study. *BJU International*, *97*, 1069–1073.

18 Generalized Anxiety Disorder

Eddie C. Erazo and Holly Hazlett-Stevens

A Brief Description of Generalized Anxiety Disorder

Generalized anxiety disorder (GAD) is a chronic psychiatric condition characterized primarily by excessive and uncontrollable worry. Although the core feature is cognitive in nature, the somatic complaints and impairment in behavioral functioning associated with worry are major components of GAD. Worry can be defined as "a cognitive process in which individuals anticipate threatening outcomes and events" (Hazlett-Stevens, 2008, p. 1). Individuals with GAD usually spend a large proportion of the day engaging in worry that is considered excessive because it is disproportionate to actual risk. In specific, negative outcomes of even the most benign situations are usually overestimated, which leads to a constant state of hypervigilance. The 12-month and lifetime prevalence rates of GAD are estimated at 3.1% and 5.7%, respectively, with an average age onset of 31 years (Kessler et al., 2005; Kessler, Chiu, Demler, & Walters, 2005). Barlow's (2002) integrative model of anxiety is the predominant model applied specifically to GAD (Roemer, Orsillo, & Barlow, 2002) and asserts that a diathesis of biological vulnerabilities (e.g., genetics) and psychological vulnerabilities (e.g., early life experiences characterized by unpredictability and lack of control) is responsible for the development of anxiety disorders. Indeed, GAD has been coined the "basic" anxiety disorder because the anxiety-provoking cognitive process underlying GAD is observed across other anxiety disorders with greater specificity, such as worry about social rejection in social anxiety disorder. Individuals who develop GAD are often intolerant of uncertainty and engage in persistent "what if?" and worst-case-scenario thinking patterns to anticipate perceived catastrophe. In addition to this attempt to thwart external catastrophes, Borkovec and colleagues' avoidance model (Borkovec, Alcaine, & Behar, 2004) further proposed that worry serves as a strategy to escape unwanted internal experiences, such as aversive imagery, physiological arousal, and difficult emotions. Content of worry can run the gamut from work performance and finances to health and relationships. In addition to overestimation of negative outcomes, individuals with GAD commonly perceive themselves as unable to cope with anticipated outcomes. Ironically, worrying yields prediction of potential negative outcomes but is often followed by anxiety and ineffective coping rather than constructive problem-solving. Worry is believed to function as an illusory attempt at gaining control within the inherent unpredictability of life; such attempts are then negatively reinforced by the absence of catastrophic outcomes.

E.C. Erazo (✉) • H. Hazlett-Stevens
Department of Psychology, University of Nevada, Reno, Reno, CA, USA
e-mail: ecerazo@gmail.com; hhazlett@unr.edu

A. Maragakis, W.T. O'Donohue (eds.), *Principle-Based Stepped Care and Brief Psychotherapy for Integrated Care Settings*, https://doi.org/10.1007/978-3-319-70539-2_18

The costs of such persistent and pervasive worry are physical symptoms, including muscle tension, fatigue, and sleep disturbance, as well as impaired functioning in work and relationship problems. To make matters worse, the costs and distress of worry can lead to a state of meta-worry in which individuals worry about the negative effects of worry despite being unable to control it. GAD is a mental disorder with excessive and uncontrollable worry as its central feature, but the associated somatic symptoms make GAD particularly relevant to primary care settings where patients often seek relief from physical symptoms. Although anxiety disorders account for an estimated $42 billion per year in direct and indirect costs in the United States, an estimated 41% of patients in primary do not receive treatment for anxiety due to lack of detection (Kroenke, Spitzer, Williams, Monahan, & Löwe, 2007), which illustrates the need for proper screening.

Effective Ways to Screen for Generalized Anxiety Disorder in the Primary Care Setting

Given the physical symptoms associated with chronic worry, it is not surprising that individuals with GAD frequently present to primary care settings with somatic complaints. Despite categorization as a mental disorder, the salience and discomfort of physical symptoms often lead patients to suspect a biological problem and seek care from medical professionals rather than mental health providers. GAD accounts for more than 50% of anxiety disorders in primary care (Wittchen & Hoyer, 2001) with a prevalence rate of 7.6% (Kroenke et al., 2007), yet subthreshold GAD prevalence rates are even higher and also involve significant impairment (Rucci et al., 2003). Annual healthcare costs are estimated to be 64%, or $2,138, higher for individuals with GAD than those without GAD (Marciniak et al., 2005; Olfson & Gameroff, 2007). The prevalence of GAD in primary care coupled with associated costs of the disorder makes screening in primary settings crucial to determining treatment needs. For example, failure to detect GAD may lead to expensive and unnecessary medical testing for physical complaints while delaying appropriate treatment.

The DSM-5 criteria for GAD are (A) excessive anxiety and worry more days than not for at least 6 months; (B) worry is experienced as difficult to control; (C) anxiety and worry are associated with at least three out of the six following symptoms, including (1) restlessness, (2) being easily fatigued, (3) difficulty concentrating, (4) irritability, (5) muscle tension, and (6) sleep disturbance; (D) the anxiety, worry, or physical symptoms cause significant distress or impairment in functioning (e.g., social or occupational); (E) the disturbance is not attributable to physiological effects of a substance or medical condition; and (F) disturbance is not better explained by another disorder (American Psychiatric Association, 2013). In order to be thorough in detection of mental disorders during the initial visit without demanding significant time from the medical team, administrative staff can have patients complete the Psychiatric Diagnostic Screening Questionnaire (Zimmerman & Mattia, 2001) in 15–20 minutes while in the waiting room before meeting with the primary care physician. The PDSQ is a 126-item measure that assesses diagnostic criteria for 13 different disorders, including GAD. The questionnaire's excellent sensitivity minimizes the chance of false negatives, which means the physician can be confident that the patient does not meet criteria for the disorder if the cutoff score is not met. If a patient meets the cutoff score for GAD and the physician suspects a psychiatric disorder from the interview, further testing can be conducted by the on-site behavioral health provider after a "warm hand-off" from the physician. In particular, the GAD-7 is a brief 7-item measure developed from a multisite, primary care study that was specifically designed to efficiently screen for GAD in primary care settings (Spitzer, Kroenke, Williams, & Löwe, 2006). Unlike the PDSQ, the GAD-7 offers both a cutoff score (10 out of a possible score of 21) for screening purposes and a severity scale ranging from mild (5) to severe (15+), which provides the clinician with greater assessment data than a dichotomous diagnosis. Between the PDSQ and the GAD-7, primary care physicians and behavioral health providers can confidently assess for the presence of GAD. These screening methods offer the advantage of time efficiency given the time constraints inherent in integrated care. However, further assessment is often necessary to specify individualized treatment targets in order to expedite treatment progress due to the varied nature of GAD complaints.

How to Further Assess for Generalized Anxiety Disorder if Screen Returns Positive

One of the major challenges of diagnosing and treating GAD is its high comorbidity with other mental disorders. Data from the large National Comorbidity Survey conducted in the United States showed that GAD was most often comorbid with major depressive disorder (39%), simple phobia (25%), social anxiety disorder (23%), and panic disorder (23%; Wittchen, Zhao, Kessler, & Eaton, 1994). Therefore, it is important for the behavioral health provider to differentially diagnose GAD as well as detect comorbid mental disorders. Although the *Anxiety and Related Disorders Interview Schedule for DSM-5* (Brown & Barlow, 2014) is the gold standard structured interview for diagnosis and differential diagnosis of anxiety disorders, the administration time (≈90 min) is prohibitive within the time constraints of brief intervention in integrated care. Fortunately, brief questionnaires that serve a similar purpose are available. One such measure is the 42-item Depression Anxiety and Stress Scales (Lovibond & Lovibond, 1995), which includes depression, anxiety, and stress subscales with five severity levels ranging from normal to extremely severe. The stress subscale assesses difficulty relaxing, nervous arousal, and irritability, and higher scores have been observed in GAD than in panic disorder and social anxiety disorder (Brown, Chorpita, Korotitsch, & Barlow, 1997), making it useful for differential diagnosis. In addition, the depression subscale would provide information about possible comorbidity of depression, which would prompt the use of a brief depression screening, such as the widely used Beck Depression Inventory-2 (Beck, Steer, & Brown, 1996).

During the clinical interview, it is important for the clinician to briefly confirm the presence of DSM-5 criteria for GAD before making a diagnosis. Due to GAD's somatic nature and high comorbidity with other disorders, an essential aspect of the interview would be to determine whether the anxiety and worry truly are *generalized* rather than situation-specific and confirm that the somatic arousal occurs predominantly during times of worry. For example, excessive worry only occurring in social situations would imply social anxiety disorder instead, and constant fatigue or muscle tension in the absence of worry may indicate the presence of a medical condition. Similarly, antecedents and consequences of worry and somatization would be important factors to assess. For instance, assessment may reveal that symptoms only occur when preceded by substances (e.g., caffeine, cigarettes). In contrast, worry may be followed by maladaptive coping strategies (e.g., alcohol, eating, behavioral avoidance), as individuals with GAD tend to cope ineffectively rather than proactively when distressed by anticipated threat. Assessment of antecedents and consequences of worry helps to confirm GAD and to place one's worry within a larger context while identifying points of intervention.

At the end of the intake session, the clinician can assign self-monitoring of worry using a diary form with columns for event/trigger, content of worry, and emotion/behavioral response. This assignment simultaneously provides the clinician with further real-world assessment of the individual's GAD-related patterns while priming the individual's awareness of causes, content, and consequences of "worry" cognitions. Finally, assigning a self-report measure of worry beliefs, such as the Consequences of Worry Scale (COWS, Davey, Tallis, and Capuzzo, 1996), may provide valuable information to elucidate the extent to which the patient holds positive or negative attitudes toward worry. In particular, the COWS helps to clarify how worry functions in the patient's life, including functional impairment, distress, and superstitions or perceived benefits. Thus, combining assessment and self-monitoring that are thorough, yet brief, sets the stage for efficient psychotherapeutic intervention.

Evidence-Based Stepped Care and Brief Psychotherapeutic Approaches

Not only is GAD the most common anxiety disorder in primary care, it is also widely considered the most difficult anxiety disorder to treat effectively due to the diffuse nature of worry (Brown, Barlow, & Liebowitz, 1994). Fortunately, there are myriad psychotherapeutic techniques for treating GAD. This chapter will focus on cognitive behavioral therapy (CBT) for GAD because it is the most widely used empirically supported treatment for anxiety. There are five core components of modern CBT for GAD: psychoeducation, applied relaxation, cognitive restructuring, behavioral activation, and mindfulness/acceptance-based techniques. In CBT for GAD, clients learn to accurately estimate the likelihood and consequences of negative outcomes, engage in problem solving instead of worry, and use acceptance and relaxation strategies to buffer excessive worry and physiological arousal. The modes of delivering CBT for GAD will be presented in a stepped care sequence, and individual components of CBT will be explained in further detail within the individual treatment format.

Bibliotherapy and eHealth

There are many self-help options for anxiety that can be used as a supplement or alternative to individual therapy. Given the minimal cost associated with self-help treatment options, these may be especially appropriate first-line approaches for mild cases or homework for moderate to severe cases, based on GAD-7 cutoff scores. Internet-based CBT, such as the freely available E-couch (http://www.ecouch.anu.edu.au) and MoodGYM (http://www.moodgym.anu.edu.au) for anxiety, has also been shown to be as effective at treating GAD as individual CBT with a 60% remission rate (Andrews, Newby, & Williams, 2015). Several self-help CBT and mindfulness-based intervention books are also available as standalone or supplemental bibliotherapy. Notable options include *Women Who Worry Too Much* (Hazlett-Stevens & Craske, 2005); *The Worry Cure* (Leahy, 2005); *Mastery of Your Anxiety and Worry, second edition* (Craske & Barlow, 2006); *Get Out of Your Mind and Into Your Life* (Hayes & Smith, 2005); *The Mindful Way Through Anxiety* (Orsillo & Roemer, 2011); and *A Mindfulness-Based Stress Reduction Workbook* (Stahl, Goldstein, Kabat-Zinn, & Santorelli, 2010), which includes audio recordings of mindfulness practices for patients to follow.

Group Therapy

Within stepped care, the level of treatment above bibliotherapy and eHealth is group therapy. CBT can be offered effectively in a group format and is an excellent treatment option for GAD patients with moderate GAD-7 scores and those who do not benefit sufficiently from self-help strategies. With the limited resources and time constraints of brief intervention in primary care, group CBT provides an efficient means of treating multiple individuals. Group CBT has been shown to be equally effective for GAD as individual CBT at less than half the cost ($646 vs. $248; Gould, Otto, Pollack, & Yap, 1997; Heuzenroeder et al., 2004). One potential advantage of group CBT over self-help and individual therapy is the social support and normalization inherent in group therapy, which may be preferred by some patients and is worth mentioning to patients when prescribing treatment. As with self-help, group therapy can also serve as an intensive supplement to individual therapy for severe cases.

Individual Therapy

The most intense form of CBT for GAD is providing individual therapy, and this option should only be reserved for moderate to severe cases, patients who do not benefit from group therapy, or if there are barriers to group therapy, such as transportation or scheduling conflicts. Even within individual therapy, self-help and group therapy remain strategies to supplement and strengthen cognitive behavioral techniques. Clinicians should approach each session with a clear agenda to maximize the use of time in 20–30 minutes sessions. Components of CBT for GAD are described in detail below within the context of individual therapy, but these are also fundamentals of self-help and group CBT for GAD. Using the five main components, the primary goals within the few sessions allotted in primary care are to (1) teach the patient why anxiety occurs and how it manifests, (2) present relaxation and acceptance techniques to manage worry and physiological arousal, (3) teach cognitive restructuring and use behavioral experiments to accurately estimate probability and consequences of negative outcomes, and (4) stimulate problem-solving for proactive coping.

Psychoeducation and self-monitoring. A primary component of CBT for GAD involves simply explaining the functional nature of anxiety, fear, and worry. Orienting patients to how anxiety promoted survival for our ancestors and has been carried over into modern society where different threats exist (e.g., social rejection) can help to de-pathologize the experience of anxiety. Similarly, explaining the Yerkes-Dodson law in which some anxiety improves performance, compared to the extremes of apathy or hyperarousal, can raise awareness of the adaptive nature of anxiety. Teaching these accessible facts to the patient combats negative beliefs about anxiety and may prevent desire to rid oneself of anxiety entirely, which is unreasonable and could lead to treatment dissatisfaction. Instead, the clinician should frame treatment as a means of decreasing anxiety to more adaptive levels and intervening early before anxiety spirals out of control, to promote effective coping.

Daily self-monitoring of an individual's specific anxiety-related thoughts, physical sensations, and behaviors as they occur provides the foundation for subsequent coping strategies. As patients systematically record their anxiety levels, any triggering internal or external events, and associated thoughts, sensations, and behaviors over the course of each day, they begin to see how anxiety is simply a process of reactions unfolding over time. Patients eventually become more aware when such anxiety spirals develop, enabling them to respond with a coping response instead of becoming increasingly anxious. Finally, it is crucial that patients are aware of their roles in therapy, including both attendance *and* effortful participation in homework. This point is especially critical in brief intervention where number (3–5) and duration (20–30 minutes) of sessions are already limited and homework is the primary means of progress, while sessions are used to review homework and introduce new practices.

Applied relaxation. Applied relaxation involves responding to anxiety with new strategies to manage or to prevent excessive physiological arousal and emotional reactivity. Patients begin with practice of specific relaxation strategies at a dedicated time and place at home. Once they develop some proficiency, patients apply their relaxation skills in response to anxiety-related triggers or cues in the course of daily life.

One of the most simple and common techniques is diaphragmatic breathing, in which the patient is instructed to focus on their breath and breathe from the "belly" rather than the chest. Breathing from the chest is more common during anxiety and contributes to tension, whereas diaphragmatic breathing uses the muscles designed for breathing and promotes relaxation. Resting one hand on the chest and one hand on the belly provides an easy form of biofeedback to focus on breathing from the diaphragm. Another applied relaxation technique is progressive muscle relaxation (PMR; Bernstein, Borkovec, & Hazlett-Stevens, 2000), which has received much empirical support in GAD treatment research. PMR teaches patients to systematically tense and release a series of muscle groups while noting associated physical sensations. Patients eventually learn to induce physical muscle relaxation quickly whenever unnecessary muscle tension is detected. A final relaxation strategy is pleasant imagery, in which the clinician prompts the patient to close his or her eyes, imagine a pleasant scene, and bring attention to the five senses. For example, a patient may imagine lying on the beach and notice the warmth of the sun on their skin, the smell of sunscreen, the taste of a tropical drink, the color of the water, and the sound of waves crashing.

When teaching relaxation, it is important that the patient understands these techniques are intended as means of coping with stressful circumstances rather than as means of escaping, avoiding, or controlling the immediate anxious experience itself. Clinicians can describe relaxation as a paradox: the harder one tries to relax, the more elusive relaxation becomes. While these relaxation techniques do not directly target worry, they allow patients to practice deployment of new coping responses and may also increase "buy-in" or willingness to try other techniques described below.

Cognitive restructuring. The underlying philosophy of CBT is that situations and events trigger automatic thoughts that lead to emotions (e.g., anxiety) and behaviors in chronological sequence. Thoughts are considered automatic because they are involuntary and informed by one's core beliefs—a stable set of beliefs about oneself, others, the world, and the future—that typically develop from early life experiences, as described in the integrative model of anxiety. Common core beliefs among patients with GAD are "I am a failure" and "I am not good enough," which engender negative predictions and perceived inability to cope. In the cognitive model, anxiety is presumed to result from distorted automatic thoughts, such as overestimation of negative outcomes and their consequences. Therefore, the primary cognitive technique within CBT is cognitive restructuring, which involves identifying the manner in which automatic thoughts are distorted by core beliefs and creating adaptive responses that promote more accurate perception of reality.

The main tool for cognitive restructuring is the thought record, with columns for recording a specific situation, thoughts/interpretations, and emotions/behaviors. Assigning a thought record early in therapy contributes to idiographic assessment of anxious thoughts and helps the patient identify specific anxiety-provoking thoughts to proceed with cognitive restructuring. For example, a patient may experience intense anxiety due to multiple negative predictions about an upcoming job interview. "Job interview" is the situation, anxiety is the emotion rated on a scale from 1 to 10, and negative predictions might include "I'll get lost and show up late. What if I don't know how to answer every question? If I don't get the job, I'll end up homeless." First, the clinician would assist the client in identifying possible distortions using a list of common categories of distorted thinking (e.g., Leahy & Holland, 2000). As in the present example, fortune telling, catastrophizing, and "what if?" thinking are among the most common distortions in GAD and may signal the presence of GAD.

Based on the plausible distortion(s), the clinician works with the patient to consider alternative outcomes, weigh evidence for and against predictions, and even question worst-case scenario if all predictions were to come true. This process is used to create adaptive responses to automatic thoughts, such as "I can trust my GPS for directions. I usually know how to answer interview questions, but I can pause to think before answering if necessary. Even if I don't get the job, it will be good practice, and I can apply for another one later. I can ask family for financial help if I need it." Then, the clinician prompts the patient to re-rate their level of anxiety from 1 to 10. While the process of cognitive restructuring is intended to promote accurate thinking, which often leads to a reduction in anxiety, it is equally important in promoting effective behavioral coping efforts.

Behavioral activation. The second major component of CBT for GAD is engaging in new and more adaptive behavioral responses. Given that patients with GAD tend to be behaviorally frozen by worry, identifying and initiating problem-solving strategies is a crucial supplement to cognitive restructuring. For GAD patients, the emotion/behavior column of the thought record usually involves anxiety, behavioral inhibition, and further worry. Avoidance of specific activities or situations, procrastination, and worry safety behaviors (such as reassurance seeking, repeated checking, calling a loved one to make sure he or she is safe, or leaving much earlier than needed for an appointment to avoid being late) are particularly common. Explicitly listing anticipated threats in the thought record and creating adaptive responses exposes instrumental behaviors that could reduce the likelihood of problematic feared outcomes. Using the job interview example, the individual can practice answering interview questions with a friend, study driving directions, and search for other available jobs. The clinician can pose the question, "What steps could you take to make this prediction less likely?" to prompt solution-focused behavioral activation instead of ineffective cognitive worry.

Similarly, CBT involves behavioral experiments aimed at testing negative predictions, promoting accurate thinking by discovering how unlikely perceived threats actually are. For example, the clinician can use a thought record to assess the patient's negative predictions of an upcoming situation, alternative neutral and positive outcomes, and their perceived likelihood (0–100%) before and after cognitive restructuring. Then, the behavioral experiment can be assigned as a homework assignment between sessions. To illustrate, a patient may be worried about requesting annual leave and being fired. Cognitive restructuring may lower perceived likelihood of being fired from 80% to 20% and likelihood of receiving leave from 10% to 50% based on evidence that others are rarely denied. A helpful approach is discussion of worst, best, and most realistic case scenarios. The patient's homework would be to request annual leave, and the result would, ideally, provide evidence against catastrophic predictions. An important note here is that the clinician must carefully consider the risk of failure and set the patient up for success while understanding that there is a calculated risk inherent in any behavioral experiment. However, even if an undesired outcome results from a patient's behavioral experiment, the clinician can explore how the patient coped with this situation and how catastrophic the outcome really was.

Stimulus control methods provide a final behavioral strategy when working with excessive and uncontrollable worry. Whenever worry is detected, patients postpone that worry to a "worry period" scheduled for a specific time and place later in the day. During the worry period, patients deliberately revisit each worry recorded and systematically work through each one using the cognitive restructuring and problem-solving strategies described above.

Mindfulness and acceptance-based techniques. Finally, a more recent addition to CBT for GAD includes interventions that promote acceptance of unwanted internal experience and cultivate mindfulness. Mindfulness can be defined as "paying attention in a particular way: on purpose, in the present moment, and nonjudgmentally" (Kabat-Zinn, 1994). Mindfulness has become a popular clinical approach through mindfulness meditation interventions such as mindfulness-based stress reduction (MBSR) and mindfulness-based cognitive therapy (MBCT). In addition, elements of these mindfulness-based interventions and of acceptance and commitment therapy (ACT) have been integrated into the acceptance-based behavior therapy for GAD (Roemer & Orsillo, 2005). Each of these interventions has received rigorous research support and is considered an evidence-based intervention for GAD.

Mindfulness practices promote a sense of intentional curiosity to one's experience, including the breath, bodily sensations, thoughts, and all five senses, in a "being" rather than "doing" mode. In contrast, psychological reactivity and rejection of one's experience may only serve to exacerbate the somatic arousal characteristic of GAD. Simple exercises to practice mindfulness in session and as homework assignment are short (5–15 minutes) periods of noticing the sensation of breathing, methodically scanning body parts for sensations, noticing the flow of thoughts, and even yoga movements. Mindfulness is readily integrated with CBT to promote nonjudgmental awareness of worry cognitions and somatic arousal. Further, given the future-oriented nature of worry, mindfulness practices are helpful in fostering present moment focus. A quick exercise that can be assigned as homework for times of anxiety is the STOP acronym. When experiencing anxiety and worry, patients Stop, Take a breath mindfully, Observe present moment experience (including thoughts and bodily sensations), and Proceed skillfully, which may involve creating a thought record or engaging in behavioral coping strategies. The ultimate aim of mindfulness practice for GAD is to build an *allowing* and *observing* relationship with one's experiences, which alleviates worry-related suffering and provides the opportunity for intentional and skillful behavioral responses.

What Does Not Work

When encountering a person struggling with excessive and uncontrollable worry, laypeople and clinicians alike may be tempted simply to reassure the person and to encourage them to stop worrying. Unfortunately, this "don't worry, be happy" approach can easily backfire, leaving the person feeling invalidated and misunderstood. Furthermore, much thought suppression research has shown that intentionally trying to stop thinking about something can ironically cause a rebound effect, characterized by an increased frequency of, and greater preoccupation with, the unwanted thought. Providing reassurance in vague or general terms (e.g., "Everything will be okay"), rather than supporting the patient in responding to his or her own worry skillfully as described above, also can undermine treatment progress. This response prevents the patient from investigating the nature and function of the worry and undermines the patient's ability to cope with the situation. Ineffective medical approaches will be discussed in the section describing the role of the primary care provider/medical team in treatment.

When to Refer to External Specialty Mental Health

Given that GAD is one of the least successfully treated mental disorders with high relapse rates (Barlow, 2002), brief intervention in primary care settings may not be sufficient to achieve remission. One simple indicator that external specialty mental health is appropriate would be a "severe" score on the GAD-7 during initial assessment. Since most CBT protocols are based on a 12–16 one hour session format, three to five 20–30 minute sessions may simply not be enough to resolve the pervasive and incapacitating worry characteristic of individuals with severe GAD. Initial self-report and clinical interview assessment is crucial to identify the combination of a severe score on the GAD-7 and severe functional impairment resulting from GAD. While a patient with a severe GAD-7 score but high social and occupational functioning may not necessarily require intensive psychotherapy, another patient with a severe GAD-7 score and severe functional impairment (e.g., social isolation, unemployment) would warrant external mental health treatment. Similarly, the high comorbidity of GAD with other mental disorders further complicates treatment, and comorbidities may indicate the need for greater resources. Indeed, research studies using internet-delivered CBT in primary care usually exclude patients whose anxiety disorder is comorbid with schizophrenia, bipolar disorder, substance abuse, and active suicidal ideation (Andrews et al., 2015). These comorbidities are appropriate exclusion criteria in primary care given the brief nature of treatment with lengthy gaps between sessions, suggesting the need for an external mental health provider.

High comorbidity of GAD with other anxiety disorders may also predict poor outcomes and serve as an indicator that a referral to external mental health is indicated. For example, a patient presenting with moderate GAD alone is more likely to respond to brief intervention than a patient with moderate GAD and comorbid panic disorder and posttraumatic stress disorder. The greater flexibility in treatment intensity offered by external mental health allows comorbid conditions to be addressed simultaneously, especially if there are shared vulnerabilities, such as a previous trauma. GAD alone is difficult to treat, which highlights the importance of assessing potential comorbid conditions during the initial visit to triage severe cases and those with complicating comorbidities to a higher level of treatment in a stepped care model.

The Role of the Primary Care Provider/Medical Team in Treatment

Despite classification as a psychiatric disorder, the primary care provider and team serve an important role in both the assessment and treatment of GAD. Administration and interpretation of the PDSQ is necessary to identify a potential GAD diagnosis, but it is crucial that the primary care provider rules out the possibility that anxiety and somatic complaints are due to a medical condition or side effects of a medication. This may be especially difficult with GAD due to the high comorbidity with other medical conditions, especially gastrointestinal problems (e.g., irritable bowel syndrome). Any clear medical explanation for GAD symptoms should be treated accordingly, but psychological treatment may still be indicated if anxiety appears to be contributing to the medical condition via psychobiological reactivity, such as inflammation.

Psychopharmacotherapy is often the preferred treatment for mental disorders in primary care settings and holds great potential for treating GAD, but a few precautions should be taken when prescribing medication. In particular, benzodiazepines were once the primary medication for anxiety, but long-term benzodiazepine is no longer recommended due to risky side effects and dependency (Berger, Edelsberg, Treglia, Alvir, & Oster, 2012). Benzodiazepines also have the potential to undermine the use of learned cognitive behavioral and relaxation strategies by promoting reliance on a pill for rapid symptom relief rather than compliance with homework. Selective serotonin reuptake inhibitors (SSRIs) and serotonin and norepinephrine reuptake inhibitors (SNRIs) are now the preferred first-line treatment for GAD (Berger et al., 2012) but are still hampered by side effects. Common side effects include sexual dysfunction, weight gain, and emotional detachment (Demyttenaere & Jaspers, 2008), which may lead patients to discontinue without notifying their physician. Indeed, attrition is often greater in studies investigating medication for GAD, compared to CBT (Mitte, 2005). While medications such as venlafaxine hydrochloride extended release (Effexor XR) are effective for GAD, high relapse rates (53.7%) have been found once medication is discontinued. In one study, 50.7% of patients prescribed with venlafaxine hydrochloride extended release improved after 6 months, but 53.7% of those randomized to receive a placebo for the next 6 months relapsed, compared to only 9.8% among those continuing to receive medication (Rickels, Etemad, Khalid-Khan, Lohoff, & Gallop, 2010).

Fortunately, not only has the combination of CBT with medication been shown to achieve effects more quickly, but also benefits were maintained without maintenance medication (Wetherell et al., 2013). This may explain why even individual CBT is more cost-effective in the long term than medication alone ($646 vs. $1153; Heuzenroeder et al., 2004). Therefore, it is important for the medical team to use appropriate medication for the duration of CBT treatment and properly plan tapering with the patient to reduce duration of side effects in therapy. A final note is the importance of the physician endorsing the psychological contribution to a patient's somatic complaints to increase psychotherapy acceptability and support mental health efforts (e.g., homework completion).

How to Assess Impact on Care/Quality Improvement Processes

Just as the GAD-7 can be used as a brief screening tool for GAD, it should be used as a standard follow-up measure to determine whether symptoms fall below threshold of GAD after treatment. The primary care staff can track decreases in GAD-7 scores and monitor the percentage of patients that have remitted to subthreshold GAD severity (<10) after four sessions, for example. Once sufficient data have been collected, the primary care setting can examine whether baseline GAD-7 scores moderate the benefit of brief treatment and determine a cutoff score that predicts treatment failure or success using a logistic regression. A baseline GAD-7 score above this cutoff indicates low chance of achieving GAD remission in the clinic. This would imply the need to refer the patient to external mental health immediately rather than attempting brief intervention first.

Given the cognitive *and* somatic nature of GAD, emphasizing the domain that fits the patient's primary complaint may enhance treatment acceptability and "buy-in." For example, minorities (e.g., Hispanics) tend to experience greater somatization of mental distress and perceive stigma with mental disorders than nonminorities (Reynolds, O'Koon, Papademetriou, Szczygiel, & Grant, 2001), which may make a somatic orientation to treatment more acceptable. With past research suggesting that greater somatization leads to greater use of and preference for medical over mental health services (Escobar et al., 1987), mental health services housed in primary care is especially well-equipped to handle this dilemma. Asking whether the patient believes GAD symptoms to be more mentally or physically caused, distressing, and problematic during the intake interview can help specify a treatment orientation. While both cognitive and relaxation strategies may still be introduced, a primary orientation can help to tailor treatment with limited sessions. Follow-up surveys, homework compliance records, and posttreatment GAD-7 scores can be used to determine whether matching presenting complaint and treatment orientation predicts treatment acceptability and improvement.

References

American Psychiatric Association. (2013). *Diagnostic and statistical manual of mental disorders* (5th ed.). Arlington, VA: American Psychiatric Publishing.

Andrews, G., Newby, J. M., & Williams, A. D. (2015). Internet-delivered cognitive behavior therapy for anxiety disorders is here to stay. *Current Psychiatry Reports*, *17*(1), 533. https://doi.org/10.1007/s11920-014-0533-1

Barlow, D. H. (2002). *Anxiety and its disorders: The nature and treatment of anxiety and panic* (2nd ed.). New York, NY: Guilford.

Beck, A. T., Steer, R. A., & Brown, G. K. (1996). *Manual for the Beck Depression Inventory-II*. San Antonio, TX: Psychological Corporation.

Berger, A., Edelsberg, J., Treglia, M., Alvir, J. M. J., & Oster, G. (2012). Change in healthcare utilization and costs following initiation of benzodiazepine therapy for long-term treatment of generalized anxiety disorder: a retrospective cohort study. *BMC Psychiatry*, *12*(1), 177. https://doi.org/10.1186/1471-244X-12-177

Bernstein, D. A., Borkovec, T. D., & Hazlett-Stevens, H. (2000). *New directions in progressive relaxation training: A guidebook for helping professionals*. Westport, CT: Greenwood.

Borkovec, T. D., Alcaine, O. M., & Behar, E. (2004). Avoidance theory of worry in generalized anxiety disorder. In R. G. Heimberg, C. L. Turk, & D. S. Mennin (Eds.), *Generalized anxiety disorder: Advances in research and practice* (pp. 3–28). New York, NY: Guilford.

Brown, T. A., & Barlow, D. H. (2014). *Anxiety and related disorders interview schedule for DSM-5 (ADIS-5L): Client interview schedule*. New York, NY: Oxford University Press.

Brown, T. A., Barlow, D. H., & Liebowitz, M. R. (1994). The empirical basis of generalized anxiety disorder. *American Journal of Psychiatry*, *151*, 1272–1280.

Brown, T. A., Chorpita, B. F., Korotitsch, W., & Barlow, D. H. (1997). Psychometric properties of the Depression Anxiety Stress Scales (DASS) in clinical samples. *Behaviour Research and Therapy*, *35*(1), 79–89.

COWS, Davey, G. C. L., Tallis, F., & Capuzzo, N. (1996). Beliefs about the consequences of worrying. *Cognitive Therapy and Research*, *20*, 499–520.

Craske, M. G., & Barlow, D. H. (2006). *Mastery of your anxiety and worry: Client workbook* (2nd ed.). New York: Oxford University Press.

Demyttenaere, K., & Jaspers, L. (2008). Bupropion and SSRI-induced side effects. *Journal of Psychopharmacology*, *22*(7), 792–804. https://doi.org/10.1177/0269881107083798

Escobar, J. I., Golding, J. M., Hough, R. L., Karno, M., Burnam, M. A., & Wells, K. B. (1987). Somatization in the community: Relationships to disability and use of services. *American Journal of Public Health*, *77*(7), 837–840.

Gould, R. A., Otto, M. W., Pollack, M. H., & Yap, L. (1997). Cognitive behavioral and pharmacological treatment of generalized anxiety disorder: A preliminary meta-analysis. *Behavior Therapy*, *28*(2), 285–305. https://doi.org/10.1016/S0005-7894(97)80048-2

Hayes, S. C., & Smith, S. (2005). *Get out of your mind and into your life: The new Acceptance and Commitment Therapy*. Oakland, CA: New Harbinger.

Hazlett-Stevens, H. (2008). *Psychological approaches to generalized anxiety disorder: A clinician's guide to assessment and treatment*. New York, NY: Springer.

Hazlett-Stevens, H., & Craske, M. G. (2005). *Women who worry too much: How to stop worry and anxiety from ruining relationships, work, and fun*. Oakland, CA: New Harbinger.

Heuzenroeder, L., Donnelly, M., Haby, M. M., Mihalopoulos, C., Rossell, R., Carter, R., … Vos, T. (2004). Cost-effectiveness of psychological and pharmacological interventions for generalized anxiety disorder and panic disorder. *The Australian and New Zealand Journal of Psychiatry, 38*(8), 602–612. https://doi.org/10.1111/j.1440-1614.2004.01423.x

Kabat-Zinn, J. (1994). *Wherever you go there you are: Mindfulness meditation in everyday life*. New York, NY: Hyperion.

Kessler, R. C., Berglund, P., Demler, O., Jin, R., Merikangas, K. R., & Walters, E. E. (2005). Lifetime prevalence of age-of-onset distributions of DSM-IV disorders in the National Comorbidity Survey Replication. *Archives of General Psychiatry, 62*, 593–602.

Kessler, R. C., Chiu, W. T., Demler, O., & Walters, E. E. (2005). Prevalence, severity, and comorbidity of 12-month DSM-IV disorders in the National Comorbidity Survey Replication. *Archives of General Psychiatry, 62*, 617–627.

Kroenke, K., Spitzer, R. L., Williams, J. B. W., Monahan, P. O., & Löwe, B. (2007). *Annals of Internal Medicine, 146*, 317–325.

Leahy, R. L. (2005). *The worry cure: Seven steps to stop worry from stopping you*. New York, NY: Harmony Books.

Leahy, R. L., & Holland, S. J. (2000). *Treatment plans and interventions for depression and anxiety disorders*. New York: Guilford.

Lovibond, S. H., & Lovibond, P. F. (1995). *Manual for the Depression Anxiety Stress Scales* (2nd ed.). Sydney: Psychology Foundation.

Marciniak, M. D., Lage, M. J., Dunayevich, E., Russell, J. M., Bowman, L., Landbloom, R. P., & Levine, L. R. (2005). The cost of treating anxiety: The medical and demographic correlates that impact total medical costs. *Depression and Anxiety, 21*, 178–184.

Mitte, K. (2005). Meta-analysis of cognitive-behavioral treatments for generalized anxiety disorder: a comparison with pharmacotherapy. *Psychological Bulletin, 131*(5), 785–795. https://doi.org/10.1037/0033-2909.131.5.785

Olfson, M., & Gameroff, M. J. (2007). Generalized anxiety disorder, somatic pain and health care costs. *General Hospital Psychiatry, 29*, 310–316.

Orsillo, S. M., & Roemer, L. (2011). *The mindful way through anxiety*. New York, NY: Guilford.

Reynolds, L. K., O'Koon, J. H., Papademetriou, E., Szczygiel, S., & Grant, K. E. (2001). Stress and somatic complaints in low-income urban adolescents. *Journal of Youth and Adolescence, 30*(4), 499–514.

Rickels, K., Etemad, B., Khalid-Khan, S., Lohoff, F. W., Rynn, M. A., & Gallop, R. J. (2010). Time to relapse after 6 and 12 months' treatment of generalized anxiety disorder with venlafaxine extended release. *Archives of General Psychiatry, 67*(12), 1274–1281. https://doi.org/10.1001/archgenpsychiatry.2010.170

Roemer, L., & Orsillo, S. M. (2005). An acceptance based behavior therapy for generalized anxiety disorder. In S. M. Orsillo & L. Roemer (Eds.), *Acceptance and mindfulness-based approaches to anxiety: Conceptualization and treatment*. New York: Springer.

Roemer, L., Orsillo, S. M., & Barlow, D. H. (2002). Generalized anxiety disorder. In D. H. Barlow (Ed.), *Anxiety and its disorders: The nature and treatment of anxiety and panic* (pp. 477–515). New York, NY: Guilford.

Rucci, P., Gherardi, S., Tansella, M., Piccinelli, M., Berardi, D., Bisoffi, G., … Pini, S. (2003). Subthreshold psychiatric disorders in primary care: Prevalence and associated characteristics. *Journal of Affective Disorders, 76*, 171–181.

Spitzer, R. L., Kroenke, K., Williams, J. B., & Löwe, B. (2006). A brief measure for assessing generalized anxiety disorder: the GAD-7. *Archives of Internal Medicine, 166*, 1092–1097.

Stahl, B., Goldstein, E., Kabat-Zinn, J., & Santorelli, S. (2010). *A mindfulness-based stress reduction workbook*. Oakland, CA: New Harbinger.

Wetherell, J. L., Petkus, A. J., White, K. S., Nguyen, H., Kornblith, S., Andreescu, C., … Lenze, E. J. (2013). Antidepressant medication augmented with cognitive-behavioral therapy for generalized anxiety disorder in older adults. *American Journal of Psychiatry, 170*(7), 782–789. https://doi.org/10.1176/appi.ajp.2013.12081104

Wittchen, H., Zhao, S., Kessler, R. C., & Eaton, W. W. (1994). DSM-III-R generalized anxiety disorder in the National Comorbidity Survey. *Archives of General Psychiatry, 51*, 355–364.

Wittchen, H. U., & Hoyer, J. (2001). Generalized anxiety disorder: Nature and course. *Journal of Clinical Psychiatry, 62*, 15–19.

Zimmerman, M., & Mattia, J. I. (2001). The Psychiatric Diagnostic Screening Questionnaire: Development, reliability and validity. *Comprehensive Psychiatry, 42*(3), 175–189. https://doi.org/10.1053/comp.2001.23126

19 Hoarding Disorder

C.W. Ong, E.B. Lee, and M.P. Twohig

A Brief Description of the Disorder or Problem

Hoarding disorder (HD) is characterized by acquiring large quantities of objects difficulty discarding, and/or keeping them organized. The diagnostic criteria identified in the *Diagnostic and Statistical Manual of Mental Disorders, Fifth Edition* (American Psychiatric Association, 2013), include (a) difficulty discarding possessions, regardless of their value; (b) a perceived need to save items and accompanying distress associated with discarding them; (c) an accumulation of items that congest active living areas; (d) hoarding that causes clinically significant distress or impairment; and (e) hoarding that is not due to another medical or mental health condition. Hoarding occurs in approximately 2–6% of the population, more often occurs among males, and is significantly more prevalent in older adults (Iervolino et al., 2009; Mueller, Mitchell, Crosby, Glaesmer, & de Zwaan, 2009; Samuels et al., 2008; Timpano et al., 2011). Hoarding symptoms usually begin early in life and are often chronic, sometimes becoming more severe over time (Tolin, Meunier, Frost, & Steketee, 2010).

C.W. Ong (✉) • E.B. Lee • M.P. Twohig
Utah State University, Logan, UT, USA
e-mail: clarissa.ong@usu.edu; eric.lee@usu.edu

Effective Ways to Screen for It in the Primary Care Setting

The two aspects of hoarding most relevant to determining the need for professional attention are clutter and functional impairment, as difficulty discarding and excessive acquisition may not be problematic in and of themselves. Indeed, many of the negative consequences linked to hoarding (e.g., inability to use living spaces, health and safety risks associated with obstructions in the home; Steketee, Frost, & Kim, 2001) tend to result from clutter rather than acquiring new items or saving possessions. Unfortunately, due to poor insight in hoarding cases, individuals have difficulty recognizing the need for help and are less likely to seek treatment (Frost, Tolin, & Maltby, 2010). Many psychometrically validated measures can be used to identify problematic hoarding in a primary care setting as part of routine screening, and oftentimes, using multiple measures simultaneously is the most reliable way to assess hoarding severity. Questions clinicians can initially use to quickly screen for hoarding include "Do you have difficulty moving around your home due to clutter?" and "Are you able to easily access entrances and exits in your home?" Both questions gauge accessibility within the home that may be compromised as a result of clutter.

Two measures have been developed for clutter and functional impairment associated with

A. Maragakis, W.T. O'Donohue (eds.), *Principle-Based Stepped Care and Brief Psychotherapy for Integrated Care Settings*, https://doi.org/10.1007/978-3-319-70539-2_19

hoarding: the Clutter Image Rating scale (CIR; Frost, Steketee, Tolin, & Renaud, 2008) and the Activities of Daily Living for Hoarding scale (ADL-H; Frost, Hristova, Steketee, & Tolin, 2013). Both scales are available online (http://www.oxfordclinicalpsych.com/view/10.1093/med:psych/9780199334940.001.0001/med-9780199334940-interactive-pdf-004.pdf [CIR]; http://www.oxfordclinicalpsych.com/view/10.1093/med:psych/9780199334940.001.0001/med-9780199334940-interactive-pdf-006.pdf [ADL-H]), are quick to administer, and measure impact of the individual's hoarding on daily functioning. The CIR is a self-report, pictorial measure of clutter containing three sets of nine color photographs. Each set of nine photographs varies in range from least cluttered (1) to most cluttered (9) and represents a common room in the home: living room, bedroom, and kitchen (Frost et al., 2008). The CIR uses a mean composite score (average across three rooms) to quantify the amount of clutter in the home. A score of 4 or greater suggests clutter severe enough to warrant clinical attention (Frost et al., 2008), though clinicians may use their judgment to determine an appropriate cutoff based on other factors in the individual's clinical presentation. In lieu of a home visit or recent photos of the individual's home, the CIR provides the closest estimate of clutter severity, as it circumvents issues associated with inaccurate or vague verbal reporting. The ADL-H is a 15-item self-report measure that assesses ability to carry out activities of daily living, such as preparing food and using the bath/shower. Items are rated from 1 to 5, with higher scores indicating greater impairment due to clutter. Again, clinicians may use their judgment as well as other aspects of the individual's presentation to interpret ADL-H scores in context. For example, a high score on the ADL-H without concomitant hoarding symptoms may suggest that someone else in the home is exhibiting hoarding behaviors that is causing difficulty for the patient.

Symptom-focused measures can be used in conjunction with the previously mentioned scales to more holistically characterize the hoarding problem. Examples include the Hoarding Rating Scale (HRS; both a self-report and clinician-rated version exist; Tolin, Frost, & Steketee, 2010; Tolin, Frost, Steketee, & Fitch, 2008) and the Saving Inventory—Revised (SI-R; self-report; Frost, Steketee, & Grisham, 2004). The HRS comprises five items spanning the dimensions of (a) difficulty discarding, (b) excessive acquisition, (c) clutter, (d) impairment, and (e) distress. Each item is rated from 0 to 8, with higher scores indicating greater severity. A score of 4 or more on difficulty discarding and clutter, as well as 4 or more on impairment or distress, has been used to indicate a HD diagnosis (Tolin et al., 2008). The brevity and flexibility of this measure make it particularly useful as a quick screening tool for a potential HD diagnosis. The SI-R is one of the most widely used self-report measures of hoarding severity, comprising 23 items across three domains: (a) difficulty discarding, (b) clutter, and (c) excessive acquisition. Each item is rated from 0 to 4, with higher scores indicating greater hoarding severity. Item scores are added up to yield a total score. The clinical cutoff score for the SI-R is 41 (Frost & Hristova, 2011). A caveat accompanying use of the SI-R is that it provides little information on the impact of hoarding on the individual due to its exclusive focus on symptoms; thus, using it with another scale, such as the ADL-H, may be more useful.

Because these measures are relatively quick to complete, clinicians could use a combination of measures to obtain a more complete picture of the individual's hoarding status without imposing a significant burden on the individual. Indeed, Frost and Hristova (2011) recommend integrating self-report, observational, and interviewer-based measures where possible and investigating the meaning of discrepant reporting across methods. For example, using the CIR and SI-R together allows for comparisons between verbal self-report of clutter and visual self-report of clutter, which may reflect individuals' level of insight into their hoarding.

How to Further Assess if a Screen Returns Positive

Using the two questions mentioned in the previous section, clinicians should be able to get an estimate of the severity of clutter in the individual's home.

Follow-up clarification questions (e.g., "How difficult is it for you to get from one room to another due to clutter?") and specific hoarding measures can then be administered if patients respond positively. If clinicians suspect that the individual's hoarding problems warrant further assessment based on results from the measures, the Structured Interview for Hoarding Disorder (SIHD; Nordsletten et al., 2013) can be used to provide a comprehensive evaluation of hoarding behaviors. The SIHD is a semi-structured instrument that corresponds closely to the DSM-5 criteria for HD and is thus the most appropriate for determining the presence of a HD diagnosis. Flexibility is incorporated in the interview, such that interviewers may come up with probes to obtain clarification from interviewees. Of clinical interest, the SIHD includes a risk assessment section containing items about potential consequences associated with severe hoarding, such as dangerous obstructions, infestations, and unhygienic conditions. The SIHD was designed to be administered in the interviewee's home environment. Even though this may be less feasible in a primary care environment, the scale developers recommend supplementing interview data with photographs of the home, clinical records, referral notes, and informant report where possible.

Evidence-Based Stepped Care and Brief Psychotherapeutic Approaches

Treatment research on HD is still in its nascent stage, with much of it focused on a cognitive behavioral treatment (CBT) protocol for HD. The content of the protocol has been largely consistent across treatment studies and typically includes five components: psychoeducation about hoarding, training decision-making, organizing, exposure, and cognitive restructuring (Frost, Steketee, & Greene, 2003). Treatment for hoarding also usually incorporates home visits (Steketee & Tolin, 2011), given the pertinence of the home environment to hoarding. Clinicians may refer to the treatment manual, *Treatment for Hoarding Disorder: Therapist Guide*, for details on how to conduct the following intervention procedures.

Educating clients about the nature of hoarding, their symptom presentation, and treatment expectations affords them a clearer understanding of their behaviors in context. The International OCD Foundation (IOCDF) provides a useful fact sheet that clinicians can use to familiarize themselves with the presentation of hoarding disorder (https://iocdf.org/wp-content/uploads/2014/10/Hoarding-Fact-Sheet.pdf). Clinicians can then work with clients to develop a case conceptualization, including its cognitive, emotional, and behavioral components, and collaboratively design a treatment plan based on this conceptualization. To understand the client's hoarding problems, clinicians can ask questions about the onset and duration of their problematic hoarding behaviors, reasons for saving, the presence of safety and/or health hazards (e.g., obstructed means of egress), previous treatment attempts, as well as treatment expectations and life goals.

Training clients in decision-making and organization entails improving their ability to categorize possessions in a useful way (e.g., all recyclables go in one bin) as well as to make considered decisions about acquiring and discarding (e.g., weighing the pros and cons of each decision). Clinicians can also help clients develop problem-solving strategies during this time, such as identifying the problem, brainstorming possible solutions, evaluating the utility of solutions, implementing a solution, assessing outcome, and repeating the process if necessary.

Exposure in HD treatment involves putting clients in situations where they are likely to acquire (e.g., yard sales) or save (e.g., asking them to discard an item) and then asking them to practice experiencing the uncomfortable emotions (e.g., anxiety, sadness, guilt) that arise. These situations are typically arranged in a hierarchy; clients start with situations that provoke less discomfort, then work their way up to more challenging situations. If clients struggle with in vivo tasks, imaginal tasks can be used when first starting with exposure exercises. For example, clients can be asked to imagine what losing a particular possession would be like and to sit with the discomfort. One of the main aspects of exposure exercises is helping clients learn that the discomfort can be tolerated, and that they can function well with the discomfort present, without giving into urges to acquire or save. It is important to note that the decision to acquire or discard ultimately rests with the client, which complicates the exposure process, because failing to discard typically does not result in much discomfort. As alluded to earlier, clinicians may need to be creative when implementing exposure practice, such as exposing clients to the *thought* of discarding, rather than discarding per se. As home visits may be difficult, discarding exposures can occur in the office if the client brings items in. During the exposure itself, clinicians should ask clients to focus on the aversive stimulus (e.g., thought of losing the belonging, feeling of sadness) and to rate the level of distress they are experiencing. The goal of exposure is typically to notice that the distress is tolerable. The brevity of treatment sessions in primary care settings means that clinicians may need to focus more on teaching clients how to do exposure exercises and assigning homework in between sessions, rather than spending sessions practicing exposure with them. If the clinician perceives a need for more intense intervention strategies, referral to a mental health professional may be indicated.

Cognitive restructuring aims to modify unhelpful beliefs about possessions by identifying and addressing problematic thinking patterns, listing the benefits and costs of hoarding, as well as differentiating between needing and wanting items. One cognitive technique commonly used in HD treatment is the downward arrow method, which involves asking clients a series of questions to reveal core beliefs that may be maintaining saving, such as "I need to always be prepared." For example, a client may experience difficulty discarding china that has not been used in years. To explore her core belief regarding saving, the clinician could ask, "What would happen if you discarded the china?" The client may then reply that she would not be able use the china at a dinner party, if she ever decided to organize one. The clinician could then follow up with several other questions to identify the underlying belief driving these thoughts (e.g., "What would happen if you did organize a dinner party and did not have the china? Where else could you find suitable crockery? What would be the worst part about not having the china?"). Eventually, the client may reveal the core belief that she always needs to be prepared. Once core beliefs are identified, clinicians can work with clients to evaluate and challenge them. Clinicians may also explore the accuracy of clients' beliefs by carefully examining them and asking questions about those beliefs. For example, the client may believe that she needs to save a piece of fabric for a future art project. In this case, the clinician may ask about the probability of that art project transpiring, how the piece of fabric might be used in the project, or if a similar piece of fabric could be acquired when the time came. Challenging clients' unhelpful beliefs in a compassionate way may aid adaptive decision-making.

In addition, motivational interviewing strategies are commonly used in CBT for HD both early in treatment to clarify the client's therapeutic goals and values and throughout treatment to enhance motivation when needed (Steketee & Tolin, 2011). Motivational interviewing techniques can be used to identify, explore, and address ambivalence about change to increase treatment adherence. For example, clients may recognize the need to change and how their hoarding is affecting family members but find it difficult to let go of their attachment to their possessions. Elucidating ambivalence, rather than direct confrontation, could help clarify different sources of clients' motivation for change, which can then be leveraged to promote behavioral change. Clinicians are recommended to read Miller and Rollnick's (2002) *Motivational Interviewing* or visit http://www.motivationalinterviewing.org/ for more information on the principles and strategies of motivational interviewing. Clients are also given homework between sessions to practice the skills they learn.

Various modes of protocol delivery have been tested, and results are promising. Both group bibliotherapy using the hoarding self-help book,

Buried in Treasures (Frost, Pekareva-Kochergina, & Maxner, 2011; Frost, Ruby, & Shuer, 2012), and an online self-help group (Muroff, Steketee, Himle, & Frost, 2010) were found to produce significant improvement in outcomes over time. Thus, such interventions requiring minimal therapist involvement may be a first option for individuals struggling with hoarding problems within a stepped care model. Group CBT for HD also appears to be helpful for symptom reduction (Muroff, Steketee, Bratiotis, & Ross, 2012) and may be recommended as a next step for individuals who do not benefit from self-guided therapy. However, further research is still needed to evaluate both the clinical and cost-effectiveness of a stepped care model for HD (Muroff, 2011). Individuals for whom these intervention methods do not work may need referrals to mental health professionals who are competent in individualized CBT for HD.

What Does Not Work

Because hoarding symptoms have been conceptualized as a symptom dimension of obsessive-compulsive disorder (OCD), researchers have used exposure-based CBT—an empirically supported treatment for OCD—for hoarding symptoms. However, research suggests that such an approach yields a poorer treatment response compared to other OCD symptom dimensions (e.g., contamination; Abramowitz, Franklin, Schwartz, & Furr, 2003). Thus, healthcare providers should recognize that HD presents differently from OCD and use evidence-based treatments that have been found to be effective for HD (described in the previous paragraphs).

When to Refer to External Specialty Mental Health

HD is a difficult disorder to treat. Standard CBT protocols are around 20 sessions (range 13–35 in published studies). This is longer than medical professions generally see clients. The treatment of hoarding often occurs at the client's home, which may not be feasible for medical professionals. Additionally, the pure amount of clutter at the client's home, along with possible hazardous material, can make clearing of the home difficult. Finally, as HD is positively correlated with age, some older clients may struggle with the physical work of clearing the home.

If bibliotherapy, web-based therapy, and a brief CBT do not have an effect on acquiring rates and removal rates after a month or so, external therapy may be suggested. The IOCDF (www.iocdf.org) maintains a directory of therapists trained to treat hoarding. If the quantity of material is high, the client may require a dumpster from the local waste management company. If the hoarded materials have reached a dangerous or toxic level, professional waste removal company—such as disaster or flood clean up—may be necessary.

The Role of the Primary Care Provider/Medical Team in Treatment

Only one open trial has investigated the use of medication in the context of HD. Among 23 patients with HD, 70% were classified as responders at the end of the 12-week venlafaxine trial based on at least a 30% decrease in hoarding symptom severity scores (UCLA Hoarding Severity Scale and SI-R) as well as a rating of at least "much improved" on the Clinical Global Impression/Improvement scale (Saxena & Sumner, 2014). Significant improvements in depression, anxiety, and overall functioning were also observed (Saxena & Sumner, 2014). Other pharmacological studies using paroxetine and sertraline among participants with an OCD diagnosis with predominant hoarding symptoms also produced similarly encouraging results (Brakoulias, Eslick, & Starcevic, 2015). However, optimism in these findings should be tempered by study limitations, such as small sample size and lack of a comparison/placebo group. Furthermore, a case series of four individuals with HD that tested the effect of extended release methylphenidate—a stimulant—on inattention and hoarding symptoms found that none of the participants chose to continue taking the medication as they felt that the adverse side effects did not outweigh its gains (Rodriguez et al., 2013). It is difficult to amalgamate these findings, given varying clinical presentations and use of different medications across studies. Nonetheless, it appears that some evidence suggests pharmacotherapy is a viable intervention for HD, and further research is needed in this area before widespread dissemination.

Furthermore, HD often co-occurs with other psychiatric conditions, in particular, major depressive disorder, generalized anxiety disorder, and social phobia. In fact, 77% of HD participants were found to have an anxiety disorder (other than OCD) and/or a mood disorder (Frost, Steketee, & Tolin, 2011). In cases where these comorbid conditions are treated with psychotropic medications, primary care providers need to be vigilant in their prescription practices, ensuring that patients do not experience long-term side effects due to consumption of multiple medications.

Because hoarding severity is linked to physical health conditions, such as hypertension, diabetes, and sleep apnea, (Ayers, Iqbal, & Strickland, 2013; Tolin, Frost, Steketee, Gray, & Fitch, 2008), it is also helpful to involve primary care providers in the assessment and treatment of individuals with HD so that comorbid physical conditions received proper care. A multidisciplinary approach may be particularly judicious in geriatric cases, as one study found that 90% of older adults with HD reported at least one medical condition relative to 44% in a nonpsychiatric comparison group (Ayers et al., 2013).

How to Assess Impact on Care/Quality Improvement Processes

The assessment procedures described in a previous section can be repeated over the course of treatment to track progress. These measures should provide insight into the amount of accumulation of items occurring, perceived need to save items, and distress and impairment caused by hoarding behavior from pre- to posttreatment. Additionally, the conspicuous nature of hoarding provides opportunities to track progress visually over time using photographs to monitor clutter and congestion where the hoarding occurs.

References

Abramowitz, J. S., Franklin, M. E., Schwartz, S. A., & Furr, J. M. (2003). Symptom presentation and outcome of cognitive-behavioral therapy for obsessive-compulsive disorder. *Journal of Consulting and Clinical Psychology*, *71*(6), 1049–1057. https://doi.org/10.1037/0022-006X.71.6.1049

American Psychiatric Association. (2013). *Diagnostic and statistical manual of mental disorders* (5th ed.). Washington, DC: Author.

Ayers, C. R., Iqbal, Y., & Strickland, K. (2013). Medical conditions in geriatric hoarding disorder patients. *Aging & Mental Health*, *18*(2), 37–41. https://doi.org/10.1080/13607863.2013.814105

Brakoulias, V., Eslick, G. D., & Starcevic, V. (2015). A meta-analysis of the response of pathological hoarding to pharmacotherapy. *Psychiatry Research*, *229*(1–2), 272–276. https://doi.org/10.1016/j.psychres.2015.07.019

Frost, R. O., & Hristova, V. (2011). Assessment of hoarding. *Journal of Clinical Psychology*, *67*(5), 456–466. https://doi.org/10.1002/jclp.20790

Frost, R. O., Hristova, V., Steketee, G., & Tolin, D. F. (2013). Activities of daily living scale in hoarding disorder. *Journal of Obsessive-Compulsive and Related Disorders*, *2*, 85–90. https://doi.org/10.1016/j.jocrd.2012.12.004

Frost, R. O., Pekareva-Kochergina, A., & Maxner, S. (2011). The effectiveness of a biblio-based support group for hoarding disorder. *Behaviour Research and Therapy*, *49*(10), 628–634. https://doi.org/10.1016/j.brat.2011.06.010

Frost, R. O., Ruby, D., & Shuer, L. J. (2012). The buried in treasures workshop: Waitlist control trial of facilitated support groups for hoarding. *Behaviour Research and Therapy*, *50*(11), 661–667. https://doi.org/10.1016/j.brat.2012.08.004

Frost, R. O., Steketee, G., & Greene, K. A. I. (2003). Cognitive and behavioral treatment of compulsive hoarding. *Brief Treatment and Crisis Intervention*, *3*(3), 323–338. https://doi.org/10.1093/brief-treatment/mhg024

Frost, R. O., Steketee, G., & Grisham, J. (2004). Measurement of compulsive hoarding: Saving inventory-revised. *Behaviour Research and Therapy*, *42*(10), 1163–1182. https://doi.org/10.1016/j.brat.2003.07.006

Frost, R. O., Steketee, G., & Tolin, D. F. (2011). Comorbidity in hoarding disorder. *Depression and Anxiety*, *28*(10), 876–884. https://doi.org/10.1002/da.20861

Frost, R. O., Steketee, G., Tolin, D. F., & Renaud, S. (2008). Development and validation of the clutter image rating. *Journal of Psychopathology and Behavioral Assessment*, *30*(3), 193–203. https://doi.org/10.1007/s10862-007-9068-7

Frost, R. O., Tolin, D. F., & Maltby, N. (2010). Insight-related challenges in the treatment of hoarding. *Cognitive and Behavioral Practice*, *17*(4), 404–413. https://doi.org/10.1016/j.cbpra.2009.07.004

Iervolino, A. C., Perroud, N., Fullana, M. A., Guipponi, M., Cherkas, L., Collier, D. A., & Mataix-Cols, D. (2009). Prevalence and heritability of compulsive hoarding: A twin study. *American Journal of Psychiatry*, *166*(10), 1156–1161. https://doi.org/10.1176/appi.ajp.2009.08121789

Miller, W. R., & Rollnick, S. (2002). *Motivational interviewing: Preparing people for change* (2nd ed.). New York, NY: The Guilford Press.

Mueller, A., Mitchell, J. E., Crosby, R. D., Glaesmer, H., & de Zwaan, M. (2009). The prevalence of compulsive hoarding and its association with compulsive buying in a German population-based sample. *Behaviour Research and Therapy*, *47*(8), 705–709. https://doi.org/10.1016/j.brat.2009.04.005

Muroff, J. (2011). Thinking outside the box: Novel delivery methods for treating hoarding. *International Journal of Cognitive Therapy*, *4*(3), 280–296. https://doi.org/10.1521/ijct.2011.4.3.280

Muroff, J., Steketee, G., Bratiotis, C., & Ross, A. (2012). Group cognitive and behavioral therapy and bibliotherapy for hoarding: A pilot trial. *Depression and Anxiety*, *29*(7), 597–604. https://doi.org/10.1002/da.21923

Muroff, J., Steketee, G., Himle, J., & Frost, R. (2010). Delivery of internet treatment for compulsive hoarding (D.I.T.C.H.) *Behaviour Research and Therapy*, *48*(1), 79–85. https://doi.org/10.1016/j.brat.2009.09.006

Nordsletten, A. E., Fernández de la Cruz, L., Pertusa, A., Reichenberg, A., Hatch, S. L., & Mataix-Cols, D. (2013). The Structured Interview for Hoarding Disorder (SIHD): Development, usage and further validation. *Journal of Obsessive-Compulsive and Related Disorders*, *2*(3), 346–350. https://doi.org/10.1016/j.jocrd.2013.06.003

Rodriguez, C. I., Bender, J., Jr., Morrison, S., Mehendru, R., Tolin, D. F., & Simpson, H. B. (2013). Does extended release methylphenidate help adults with hoarding disorder? A case series. *Journal of Clinical Psychopharmacology*, *33*(3), 444–447. https://doi.org/10.1097/JCP.0b013e318290115e

Samuels, J. F., Bienvenu, O. J., Grados, M. A., Cullen, B., Riddle, M. A., Liang, K. Y., ... Nestadt, G. (2008). Prevalence and correlates of hoarding behavior in a community-based sample. *Behaviour Research and Therapy*, *46*(7), 836–844. https://doi.org/10.1016/j.brat.2008.04.004

Saxena, S., & Sumner, J. (2014). Venlafaxine extended-release treatment of hoarding disorder. *International Clinical Psychopharmacology*, *29*, 266–273. https://doi.org/10.1097/YIC.0000000000000036

Steketee, G., Frost, R. O., & Kim, H.-J. (2001). Hoarding by elderly people. *Health & Social Work*, *26*(3), 176–184. https://doi.org/10.1093/hsw/26.3.176

Steketee, G., & Tolin, D. F. (2011). Cognitive-behavioral therapy for hoarding in the context of contamination fears. *Journal of Clinical Psychology*, *67*(5), 485–496. https://doi.org/10.1002/jclp.20793

Timpano, K. R., Exner, C., Glaesmer, H., Rief, W., Keshaviah, A., Brähler, E., & Wilhelm, S. (2011). The epidemiology of the proposed DSM-5 hoarding disorder: Exploration of the acquisition specifier, associated features, and distress. *Journal of Clinical Psychiatry*, *72*(6), 780–786. https://doi.org/10.4088/JCP.10m06380

Tolin, D. F., Frost, R. O., Steketee, G., Gray, K. D., & Fitch, K. E. (2008). The economic and social burden of compulsive hoarding. *Psychiatry Research, 160*(2), 200–211. https://doi.org/10.1016/j.psychres.2007.08.008

Tolin, D. F., Frost, R. O., & Steketee, G. (2010). A brief interview for assessing compulsive hoarding: The Hoarding Rating Scale-Interview. *Psychiatry Research*, *178*(1), 147–152. https://doi.org/10.1016/j.psychres.2009.05.001

Tolin, D. F., Frost, R. O., Steketee, G., & Fitch, K. E. (2008). Family burden of compulsive hoarding: Results of an internet survey. *Behaviour Research and Therapy*, *46*(3), 334–344. https://doi.org/10.1016/j.brat.2007.12.008

Tolin, D. F., Meunier, S. A., Frost, R. O., & Steketee, G. (2010). Course of compulsive hoarding and its relationship to life events. *Depression and Anxiety*, *27*(9), 829–838. https://doi.org/10.1002/da.20684

20 Insomnia

Karen Kersting

A Brief Description of Sleep Disturbance and Insomnia

Primary insomnia, defined as difficulty initiating or maintaining sleep three nights per week for at least 3 months with related distress, is estimated to occur in 10–15% of primary care patients (American Psychiatric Association, 2013, pp. 362–368; Ram, Seirawan, Kumar, & Clark, 2010). A much larger proportion of the population, up to 50%, experience at least occasional inability to sleep, if not fully established insomnia, making sleep problems a major source of distress for the U.S. primary care population. The number of primary care visits in the United States that included insomnia as a reason for the medical visit increased by 13% from 1999 to 2010, and the number of prescriptions for sleep medications increased by 293% (Ford et al., 2014). With this large increase in mind, as well as concerns about routine use of sleep medications, behavioral interventions are an attractive alternative.

Behavioral treatments for sleep problems, including sleep hygiene, stimulus control, sleep restriction, and relaxation, have been shown to be as effective and longer-lasting than medication approaches (Morin et al., 2014). First-line treatment for sleep problems includes psychoeducation and goal setting related to sleep hygiene procedures including setting regular wake times, avoiding daytime napping, creating a relaxing set of pre-bed behaviors, and sleeping in a quiet, dark, and cool environment.

Effective Ways to Screen for Sleep Problems and Insomnia in the Primary Care Setting

Screening for sleep problems including insomnia in the primary care setting most often starts with a primary care provider (PCP) or behavioral health consultant (BHC) inquiring about the quality of a patient's sleep or responding to a patient's report of poor sleep. BHCs working in integrated settings should include basic questions about sleep duration and quality in their standard initial, functional assessments of patients. In some cases, initial information about a sleep problem comes from a response to a sleep question on a depression screener like the Patient Health Questionnaire-9 (PHQ-9; Kroenke, Spitzer, & Williams, 2001), which specifically asks about distress related to trouble "falling asleep or staying asleep, or sleeping too much."

With sleep flagged as a patient concern, the next stage of screening is taking a brief, recent sleep history of the patient, with the goal of gaining a clear understanding of what the patient means when he says he is "not sleeping well." This initial detective work using a series of simple questions

K. Kersting, Ph.D.
Department of Family and Community Medicine, Medical College of Wisconsin, Milwaukee, WI, USA
e-mail: kkersting@mcw.edu

A. Maragakis, W.T. O'Donohue (eds.), *Principle-Based Stepped Care and Brief Psychotherapy for Integrated Care Settings*, https://doi.org/10.1007/978-3-319-70539-2_20

about the patient's sleep experience provides a road map for further assessment and intervention.

Initial questions for a functional assessment of a reported sleep problem typically include:

- What time do you get into bed? And is that when you close your eyes to try to go to sleep?
- How long does it take you to get to sleep after closing your eyes?
- Do you know what's keeping you from falling asleep?
- What do you do when you can't fall asleep?
- Once you're asleep, do you often wake up before morning?
- Do you know what's waking you up?
- Are you usually able to fall back asleep?
- Do you wake up too early?
- What time do you get out of bed?
- How many nights a week do you have difficulty with sleep?
- Do you take naps during the day? If so, how often? And for how long?
- Is your sleep significantly different on the weekends or non-work days?
- How long have you had this problem with your sleep?

With these questions answered, the provider can do some basic math on how much sleep the patient is getting on an average night. For example, if the patient reports getting into bed at 10 p.m., taking about 2 hours to get to sleep, waking for about an hour in the night, and getting out of bed at 7 a.m., the clinician determines that the patient is getting about 6 hours of sleep per night. This number helps define the problem, as does information about the distress the patient describes related to not being able to initiate or continue sleep. Notably, the clinician is likely to get a much better sense of the patient's sleep concern by asking these specific questions, than they would by simply asking the patient "How much sleep do you usually get?" Retrospective patient reports of sleep like these, without careful recording of sleep and wake times in a sleep journal, tend to be imprecise but will help give the PCP or BHC a general understanding of the patient's distress related to sleep.

From these questions, the provider can figure out what the patient is describing when he or she reports poor sleep. Many patients report poor sleep that is directly related to a behavioral problem and is actually quite different than what we typically think of as insomnia. Answers to these questions also help the clinician understand if there is a related mental health issue undermining sleep. For example, patients with an anxiety disorder often report difficulty falling asleep due to racing thoughts or uncontrolled worry. This symptom report may be the first indication of a mood or anxiety disorder that deserves treatment and may, in fact, be the primary cause of the sleep problem.

In addition to a functional assessment of sleep, a self-report measure can be helpful for identifying insomnia in a primary care setting. The Insomnia Severity Index (ISI; Bastien, Vallières, & Morin, 2001) assesses sleep impairment with seven items that ask the patient to rate the severity of his or her difficulty falling asleep, staying asleep, and waking up too early and inquire about satisfaction with sleep, interference with daily functioning, noticeable impairment, and worry about sleep. Smith and Trinder (2001) found that the ISI is able to identify those with and without insomnia with a sensitivity of 94% and specificity of 94%, and Smith and Wegener (2003) determined that the measure is valid.

How to Further Assess if a Screen Returns Positive

Once a patient has screened positive for insomnia or a related sleep problem, additional questions about specific problematic behaviors can help the clinician see the likely causes of a sleep disturbance, such as watching TV in the bedroom, using smartphones or tablet computers in bed, sleeping in an uncomfortable bed, and lack of daytime exercise. Understanding factors that may be impacting sleep will help the clinician outline specific strategies that the patient can use to improve sleep.

Behaviors

- What is your routine before bed?
- Is there a TV in your bedroom?
- When you wake up at night, do you know the time by looking at a clock or are you picking up a smartphone?
- Is your bed comfortable?

- Is your bedroom quiet?
- Is your bedroom dark?
- Is your bedroom at a comfortable temperature?
- Are there pets in your bed waking you up in the night?
- If you sleep with a partner, does he or she affect your sleep?
- Do you take sleep medications or supplements before bed?
- How much alcohol do you consume? Are you using it to help you fall asleep?
- Do you use tobacco?
- How much caffeine do you consume? How much coffee or caffeinated soda do you drink? When do you consume it?
- Do you exercise during the day? What time? Do you break a sweat?
- Is there anything you are particularly worried or stressed about that is keeping you awake?

The clinician should also aim to briefly assess the *consequences* of a sleep problem.

Consequences

- Do you feel rested when you wake up?
- Do you struggle to get out of bed in the morning?
- Do you feel sleepy during the day?
- Any difficulty concentrating?
- Does feeling sleepy or tired affect your performance at school or work?

And, finally, a few more questions will help rule out other disorders that can affect sleep, including sleep apnea, restless leg syndrome, and teeth grinding.

Rule-Outs

- Do you snore at night?
- Do you wake up with a headache?
- Have you been told by someone else that you gasp for air during the night?
- Are there sensations in your legs that make it hard to fall asleep or stay asleep?

Additional measures, more commonly used in specialty sleep clinics, can also be used in primary care. These include the Multidimensional Fatigue Inventory (MFI; Smets, Garssen, Bonke, & De Haes, 1995), the Dysfunctional Beliefs and Attitudes about Sleep Scale revised version (DBAS-10; Espie, Inglis, Harvey, & Tessier, 2000), and the Epworth Sleepiness Scale (Hauri, 1993). A detailed sleep diary may also be used at this point: Patients are asked to log 2 weeks' worth of data including bedtime, sleep latency (minutes between bedtime and sleep), number and duration of awakenings, total time spent in bed, total sleep time, and daytime napping.

Detailed recommendations on the type of comprehensive sleep assessment often conducted in specialty sleep clinics are available (i.e., Schutte-Rodin, Broch, Buysse, Dorsey, & Sateia, 2008), and the book *Integrated Behavioral Health in Primary Care* (Hunter, Goodie, Oordt, & Dobmeyer, 2017) provides excellent guidelines for evaluation in the primary care setting.

Evidence-Based Stepped Care and Brief Psychotherapeutic Approaches to Treating Sleep Problems and Insomnia

An overall program of stepped care for insomnia treatment in a specialty sleep clinic was recently evaluated by Vincent and Walsh (2013) and included Step 1, a 6-week computerized treatment; Step 2, a single session consultation with a staff psychologist; Step 3, a manualized 6-week cognitive behavioral group treatment; and Step 4, highly tailored, multi-week psychotherapy provided by a psychologist. These authors found that stepped care resulted in a 69% improvement in efficiency and that low-intensity treatment was often sufficient for people who were young and employed as well as for those who reported better sleep at treatment initiation. With this evidence in mind, the following section offers recommendation for stepped care in the primary care setting.

Psychoeducation and Problem-Solving

Based on the patient's report of their sleep problem, the PCP or BHC may identify a straightforward behavioral cause for lack of sleep. For example, an older adult patient who is retired, with little structured activity during the day, may be napping on and off much of the day, causing a lack of sleep drive at night and related difficulty initiating and sustaining sleep. For this patient, appropriate first-stage interventions would include psychoeducation about how sleep quality decreases as people age to normalize their sleep experience and a discussion of strategies to decrease daytime napping and increase daytime physical activity. Alternately, the patient may report that she likes daytime napping, doesn't mind being awake at night, and doesn't feel able to increase daily activity, which could lead to a discussion of the pros and cons of changing her sleep schedule and making an informed decision about her sleep pattern.

Patients may also report sleep problems that are primarily lack of access to sleep. For example, a patient who is a parent gets up at 6 a.m. to get children ready for school and get herself to work and then stays up until 2 a.m. waiting for her partner to get home from a second shift job, leaving only a 4 hour window for sleep. For this patient, a first-stage intervention would include problem-solving related to creating more time for sleep and negotiating responsibilities with a domestic partner.

For true insomnia, treatment in the primary care setting starts with strategies for reducing behaviors that interfere with sleep. The clinician discusses sleep hygiene, stimulus control, sleep restriction, and relaxation behaviors with the patient, focusing on those relevant to the problems identified in the patient's functional assessment. The following core principles for insomnia treatment are fundamental to empirically supported cognitive behavioral treatments including CBTI (Edinger and Carney, 2014; Morin et al., 2006). CBT for insomnia has been shown to be beneficial for about 75% of patients with chronic primary insomnia, with about 50% reductions of sleep latency and unwanted awakenings (Morin, Colecchi, Stone, Sood, & Brink, 1999).

Stimulus Control

Stimulus control refers to conditioning a patient to associate sleep with being in bed and to stop associating the bed with other behaviors like watching TV, lying awake, and worrying. Key instructions include:

- *Use the bed and bedroom only for sleep and sex*: Do not read, eat, watch TV, listen to music, or use your smartphone in bed.
- *Get into bed only when sleepy and ready to go to sleep*: Your goal is to avoid lying awake in bed, so you don't want to get into bed until you are "hungry" for sleep.
- *Get out of bed when you've been unable to sleep for 15 min or more*: As part of avoiding spending time in bed awake, you need to get out of bed and, ideally, leave the bedroom when you are unable to sleep. Engage in a calming activity when out of bed like reading a book, folding laundry, or crossword puzzles, until you feel sleepy. Keep lights relatively dim and avoid light coming from screens, tablets, and phones. Get up again if you can't fall asleep the next time you try.
- *Set up a traditional clock in your room*: This will allow you to check the time when trying to fall asleep or when you wake up in the night *without* reaching for your smartphone.

Sleep Hygiene

Keep a regular sleep schedule: Get out of bed at the same time every day, including weekends and non-work days. This will help set your circadian so that your body knows to wake and sleep at the same times every day. Keep the same wake time even if you struggle to sleep that night or a life circumstance interferes with your normal bedtime.

Avoid caffeine, alcohol, and nicotine before bed: Caffeine disturbs sleep, and this effect may becomes more prolonged with age; it should be avoided for 6–8 hours before bedtime. Though alcohol can make falling asleep feel easier, it disrupts the sleep cycle potentially resulting in nighttime awakenings and poor-quality sleep; it should be avoided for 4 hours before sleep. Nicotine can keep you awake; avoid smoking shortly before bed and during the night.

Avoid napping: Think of going to bed like getting ready for Thanksgiving dinner; you want to show up *hungry* for sleep. Napping is like snacking before a meal. If you must nap, do so at least 6 hours before planning to go to bed for the night and keep naps short, no more than 15–30 min.

Exercise, but not before bed: A healthy amount of exercise can tire out the body and improve sleep. However, exercise in the 2 hours before bed can interfere with sleep.

Eat healthy: Choose a healthy diet and avoid large meals in the 2–3 hours before going to bed.

Set your bedroom up for sleep: Make sure your bedroom is quiet, dark, and at a comfortable, but slightly cool, temperature. Sleep masks and earplugs can help with light and sound, as can room-darkening shades.

Allow yourself time to relax before bed: Take at least an hour to unwind in whatever way works for you. Engage in relaxing activities and routines. Try methods for physical relaxation including breathing exercises, gentle yoga and stretching, and progressive muscle relaxation—all abundantly available to patients online.

Clinicians may want to use a checklist of stimulus control or sleep hygiene strategies to go over with the patient; several are available including online or from primary care integration texts (e.g., Hunter et al., 2017). It's useful to go over this list in session as part of the feedback and intervention provided to the patient. Mark each item on the list that may be a problem for the patient and write down what the patient plans to do instead.

After behavioral goals have been identified, the clinician may want to review with the patient their reasons for wanting to improve sleep, including ameliorating the consequences of poor sleep such as daytime sleepiness and poor concentration, identify and problem-solve any barriers to initiating new behaviors, and establish a plan for clinician follow-up of patient progress.

Sleep Restriction

When sincerely attempted sleep hygiene and stimulus control measures fail to produce improved sleep, sleep restriction may be an appropriate next step. In sleep restriction, a patient restricts their sleep window, or the amount of time allowed for sleep, to the number of hours they are currently able to sleep (Spielman, Saskin & Thorpy, 1987). This number of hours is generated through self-report/functional assessment of the patient's sleep or by keeping a simple sleep diary with sleep and wake times. The patient is instructed to keep their standard daily wake time in place but to get into bed late enough to only allow for the number of hours of sleep they currently achieve. For example, if a patient is getting only 5.5 hours of sleep a night amid difficulty falling asleep and nighttime awakenings, you would limit their sleep window to 5.5 hours. If their wake time is 7 a.m., they would wait to get into bed until 1:30 a.m. The patient is instructed to adhere carefully to this schedule every night, as well as previously discussed sleep hygiene and stimulus control behaviors, until she is able to sleep for 90% of the sleep window. After achieving this "sleep efficiency," the patient may only then start adding to 15- to 20-min blocks of sleep to the sleep window. The patient is instructed to continue to adjust until their sleep window becomes too long to maintain 85% sleep efficiency, at which point they have established the proper sleep window for their sleep cycle. Importantly, clinicians should seek appropriate training to support patients through the process of sleep restriction, but, if available, this treatment is an asset to primary care patients and providers.

Relaxation

If patients report difficulty sleeping due to arousal, anxiety, worry, or physical tension, relaxation techniques, similar to those presented in Chapter 18, can be introduced. Additionally, if worry is the main driver of the sleep problem, the patient may benefit from keeping a worry log or engaging other cognitive strategies for managing repetitive thought.

Self-Guided and Online Interventions

Self-help cognitive behavioral therapy (CBT) for insomnia includes many of the same behavioral interventions described above and is an effective treatment for insomnia (Ho et al., 2015). Ho's 2015 meta-analysis of 20 studies found that self-help programs presented through written materials, and those presented through online methods, were equality effective and dropout rates were similar to those of traditional, in-person CBT. This analysis is an excellent resource for matching self-help options with primary care populations.

Group Interventions

Group delivery of cognitive behavioral therapy for insomnia is a natural extension of initial psychoeducation and self-help offerings, as it provides more intensive instruction while limiting costs and provider time by serving multiple patients at once. A meta-analysis of eight randomly controlled trials of group therapy for insomnia showed medium to large effect sizes for sleep onset latency, sleep efficiency, and awakenings after sleep onset (Koffel, Koffel, & Gehrman, 2015). The authors suggest that group therapy for insomnia be considered an important aspect of stepped care for sleep problems and provide a useful resource for selecting a group modality.

Brief Individual Therapy

Beyond psychoeducation, self-guided interventions, and group therapies, brief individual therapy for insomnia may be helpful to patients who did not improve with previous steps and for those with more severe, long-standing sleep problems (Vincent & Walsh, 2013). Individual therapy will include previously discussed components of cognitive behavioral interventions, with increased emphasis on challenging dysfunctional beliefs. One example of a manualized brief individual therapy protocol is brief behavioral treatment for insomnia (BBTI) developed by Troxel, Germain, and Buysse (2012). This treatment includes four sessions, two of which may be phone sessions, has an explicit behavioral focus, and uses concise delivery for ease of training a variety of clinicians. BBTI has demonstrated efficacy in treating older adults with insomnia (Buysse et al., 2011).

What Does Not Work

Sleep medications: Sleep medications are popular with patients and often prescribed in primary care settings. Though these medications may be helpful for some patients, it's useful to talk with patients about limiting long-term use of sleep medications. Behavioral interventions should be encouraged over reliance on sleep medications, as they have been shown to work for 70–80% of patients diagnosed with insomnia (Hunter et al., 2017). It may also be helpful to provide PCPs with information about the effectiveness of behavioral interventions for sleep, as a reminder that these interventions are a viable alternative to sleep medications and should be recommended to patients.

Simply setting an earlier bedtime: Sleep problems cause patients to be more tired during the day and feel in need to increased sleep. This can lead patients to simply work toward spending more time in bed by going to bed earlier. As discussed above, spending time in bed unable to sleep can make sleep problems worse, so, somewhat counterintuitively to patients and even some clinicians, an earlier bedtime alone will not improve sleep.

When to Refer to External Specialty Mental Health

When the functional assessment of the sleep problem doesn't clearly identify specific problematic behaviors or if the patient takes steps to improve their sleep hygiene and stimulus control but still has difficulty initiating and maintaining sleep, it may be useful to refer the patient to specialty mental health services, specifically a clinical health psychologist who specializes in cognitive behavioral therapy for insomnia (CBTi).

If the patient reports snoring, morning headaches, gasping for breath in the night, and/or unusual physical sensations during sleep, he or she should be considered for referral to sleep clinic for further evaluation potentially including polysomnography.

The Role of the Primary Care Provider/Medical Team in Treatment

As discussed above, the PCP and the medical team are often an essential part of identifying sleep problems in primary care patients. Following assessment and intervention by a BHC, the medical team can support treatment for sleep problems and insomnia through familiarity with the behavioral recommendations and support of the plan. For example, a PCP should be aware of the recommendations made by the BHC and discuss them briefly with the patient at any follow-up appointments, making sure to support their utility and the patient's ongoing compliance.

How to Assess Impact on Care/ Quality Improvement Processes

Demonstrating the impact of behavioral treatment for sleep problems can be challenging because treatment is often brief (one to two sessions) and patients may not return if their symptoms quickly improve. That said, the Insomnia Severity Index discussed above is a good tool for tracking change in symptoms, as is the patient's self-report of the number of hours of sleep per night. Even when the patient fails to return for follow-up sessions with a BHC, outcomes can be tracked through subsequent PCP visits either by noting the patient's reports of improved sleep or the absence of symptom report.

References

American Psychiatric Association. (2013). *Diagnostic and statistical manual of mental disorders (DSM-5®)*. Arlington, VA: American Psychiatric Publishing.

Bastien, C. H., Vallières, A., & Morin, C. M. (2001). Validation of the Insomnia Severity Index as an outcome measure for insomnia research. *Sleep Medicine*, *2*(4), 297–307.

Buysse, D. J., Germain, A., Moul, D. E., Franzen, P. L., Brar, L. K., Fletcher, M. E., ... Monk, T. H. (2011). Efficacy of brief behavioral treatment for chronic insomnia in older adults. *Archives of Internal Medicine*, *171*(10), 887–895.

Edinger, J. D., & Carney, C. E. (2014). *Overcoming insomnia: A cognitive-behavioral therapy approach, therapist guide*. Oxford: Oxford University Press.

Espie, C. A., Inglis, S. J., Harvey, L., & Tessier, S. (2000). Insomniacs' attributions: Psychometric properties of the Dysfunctional Beliefs and Attitudes about Sleep Scale and the Sleep Disturbance Questionnaire. *Journal of Psychosomatic Research*, *48*(2), 141–148.

Ford, E. S., Wheaton, A. G., Cunningham, T. J., Giles, W. H., Chapman, D. P., & Croft, J. B. (2014). Trends in outpatient visits for insomnia, sleep apnea, and prescriptions for sleep medications among US adults: Findings from the National Ambulatory Medical Care Survey 1999–2010. *Sleep*, *37*(8), 1283–1293.

Hauri, P. J. (1993). Consulting about insomnia: A method and some preliminary data. *Sleep*, *16*, 344–350.

Ho, F. Y. Y., Chung, K. F., Yeung, W. F., Ng, T. H., Kwan, K. S., Yung, K. P., & Cheng, S. K. (2015). Self-help cognitive-behavioral therapy for insomnia: A meta-analysis of randomized controlled trials. *Sleep Medicine Reviews*, *19*, 17–28.

Hunter, C. L., Goodie, J. L., Oordt, M. S., & Dobmeyer, A. C. (2017). *Integrated behavioral health in primary care: Step-by-step guidance for assessment and intervention* (2nd ed.). Washington, DC: American Psychological Association.

Kroenke, K., Spitzer, R. L., & Williams, J. B. (2001). The Phq-9. *Journal of General Internal Medicine*, *16*(9), 606–613.

Koffel, E. A., Koffel, J. B., & Gehrman, P. R. (2015). A meta-analysis of group cognitive behavioral therapy for insomnia. *Sleep Medicine Reviews*, *19*, 6–16.

Morin, C. M., Bootzin, R. R., Buysse, D. J., Edinger, J. D., Espie, C. A., & Lichstein, K. L. (2006). Psychological and behavioral treatment of insomnia: Update of the recent evidence (1998-2004). *Sleep*, *29*(11), 1398.

Morin, C. M., Colecchi, C., Stone, J., Sood, R., & Brink, D. (1999). Behavioral and pharmacological therapies for late-life insomnia: A randomized controlled trial. *JAMA*, *281*(11), 991–999.

Morin, C. M., Drake, C. L., Harvey, A. G., Krystal, A. D., Manber, R., Riemann, D., & Spiegelhalder, K. (2014). Insomnia disorder. *Nature Reviews. Disease Primers*, *1*, 15026–15026.

Ram, S., Seirawan, H., Kumar, S. K., & Clark, G. T. (2010). Prevalence and impact of sleep disorders and sleep habits in the United States. *Sleep and Breathing*, *14*(1), 63–70.

Schutte-Rodin, S., Broch, L., Buysse, D., Dorsey, C., & Sateia, M. (2008). Clinical guideline for the evaluation and management of chronic insomnia in adults. *Journal of Clinical Sleep Medicine*, *4*(5), 487–504.

Smets, E. M. A., Garssen, B., Bonke, B. D., & De Haes, J. C. J. M. (1995). The Multidimensional Fatigue Inventory (MFI) psychometric qualities of an instrument to assess fatigue. *Journal of Psychosomatic Research*, *39*(3), 315–325.

Smith, M. T., & Wegener, S. T. (2003). Measures of sleep: The Insomnia Severity Index, Medical Outcomes Study (MOS) Sleep Scale, Pittsburgh Sleep Diary (PSD), and Pittsburgh Sleep Quality Index (PSQI). *Arthritis Care & Research*, *49*(S5), S184–S196.

Smith, S., & Trinder, J. (2001). Detecting insomnia: Comparison of four self-report measures of sleep in a young adult population. *Journal of Sleep Research*, *10*(3), 229–235.

Spielman, A. J., Saskin, P., & Thorpy, M. J. (1987). Treatment of chronic insomnia by restriction of time in bed. Sleep, *10*(1), 45–56.

Troxel, W. M., Germain, A., & Buysse, D. J. (2012). Clinical management of insomnia with brief behavioral treatment (BBTI). *Behavioral Sleep Medicine*, *10*(4), 266–279.

Vincent, N., & Walsh, K. (2013). Stepped care for insomnia: An evaluation of implementation in routine practice. *Journal of Clinical Sleep Medicine*, *9*(3), 227.

21 Low Sexual Desire Disorder

Rory Newlands and William T. O'Donohue

The aim of this chapter is to help health-care professionals understand low sexual desire disorder ("LSDD")—the most common sexual dysfunction affecting both women and men (Simons & Carey, 2001)—assess for problems of sexual desire, and implement empirically supported interventions for LSDD. With research advances and widespread marketing for "the little blue pill," sexual dysfunction has become increasingly visible. Despite increased public awareness, sexual dysfunction—particularly low desire—remains enigmatic and surrounded by stigma. Between 70 and 90% of Americans experiencing sexual dysfunction receive no treatment (Shifren et al., 2009). Many factors account for this treatment failure, including patients' embarrassment talking about sexual issues (Montgomery, 2008), clinicians' discomfort with the subject matter, and the low priority given to sexual medicine in the training of health-care professionals (Coleman et al., 2013).

R. Newlands (✉) • W.T. O'Donohue
Department of Clinical Psychology,
University of Nevada, Reno, NV, USA
e-mail: rorynewlands@gmail.com;
williamodonohue@yahoo.com

Low Sexual Desire Disorder

Low sexual desire disorder is a construct previously listed in the DSM-IV as hypoactive sexual desire disorder ("HSDD"). For female patients, the DSM-5 (2013) merged HSDD with arousal disorders for a diagnosis of female sexual interest/arousal disorder ("FSIAD"). The decision to combine female desire and arousal was based on the high comorbidity of the two disorders and on findings that most women, when viewing their sexuality, rarely differentiate arousal and desire as distinct processes (Brotto, Heiman, & Tolman, 2009). However, correlations between female arousal and desire/interest ranging from 0.52 to 0.85 (Brotto, 2010) also support the existence of independent constructs. For male patients, the DSM-5 diagnosis of male hypoactive sexual desire disorder ("MHSDD") covers LSDD.

Prevalence

For women, LSDD is the most common sexual difficulty encountered across all ages (Kingsberg & Woodard, 2015; Shifren et al., 2009; Simons & Carey, 2001). Estimates suggest that, roughly, between 10 and 20% of Western women experience problems with LSDD (Simons & Carey, 2001), although these prevalence rates vary with age.

A. Maragakis, W.T. O'Donohue (eds.), *Principle-Based Stepped Care and Brief Psychotherapy for Integrated Care Settings*, https://doi.org/10.1007/978-3-319-70539-2_21

What Is "Normal" Versus Low Sexual Desire?

Sexual desire can be defined as the culmination of three distinct elements: drive, motivation, and responsiveness (Bitzer, Giraldi, & Pfaus, 2013). *Drive*, the biological component of desire, is largely controlled by the neuroendocrine process (Kingsberg & Rezaee, 2013). *Motivation* entails cognitive, interpersonal, and emotional processes, such as rewards, incentives, mood, and individual learning history (Bitzer et al., 2013; Kingsberg & Rezaee, 2013). The motivation element of desire, not entirely sexual, may be driven by a longing to be intimate, to feel wanted or desirable, or to satisfy a partner, among other reasons (Bitzer et al., 2013). *Responsiveness* refers to the ability of sexual stimuli to prompt sexual behaviors, desire, arousal, and pleasure in an individual (Bitzer et al., 2013). The responsiveness element of desire encompasses both the physiological and cognitive/behavioral realms, such as sexual expectancies and sexual scripts (Bitzer et al., 2013). Low sexual desire has been described as an absent or diminished interest in sex, sexual activity, or sexual fantasies, failure to respond to sexual stimuli, or feeling detached or empty despite being in a good quality relationship (Kingsberg & Woodard, 2015). Although examining sexual desire through the tripartite lens of drive, motivation, and responsiveness provides a more robust understanding, there is no unified theory that accounts for the observed variability in desire (Bitzer et al., 2013).

The Sexual Response Cycle

Desire is not the only aspect of sexuality lacking a coherent theory; there also is no single model of the sexual response cycle that accounts for the multifaceted and idiographic nature of sex, sexuality, and sexual response (Sand & Fisher, 2007).

The Masters and Johnson model of the sexual response (MJSR) cycle developed by Masters and Johnson is the first model of the human sexual response cycle, which they conceptualized as a linear model with distinct phases (Masters & Johnson, 1966). This linear model presumes that individuals move in a steplike fashion from one discrete phase to the next (desire → arousal → orgasm → resolution), and thus "normal" sexual functioning requires the individual to graduate from one phase before moving on to the next. Critics argue that this overly simplistic model does not adequately integrate the different facets of sexual functioning (Basson, 2001, 2007; Gehring, 2003). In response to these deficits, Basson developed a circular model of sexual responding (Basson, 2001).

The Basson model of the sexual response cycle (BSRC). The transition from the linear MJSR model to the circular BSRC model resulted in a paradigm shift in which no aspect of sexual response is the initiating step (Basson, 2001; Bitzer et al., 2013). In this transactional model, each phase—consisting of both sexual and nonsexual components—is interconnected to and impacted by the previous phase (Basson, 2001; Bitzer et al., 2013). The circular Basson model allows for a superior understanding of sexual functioning and desire because it considers and includes contextual features (psychological factors, relationship quality, culture, etc.) and the concept of receptive/responsive desire (the notion that—particularly for women—sexual engagement often starts from a position of neutrality) (Basson, 2001; Kingsberg & Rezaee, 2013).

Etiology

The many factors implicated in the etiology of LSDD, including psychological, interpersonal, and physiological, complicate the challenge of defining and treating low sexual desire disorder. Furthermore, the factors contributing to and maintaining LSD can vary drastically from one individual to the next (Wincze & Weisberg, 2015).

Psychological factors. In LSDD for women, all these factors have been implicated: depression, a history of sexual abuse and trauma, increased psychological distress, distraction, anxiety, poor body image, negative beliefs about sex, substance abuse (Brotto, Bitzer, Laan, Leiblum, & Luria, 2010) and, compared to women without LSDD, weaker positive associations with sexual stimuli (Brauer et al., 2012). The most common reasons that women cite for their lack of desire are fatigue and perceived stress (Ellison, 2006). For men, several psychological factors have been implicated in the development and maintenance of LSDD: depression, anxiety, work-related stress, fatigue, restrictive attitudes toward sex, guilt surrounding sex, and sexual performance anxiety (Carvalheira, Træen, & Štulhofer, 2014; McCabe & Connaughton, 2014).

Interpersonal factors. For women, these interpersonal factors have been associated with LSDD: poor dyadic adjustment, dissatisfaction with conflict resolution, and feelings of emotional distance from partner (Trudel, Boulos, & Matte, 1993). For men and women, all these factors are related to LSDD: poor communication about sex (Metz & Epstein, 2002), being in a long-term relationship (Carvalheira et al., 2014), not finding one's partner attractive, and overall relationship dissatisfaction (Carvalheira et al., 2014; Trudel et al., 1993). Research has also found that sexual dysfunction in one partner may contribute to the development of LSD in the other partner (Fisher, Rosen, Eardley, Sand, & Goldstein, 2005; McCabe & Connaughton, 2014). In such cases, research has shown that treatment of the male partner resulted in an increase in the female partner's sexual desire (Goldstein et al., 2005).

Biological and physiological factors. These factors contribute to LSDD: chronic illness (hypothyroidism, diabetes, multiple sclerosis, STIs, etc.), medications (e.g., SSRIs), and hormonal changes. (See Bitzer et al., 2013 for a review.) Medical treatments for LSD, typically those targeting hormones, have received more attention than psychological treatments (Balzer, 2012), despite the low parlance of known hormonal causes (Gehring, 2003). While research has repeatedly found that low testosterone levels correlate with low levels of sexual desire, testosterone replacement therapy has been found to increase sexual desire only in men with lower than normal levels of testosterone (Corona, Rastrelli, Forti, & Maggi, 2011). The FDA recently approved the drug flibanserin for the treatment of LSDD in women (FDA, 2015), but such treatments have been associated with negative and life-threatening side effects such as increased risk for breast cancer, strokes, high blood pressure, and blood clots (Davis et al., 2008; FDA, 2015). Patients and practitioners may be swayed by the ease of implementing hormonal interventions, but scant evidence exists for a biological basis of LSDD in healthy, premenopausal women (Stuart, Hammond, & Pett, 1987); research suggests instead that, for women, psychosocial factors are more predictive of desire problems than are biological factors (Corona et al., 2004).

Screening in a Primary Care Setting

Sexual health is often neglected due to time constraints and/or reluctance of the patient or health-care provider to initiate the topic (Montgomery, 2008). However, any office visit can include brief assessments for sexual dysfunction. To put the patient and yourself at ease when discussing sexual health, these steps are recommended:

1. Broach the topic in a confident and neutral manner. Research has shown women are less likely to divulge sexual problems when they perceive the health-care provider is uncomfortable, hesitant, or disengaged (Buster, 2013).
2. Be culturally sensitive and aware of relevant idiographic variables when taking an individual's sexual history.
3. Normalize the importance of sexual health (e.g., present rates of sexual dysfunction, discuss role of sexual health in the context of psychological, physical, and relationship health).
4. Ask open-ended questions regarding sexual health and functioning.
5. If the patient expresses concerns, delineate which aspect of the sexual response cycle is causing those concerns.

See Table 21.1, *Helpful Assessment Questions*. Asked in the initial screening, these questions can help to determine the key concern and can also aid in treatment decisions (Kingsberg & Rezaee, 2013). Note: Patient distress around a sexual problem *must* be present for a diagnosis of sexual dysfunction (Basson et al., 2000).

In addition to structured interviews, several self-report scales have been developed and validated for detecting sexual dysfunction. Self-report scales are relatively simple tools that promote discussion while providing practitioners with a clearer understanding of the patient's issues. It is recommended that self-report scales be used in conjunction with a structured or semi-structured interview, as self-reporting allows women to relay their experiences in a more comfortable manner (Kingsberg & Rezaee, 2013).

Table 21.1 Helpful assessment questions

1. How would you describe the problem(s)?
2. How long has (have) the problem(s) lasted? (Note: The DSM-5 requires a minimum of 6 months to meet the criteria for sexual dysfunction.)
3. Did the problem(s) occur suddenly or was the onset gradual?
4. Does the problem occur across all situations and partners? Or only in specific situations/with specific partners?
5. Did anything trigger or contribute to the development of the problem(s)?
6. Are there any nonsexual problems with your sexual partner(s)?
7. Can you think of any current life stressors that may be related to the problem(s)?
8. Are you experiencing any emotions that could contribute to the problem(s)? (e.g. stress, anxiety, resentment, fear, guilt, sadness, etc.)
9. Are you unhappy with your weight or physical appearance?
10. Are you experiencing any physical health problems, such as pain, chronic illness, fatigue, etc.?
11. Do you experience any issues with desire, arousal, or orgasm? (Note: You may need to explicate what is meant by desire vs. arousal.)
12. Do you have a history of sexual, physical, or emotional abuse?
13. Does your partner have any sexual problems?

From Basson et al. (2000)

See Kingsberg and Rezaee (2013) or Wincze and Weisberg (2015) for suggested self-reporting options.

Arriving at a diagnosis of LSDD is only one step in the assessment process. It is crucial to determine if the sexual dysfunction is the primary problem or if it is secondary to other aspects of sexual functioning and side effects of medicine, substance use, disease, or some other psychological disorders. Therefore, a thorough evaluation of the patient's psychological, medical, and medication history is required (Latif & Diamond, 2013). In some cases, such as those where no psychosocial risk factors are present, physical examination and/or laboratory evaluation may be necessary (Latif & Diamond, 2013). However, laboratory evaluation is rarely helpful and should only be a last resort when the interview and physical examination are unable to detect contributing and maintaining factors (Kingsberg & Woodard, 2015).

Evidence-Based Steeped Care and Brief Psychotherapeutic Approaches

The complexity and interactions of etiological factors, along with the dearth of empirically supported treatments, all make treatment of LSDD challenging (Balzer, 2012). Treatments must focus on the history of the individual experiencing the problem while simultaneously accounting for the roles the relationship plays in maintaining the dysfunction (Balzer, 2012). A solid understanding of the different idiographic factors contributing to the problem (psychological, interpersonal, physical, etc.), coupled with a stepped-care approach, can simplify treatment.

Level 1: Psychoeducation and Bibliotherapy

Using the stepped-care framework, the practitioner begins with the least invasive treatments to maximize time and resources while reducing costs and possible risks that accompany more intensive treatments (Bower & Gilbody, 2005). Once it is clear that low sexual desire is the patient's primary problem, rather than a side effect of another condition, the first step is to address general issues associated with health and overall well-being, such as sleep hygiene, diet, substance abuse, and exercise. Many patients also benefit from education about sexual anatomy and physiology as well as "normal" sexual functioning, as representations in the media are often skewed, perpetuating maladaptive behaviors and attitudes regarding sex (Kingsberg & Woodard, 2015).

Although simply providing psychoeducation on sexual functioning can ameliorate patient distress, many patients require additional care. Bibliotherapy for sexual dysfunction in general has been found to be equivalent to therapist-administered treatment and has demonstrated larger effect sizes than for other health problems (Marrs, 1995). Balzer (2012) evaluated the efficacy of bibliotherapy for the treatment of LSDD in women, comparing the effectiveness of two self-help books to each other and to a wait list control. The books were *A Tired Woman's Guide to Passionate Sex* (Mintz, 2009) and *Reclaiming Your Sexual Self: How You Can Bring Desire Back into Your Life* (Hall, 2004). Compared to the control group, both treatment groups evidenced significant gains on self-rated sexual desire, sexual satisfaction, arousal, and overall sexual functioning (Balzer, 2012).

Level 2: Group Psychotherapy or Guided Self-Help

Many patients need more intensive treatments (e.g., those who do not show improvements in desire after Level 1 interventions or those presenting with many contributing etiological factors). Unfortunately, there are few Level 2 treatments for LSDD. However, Brotto, Basson, and Luria (2008) adapted and evaluated a three-session mindfulness-based group psychoeducation (PED) intervention for women with LSDD and/or sexual arousal dysfunction. The intervention integrated fundamentals of CBT, mindfulness, psychoeducation, sex therapy, and marital therapy and also addressed body image distortion, depression, harmful beliefs about sexuality, and relationship problems, all of which have been linked with LSDD (Brotto et al., 2008).

Positive results were found for different aspects of sexual functioning, including increased desire and decreased distress; additionally, women with a history of sexual abuse showed greater improvements than those with no such history (Brotto et al., 2008). However, because no control group was used, conclusions are still tentative. PED does appear to be promising for the treatment of LSDD given that distraction (due to body image distortion, depression, harmful beliefs, etc.) has been shown to be hurtful to female sexual functioning (Dove, Michael, & Wiederman, 2000).

Level 3: Brief Individual Psychotherapy

Unfortunately, no true "brief" individual therapies (i.e., three to five sessions) have been developed or evaluated for the treatment of LSDD. However, Brotto and colleagues' (Brotto et al., 2008) PED may offer promise in this arena. There is no theoretical reason why their group PED treatment could not be adapted to an individual, although this application remains to be explored in future studies. Brotto and Luria (2014) posit that using CBT to combat maladaptive thoughts and beliefs, in conjunction with mindfulness-based interventions—which increase acceptance and awareness and help cultivate nonjudgmental attitudes—offers great potential for the treatment of LSDD.

The shortage of Level 3 interventions for LSDD requires practitioners to develop creative treatment plans for patients who require this level of help. Given the success of group PED for the treatment of LSDD (Brotto & Luria, 2014), it is recommended that practitioners tailor group PED for the individual patient by delivering the original intervention and then spending additional time on certain segments or adding treatment ingredients (see Table 21.2) relevant to the patient's presentation.

Table 21.2 Key treatment ingredients

Normalizing sexual dysfunction	Despite the prevalence of SD, many patients feel immense embarrassment. Therefore normalizing the problem and providing patients with hope regarding their prognosis help to ameliorate distress regarding SD
Removing blame	Many patients blame their partners or themselves for their SD. By removing blame, patients can focus on strengthening communication and their relationship
Correcting maladaptive beliefs about sex and sexuality	Misinformation regarding "appropriate" sexual behaviors abounds. For instance, the belief "men should always be interested in sex" may incite feelings of rejection if the male partner is not interested in sex, which may then contribute to the development of LSDD
Identifying all the variables involved in patient's SD	Oftentimes patients neglect the complexity of their SD and attribute it to a single cause (typically a medical one). Highlighting the interplay of historical and contextual factors in the development and presentation of SD aids both patient and practitioner in the treatment of SD
Creating an environment conducive to sex	Certain environments (e.g., lack of privacy, bright lights, pets, etc.) can interfere with sexual functioning. Simple changes to create an environment conducive to sex can aid greatly in the treatment of SD
Improving communication	Communication patterns that invalidate, avoid, and deflect can lead to resentment, lack of intimacy, and other negative feelings that then contribute to the development and maintenance of LSDD. Thus addressing issues in couple communication is important in the treatment of LSDD
Sensate focus	This key ingredient of sex therapy aims to train the individual to focus on experiencing sensations in the moment, rather than focusing on anticipated outcomes, and in this regard is similar to mindfulness approaches. Additionally, this strategy can increase sexual communication
Exercise	Exercise ameliorates depression, anxiety, and other chronic illness, and has also been found to positively impact body image, which is implicated in LSDD. Exercise enhances sexual desire (White et al., 1990). Furthermore, exercise has been shown to hinder the sexual-suppressing effects of anti-depressants (Lorenz & Meston, 2012)

Adapted from Wincze and Weisberg (2015); *SD* sexual dysfunction

Level 4: Long-Term or Biomedical Interventions—When to Refer Out

Given the many etiological factors that can play a role in the development and maintenance of LSDD, as well as the frequent comorbidity with other psychological and physiological disorders, many patients will require more intensive long-term treatments. Ideally, the decision to implement such treatments would occur after the initial assessment. However, it may not become apparent that a patient requires a Level 4 intervention until after a lower-level treatment has begun, hence the importance of a comprehensive assessment to understand the level of complexity involved in the manifestation of LSDD.

While no hard and fast rules exist for determining which level of intervention is appropriate for which client, considering the following factors can help: (1) typically, the need for higher-level interventions increases as the number of etiological factors increases (particularly if there are several risk factors in all three domains—i.e., bio-/physiological, psychological, interpersonal); (2) low levels of androgens in men indicate the implementation of a biomedical intervention (Wincze & Weisberg, 2015), although hormonal causes are rare for LSDD in premenopausal women (Gehring, 2003); (3) if LSDD is lifelong, rather than acquired, and/or occurs across multiple partners, a higher-level intervention may be warranted; (4) if the partner of the patient is unwilling to participate in the treatment process, a higher-level intervention will be likely required; and (5) if the client comes from a culture with many taboos surrounding sex and sexuality, short-term interventions may be ineffective.

What Does Not Work

When faced with treating a sexual dysfunction, some practitioners may think that sex therapy is the obvious treatment choice, given that it has shown considerable success in the treatment of many sexual dysfunctions (Hawton, 1985). Unfortunately, sex therapy has not demonstrated much success for patients suffering from LSDD (Hawton, 1985; Kingsberg & Rezaee, 2013). Treating LSDD with traditional sex therapy fails to account for and address many of the disorder's contributing psychological and interpersonal factors (Basson, 2006). However, some elements of sex therapy can have a place in the treatment of LSDD. For instance, the principle of *sensate focus*—intended to enhance participants' sexual awareness, preferences, and intimacy while reducing anxiety via graded exposure (Masters & Johnson, 1970)—remains an important tool in the treatment of LSDD.

The Role of the Primary Care Provider/Medical Team in Treatment

Because psychological and interpersonal factors play a key role in the genesis and maintenance of LSDD (Kingsberg & Rezaee, 2013), psychotherapy tends to be the optimal treatment. However, the medical team is an important component in the treatment process. A thorough medical work-up can determine the presence of general medical conditions or substances that can account for or contribute to LSDD (Montgomery, 2008), dramatically altering treatment decisions. Given the high comorbidity of LSDD with certain medical conditions and medications (Montgomery, 2008), the medical team and behavioral health specialist (BHS) must stay in close communication throughout the treatment process to provide the patient with comprehensive holistic care. Effective communication between the medical team and the BHS helps each to ensure that the patient is adhering to the treatment regimen laid out by the other.

Quality Improvement

Quality improvement (QI), the process of increasing treatment efficiency and patient satisfaction, plays an important role in improving the understanding and treatment of LSDD. One of the biggest challenges in treating LSDD is creating an environment in which patients are comfortable talking about sex and sexual problems. Health-care professionals must be comfortable, sensitive, and knowledgeable when discussing sexual health. To accomplish this goal in integrated care settings, because sexual health tends to be glossed over in the education of health-care professionals (Kingsberg & Rezaee, 2013), sites should provide additional training to their staff regarding sexuality and sexual health. Because not all patients are comfortable talking about sexual health (Montgomery, 2008), using self-report questionnaires such as the Female Sexual Functioning Index (FSFI; Rosen et al., 2000) may open the channels of communication. Given the sensitive nature of sexual desire, it is also important for researchers and clinicians to gain a more thorough understanding of the role that culture and religion play in the development, assessment, and treatment of LSDD, as research has begun to highlight the significance of cultural differences (Kingsberg & Rezaee, 2013). Additionally, the paucity of empirically supported Level 2 and 3 treatments calls for greater research efforts in this area. Specifically, given the success of Brotto et al. (2008) use of the Level 2 PED treatment, clinicians and patients would benefit from research regarding the efficacy of an adapted PED protocol for brief individual psychotherapy. To ultimately improve assessment and treatment of LSDD, it is paramount that the channels of communication remain open between practitioners, researchers, and patients.

References

Balzer, A. M. (2012). *Efficacy of bibliotherapy as a treatment for low sexual desire in women*. Columbia: Doctoral dissertation, University of Missouri.

Basson, R. (2001). Using a different model for female sexual response to address women's problematic low sexual desire. *Journal of Sex & Marital Therapy, 27*(5), 395–403.

Basson, R. (2006). Sexual desire and arousal disorders in women. *New England Journal of Medicine, 354*(14), 1497–1506.

Basson, R. (2007). Sexual desire/arousal disorders in women. In S. Leiblum (Ed.), *Principles and practice of sex therapy* (pp. 25–53). New York: Guilford Press.

Basson, R., Berman, J., Burnett, A., Derogatis, L., Ferguson, D., Fourcroy, J., … Leiblum, S. (2000). Report of the international consensus development conference on female sexual dysfunction: Definitions and classifications. *The Journal of Urology, 163*(3), 888–893.

Bitzer, J., Giraldi, A., & Pfaus, J. (2013). Sexual desire and hypoactive sexual desire disorder in women. Introduction and overview. Standard operating procedure (SOP Part 1). *The Journal of Sexual Medicine, 10*(1), 36–49.

Bower, P., & Gilbody, S. (2005). Stepped care in psychological therapies: Access, effectiveness and efficiency. *The British Journal of Psychiatry, 186*(1), 11–17.

Brauer, M., van Leeuwen, M., Janssen, E., Newhouse, S. K., Heiman, J. R., & Laan, E. (2012). Attentional and affective processing of sexual stimuli in women with hypoactive sexual desire disorder. *Archives of Sexual Behavior, 41*(4), 891–905.

Brotto, L., & Luria, M. (2014). Sexual interest/arousal disorder in women. In Y. M. Binik & K. S. K. Hall (Eds.), *Principles and practice of sex therapy* (5th ed., pp. 17–41). New York: Guilford Press.

Brotto, L. A. (2010). The DSM diagnostic criteria for hypoactive sexual desire disorder in women. *Archives of Sexual Behavior, 39*(2), 221–239.

Brotto, L. A., Basson, R., & Luria, M. (2008). Original research—Psychology: A mindfulness-based group psychoeducational intervention targeting sexual arousal disorder in women. *Journal of Sexual Medicine, 5*(7), 1646–1659.

Brotto, L. A., Bitzer, J., Laan, E., Leiblum, S., & Luria, M. (2010). Women's sexual desire and arousal disorders. *Journal of Sexual Medicine, 7*(1pt2), 586–614.

Brotto, L. A., Heiman, J. R., & Tolman, D. L. (2009). Narratives of desire in mid-age women with and without arousal difficulties. *Journal of Sex Research, 46*(5), 387–398.

Buster, J. E. (2013). Introduction: Sexual health matters!. *Fertility and sterility, 100*(4), 897. https://doi.org/10.1016/j.fertnstert.2013.08.019.

Carvalheira, A., Træen, B., & Štulhofer, A. (2014). Correlates of men's sexual interest: A cross-cultural study. *The Journal of Sexual Medicine, 11*(1), 154–164.

Coleman, E., Elders, J., Satcher, D., Shindel, A., Parish, S., Kenagy, G., … Lunn, M. R. (2013). Summit on medical school education in sexual health: Report of an expert consultation. *The Journal of Sexual Medicine, 10*(4), 924–938.

Corona, G., Mannucci, E., Petrone, L., Giommi, R., Mansani, R., Fei, L., … Maggi, M. (2004). Psychobiological correlates of hypoactive sexual desire in patients with erectile dysfunction. *International Journal of Impotence, 16*(3), 275–281.

Corona, G., Rastrelli, G., Forti, G., & Maggi, M. (2011). Update in testosterone therapy for men (CME). *The Journal of Sexual Medicine, 8*(3), 639–654.

Davis, S. R., Moreau, M., Kroll, R., Bouchard, C., Panay, N., Gass, M., … Koch, H. (2008). Testosterone for low libido in postmenopausal women not taking estrogen. *New England Journal of Medicine, 359*(19), 2005–2017.

Dove, L., Michael, W., & Wiederman, N. (2000). Cognitive distraction and women's sexual functioning. *Journal of Sex & Marital Therapy, 26*(1), 67–78.

Ellison, C. (2006). *Women's sexualities: Generations of women share intimate secrets of sexual self-acceptance*. Oakland, CA: New Harbinger Publications.

Fisher, W. A., Rosen, R. C., Eardley, I., Sand, M., & Goldstein, I. (2005). Sexual experience of female partners of men with erectile dysfunction: The female experience of men's attitudes to life events and sexuality (FEMALES) study. *The Journal of Sexual Medicine, 2*(5), 675–684.

Gehring, D. (2003). Couples therapy for low sexual desire: A systemic approach. *Journal of Sex & Marital Therapy, 29*(1), 25–38.

Goldstein, I., Fisher, W. A., Sand, M., Rosen, R. C., Mollen, M., Brock, G., … Derogatis, L. R. (2005). Women's sexual function improves when partners are administered Vardenafil for erectile dysfunction: A prospective, randomized, double-blind, placebo-controlled trial. *The Journal of Sexual Medicine, 2*(6), 819–832.

Hall, K. (2004). *Reclaiming your sexual self: How you can bring desire back into your life*. Hoboken, NJ: Wiley.

Hawton, K. (1985). *Sex therapy: A practical guide* (p. 273). Oxford, UK: Oxford University Press.

Kingsberg, S. A., & Rezaee, R. L. (2013). Hypoactive sexual desire in women. *Menopause*, *20*(12), 1284–1300.

Kingsberg, S. A., & Woodard, T. (2015). Female sexual dysfunction: Focus on low desire. *Obstetrics & Gynecology*, *125*(2), 477–486.

Latif, E. Z., & Diamond, M. P. (2013). Arriving at the diagnosis of female sexual dysfunction. *Fertility and Sterility*, *100*(4), 898–904.

Lorenz, T. A., & Meston, C. M. (2012). Acute exercise improves physical sexual arousal in women taking antidepressants. *Annals of Behavioral Medicine*, *43*(3), 352–361.

Marrs, R. W. (1995). A meta-analysis of bibliotherapy studies. *American Journal of Community Psychology*, *23*(6), 843.

Masters, W., & Johnson, V. E. (1966). *Human sexual response*. Boston, MA: Little Brown.

Masters, W. H., & Johnson, V. E. (1970). *Human sexual inadequacy*. Boston, Little, Brown.

McCabe, M. P., & Connaughton, C. (2014). Psychosocial factors associated with male sexual difficulties. *Journal of Sex Research*, *51*(1), 31–42.

Metz, M. E., & Epstein, N. (2002). Assessing the role of relationship conflict in sexual dysfunction. *Journal of Sex & Marital Therapy*, *28*(2), 139–164.

Mintz, L. B. (2009). *A tired woman's guide to passionate sex: Reclaim your desire and reignite your relationship*. Avon, MA: Adams Media.

Montgomery, K. A. (2008). Sexual desire disorders. *Psychiatry (Edgmont)*, *5*(6), 50–55.

Rosen, C., Brown, J., Heiman, S., Leiblum, C., Meston, R., Shabsigh, D., … D'Agostino, R. (2000). The Female Sexual Function Index (FSFI): A multidimensional self-report instrument for the assessment of female sexual function. *Journal of Sex & Marital Therapy*, *26*(2), 191–208.

Sand, M., & Fisher, W. A. (2007). Women's endorsement of models of female sexual response: The nurses' sexuality study. *The Journal of Sexual Medicine*, *4*(3), 708–719.

Shifren, J. L., Johannes, C. B., Monz, B. U., Russo, P. A., Bennett, L., & Rosen, R. (2009). Help-seeking behavior of women with self-reported distressing sexual problems. *Journal of Women's Health*, *18*(4), 461–468.

Simons, J. S., & Carey, M. P. (2001). Prevalence of sexual dysfunctions: Results from a decade of research. *Archives of Sexual Behavior*, *30*(2), 177–219.

Stuart, F. M., Hammond, D. C., & Pett, M. A. (1987). Inhibited sexual desire in women. *Archives of Sexual Behavior*, *16*(2), 91–106.

Trudel, G., Boulos, L., & Matte, B. (1993). Dyadic adjustment in couples with hypoactive sexual desire. *Journal of Sex Education and Therapy*, *19*(1), 31–36.

U.S. Food and Drug Administration. (2015). Retrieved June 30, 2016, from http://www.fda.gov/NewsEvents/Newsroom/PressAnnouncements/ucm458734.htm

White, J. R., Case, D. A., McWhirter, D., & Mattison, A. M. (1990). Enhanced sexual behavior in exercising men. *Archives of Sexual Behavior*, *19*(3), 193–209.

Wincze, J. P., & Weisberg, R. B. (2015). *Sexual dysfunction: A guide for assessment and treatment* (pp. 63–172). New York, NY: Guilford Publications.

22 Medical Treatment Adherence

Lauren Ostarello, Morgan Wright, and Thomas J. Waltz

Introduction

Advancements in healthcare have resulted in many promising medical and behavioral treatments to address a variety of acute and chronic medical conditions through outpatient services. Inherent in many of these approaches is the need for patients to independently monitor and manage these regimens. Historically, this area of patient engagement has been discussed in terms of treatment adherence and nonadherence. We refer to self-management in this chapter because it is more descriptive of what care systems aim to have patients do when clinicians intervene to improve treatment adherence.

While self-management needs will vary by clinical presentation, there are two broad categories of self-management activities patients need to effectively adhere to treatments for their medical conditions. The first category involves effective engagement with the care system and includes (a) making and keeping appointments with primary and specialty care providers; (b) communicating with providers about one's health, health priorities, and healthcare preferences; and (c) obtaining the foundational knowledge, skills, and other resources necessary for self-management activities to be implemented. The second category builds off of the first and involves (d) the establishment of effective routines and material supports so that the mechanics of the care plan can be integrated into daily life and (e) skills and social-emotional supports to cope with the negative affect and effort involved in managing medical conditions. Effective medical treatment of self-management is likely to occur when all five elements discussed above operate at their full potential.

Effective Ways to Screen for Adherence in the Primary Care Setting

The importance of prescribed medications and behavioral recommendations for positive health outcomes is well known, yet follow-up assessment of self-management practices is relatively uncommon (IOM, 2003). To obtain information that accurately reflects self-management practices, direct and frequent measurement of behavior is required. There is no single "gold standard" method for assessing treatment adherence or the implementation of self-management routines. There are a range of assessment tools available depending on the health condition, outcome of interest, care system resources, and patient willingness and ability to engage in adherence

L. Ostarello (✉) • M. Wright • T.J. Waltz
Department of Psychology, Eastern Michigan University, Ypsilanti, MI, USA
e-mail: lostarel@emich.edu; mwrigh57@emich.edu; twaltz1@emich.edu

A. Maragakis, W.T. O'Donohue (eds.), *Principle-Based Stepped Care and Brief Psychotherapy for Integrated Care Settings*, https://doi.org/10.1007/978-3-319-70539-2_22

monitoring. Assessment of treatment adherence can be conducted using institutional records and direct monitoring by patients.

Screeners embedded in care routines. There are many methods for screening patients to identify those who may have difficulties adhering to treatment regimens. Care systems with mature electronic record systems can utilize measurement-based care routines to identify patients for whom adherence concerns may be contributing to poor or suboptimal outcomes. Somatic care variables that may be routinely updated in the medical record as part of care encounters include prescription refill timing, blood panel results, HbA1c levels, weight, blood pressure, spirometry, etc. Psychosocial measures that are part of routine clinical screening may also indicate increased risk for poor self-management. For example, depression is associated with a threefold increase in noncompliance with medical routines (DiMatteo, Lepper, & Croghan, 2000). Measures such as the Patient Health Questionnaire come in 2- and 9-item versions to support a stepped approach to screening for depression (Arroll et al., 2010; Manea et al., 2016). Worsening or continued poor performance on these measures can be used to identify patients in need of a follow-up assessment to determine whether supplemental intervention is warranted to increase self-management of care.

Patient Activation Measure (PAM). The PAM is a tool that can be used to identify patients at risk for poor adherence on the basis of their self-reported knowledge, skills, and self-confidence related to managing their health. Scores on the PAM fall under four levels. Level 1 scores reflect that the patient does not believe they have an active or important role in managing their health condition. Level 2 reflects that the patient lacks confidence and knowledge to take action. Level 3 scores reflect that the client is beginning to take action on their health condition. Finally, Level 4 scores reflect that the patient is able to maintain health-related behaviors over time. Higher scores on the PAM are associated with better health outcomes, better care experiences, and reduced care costs (Greene, Hibbard, Sacks, Overton, & Parrotta, 2015; Hibbard & Greene, 2013). Most self-management routines for health conditions presume the patient would score at Level 4 on the PAM, and these are the patients best prepared to benefit from "care as usual." Patients with PAM scores at Levels 1 through 3 will benefit from tailored supports from a case manager, behavioral health provider, or other relevant supports related to the challenges identified by the measure.

Self-monitoring. Self-monitoring is an assessment tool that can be utilized to record both subjective and objective measures of behavior, ideally in "real time." This type of assessment eliminates the need for patients to retrospectively report treatment engagement and decreases the risk of bias the closer the self-monitoring recordings occur to the events of interest. Moreover, behaviors that are difficult to assess objectively, such as diet and exercise adherence, can be relatively easily and accurately recorded using self-monitoring. The data provided by self-monitoring can be used to evaluate patterns of treatment adherence over time and help identify barriers to effective self-management.

Self-monitoring can be used to record various aspects of treatment-related behavior. Frequency count data can be collected when practitioners are interested in evaluating how often a behavior occurs. For example, a practitioner might instruct a patient to record each time they exercise throughout the week. Duration can be used to measure how long a behavior occurs. This might be useful to determine the total number of minutes a patient exercises. Self-ratings can be used to measure subjective states, such as mood, pain, or symptoms. These ratings can be recorded at predesignated times or when specific behaviors occur. Methods for recording self-monitoring data range in technology from pencil-and-paper tally systems to mobile applications.

There are many variables that impact the accuracy of self-monitored data. The more well defined the treatment-related behavior or health outcome variable is, the more accurate the record. In general, patients benefit from direct and systematic training regarding the self-monitoring routine. The highest standard of training, behavioral skills rehearsal, includes:

(a) Providing the patient with a verbal description of the variable(s) to be monitored, how the monitoring routine is to be executed, and the rationale for including these variables,
(b) Provide the patient with a written description of item (a).
(c) The clinician demonstrates how to complete the self-monitoring routine using the same materials the patient will use.
(d) The patient is required to practice the self-monitoring routine while under the supervision of the clinician.
(e) The clinician provides both positive and corrective feedback each time the patient rehearses the skill.
(f) Practice and feedback cycles are repeated until the client has mastered the self-monitoring routine.

Other variables influencing the accuracy of self-monitored data include regular fidelity checks for accuracy and compliance with monitoring routines and basing positive feedback on reporting accurate data rather than positive outcomes. Korotitsch and Nelson-Gray (1999) provide an extended discussion of variables influencing self-monitoring in a clinical context, and we highly recommend behavioral healthcare providers review this reference.

Mobile applications allow patients to monitor treatment-related behavior and subjective experiences as they occur without creating a significant burden on daily activities. Mobile applications are becoming increasingly common to track a variety of treatment-related variables such as symptoms, engagement in treatment, and medication management and can be used to monitor additional outcomes of interest such as weight, caloric intake, and blood glucose levels. Some features of mobile applications allow patients to be reminded to record their behavior at specific time intervals, reducing the impact of memory-based error.

Overall, self-monitoring can be a useful tool for assessing treatment adherence. Self-monitoring has also been identified as an intervention to increase self-management of care routines (Johnston et al., 2016). The act of self-monitoring may increase patients' awareness of treatment engagement and may subsequently increase patients' adherence to the prescribed regimen. Although self-monitoring can provide frequent, direct measures of treatment engagement, it may be burdensome for patients to log several behaviors over extended periods of time. To reduce this burden, practitioners should design recording systems that can be easily implemented and consider limiting the number of behaviors and frequency of recording to the elements necessary to support a patient. For self-monitoring to be sustained, patients need to find the information they gather to be a valuable asset for understanding the relationship between self-management behaviors, other variables that are recorded, and their link with a patient's health goals (Mann, De Ridder, & Fujita, 2013). How to support effective goal setting will be discussed later in this chapter.

Clinical interview. While the medical record-based and client-report-based methods described above are useful adherence assessment and monitoring tools, all members of the treatment team should be on the lookout for potential barriers to self-management aspects of the treatment plan. Curiosity, empathy, and a collaborative stance should guide these interactions to facilitate barrier disclosures as many patients may experience shame or other negative affect when discussing nonadherence. When the interview focuses on person-environment fit variables that impact adherence, patients often find this discussion to be easier to participate in than discussions that focus exclusively on internal attributions (i.e., personality characteristics). A candid and compassionate discussion of the what, where, and when features of barriers to effective self-management is the first step in taking a collaborative problem-solving approach to addressing these barriers.

What to Do If a Screen Returns Positive

Since treatment adherence is essential to effective healthcare delivery, it is important to determine patients' perceived and real barriers to self-management. It should be assumed that nonadherence to a medical regimen is due to a patient's life context rather than a lack of motivation or some inherent flaw within the patient. This focuses the post-screening inquiry on aspects of the patient's life that can be directly influenced by the clinician and the patient. Patients may attribute their difficulties to broad barriers such as lack of time or motivation; however, these attributions often reflect socially conventional reasons for nonadherence. Additional assessment is required to obtain an adequate picture of the multiple variables influencing time management or life factors impacting the report of motivational status.

While a wide range of barriers to self-management have been documented in the literature, there is significant variation in how these barriers are defined and measured. Many theoretical models have been developed to more clearly understand and predict treatment nonadherence but have failed to provide clarification into how to evaluate and improve the effects of these barriers on adherence (Christensen, 2004). In general, barriers to treatment adherence tend to be quite ideographic (Gellad, Grenard, & McGlynn, 2009). Conceptualization of barriers to treatment adherence from a contextual behavioral framework may be particularly useful for identifying and improving the impact of barriers on treatment-related behavior. A contextual behavioral framework aims to understand patients' interaction with the treatment in the context of their lives and avoids placing blame on the patient or attributing nonadherence to internal factors that are not amenable to change (e.g., intentions and motivation are not directly changed; these are always influenced by some change in the patient's context). Rather, providers should focus on identifying specific contextual barriers surrounding the patient's actual experiences and care management behaviors. Once barriers to self-management have been identified, these barriers should be systematically targeted, and appropriate modifications to the treatment regimen should be considered if necessary. Table 22.1 provides suggestions for assessing specific barriers to effective self-management and offers intervention strategies for the integrated primary care team to deliver.

Self-management barriers may manifest in a variety of ways in patients' lives. Patients may lack education about their medical regimen or may have doubts about features of the prescribed regimen. Patients may have insufficient economic or material resources making it difficult for them to attend appointments or purchase medications. Moreover, it may be difficult for patients to incorporate a new or complex regimen into their current environment. For example, patients might have difficulties remembering to take their medication or may have activities or conflicts in their lives that interfere with their ability to develop habits related to the medical regimen. In general, it may be difficult for patients to establish and maintain habit inertia. Furthermore, patients may be unable to fulfill social roles as a result of their medical condition or treatment regimen and may have social support systems that are unsupportive of treatment-related behavior. Some barriers to self-management may be the result of skills deficits. For example, patients may have communication skills deficits preventing them from being able to effectively inform practitioners about their concerns, treatment/medication side effects, or their uncertainty regarding the treatment plan. Undetected cognitive impairment and psychological problems such as depression may impact patients' abilities to engage in the prescribed medical regimen and may therefore result in poorer self-management. If your screening assessments and interview do not point clearly to any of the barriers described in Table 22.1, have the client demonstrate the self-management related skill(s) during the clinical encounter. Skills demonstration and observation

Table 22.1 Assessment and interventions for barriers to medical treatment nonadherence

Barrier	Assessment	Stepped-care interventions
Resources • Material • Economic	Verbal self-report • How reliable is your transportation? • Does transportation ever impact your ability to engage in your medical treatment? • How do co-pays impact your ability to receive medical care? • What types of practical obstacles tend to interfere with your ability to follow through with your care plan?	CM • Facilitate problem-solving to ameliorate resource barriers • Connect patient to resource aid programs
Uncertainty	Verbal self-report • How confident are you that your medical condition will improve if you closely follow the treatment? • Do you think that anything you do to manage this medical condition actually matters? • Do you feel like you have a good understanding of what your medical condition is and what that means?	Nurse/medical assistant/physician • Characterize the medical condition, prognosis, and treatment response of the medical condition in terms the client can understand. Ensure written materials are understood • After answering the patient's questions, have the patient explain to you the informational features that were the previous source of uncertainty • Reconcile sources of apparent conflicting information, and provide the patient with a coherent, integrated summary
Mental health status	Self-report measures • PHQ-2/9, GAD-7, PRIME-MD Verbal self-report • Do your depression/anxiety* symptoms ever impact your ability to engage in your medical regimen? * Use terms the client identifies with. For example, "nerves," "mood," "irritability," "stubbornness," etc.	BHP • Motivational interviewing[a] • Brief Acceptance and Commitment Therapy[b] • Brief Cognitive Behavior Therapy[c] • Problem-solving treatment for primary care[d] • May provide self-help resources SMH • BHP should refer to SMH when symptoms can be better addressed with longer-term care
Executive functioning/ initiation difficulties/ mental status	Verbal self-report • Are there periods during the day where you don't know where your time went? • Are there periods during the day where you're not able to concentrate and you think you should? • Tell me about your sleep (e.g., latency, duration, frequency of waking, etc.) • Are there any side effects of this regimen? • Executive function screening measures: BRIEF, RBANS, SLUMS, MMSE	BHP • Follow up to identify if neuropsychology referral is necessary to gain better understanding of deficits to implement appropriate accommodations so that problem-solving can occur PC • Rule out delirium or adverse medical events (e.g., medications)

(continued)

Table 22.1 (continued)

Barrier	Assessment	Stepped-care interventions
Communication skills	Verbal self-report • When your physician comes in, what do you tell them? • Role-play: I'm the physician, what do you say to me when I walk in? (Do they know what to tell the physician? See problem-solving manual[df] for more guidance on how to identify the problem, talk about it, etc.)	BHP • Communication skills rehearsal: How to talk to help physician gain better understanding
Skills deficits	Verbal self-report • Can you do X? • Has anyone observed you engage in the skill and given feedback about how to complete the skill? Who was that person? • Please demonstrate the skill.	BHP (or medical team member trained in behavioral skills training) • Behavioral skills training[e] (rather than information training)
Problems with arranging effective supports	Verbal self-report • Do you have difficulty remembering/managing complex routines? • Do you receive a bubble pack? • What kinds of prompts do you use to remind yourself to engage with your medical regimen? • Do you use/know how to use the reminders on your phone?	CM • Provide access to instrumental support (e.g., bubble packs) CM or BHP • Technical interventions (e.g., setting alarm reminders on cell phone)
Habit/inertia	Verbal self-report • How do your existing routines allow you to do X related to your health condition? • How does your medical condition impact your existing routines? • How do your existing routines allow you to engage in your medical treatment? Written self-report (e.g., diaries, self-monitoring)	BHP • Behaviorally focused problem-solving SMH • BHP should refer to SMH when rigidity is too excessive to be addressed in integrated setting
Competing incentives • Values conflict • Cost/benefit perception	Verbal self-report • Do you have any pressing issues in your life that impact your ability to engage in medical treatment? • How do your medical care needs interfere with your other life priorities? • Are there emotional costs to engaging in medical care that you don't think others would understand? • What kind of emotional stressors show up in relation to your medical care? • What kinds of thoughts or emotions come up when you're thinking about engaging in medical care? • Do these thoughts ever become reasons not to engage in the treatment? • Is there anything that is unacceptable about the current treatment? • Are you experiencing any side effects from your treatment that make other parts of your life more difficult?	BHP • Motivational interviewing[a] • Brief Acceptance and Commitment Therapy[b] • Brief Cognitive Behavior Therapy[c] (e.g., cost-benefit two column technique) SMH • BHP should refer patient to SMH if emotional barriers are greater than what can be addressed in integrated setting PC • Medication review. Consider pharmacy consult

Table 22.1 (continued)

Barrier	Assessment	Stepped-care interventions
Social support system • Isolation • Skills challenges and adversity	Verbal self-report • How has your health condition impacted social relationships? • How does your health condition impact your ability to fulfill your social roles?	BHP • Assess whether needs would be better met by support group (address isolation) • Social problem-solving skills[f] SMH • Longer-term social problem-solving therapy[f]

Abbreviations for assessments: *BRIEF* Behavior Rating Inventory of Executive Function, *RBANS* Repeatable Battery for Neuropsychological Status, *SLUMS* the Saint Louis University Mental Status, *MMSE* Mini Mental Status Examination

Abbreviations for stepped-care interventions: *BHP* behavioral health provider, *CM* case manager, *PC* primary care provider, *SMH* specialty mental health

Note. Motivational and psychosocial treatments noted above include

[a]Motivational interviewing (Rollnick et al., 2008)

[b]Focused acceptance and commitment therapy (Strosahl et al., 2012)

[c]Brief cognitive behavior therapy (Cully & Teten, 2008)

[d]Problem-solving therapy for primary care (Hegel & Arean, 2003)

[e]Behavioral skills training (Parsons et al., 2012)

[f]Social problem-solving skills (Nezu, Nezu, & D'Zurilla, 2013)

often help the clinician and patient better define and describe the types of barriers present.

Not all patients can readily identify the types of barriers that contribute to their poor self-management of their care. If a patient has difficulties describing the barriers contributing to poor self-management, it is often helpful to ask the patient to provide a narrative of their daily schedule including their engagement in the medical regimen to determine where barriers might arise. Practitioners should ask questions about how various environmental factors influence the patient's ability to engage in the medical regimen. There are often specific considerations that need to be taken into account for specific treatments and populations. O'Donohue and Levensky (2006) provide a practical review of considerations for several treatments and populations. This chapter focuses on broad factors to consider for supporting treatment adherence as a detailed review of strategies, for individual treatments and populations is beyond the scope of the chapter.

From Positive Screen to SMART Goals

Identifying the most appropriate stepped care option for an individual with a positive screen for poor treatment adherence depends largely on the care plan's goals and the likely barriers to meeting those goals. Goals and the goal-setting process can serve an important motivational function in support of self-management of health-related behavior. While there have been no randomized controlled trials regarding goal setting as a stand-alone intervention for adherence, it is an integral component of all treatment planning, and healthcare providers and their patients will benefit from what is known in this research domain. A separate intervention, motivational interviewing, will be briefly discussed in a later section for those patients that are ambivalent with respect to setting adherence and self-management-related goals.

Goal setting often begins with identifying a superordinate goal, or value statement, that is relatively brief and high in affect and orients the individual to the purpose and inspiration behind more specific goals that will follow: "Maintaining my health so I can be there when my family needs me"; "Regaining my mobility and independence," and "Participate more fully in my relationships, with patience and kindness." Superordinate goals and values serve a motivational function, but more specific goals need to follow for effective action to be supported. Latham (2003) popularized SMART as a heuristic for effective goal setting: specific, measureable, attainable, realistic, and timely.

When setting specific goals, approach goals (i.e., goals that focus on desired outcomes) are more effective than avoidance goals (i.e., goals that focus on avoiding future adverse medical outcomes) (Mann et al., 2013). There is also evidence that it is important for individuals to actively participate in developing the narrative that outlines the specific of a goal. This is associated with greater willingness to collaboratively problem-solve with others in order to meet expectations of the goal (Locke & Latham, 2002). While an aim of collaborative care is to have patients actively participate in their treatment planning, many individuals quickly acquiesce to the judgment of the professional authorities on the treatment team. While healthcare providers may make suggestions regarding how to frame a specific goal, it is important to ask the client how they would describe the specifics of the goal using their own words.

Goals need to be measurable, and a system for regular and frequent progress monitoring needs to be established. Feedback is essential if a patient is to adjust their behavior to be more in-line with goals. Progress monitoring must involve a scheme for recording key data related to the goal as "trying to pay attention," and other non-recorded monitoring schemes are not effective (Harkin et al., 2016). It is important that the data collected in relation to the goal can meaningfully inform goal progress. Is the aim of the goal to meet a certain performance standard or outcome? Is the aim of the goal to develop and master certain health-related skills? Mastery goals (aka, learning or process goals) are often more effective, especially when engagement is more important than achieving a specific outcome (e.g., developing a walking routine versus losing 20 pounds) (Mann et al., 2013).

That health-related goals need to be attainable does not mean these goals should be easy. At the other extreme, near-impossible goals risk being abandoned. Goals in the "Goldilocks" zone of difficulty require high levels of effort and performance. If a goal is personally meaningful, specific, and measurable, the patient can develop an important sense of self-efficacy when positively monitoring their progress toward a difficult goal (Locke & Latham, 2002). The specificity of the goal is important because aspirational goals to "do my best" lack the specificity needed to support higher levels of effort and performance. It is also important to assess for skills deficits and ineffective problem-solving strategies in relation to difficult goals. When performance quickly breaks down, a difficult goal can be experienced as unattainable. Mastery or learning-based goals can be an important route to take when skills deficits and developing more effective problem-solving strategies are important components of the skills needed to achieve a difficult goal.

To determine whether or not a goal is realistic, a provider needs to know important information about a patient's medical condition and their history. What counts as a realistic goal for a patient with a history of high-intensity athletic training versus a patient with no athletic background may differ substantially. It is important to explore a patient's background for historical evidence that they have the skills and resilience needed for the level of goal that is set. Most goals point to temporally distant outcomes (e.g., health and wellness), and these types of outcomes are easily undermined by more temporally proximal competing outcomes (e.g., unhealthy foods, medication side effects, pain, other life obligations) (Bickel & Vuchinich, 2000). It is important to prospectively discuss with patients how their multiple life goals and obligations are likely to interact with treatment plan goals for adherence. Planning for how to handle goal conflicts and setbacks and determining appropriate intervals for revisiting the goal-setting process can all be important parts of guarding against the abandonment of goals secondary to setbacks that make goals appear unrealistic (Mann et al., 2013).

The final component of a SMART goal is timeliness. Effective goals specify when key actions should be accomplished. Developing routines for adhering to the goal, measuring performance, and monitoring goal progress is essential for developing resilient health-related habits (Gardner, Lally, & Wardle, 2012). Enforcing the timeliness features of a goal by making public commitments or using some other public forum for reporting engagement that increases accountability for goal-related activities is one of the most effective strategies for enhancing commitment to goals (Locke & Latham, 2002). Social supports around adherence goals should reflect the timeliness needs of the patient and their care routine.

Evidence-Based Stepped Care and Brief Psychotherapeutic Approaches

The most successful interventions for improving self-management attend to the unique health presentations and personal characteristics of each patient (McDonald, Garg, & Haynes, 2002). Thus, clinicians need to be aware of health condition-specific challenges (e.g., cognitive and emotional challenges with thyroid conditions) as well as material resource barriers related to accessing appropriate care (e.g., high co-pays, transportation difficulties, expensive equipment) for those specific conditions. Table 22.1 provides a brief description of interventions for each of the barriers covered there. This section will discuss details regarding three broad areas of intervention: technical interventions, provider-patient communication, and brief therapeutic approaches used by behavioral health providers.

Technical interventions. Technical interventions can be useful in addressing barriers such as scheduling and attending appointments, reducing the complexity of medical treatment regimens, and remembering to take medications. For instance, a meta-analysis by Macharia, Leon, Rowe, Stephenson, and Haynes (1992) found that significantly more appointments were attended when preceded by a postal mail or telephone reminder. Similarly, a review by van Eijken, Tsang, Wensing, de Smet, and Grol (2003) found evidence that automated telephone reminders successfully increased medication self-management in elderly people. Phone, text, and app-based technologies can be used to prompt treatment engagement. More advanced technologies effectively engage social networks so that positive social feedback is recruited to support effective engagement—a significant innovation that goes beyond reminder-based systems by mobilizing natural social supports for self-management and treatment adherence.

Consulting with pharmacists to facilitate problem-solving on how to simplify medication regimens, or addressing treatment-interfering side effects can be a useful first step in reducing medication compliance barriers. In addition, technical adherence interventions have been developed primarily to simplify medication regimens to improve the likelihood of compliance. Simplifying medication regimens either by reducing the number of different medications taken per day or reducing the number of times per day medications have to be taken has been shown to increase medication compliance for a wide range of health conditions. Arranging services so pill boxes or blister packaging organize medications also improves self-management. Technology involving smart containers and smart pills represents new opportunities for monitoring and prompting self-management behaviors for medications, but these are not yet widely available.

Physician-patient communication. Effective communication by the physician or anyone else on the medical team involved in interacting with the patient can significantly impact medical treatment adherence (Martin, Williams, Haskard, & DiMatteo, 2005). Research has shown that the even though patients generally are able to communicate their concerns to physicians within the first 30 seconds of their encounter, they are interrupted by the physician after an average of 23.1 s (Marvel, Epstein, Flowers, & Beckman, 1999). Moreover, a meta-analysis found a positive relationship between physician communication and patient adherence to treatment in that patients of physicians with poor communication skills were 1.47 times more likely to be nonadherent, while clients of physicians with adequate communication skills were 2.16 times more likely to be adherent (Haskard-Zolnierek & DiMatteo, 2009). In addition to improved adherence, good physician communication skills have been shown to increase patients' satisfaction with care and are associated with improved patient health status. Key skills for providers include training in the effective use of verbal (e.g., patient-centered) and nonverbal (e.g., tone, body language) communication, willingness to discuss client affect, ability to collaboratively problem-solve with patients to address task-relevant difficulties, and actively involving patients in the creation of their treatment plan.

There are resources available to help providers assess their communication skills and routines to develop better integrated, patient-centered care. For example, the Kalamazoo Consensus Statement (Makoul, 2001) outlines essential sets of communication tasks in medical encounters. Assessment tools have been developed with behavioral anchors for nine domains of communication that can be used as a self-assessment guide for clinicians (Peterson, Calhoun, & Rider, 2014). While this assessment tool has been used in medical resident education, it is well suited for ongoing professional development efforts in integrated care settings.

Brief therapeutic approaches. Behavioral health specialists can use a variety of evidence-based strategies that have been adapted for integrated care settings. Motivational interviewing utilizes techniques to help patients identify their motivations for treatment adherence-related behavior change (Rollnick, Miller, & Butler, 2008). This approach was developed to help patients move from being ambivalent toward treatment to developing personalized treatment goals without the use of social coercion that increases the probability of patient disengagement from care. The communication skills covered in this approach are useful for all members of a care team, and there is preliminary evidence that this approach supports more effective treatment engagement by patients in multiple health areas (Martins & McNeil, 2009).

There are several other behavioral therapies that commonly include adherence within their treatment goals, but to our knowledge, none have primary care-based RCTs that focus on treatment adherence as a primary outcome. Acceptance and commitment therapy has been adopted for use in primary care settings and focuses on addressing thoughts and feelings that serve as barriers to effective action and clarifying one's goals and values so actions taken are connected with a deeper sense of purpose (Strosahl, Robinson, & Gustavsson, 2012). Cognitive behavior therapy represents a skills and solution-focused approach that is readily applied to a wide variety of clinical and subclinical emotional and behavioral disturbances that may interfere with self-management efforts and support the development of care plan consistent habits (Cully & Teten, 2008). Another specific form of behavior therapy, problem-solving therapy, has been adopted for addressing depression in the primary care setting (Mynors-Wallis, 2012; Oxman, Hegel, Hull, & Dietrich, 2008). Robinson (2005) provides useful guidance regarding the process of adapting evidence-based therapies to the primary care setting from a stepped-care perspective.

Patients with skills deficits can benefit from behavioral skills training which utilizes patient education, modeling, and skills rehearsal to resolve such deficits. For example, a behavioral health specialist (or other members or the integrated care team) can engage in brief behavioral skills training with a diabetic patient by first providing information and education on the function and importance of insulin injections, modeling how to administer an injection, watching the patient engage in this behavior, and then providing the patient feedback on their performance. A more detailed description on behavioral skills training can be found in Parsons, Rollyson, and Reid (2012).

What Does Not Work

Traditional psychoeducation that is provided in most clinical settings is often effective at improving knowledge but has no effect or short-lived effects on treatment adherence. Similarly, educational interventions consisting of teaching patients about their illness (or disease process) and the importance of adhering to treatment recommendations, as well as the mode in which educational interventions are delivered (e.g., individual versus group education, in writing, face to face contact, etc.), have been shown to have no effect to modest effects when used as a stand-alone treatment mode. Most studies focusing on patient education fail to provide sufficient detail on the educational intervention provided rendering it difficult to evaluate the quality of these studies. Overall, while education regarding the individual's health condition may be a necessary component of care, education is rarely sufficient in and of itself to maintain adherence to a care regimen.

Another category of ineffective interventions is rooted in folk psychological approaches to motivating behavior change: placing blame and shame onto the patient, equating self-management failure with moral failure, and attributing nonadherence to pejorative internal attributes that are not amenable to change (e.g., laziness or stupidity). Similarly, when a health professional or family member declares that the patient needs to "accept responsibility" for their medical condition and comply with a self-management routine, they are essentially invoking a moral failure argument. These arguments have been historically associated with interfering with effective responses to health conditions by society (Herek, Capitanio, & Widaman, 2003). While these approaches may give the health professional or family member a comforting sense of righteousness, there is no evidence that such approaches improve treatment adherence. Negatively valent language regarding health conditions can function to identify patients as being deviant from the majority group in culture, and this type of labeling can be stigmatizing. Stigmatizing language has been associated with delays in seeking healthcare, dysfunctional coping, and poor treatment adherence across a variety of conditions (Kamaradova et al., 2016; Livingston & Boyd, 2010). It is important to note that patients identify healthcare providers as one of the most common sources of stigmatization, and providers tend to spend less time in appointments with stigmatized groups (Puhl & Brownell, 2010; Puhl & Heuer, 2010). This suggests that minimizing the use of stigmatizing language can be as important for its effects on the care team as it is for its effects on the patient.

A contextual behavioral approach holds the fundamental assumption that all behavior, including poor self-management, makes sense given the patient's history and current context. Folk psychological interpretations of adherence failures commonly place the problem inside the person and thus distract the treatment team from gathering the relevant contextual information to understand why adherence is insufficiently supported and other competing behaviors are supported. The training behavioral health providers receive aims to provide them with the skills and sufficient background to help them identify these contextual variables with the help of the client.

When to Refer to External Specialty Mental Health

Medical treatment adherence for many conditions is difficult independent of whether a patient has or is likely to have a mental health diagnosis. While mental health presentations can serve as barriers to effective self-management, clinicians need to be aware of the risk of holding a diagnostic overshadowing bias that too quickly attributes adherence problems to mental health. Such a bias cuts short the adequate consideration of the myriad of other variables that may be impacting adherence. A successful course of treatment for depression in specialty mental healthcare may lessen one contributing factor to poor adherence, but other barriers may still remain.

When mental health concerns are present, consult with the behavioral health provider regarding the availability of primary care-based mental health services for the concern before automatically referring the patient to specialty care. The behavioral health provider will be able to determine whether an appropriate primary care-based intervention is available for the patient. There is increasing evidence that a wide variety of clinical presentations can effectively be treated through primary care-based mental health services (Woltmann et al., 2012). There are, however, clinical presentations (e.g., PTSD as the primary concern) for which the best care resides in specialty care settings as the course of evidence-based treatment involves parameters that would shift the behavioral health provider's role away from integrated care and toward colocated care (e.g., 90- to 120-min psychotherapy sessions). Individuals with severe emotional disturbances with poor response to less intense interventions are the typical candidates for specialty mental health referral. In addition, there are many patients that experience adherence difficulties secondary to having a complex or dysfunctional social support system. Specialty mental health services can be an important resource for these patients to develop the skills necessary to navigate and manage this complexity.

The Role of the Primary Care Provider/Medical Team in Supporting Treatment Adherence

There are aspects of ordinary care that decrease the likelihood of a primary care provider adequately supporting treatment adherence. Practice pressures for expediency commonly result in patients being allocated only brief periods of time to speak uninterrupted (Marvel et al., 1999; Rhoades, McFarland, Finch, & Johnson, 2001). Furthermore, 50% of patients leave the treatment encounter not understanding what they were told by their physician (Roter & Hall, 1989). Poor communication from the patient to the provider and from the provider to the patient can increase the role uncertainty plays as a barrier to treatment adherence. This uncertainty is compounded when patients experience the treatment directives they receive from multiple care providers as being inconsistent (e.g., consider a diabetic where Provider A recommends a low glycemic diet and Provider B recommends a diet low in saturated fats, trans fats, cholesterol, and sodium due to the increased risk of heart disease and stroke for this population). It is important for good interprofessional communication to be present on a care team so that each point of care is able to help the patient understand how the multiple elements of a treatment plan come together.

Miller and colleagues (Miller, Duncan, Brown, Sorrell, & Chalk, 2006) have developed an extremely brief tool for assessing clinician-patient working alliance in psychotherapy encounters that is also applicable to primary care encounters. Their working alliance assessment involves four questions: (1) To what degree did you feel, heard, and understood today? (2) To what degree did we work on the issues that you wanted to work on today? (3) How well did my approach, the way I worked, make sense and fit for you? (4) How would you rate how things were in today's session overall? The use of these questions at every encounter has been demonstrated to improve patient retention and treatment engagement. These brief questions seem well suited to assessing patient-care provider working alliance in integrated primary care.

The Institute for Healthcare Improvement has developed a toolkit to help healthcare teams improve patient self-management that provides resources for building effective skills for the care team members as well as patient supports before, during, and after the care encounter (Schaefer, Miller, Goldstein, & Simmons, 2009). Members of the medical team should find this to be a rich resource.

How to Assess Impact on Care/Quality Improvement Process

Self-management is a common component for most health conditions, and there are often specific features that need to be accounted for (e.g., education, skills) related to each condition. While there are quality improvement assessment processes that include evaluation of the self-management supports for specific health conditions, multimorbidity is common. This points to the need for a system assessment tool that captures the breadth of the self-management needs in primary care. The Primary Care Resources and Supports for Chronic Disease Self-Management (PCRS) is a care team-level assessment that was designed to facilitate quality improvement for self-management support in primary care (Brownson et al., 2007). This tool is intended to be used quarterly or semiannually to monitor and guide efforts to support self-management and has two primary sections. The first section of the PCRS concerns "patient support" and includes the following characteristics: individualized assessment, self-management education, goal setting, problem-solving skills, emotional health, patient involvement in decision-making, social support, and links to community resources. The second section of the PCRS concerns "organizational support" and includes the following characteristics: continuity of care, coordination of referrals, ongoing quality improvement, system for documentation, patient input, integration of self-management into primary care, team approach, staff education, and training. The PCRS has team members that independently rate each of the characteristic areas in terms of their current quality (1 is not done or does not exist; 10 is done, supported, incentivized, and sustainment monitored by ongoing quality improvement processes). Team member scores are aggregated and discussed. Low scores point to opportunities for improvement, and discrepant scores tend to identify areas where improved team communication can increase self-management support. Currently, there is only one study describing the use of the PCRS in an integrated health learning collaborative. All sites reported progress on multiple elements of the PCRS and satisfaction with using this tool (Vannoy et al., 2011). More research is needed to determine whether this tool reliably produces positive effects.

At the patient level, there are several opportunities for assessing the impact of quality improvement efforts at facilitating self-management skills and supports. Passively, care systems can look at appointment attendance rates, prescription refill rates, and variables routinely gathered as part of somatic care (e.g., HbA1c, blood pressure) to evaluate patient engagement and health-related outcomes. If monitoring somatic variables is impractical or too costly for a specific clinical problem, the PAM, discussed earlier, is a tool that can capture changes in patients taking more active roles in managing their medical conditions. Interventions that improve self-management should also improve patient satisfaction with care.

References

Arroll, B., Goodyear-Smith, F., Crengle, S., Gunn, J., Kerse, N., Fishman, T., … Hatcher, S. (2010). Validation of PHQ-2 and PHQ-9 to screen for major depression in the primary care population. *Annals of Family Medicine*, *8*(4), 348–353. https://doi.org/10.1370/afm.1139

Bickel, W. K., & Vuchinich, R. E. (Eds.). (2000). *Reframing health behavior change with behavioral economics*. Mahwah, NJ: Lawrence Erlbaum Associates.

Brownson, C. A., Miller, D., Crespo, R., Neuner, S., Thompson, J., Wall, J. C., … Glasgow, R. E. (2007). A quality improvement tool to assess self-management support in primary care. *The Joint Commission Journal on Quality and Patient Safety*, *33*, 408–416. https://doi.org/10.1016/S1553-7250(07)33047-X

Christensen, A. J. (2004). *Patient adherence to medical treatment regimens: Bridging the gap between behavioral science and biomedicine*. New Haven: Yale University Press.

Cully, J. A., & Teten, A. L. (2008). *A therapist's guide to brief cogntive behavioral therapy*. Houston: Department of Veterans Affairs South Central MIRECC.

DiMatteo, M. R., Lepper, H. S., & Croghan, T. W. (2000). Depression is a risk factor for noncompliance with medical treatment. *Archives of Internal Medicine*, *160*, 2101–2107.

Gardner, B., Lally, P., & Wardle, J. (2012). Making health habitual: The psychology of 'habit formation' and general practice. *British Journal of General Practice*, *62*, 664–666. https://doi.org/10.3399/bjgp12X659466

Gellad, W. F., Grenard, J., & McGlynn, E. A. (2009). *A review of barriers to medication adherence: A framework for driving policy options*. Santa Monica, CA: RAND Corporation.

Greene, J., Hibbard, J. H., Sacks, R., Overton, V., & Parrotta, C. D. (2015). When patient activation levels change, health outcomes and costs change, too. *Health Affairs*, *34*(3), 431–437. https://doi.org/10.1377/hlthaff.2014.0452

Harkin, B., Webb, T. L., Chang, B. P. I., Prestwich, A., Conner, M., Kellar, I., … Sheeran, P. (2016). Does monitoring goal progress promote goal attainment? A meta-analysis of the experimental evidence. *Psychological Bulletin*, *142*, 198–229.

Haskard-Zolnierek, K. B., & DiMatteo, M. R. (2009). Physician communication and patient adherence to treatment: A meta-analysis. *Medical Care*, *47*(8), 826–834. https://doi.org/10.1097/MLR.0b013e31819a5acc

Hegel, M., & Arean, P. (2003). *Problem-solving treatment for primary care: A treatment manual for depression*. Lebanon, NH: Project IMPACT.

Herek, G. M., Capitanio, J. P., & Widaman, K. F. (2003). Stigma, social risk, and health policy: Public attitudes toward HIV surveillance policies and the social construction of illness. *Health Psychology*, *22*, 533–540.

Hibbard, J. H., & Greene, J. (2013). What the evidence shows about patient activation: Better health outcomes and care experiences; fewer data on costs. *Health Affairs, 32*(2), 207–214.

IOM. (2003). In K. Adams & J. M. Corrigan Eds (Eds.), *Priority areas for national action: Transforming health care quality*. Washington, DC: The National Academies Press.

Johnston, N., Bodegard, J., Jerström, S., Åkesson, J., Brorsson, H., Alfredsson, J., … Varenhorst, C. (2016). Effects of interactive patient smartphone support app on drug adherence and lifestyle changes in myocardial infarction patients: A randomized study. *American Heart Journal, 178*, 85–94.

Kamaradova, D., Latalova, K., Prasko, J., Kubinek, R., Vrbova, K., Mainerova, B., … Tichackova, A. (2016). Connection between self-stigma, adherence to treatment, and discontinuation of medication. *Patient Preference and Adherence, 10*, 1289–1298.

Korotitsch, W. J., & Nelson-Gray, R. O. (1999). An overview of self-monitoring research in assessment and treatment. *Psychological Assessment, 11*(4), 415–425.

Latham, G. P. (2003). Goal setting: A five-step approach to behavior change. *Organizational Dynamics, 32*, 309–318.

Livingston, J. D., & Boyd, J. E. (2010). Correlates and consequences of internalized stigma for people living with mental illness: A systematic reivew and meta-analysis. *Social Science and Medicine, 70*, 2150–2161.

Locke, E. A., & Latham, G. P. (2002). Building a practically useful theory of goal setting and task motivation: A 35-year odyssey. *American Psychologist, 57*, 705–717.

Macharia, W. M., Leon, G., Rowe, B. H., Stephenson, B. J., & Haynes, R. B. (1992). An overview of interventions to improve compliance with appointment keeping for medical services. *Journal of the American Medical Association, 267*, 1813–1817.

Makoul, G. (2001). Essential elements of communication in medical encounters: The Kalamazoo Consensus Statement. *Academic Medicine, 76*, 390–393.

Manea, L., Gilbody, S., Hewitt, C., North, A., Plummer, F., Richardson, R., … McMillan, D. (2016). Identifying depression with the PHQ-2: A diagnostic meta-analysis. *Journal of Affective Disorders, 203*, 382–395. https://doi.org/10.1016/j.jad.2016.06.003

Mann, T., De Ridder, D., & Fujita, K. (2013). Self-regulation of health behavior: Social psychological approaches to goal setting and goal striving. *Health Psychology, 32*, 487–498.

Martin, L. R., Williams, S. L., Haskard, K. B., & DiMatteo, M. R. (2005). The challenge of patient adherence. *Therapeutics and Clinical Risk Management, 1*(3), 189–199.

Martins, R. K., & McNeil, D. W. (2009). Review of motivational interviewing in promoting health behaviors. *Clinical Psychology Review, 29*, 283–293.

Marvel, M. K., Epstein, R. M., Flowers, K., & Beckman, H. B. (1999). Soliciting the patient's agenda: Have we improved? *Journal of the American Medical Association, 281*(3), 283–287. https://doi.org/10.1001/jama.281.3.283

McDonald, H. P., Garg, A. X., & Haynes, R. B. (2002). Interventions to enhance patient adherence to medication prescriptions: Scientific review. *Journal of the American Medical Association, 288*(22), 2868–2879. https://doi.org/10.1001/jama.288.22.2868

Miller, S. D., Duncan, B. L., Brown, J., Sorrell, R., & Chalk, M. B. (2006). Using formal client feedback to improve retention and outcome: Making ongoing, real-time assessment feasible. *Journal of Brief Therapy, 5*, 5–22.

Mynors-Wallis, L. (2012). *Problem-solving treatment for anxiety and depression: A practical guide*. Oxford, UK: Oxford University Press.

Nezu, A. M., Nezu, C. M., & D'Zurilla, T. J. (2013). *Problem solving therapy: A treatment manual*. New York: Springer.

O'Donohue, W. T., & Levensky, E. R. (Eds.). (2006). *Promoting treatment adherence: A practical handbook for health care providers*. Thousand Oaks, CA: Sage Publications.

Oxman, T. E., Hegel, M. T., Hull, J. G., & Dietrich, A. J. (2008). Problem-solving treatment and coping styles in primary care for minor depression. *Journal of Consulting and Clinical Psychology, 76*, 933–943.

Parsons, M. B., Rollyson, J. H., & Reid, D. H. (2012). Evidence-based staff training: A guide for practitioners. *Behavior Analysis in Practice, 5*, 2–11.

Peterson, E. B., Calhoun, A. W., & Rider, E. A. (2014). The reliability of a modified Kalamazoo consensus statement checklist for assessing the communication skills of multidisciplinary clinicians in the simulated environment. *Patient Education and Counseling, 96*, 411–418.

Puhl, R. M., & Brownell, K. D. (2010). Confronting and coping with weight stigma: An investigation of overweight and obese adults. *Obesity, 14*, 1802–1815.

Puhl, R. M., & Heuer, C. A. (2010). Obesity stigma: Important considerations for public health. *American Journal of Public Health, 100*, 1019–1028.

Rhoades, D. R., McFarland, K. F., Finch, W. H., & Johnson, A. O. (2001). Speaking and interruptions during primary care office visits. *Family Medicine, 33*, 528–532.

Robinson, P. (2005). Adapting empirically supported treatments to the primary care setting: A template for success. In W. T. O'Donohue, M. Byrd, N. A. Cummings, & D. Henderson (Eds.), *Behavioral integrative care: Treatments that work in the primary care setting* (pp. 53–71). New York: Brunner-Routledge.

Rollnick, S., Miller, W. R., & Butler, C. C. (2008). *Motivational interviewing in health care: Helping patients change behavior*. New York: The Guilford Press.

Roter, D. L., & Hall, J. A. (1989). Studies of doctor-patient interaction. *Annual Review of Public Health, 10*, 163–180.

Schaefer, J., Miller, D., Goldstein, M., & Simmons, L. (2009). *Partnering in self-management support: A toolekit for clinicians*. Cambridge, MA: Institute for Healthcare Improvement. Retrieved from www.IHI.org

Strosahl, K., Robinson, P. J., & Gustavsson, T. (2012). *Brief interventions for radical change: Principles & practice of focused acceptance and commitment therapy*. Oakland, CA: New Harbinger.

van Eijken, M., Tsang, S., Wensing, M., de Smet, P. A. G. M., & Grol, R. P. T. M. (2003). Interventions to improve medication compliance in older patients living in the community: A systematic review of the literature. *Drugs & Aging*, *20*, 229–240.

Vannoy, S. D., Mauer, B., Kern, J., Girn, K., Ingoglia, C., Campbell, J., … Unützer, J. (2011). A learning collaborative of CMHCs and CHCs to support integration of behavioral health and deneral medical care. *Psychiatric Services*, *62*, 753–758.

Woltmann, E., Grogan-Kaylor, A., Perron, B., Georges, H., Kilbourne, A. M., & Bauer, M. S. (2012). Comparative effectiveness of collaborative chronic care models for mental health conditions across primary, specialty, and behavioral health care settings: Systematic review and meta-analysis. *American Journal of Psychiatry*, *169*(8), 790–804. https://doi.org/10.1176/appi.ajp.2012.11111616

23 Neurocognitive Disorders

Claudia Drossel and Rachel VanPutten

A Brief Description of Neurocognitive Disorders

Most individuals with difficulties in decision-making, reasoning, attending, remembering, or problem-solving receive healthcare services from primary care physicians. For this reason, primary care is uniquely positioned to lead efforts in the early detection and management of cognitive loss and the prevention or reduction of associated behavioral and emotional changes. As defined by the current diagnostic criteria (American Psychiatric Association, 2013), neurocognitive disorders (NCDs) are a clinical syndrome that entails an observable change in cognition, resulting in either subtle difficulties amenable to compensatory strategies ("mild" NCDs) or significant disruption of activities of daily living ("major" NCDs, formerly called dementia). Of note, to make a diagnosis of NCD, delirium must be ruled out (Inouye, Westendorp, & Saczynski, 2014). A wide range of neurological conditions—among them are Alzheimer's or Lewy body disease, frontotemporal lobar degeneration, vascular diseases, neoplasms, endocrine or immune conditions, trauma, or substance use—may underlie cognitive decline. Frequently multiple etiologies, some of which could be reversible, are involved in one clinical presentation.

While age is a dominant risk factor for progressive neurodegenerative diseases, such as Alzheimer's disease, other risk factors for cognitive decline are exogenous (e.g., history of brain trauma or exposure to neurotoxins), endogenous (e.g., autoimmune or endocrine diseases), and behavioral (e.g., tobacco or other substance use, sedentary behavior). Decreasing prevalence rates of NCDs suggest modifiability of risk through health promotion in midlife (Baumgart et al., 2015).

Early detection of neurodegenerative processes within the scope of primary care services allows the primary care team to initiate proper rule-outs, differential diagnoses, and interventions as indicated. It also gives individuals and families an opportunity to receive information, complete important life tasks, and plan for future care with appropriate support, while the cognitive decline is subtle, and the prospective care recipient still participates in decision-making.

When a major NCD due to a progressive neurodegenerative disease is probable, specialized knowledge and skills related to the management of cognitive decline and its impact on everyday life can prevent the behavioral and emotional changes that constitute the main reasons for institutionalization. However, family members, most commonly wives and daughters, typically assume

C. Drossel (✉) • R. VanPutten
Department of Psychology, Eastern Michigan University, Ypsilanti, MI, USA
e-mail: cdrossel@emich.edu; rarmstr9@emich.edu

A. Maragakis, W.T. O'Donohue (eds.), *Principle-Based Stepped Care and Brief Psychotherapy for Integrated Care Settings*, https://doi.org/10.1007/978-3-319-70539-2_23

care responsibilities without being equipped by providers to understand the gradual loss of complex skill sets that characterize slow decline. Everyday stepwise tasks such as cooking, managing finances, driving, or using electronic devices progressively require more external supports for smooth execution. The individual with NCD may catch him or herself "drawing blanks" while performing tasks that used to seem automatic, go through a period of struggle, and eventually withdraw from the activity. Associated with the decline in the completion of tasks of daily living are perceptual, cognitive, and language alterations that are imperceptible initially and difficult to characterize by laypersons (see Table 23.1 for domains of functioning and examples).

Table 23.1 Domains of functioning

Domain potentially affected by NCD
Perception
Olfaction
Visuospatial skills
Perceptual disturbances, involving multiple aspects of vision (e.g., color, depth, motion) and binaural hearing
Attention
Complex attention (e.g., divided or selective attention)
Sustained attention
Simple attention
Processing speed
Executive functioning
Planning, organizing
Sequencing, yet flexibly switching strategies when appropriate to context
Problem-solving
Initiating and stopping actions appropriate to context
Language
Fluency/word-finding
Categorizing
Reasoning
Verbal and nonverbal memory
Immediate memory (e.g., repeating back a story)
Delayed memory (e.g., repeating that story after 20 min)
Episodic memory (personal history)
Motor skills
Fine (e.g., finger tapping)
Gross (e.g., gait)

Most laypersons focus on memory loss, yet other, marked deficit clusters may distinguish different NCDs (e.g., impulsivity and frontotemporal lobar degeneration, perceptual disturbances and Lewy body disease), and NCDs affect individuals uniquely—depending on personal strengths and weaknesses. For example, a person with uncorrected hearing loss or a poorly managed medical condition may present with steeper declines in functioning than predicted by the neurodegenerative disease alone ("excess disability"; Kahn, 1965). Alternatively, a person who worked as an architect for most of her life may have relatively preserved visuospatial skills, even when a rapid decline in that domain would be predicted by the type of NCD (e.g., Lewy body disease). Lastly, a person who has a history of alcohol use may increase his or her consumption as cognitive skills decline, thereby exacerbating the effects of the neurodegenerative process. Families living with a NCD must learn how the family member is affected, what coping skills he or she brings to the situation, and how psychosocial and medical history intersect with current circumstances to create the person's response to cognitive loss.

The highly personal nature of NCDs creates heterogeneous presentations, and brief assessments are available for use by a behavioral health specialist who can pinpoint idiosyncratic strengths and weaknesses. Based upon a clinical interview and brief assessment measures (see Table 23.2 for examples, and Burns, Lawlor, & Craig, 2004), behavioral health specialists can provide families with information that is directly relevant to the person about whom they care, monitor potential progression of the disease, and prevent excess disability through appropriate and individually tailored interventions.

Screening for Early Detection

Brief assessments of instrumental activities of daily living may detect early difficulties in functioning. These measures rely on accurate proxy reporting to pinpoint changes in the execution of complex everyday behaviors, such as cooking, or financial and medication management. Next, cognitive

Table 23.2 Examples of brief assessment measures

Goal/target/title and reference
Screening
Person with NCD
Montreal Cognitive Assessment (Julayanont & Nasreddine, 2017; Nasreddine et al., 2005)
Detailed assessment
Person with NCD
Cognition
Mattis Dementia Rating Scale-2 (Jurica et al., 2002)
Functional status
Direct Assessment of Functional Status (Loewenstein et al., 1989)
Instrumental Activities of Daily Living Scale (Lawton & Brody, 1969)
Emotion and behavior
Cornell Scale for Depression in Dementia (Alexopoulos, Abrams, Young, & Shamoian, 1988)
Revised Memory and Behavior Problems Checklist (Teri et al., 1992)
Quality of Life in Alzheimer's Disease (Logsdon, Gibbons, McCurry, & Teri, 1999)
Adherence to health promotion and disease prevention (see Chap. 22)
Comorbidities
Charlson Comorbidity Index (via record review) (Charlson, Pompei, Ales, & MacKenzie, 1987)
Care partner knowledge
Short Sense of Competence Questionnaire (Vernooij-Dassen et al., 1999)
Alzheimer's Disease Knowledge Scale (Carpenter, Balsis, Otilingam, Hanson, & Gatz, 2009)
Care partner functional status
Symptom Checklist 90 Revised (Derogatis, 1996)
Center for epidemiological studies depression scale (Radloff, 1977)
Ways of Coping Checklist Revised (Vitaliano, Russo, Carr, Maiuro, & Becker, 1985)
Pittsburgh Sleep Quality Index (Buysse, Reynolds, Monk, Berman, & Kupfer, 1989)
Short Form Health Survey (Ware & Sherbourne, 1992)
Risk and safety concerns
Risk Appraisal Measure (Czaja et al., 2009)

screening instruments are freely available and take approximately 10 min to administer (Larner, 2017). Note that performance below a certain cutoff score does not necessarily suggest the presence of a neurodegenerative disease. Instead, further assessment is indicated to pinpoint why performance did not match the range expected.

Upon completion of screening, the unknown etiology of the problem and the need for further assessment should be stressed to the individual and his or her care partner. For example, sleep disorders, medication effects or polypharmacy, depression, or unmanaged medical conditions and delirium can affect performance on screening instruments. For this reason, the second step in the process may include targeted assessment of sleep, depression, or delirium, medication review by the team pharmacist with a special focus on the regimen's potential impact on cognition, or—if no other factor has been identified—referral to specialty care including cognitive disorder clinics or neurology. A recent review of referrals to a specialty clinic for cognitive disorders (Cannon & Larner, 2016) noted common scoring and reporting errors in primary care, indicating a need for more training of primary care providers.

Detailed Assessment

When decline is progressive, the following domains—also listed in Table 23.2—should be monitored throughout the duration of care. For comprehensive assessment strategies, please refer to Mast (2011).

Cognition

When a major NCD is present and neuropsychological evaluation is not available or accessible, instruments such as the Mattis Dementia Rating Scale 2 (Jurica, Leitten, & Mattis, 2002) take about 20 min to administer and give providers and care partners an overview of strengths and weaknesses across domains. Additionally, the testing process itself contains important information (e.g., how does the person respond to demand, do strong social skills mask cognitive difficulties, does anxiety interfere with testing performance, does the person give up on tasks easily, does the person have insight into performance failures). As testing is not done for diagnostic purposes but to inform intervention, upon the instrument's standard administration, tasks may be modified to determine whether compensatory techniques might lead to successful performance (Boosman, Bovend'Eerdt, Visser-Meily, Nijboer, & van Heugten, 2016). With the examinee's permission, care partners may be present during testing, instructed to be a "fly on the wall," and sitting out of the line of vision (i.e., behind the examinee). For many care partners, observing the person's responses puts them in touch with deficits and functions as a motivational intervention, increasing the likelihood of adhering to recommendations for specific care strategies, including compensatory measures and home safety considerations.

Functional Status

Assessments of adaptive functioning pertaining to both instrumental and basic activities of daily living tend to rely on proxy reports, particularly as individuals with NCDs frequently overstate their abilities. Because caregivers often attribute withdrawal from activities to personality factors rather than skill deficits, they also may not characterize the person's ability correctly, and safety concerns can arise. For this reason, particularly when deficits are in the mild to moderate range, it is useful to ask the person with NCD to demonstrate skills (e.g., "What is your daughter's name," "What time is it," "Can you show me how you would call your care partner using your cell phone," "Could you give me change for a dollar," "Can you show me how to balance this checkbook?") (Ala, Berck, & Popovich, 2005; Loewenstein et al., 1989). The skills selected for demonstration must have been part of the individual's baseline repertoire. Referral for a driving evaluation, also including a road test, is recommended.

Emotion and Behavior

Rather than being an inevitable part of NCDs, emotional and behavioral changes can be understood by examining the psychosocial context in which they occur. They do not come "out of the blue" and can be predicted with individualized assessment across time: Under what circumstances are emotional and behavioral changes most likely? What happens before and after their occurrence? How are others responding to the individual's difficulties? What management strategies have been implemented? Behavior monitoring forms for care partners, focusing on a description of the behavioral problem, its antecedents, and its consequences ("ABC" forms) are easily generated, can be assigned for completion between sessions, and facilitate individualized pattern detection. They are also available in manuals (see "Evidence-Based Stepped Care" section below).

In terms of the emotional sequelae of cognitive decline, withdrawal from activities, worry, and social disengagement are most common. Access to meaningful events tends to decrease as cognitive losses increase; thus, meaningful activity based upon the person's history and preferences always should be assessed.

Health Promotion and Disease Prevention

To optimize cognitive functioning, promote health, and prevent both onset of novel conditions and worsening of existing ones, the following basic care routines should be assessed and, if lacking, implemented: sleep (Cipriani, Lucetti, Danti, & Nuti, 2015); nutrition, hydration, and voiding; regular exercise; and monitoring and correction of sensory loss when indicated (note that a person may lose the ability to hear and need hearing aids, or need less complex glasses) (Bernat et al., 1996). Chronic disease management is detailed below.

Management of Comorbidities and Medication Effects

Even when language is still fluent, individuals with NCDs may have lost their ability to describe or explain their own behavior or physical status. As care partners and healthcare providers primarily rely on self-reports, this loss of self-descriptive repertoire puts individuals with NCDs in precarious situations: About 40% of community-dwelling individuals with NCD may have undetected acute illnesses, poorly managed or undetected chronic diseases (Hodgson, Gitlin, Winter, & Czekanski, 2011), or undiagnosed cancer (Magaki, Yong, Khanlou, Tung, & Vinters, 2014). Care partners' tendency to prioritize and focus on cognitive, behavioral, and emotional changes to the exclusion of other comorbid conditions (e.g., hypertension, diabetes), or leave chronic disease management and medication administration to the person with a NCD, exacerbates already deficient or poorly coordinated care. Thus, any report of uncharacteristic or abrupt behaviors and/or emotions must be understood as a potential signal of pain or discomfort that the person with NCD may not be able to report, requiring a physiological workup (e.g., for urinary tract infection, toothache, etc.) and/or a medication review. In routine clinical practice, it is not unusual to detect severe, albeit unreported, acute medical conditions (e.g., fractures, gastric bleeding), poorly managed or unmanaged chronic conditions (e.g., rheumatoid arthritis, diabetes), or adverse medication effects signaled by behavioral and emotional changes. Because of an already compromised central nervous system and sometimes multiple comorbid conditions, each newly emerging symptom should prompt a medication review by a geriatric pharmacist. Notably, NCDs are a risk factor for delirium, and delirium superimposed on a NCD should also be considered and addressed (Fong, Davis, Growdon, Albuquerque, & Inouye, 2015).

Care Partner Health

Lastly, as individuals with NCD must rely on care partners for even basic tasks of daily living, such as personal care and dressing, for advocacy, and for care coordination, care partner functional status should be assessed (see Table 23.2). Beach et al. (2005) suggest that care partner physical and cognitive decline and depression are the most common correlates of harmful caregiving behavior, for which individuals with NCDs are at increased risk particularly when decline is moderate to severe. In addition to self-report instruments for care partner mood and sleep, brief measures can indicate whether the care partner takes the care recipient's behavior personally and attributes it to intention rather than neurodegenerative disease or whether wishful thinking presents a barrier to effective care (e.g., reluctance to find and utilize appropriate respite services or to solicit and structure assistance from other family members or friends).

Many care partners incur a loss of wages or terminate employment to care for a family member. Because emotional and instrumental stressors of caregiving and sleep deprivation result in adverse mental and physical health consequences, proactive problem-solving is tantamount. Not only care skills but also health behaviors should be monitored: It is not unusual for care partners to neglect their own healthcare, including chronic disease management, while prioritizing the care recipient's.

The results of the detailed assessment should lead to a behavioral treatment plan that is useful to the individual and his or her family. The treatment plan pinpoints clear areas for improvement and scaffolds both care recipient and care partner everyday functioning, including health promotion and disease prevention. A focus on engagement in meaningful activities and related compensatory strategies, including home modifications for safety, should be central to the treatment recommendations.

Evidence-Based Stepped Care/ Brief Psychotherapy

The goal of interventions with the person with NCD and his or her care partner(s) is to preserve repertoires, prevent excess disability, and optimize quality of life. In general, all individuals with NCDs and their families should be referred to community agencies for general support and education (e.g., such as the Alzheimer's Association, the National Stroke Association, the Lewy Body Dementia Association, or the National Parkinson Foundation). Some individuals and families may welcome books or other educational materials (see Patient Resources below). Two types of groups tend to be offered in the community: Emotional support groups are typically relatively unstructured and allow scattered session attendance. They might provide useful sharing experiences. However, care partners should attend community skills groups consisting of a fixed number of sessions with a training sequence, typically provided by hospitals, university-affiliated clinics, or specialized community partners.

The next step for implementation is tailored education, based upon the brief detailed assessment as described above. Generalization of the information the family may already have received by other agencies or through reading is facilitated by supporting the family in applying this basic information to the individual situation.

If necessary, brief interventions are easily deliverable within the primary care settings and implemented by behavioral health specialists in collaboration with nurses, nurse practitioners, or social workers (Callahan et al., 2006; Fortinsky et al., 2014; Guerriero Austrom et al., 2004). These interventions can also be thought of as "stepped care," with the following priorities:

1. *Reinforcing adherence.* As outlined above, basic health promotion and disease prevention and the management of chronic diseases are the foundation of proper care. For example, if a care recipient's diabetes is poorly managed, behavioral health specialists' emphasis on the intersection of physical health with emotion, behavior, and cognition—using examples that the family has provided, such as increased restlessness when blood sugar levels are high or confusion when they are low—will help family members adhere to medical regimens and alert the primary care team to unexpected, uncharacteristic, or abrupt changes in functioning.
2. *Outlining compensatory strategies* specific to cognitive deficits (Buchanan, Christenson, Houlihan, & Ostrom, 2011). Most care partners do not know how to conduct task analyses to pinpoint where performances break down, and thus they fail to provide prompts allowing for semi-independent task performance (e.g., gluing a red dot on the microwave start button permits the person with NCD to reheat coffee). Mihailidis and colleagues (Mihailidis, Boger, Craig, & Hoey, 2008) provide an example of an automated prompting system, designed to further increase independence from care partners. Through insufficient or excessive prompting, by correcting a person with NCD who may not retain the accurate information, or by relying on unanswerable "W" questions (where, when, why, what) for conversation, care partners may inadvertently quench attempts to ask for help or engage in social interaction. For this reason, communication strategies are among the compensatory techniques.
3. *Promoting engagement in meaningful activity*, considering the person's abilities, history, and preferences. Preserving dignity and respect and generating continuity with life roles are tantamount when programming activities. Notably, the myth that individuals with NCDs "regress to their childhood" often leads to infantilization (Salari, 2006), including activity planning that is inappropriate for adults. For example, a 70-year-old adult with NCD who has a history with cars (repairing them, watching NASCAR races, collecting specialty vehicles) may appreciate greeting people as a volunteer in a car museum or spending time there. Alternatively, she may enjoy organizing ratchets in a toolbox. It would be inappropriate to provide this

individual with children's toy cars or children's coloring books with cars.

4. *Addressing emotional and behavioral changes nonpharmacologically* as first-line interventions. As pointed out earlier, behavior can be understood in its context (assessing antecedents and consequences), even when cognitive decline is severe. Systematic assessment of behavior and its context leads to psychosocial interventions that are individually tailored. For example, refusal (e.g., to attend appointments, participate in activities, or allow respite) is common, but saying "no" to requests may be a function of very different contextual variables: (1) Comprehension may be lacking, such that "get ready to go to Mary's house" may be too vague of a suggestion. "Please put on your coat" might be a sufficient first step to make a request clear and effective. (2) Refusal may provide access to preferred events (e.g., spending time with family and not at the day center) or avoid aversive events (e.g., infantilization at the day center). (3) Refusal may result in the avoidance of situations that are too complex or overwhelming (e.g., social gatherings with multiple people in one conversation rather than one-on-one interactions). Note that interventions would be different in each example. While none would involve medications as a solution, many would require close collaboration with family members and some with staff (e.g., at day centers). Please see Fisher, Drossel, Yury, and Cherup (2007) for a brief introduction to systematic, contextual problem-solving and McCurry and Drossel (2011) for a step-by-step manual. Additionally, intervention manuals for Project REACH (Burgio et al., 2009) are available online and include contextual problem-solving components ("REACH II: Resources for Enhancing Alzheimer's Caregiver Health II").
5. *Planning and implementing respite*, building a social support network, if possible involving other family members in some of the care tasks (e.g., advocacy, interaction with agencies, medical visits).
6. *Assessing and intervening on care partner barriers* to implementing (1–5). Barriers may include limited resources (e.g., finances, time, access, etc.), a lack of knowledge and/or skill deficits, and preexisting psychological problems, such as depression, anxiety, or substance use.

What Does Not Work

A wait-and-see stance. Primary care providers may not initiate the management of NCD because of a lack of training in geriatrics (Khanassov, Vedel, & Pluye, 2014). At the same time, many families indicate they will "cross the bridge when they get to it," indicating that if cognitive decline is subtle, they will avoid education and training and sometimes diagnostic procedures. When such avoidance is present, it should become the focus of intervention—either at the team or at the patient level. If reluctance to adopt the care role continues, barriers should be reassessed and alternative options for care explored, to avoid the risk of neglect.

An exclusive focus on care partner well-being. Health professionals often provide care partners of individuals with NCDs with the needed recommendations for self-care and stress management to promote sustainable routines but fail to address skill deficits. Skill deficits on the care partner side may include ineffective task or time management, absence of routines (e.g., bedtime and waking), unproductive attempts at helping that lead to premature dependence, lacking interpersonal skills for soliciting social support, or lack of distress tolerance skills. Care partner knowledge and skill should be assessed first to determine whether the amelioration of these skill deficits may contribute to decreased stress.

Relying on medications for NCD. In general, because of an already compromised nervous system, advanced age, a frequent need for multiple medications to manage comorbidities such as diabetes and hypertension, and complex drug interactions, approaches to medications should be conservative (for a list of inappropriate medications for older adults, see Campanelli, 2012). Many progressive neurodegenerative diseases, such as Alzheimer's or Lewy body, have no cure, and there currently are no medications that stop disease progression. Disease-slowing medications have frequent systemic adverse effects (American Geriatrics Society (AGS) Choosing Wisely Workgroup, 2014). Finally, to emphasize, nonpharmacological interventions are first-line interventions for behavioral and emotional difficulties. When psychotropic medications are used, the person with NCD should be closely monitored for adverse events (Goldberg & Ernst, 2012), such as sedation and worsening of confusion but also restlessness and increased risk of falls. If a person with NCD must be hospitalized, physical restraint should be avoided (AGS Choosing Wisely Workgroup, 2014).

When to Refer to Specialty Treatment

Because of the complexity and heterogeneity of NCDs, the involvement of specialty services is recommended (e.g., neurologist, neuropsychologist, geriatrician, geriatric pharmacist). If a social worker is not part of the care team, referral to social work agencies may be indicated to locate resources, including respite care, to implement home-based interventions, or to address financial constraints secondary to caregiving. Unless individuals receive routine care in a geriatric primary care setting—itself a specialty context—the involvement of specialty care for the person with NCD tends to be sporadic and brief, and care coordination rests upon the care partner with the primary care team's support.

A referral to geropsychology with specialization in NCD is indicated when significant barriers to proper care have been detected and when interventions are longitudinal and extensive, e.g., with implementation in community setting, such as day centers.

Referral to specialized mental health treatment also should be initiated when the care partner has a preexisting condition that is poorly managed or has not been addressed or when care partner difficulties exceed the resources of primary care. Indeed, the person with NCD might have emotionally and instrumentally supported an adult child with severe psychological difficulties who now is struggling to provide care or who hesitates to access available resources because of stigma or other barriers. In this case, immediate referral of that care partner to mental health specialty providers is indicated.

The Role of the PCP and the Team

The primary care team has a unique opportunity to initiate early diagnosis and deliver education and management techniques that can contribute to increased quality of life of individuals with NCDs and their families, prevention or postponement of institutionalization, as well as decreased morbidity, mortality, and healthcare costs. As pointed out above, the primary care team coordinates specialty care and monitors progress of overall treatment. The behavioral health specialist may advocate for the care partner and the person with NCD within the team and communicate with specialty care providers: Particularly if adults are older, they may not receive an opportunity to voice their concerns to providers, and the behavioral health specialist's role may be to arrange effective interactions (e.g., providing information in writing to the specialty provider prior to the visit, making lists of concerns, role-playing). As individuals with NCDs rely upon care partners for assistance with activities of daily living, including adherence to the medical regimen and acute as well as chronic disease management (Sloane et al., 2017), an essential role of the primary care team is to support the care partner, considering him or her a service provider within the extended care team.

Assessing Impact

Because of the heterogeneity of adults with NCDs, outcome measures specifically designed for NCDs in primary care are not available. However, considering both quality improvement efforts in neurology which focus on NCDs regardless of age (Odenheimer et al., 2013), and efforts to improve the primary care of vulnerable adults age 65 and older (Sloss et al., 2000; Wenger, Roth, Shekelle, & the ACOVE Investigators, 2007), among whom individuals with NCDs are a subset, the following outcome measures can be suggested (percentage of patients):

1. Documentation of baseline assessment of cognitive ability and functional status
   (a) Annual evaluations for changes
2. Identification of individuals with cognitive complaints
   (a) Proper rule-out and diagnoses
3. If a NCD is present,
   (a) Behavioral activation/meaningful activities to prevent depression
   (b) Ongoing monitoring of emotional and behavioral changes
   (c) Basic caregiver education and general skills training
      i. Health promotion: Sleep; nutrition, hydration, and voiding; regular exercise; and monitoring and correction of sensory loss
      ii. Adherence to treatment regimens for comorbid conditions
      iii. Addressing safety concerns, including substance use, wandering, falls, driving, and firearms
   (d) Advanced caregiver skills training: Access to first-line nonpharmacological interventions for emotional and behavioral changes
   (e) Regular medication reviews
   (f) Advance care planning
   (g) Referral to palliative care
   (h) Monitoring of hospitalizations, with special attention to those involving restraint (American Geriatrics Society (AGS) Choosing Wisely Workgroup, 2014)
   (i) Assessing risk of abuse, exploitation, or neglect (Lachs & Pillemer, 2015)

Healthcare utilization and associated healthcare costs of individuals with NCD are disproportionately high compared to those of age and gender-matched peers and to those with similar chronic illnesses (Alzheimer's Association, 2017): Individuals with NCDs have an increased risk of hospitalization, a higher number of hospital admissions, and longer stays. A proportion of hospitalizations and institutionalizations could be prevented if effective primary care services were rendered (Parmar et al., 2014).

Patient Resources

Alzheimer's Disease Education and Referral (ADEAR) Center. (2010). *Home safety for people with Alzheimer's disease* (NIH Publication No. 02-5179). Retrieved July 17, 2017, from https://www.nia.nih.gov/sites/default/files/home_safety_for_people_with_alzheimers_disease.pdf

Bell, V., & Troxel, D. (2012). *A dignified life, revised and expanded: The best friends™ approach to Alzheimer's care: A guide for care partners*. Deerfield Beach, FL: Health Professions Press.

McCurry, S. (2006). *When a family member has dementia: Steps to becoming a resilient caregiver*. Westport, CT: Praeger.

References

Ala, T. A., Berck, L. G., & Popovich, A. M. (2005). Knowledge of personal information and caregiver awareness in Alzheimer's disease. *American Journal of Alzheimer's Disease and Other Dementias, 20*(2), 119–125.

Alexopoulos, G. A., Abrams, R. C., Young, R. C., & Shamoian, C. A. (1988). Cornell scale for depression in dementia. *Biological Psychiatry, 23*, 271–284. https://doi.org/10.1016/0006-3223(88)90038-8

Alzheimer's Association. (2017). 2017 Alzheimer's disease facts and figures. *Alzheimer's & Dementia, 13*(4), 325–373. https://doi.org/10.1016/j.jalz.2017.02.001

American Geriatrics Society (AGS) Choosing Wisely Workgroup. (2014). American Geriatrics Society identifies another five things that healthcare providers and patients should question. *Journal of the American Geriatrics Society, 62*(5), 950–960. https://doi.org/10.1111/jgs.12770

American Psychiatric Association. (2013). *Diagnostic and statistical manual of mental disorders: DSM-5* (5th ed.). Washington, DC: Author.

Baumgart, M., Snyder, H. M., Carrillo, M. C., Fazio, S., Kim, H., & Johns, H. (2015). Summary of the evidence on modifiable risk factors for cognitive decline and dementia: A population-based perspective. *Alzheimer's & Dementia, 11*(6), 718–726. https://doi.org/10.1016/j.jalz.2015.05.016

Beach, S. R., Schulz, R., Williamson, G., Miller, L. S., Weiner, M. F., & Lance, C. E. (2005). Risk factors for potentially harmful informal caregiver behavior. *Journal of the American Geriatrics Society, 53*(2), 255–261. https://doi.org/10.1111/j.1532-5415.2005.53111.x

Bernat, J. L., Beresford, H. R., Celesia, G. G., Cranford, R. E., McQuillen, M. P., Pellegrino, T. R., … Wichman, A. (1996). Ethical issues in the management of the demented patient: The American Academy of Neurology Ethics and Humanities Subcommittee. *Neurology, 46*(4), 1180–1183. https://doi.org/10.1212/WNL.46.4.1180

Boosman, H., Bovend'Eerdt, T. J. H., Visser-Meily, J. M. A., Nijboer, T. C. W., & van Heugten, C. M. (2016). Dynamic testing of learning potential in adults with cognitive impairments: A systematic review of methodology and predictive value. *Journal of Neuropsychology, 10*(2), 186–210. https://doi.org/10.1111/jnp.12063

Buchanan, J. A., Christenson, A., Houlihan, D., & Ostrom, C. (2011). The role of behavior analysis in the rehabilitation of persons with dementia. *Behavior Therapy, 42*(1), 9–21. https://doi.org/10.1016/j.beth.2010.01.003

Burgio, L. D., Collins, I. B., Schmid, B., Wharton, T., McCallum, D., & DeCoster, J. (2009). Translating the REACH caregiver intervention for use by area agency on aging personnel: The REACH OUT program. *The Gerontologist, 49*(1), 103–116. https://doi.org/10.1093/geront/gnp012

Burns, A., Lawlor, B., & Craig, S. (2004). *Assessment scales in old age psychiatry* (2nd ed.). London, UK: CRC Press.

Buysse, D. J., Reynolds, C. F., Monk, T. H., Berman, S. R., & Kupfer, D. J. (1989). The Pittsburgh sleep quality index: A new instrument for psychiatric practice and research. *Psychiatry Research, 28*(2), 193–213. https://doi.org/10.1016/0165-1781(89)90047-4

Callahan, C. M., Boustani, M. A., Unverzagt, F. W., Austrom, M. G., Damush, T. M., Perkins, A. J., … Hendrie, H. C. (2006). Effectiveness of collaborative care for older adults with Alzheimer disease in primary care: A randomized controlled trial. *JAMA, 295*(18), 2148–2157. https://doi.org/10.1001/jama.295.18.2148

Campanelli, C. M. (2012). American Geriatrics Society updated beers criteria for potentially inappropriate medication use in older adults. *Journal of the American Geriatrics Society, 60*(4), 616–631. https://doi.org/10.1111/j.1532-5415.2012.03923.x

Cannon, P., & Larner, A. J. (2016). Errors in the scoring and reporting of cognitive screening instruments administered in primary care. *Neurodegenerative Disease Management, 6*(4), 271–276. https://doi.org/10.2217/nmt-2016-0004

Carpenter, B. D., Balsis, S., Otilingam, P. G., Hanson, P. K., & Gatz, M. (2009). The Alzheimer's disease knowledge scale: Development and psychometric properties. *The Gerontologist, 49*(2), 236–247. https://doi.org/10.1093/geront/gnp023

Charlson, M. E., Pompei, P., Ales, K. L., & MacKenzie, C. R. (1987). A new method of classifying prognostic comorbidity in longitudinal studies: Development and validation. *Journal of Chronic Diseases, 40*(5), 373–383. https://doi.org/10.1016/0021-9681(87)90171-8

Cipriani, G., Lucetti, C., Danti, S., & Nuti, A. (2015). Sleep disturbances and dementia. *Psychogeriatrics, 15*, 65–74. https://doi.org/10.1111/psyg.12069

Czaja, S. J., Gitlin, L. N., Schulz, R., Zhang, S., Burgio, L. D., Stevens, A. B., … Gallagher-Thompson, D. (2009). Development of the risk appraisal measure (RAM): A brief screen to identify risk areas and guide interventions for dementia caregivers. *Journal of the American Geriatrics Society, 57*(6), 1064–1072. https://doi.org/10.1111/j.1532-5415.2009.02260.x

Derogatis, L. R. (1996). *SCL-90-R: Symptom Checklist-90-R: Administration, scoring, and procedures manual*. Minneapolis, MN: NCS Pearson.

Fisher, J. E., Drossel, C., Yury, C., & Cherup, S. (2007). A contextual model of restraint-free care for persons with dementia. In P. Sturmey (Ed.), *Functional analysis in clinical treatment* (pp. 211–237). Burlington, MA: Academic Press/Elsevier.

Fong, T. G., Davis, D., Growdon, M. E., Albuquerque, A., & Inouye, S. K. (2015). The interface between delirium and dementia in elderly adults. *Lancet Neurology, 14*, 823–832. https://doi.org/10.1016/S1474-4422(15)00101-5

Fortinsky, R. H., Delaney, C., Harel, O., Pasquale, K., Schjavland, E., Lynch, J., … Crumb, S. (2014). Results and lessons learned from a nurse practitioner-guided dementia care intervention for primary care patients and their family caregivers. *Research in Gerontological Nursing, 7*(3), 126–137. https://doi.org/10.3928/19404921-20140113-01

Goldberg, J. F., & Ernst, C. L. (2012). *Managing the side-effects of psychotropic medications*. Arlington, VA: American Psychiatric Association.

Guerriero Austrom, M., Damush, T. M., West Hartwell, C., Perkins, T., Unverzagt, F., Boustani, M., … Callahan, C. M. (2004). Development and implementation of nonpharmacologic protocols for the management of patients with Alzheimer's disease and their families in a multiracial primary care setting. *The Gerontologist, 44*(4), 548–553. https://doi.org/10.1093/geront/44.4.548

Hodgson, N., Gitlin, L. N., Winter, L., & Czekanski, K. (2011). Undiagnosed illness and neuropsychiatric behaviors in community-residing older adults with dementia. *Alzheimer Disease and Associated Disorders, 25*(2), 109–115. https://doi.org/10.1097/WAD.0b013e3181f8520a

Inouye, S. K., Westendorp, R. G., & Saczynski, J. S. (2014). Delirium in elderly people. *Lancet, 383*, 911–922. https://doi.org/10.1016/S0140-6736(13)60688-1

Julayanont, P., & Nasreddine, Z. S. (2017). Montreal Cognitive Assessment (MoCA): Concept and clinical review. In A. J. Larner (Ed.), *Cognitive screening instruments: A practical approach* (2nd ed., pp. 139–195). Cham, CH: Springer International Publishing.

Jurica, P. J., Leitten, C. L., & Mattis, S. (2002). *Dementia Rating Scale-2 (DRS-2) professional manual*. Odessa, FL: Psychological Assessment Resources.

Kahn, R. S. (1965). *Comments*. Retrieved from Philadelphia

Khanassov, V., Vedel, I., & Pluye, P. (2014). Case management for dementia in primary health care: A systematic mixed studies review based on the diffusion of innovation model. *Clinical Interventions in Aging, 9*, 915–928. https://doi.org/10.2147/CIA.S64723

Lachs, M. S., & Pillemer, K. A. (2015). Elder abuse. *New England Journal of Medicine, 373*(20), 1947–1956. https://doi.org/10.1056/NEJMra1404688

Larner, A. J. (Ed.). (2017). *Cognitive screening instruments: A practical approach* (2nd ed.). Cham, CH: Springer International Publishing.

Lawton, M. P., & Brody, E. M. (1969). Assessment of older people: Self-maintaining and instrumental activities of daily living. *The Gerontologist, 9*(3_Part_1), 179–186. https://doi.org/10.1093/geront/9.3_Part_1.179

Loewenstein, D. A., Amigo, E., Duara, R., Guterman, A., Hurwitz, D., Berkowitz, N., … Eisdorfer, C. (1989). A new scale for the assessment of functional status in Alzheimer's disease and related disorders. *Journal of Gerontology, 44*(4), P114–P121.

Logsdon, R. G., Gibbons, L. E., McCurry, S. M., & Teri, L. (1999). Quality of life in Alzheimer's disease: Patient and caregiver reports. *Journal of Mental Health and Aging, 5*(1), 21–32.

Magaki, S., Yong, W. H., Khanlou, N., Tung, S., & Vinters, H. V. (2014). Comorbidity in dementia: Update of an ongoing autopsy study. *Journal of the American Geriatrics Society, 62*(9), 1722–1728. https://doi.org/10.1111/jgs.12977

Mast, B. T. (2011). *Whole person dementia assessment*. Baltimore, MD: Health Professions Press.

McCurry, S., & Drossel, C. (2011). *Treating dementia in context: A step-by-step guide to working with individuals and families*. Washington, DC: American Psychological Association.

Mihailidis, A., Boger, J. N., Craig, T., & Hoey, J. (2008). The COACH prompting system to assist older adults with dementia through handwashing: An efficacy study. *BMC Geriatrics, 8*(1), 28. https://doi.org/10.1186/1471-2318-8-28

Nasreddine, Z. S., Phillips, N. A., Bédirian, V., Charbonneau, S., Whitehead, V., Collin, I., … Chertkow, H. (2005). The Montreal Cognitive Assessment, MoCA: A brief screening tool for mild cognitive impairment. *Journal of the American Geriatrics Society, 53*(4), 695–699. https://doi.org/10.1111/j.1532-5415.2005.53221.x

Odenheimer, G., Borson, S., Sanders, A. E., Swain-Eng, R. J., Kyomen, H. H., Tierney, S., … Johnson, J. (2013). Quality improvement in neurology: Dementia management quality measures. *Neurology, 81*(17), 1545–1549. https://doi.org/10.1212/WNL.0b013e3182a956bf

Parmar, J., Dobbs, B., McKay, R., Kirwan, C., Cooper, T., Marin, A., & Gupta, N. (2014). Diagnosis and management of dementia in primary care: Exploratory study. *Candian Family Physician, 60*(5), 457–465.

Radloff, L. (1977). The CES-D Scale: A self-report depression scale for research in the general population. Applied Psychological Measurement, 1, 385–401. doi:10.1177/014662167700100306

REACH II: Resources for Enhancing Alzheimer's Caregiver Health. Retrieved from http://www.edc.gsph.pitt.edu/reach2/public/manuals.html

Salari, S. M. (2006). Infantilization as elder mistreatment: Evidence from five adult day centers. *Journal of Elder Abuse & Neglect, 17*(4), 53–91. https://doi.org/10.1300/J084v17n04_04

Sloane, P. D., Schifeling, C. H., Beeber, A. S., Ward, K. T., Reed, D., Gwyther, L. P., … Zimmerman, S. (2017). New or worsening symptoms and signs in cmmunity-dwelling persons with dementia: Incidence and relation to use of acute medical services. *Journal of the American Geriatrics Society, 65*(4), 808–814. https://doi.org/10.1111/jgs.14672

Sloss, E. M., Solomon, D. H., Shekelle, P. G., Young, R. T., Saliba, D., MacLean, C. H., … Wenger, N. S. (2000). Selecting target conditions for quality of care improvement in vulnerable older adults. *Journal of the American Geriatrics Society, 48*(4), 363–369. https://doi.org/10.1111/j.1532-5415.2000.tb04691.x

Teri, L., Truax, P., Logsdon, R., Uomoto, J., Zarit, S., & Vitaliano, P. P. (1992). Assessment of behavioral problems in dementia: The revised memory and behavior problems checklist. *Psychology and Aging, 7*(4), 622–631. https://doi.org/10.1037/0882-7974.7.4.622

Vernooij-Dassen, M. J. F. J., Felling, A. J. A., Brummelkamp, E., Dauzenberg, M. G. H., van den Bos, G. A. M., & Grol, R. (1999). Assessment of caregiver competence in dealing with the burden of caregiving for a dementia patient: A short sense of competence questionnaire (SSCQ) suitable for clinical practice. *Journal of the American Geriatrics Society, 47*(2), 256–257. https://doi.org/10.1111/j.1532-5415.1999.tb04588.x

Vitaliano, P. P., Russo, J., Carr, J. E., Maiuro, R. D., & Becker, J. (1985). The ways of coping checklist: Revision and psychometric properties. *Multivariate Behavioral Research, 20*(1), 3–26. https://doi.org/10.1207/s15327906mbr2001_1

Ware, J. E., & Sherbourne, C. D. (1992). The MOS 36-item short-form health survey (SF-36): I. Conceptual framework and item selection. *Medical Care, 30*(6), 473–483.

Wenger, N. S., Roth, C. P., Shekelle, P., & the ACOVE Investigators. (2007). Introduction to the assessing care of vulnerable elders-3 quality indicator measurement set. *Journal of the American Geriatrics Society, 55*, S247–S252. https://doi.org/10.1111/j.1532-5415.2007.01328.x

24 Obesity

Sarah M. Lindeman and Alexandros Maragakis

The rise in obesity rates seen over the course of the last three decades has received significant attention from healthcare professionals and government officials (Centers for Disease Control and Prevention (CDC), 2015a). Results from the National Health and Nutrition Examination Survey have shown a rise in adult prevalence rates from approximately 23% in the 1988–1994 survey to an estimated 34% in the 2005–2006 survey (CDC, 2015a). In addition, 10–15% of children meet the criteria for obesity (Mitchell, Catenacci, Wyatt, & Hill, 2011). These staggering rates are accompanied by increased risk of developing a wide range of diseases and health problems, such as cardiovascular disease, diabetes, cancer, sleep apnea (pauses in, or shallow, breathing while sleeping), and reproductive issues (CDC, 2015b; National Heart, Lung, and Blood Institute (NHLBI), 2012). Due to these health complications, healthcare costs for obese patients are approximately $1,429 per year more than nonobese patients (CDC, 2015b). As prevalence rates for obesity remain alarmingly high, the need for healthcare providers to understand effective treatment options for this disease continues to grow. Fortunately, a large body of research regarding this topic provides substantial information to inform the treatment of patients with obesity.

Effective Ways to Screen in the Primary Care Setting

Patients whose body weight exceeds a healthy range for their height meet the criteria for being either overweight or obese (CDC, 2012). Body mass index (BMI) is an affordable, commonly used method for screening that uses the ratio between a person's weight (kilograms) and their height (meters) to calculate a BMI score ($BMI = kg/h^2$). Scores ranging from 18.5 to 24.9 are considered to be within a normal range, while scores from 25.0 to 29.9 are overweight, and scores at or above 30 are considered to be obese (CDC, 2012). While the use of BMI scores are convenient and affordable, it is important to note that this method of screening is not intended for diagnostic purposes as it does not take body composition into consideration. Rather, this score is correlated with more costly and/or time-consuming measures that assess adiposity more directly, such as bioelectrical impedance, underwater weighing, skinfold measurements, and

S.M. Lindeman, M.S.
Department of Psychology and Counseling, University of Central Arkansas, Conway, AR, USA
e-mail: sarah-lindeman@hotmail.com

A. Maragakis, Ph.D. (✉)
Eastern Michigan University, Ypsilanti, MI, USA
e-mail: amaragak@emich.edu

A. Maragakis, W.T. O'Donohue (eds.), *Principle-Based Stepped Care and Brief Psychotherapy for Integrated Care Settings*, https://doi.org/10.1007/978-3-319-70539-2_24

dual-energy x-ray absorptiometry (CDC, 2012). For patients whose BMI falls within a potentially unhealthy range, skinfold measurements are the most affordable option for confirmation of a high body fat percentage.

How to Further Assess If a Screen Returns Positive

Due to the increased risk of developing other chronic diseases, upon receipt of a positive screen for obesity, clinicians should consider the use of additional screens to ensure the earliest detection of other illnesses, such as cardiovascular disease and diabetes (CDC, 2015b; National Heart, Lung, and Blood Institute (NHLBI), 2012). In such cases, early detection is essential for the prevention of further damage to the body. For example, when undetected, high levels of blood sugar caused by diabetes can lead to damage of the blood vessels and organs, alongside a range of other health complications, making the early detection of the disease imperative (National Health Service, 2014). As such, the detection of obesity alone is not sufficient for patients who are obese. Instead, the detection of obesity indicates the need to assess for the presence of those diseases which obese patients are at increased risk of developing.

Stepped Care and Evidence-Based, Brief Interventions

The treatment of obesity is accomplished via a reduction in body fat and is achieved through weight loss, a process whereby individuals expend more energy than they consume, thus achieving a caloric deficit that leads to a breakdown of body fat for energy expenditure (CDC, 2015c). Fortunately, even a modest weight loss (5–10% of body fat) can improve blood sugar levels, reduce cholesterol, and lower blood pressure (CDC, 2015c). The lifestyle changes required to lose weight are (1) decrease caloric intake (dietary change), (2) increase caloric expenditure (physical activity), or ideally, (3) both. Wellness checks provide an opportune time to detect and begin the treatment process for obesity, but providing directions regarding the aforementioned three options for losing weight are often insufficient to produce change. A range of environmental barriers provide challenges for patients attempting to alter their lifestyle, including large restaurant portion sizes, sedentary employment, easy access to processed food, and exposure to unhealthy food advertisements (American Heart Association, 2016). Fortunately, research regarding the treatment of obesity has provided support for interventions that can be used to enhance the effectiveness of physician advice. For example, the use of a behavioral intervention for long-term maintenance of weight loss has been shown to be more effective than nutritional education alone (Gormally & Rardin, 1981). The following subsections introduce evidence-based principles that healthcare professionals can apply during treatment to improve outcomes for patients.

Stepped Care

Due to the high prevalence rates of obesity worldwide (Mitchell et al., 2011), the need for affordable treatment is of utmost importance to minimize healthcare costs and prevent excessive burdens on healthcare professionals. As such, a stepped-care approach is an ideal strategy for the treatment of obesity. In this approach, treatment begins with the least invasive, lowest-cost treatment option. If weight loss is attained via this approach, an increase in intervention intensity is unnecessary. Increasing the intensity is only required for those patients who do not respond to their current treatment step. Each subsequent step follows the same guidelines, whereby the next step is not taken if the patient is responsive to the currently implemented step (Carels et al., 2012). Levels of invasiveness for the treatment of obesity range from self-help or educational interventions to bariatric surgery (Carels et al., 2009; Gormally & Rardin, 1981; Marek, Heinberg, Lavery, Merrell Rish, & Ashton, 2016).

As healthcare systems move toward stepped-care programs, research regarding their effectiveness emerges in support of this approach, such as a stepped-care approach whereby obese patients who did not respond to a self-help intervention were stepped up to a weekly group intervention. After being stepped up, comparisons between those who responded to self-help and thereby remained in the self-help step and the stepped-up group intervention placements showed equivalent weight loss outcomes (Carels et al., 2009). These results indicate that a stepped approach has the potential to save resources by identifying and appropriately increasing treatment for those who do not achieve weight loss via a self-help program rather than assigning all patients to more intensive treatments. Such resource savings were achieved by Jakicic and colleagues (2012) when comparisons were made between the effectiveness of standard behavioral and stepped-care weight loss interventions. While the mean weight loss of the standard behavioral group was higher, implementing a stepped approach beginning with self-help reduced treatment costs while producing clinically significant weight loss.

Implementing a stepped-care approach has the potential to save resources; however, this approach is not guaranteed to produce positive results for all patients. While some may experience benefits from this approach, others may not achieve weight loss even after being stepped up (Carels et al., 2012). As such, it is important that clinicians remain up to date regarding evidence-based practices and referral appropriateness for healthcare settings to ensure that practices are being refined as research arises to improve the stepped-care process. The following subsections describe brief, evidence-based interventions for improving patient weight loss outcomes.

Online Interventions

The topic of obesity has led to the creation of multiple commercial and open-source online programs that have been shown to be effective at helping individuals with weight loss. These programs, like the commercial product Weight Watchers (https://www.weightwatchers.com) or the open-source program Livestrong.com (www.livestrong.com), provide users with information and tools that focus on multiple components of weight loss. For example, the website Livestrong.com provides users with information about nutrition (i.e., various recipes for different meals and dietary restrictions), exercise (i.e., various types of workouts and what muscle groups they target), and access to various articles about topics such as ways to increase healthy eating and exercise and potential pitfalls when losing weight. Furthermore, there are functions like the "tracker" that allows a user to input their weight, height, and desired weight loss goal that will create a target goal for daily caloric intake. From there, users can track their food intake and workouts online and track their progress. For those who have easy access to the internet, these programs provide a very cheap (i.e., free to a few dollars a day) and accessible way to obtain effective treatment at losing weight.

Group-Based Psychoeducation

Psychoeducation around basic nutritional intake and weight loss/calorie goals has been shown to be an effective way in helping patient's loss weight. For example, a five-session psychoeducation program that covered the basic nutritional information (e.g., recommended fruit/vegetable intake) and allowed for patients to ask questions in areas that they required further elaboration resulted in significant weight loss in comparison to treatment as usual. Furthermore, this psychoeducational approach produced similar outcomes to individual sessions that used motivational interviewing techniques (Barnes, White, Martino, & Grilo, 2014).

Motivational Interviewing

Motivational interviewing (MI) involves a positive, collaborative engagement with patients that promotes intrinsic motivation to change. Rather than educating and urging clients to alter their unhealthy behaviors, the developers of MI explain that patients are often already aware of a need for change and are struggling with ambivalent feelings regarding the next steps to take. When clinicians discuss the need to make a change, patients will often present reasons not to change, producing a scenario that is not ideal for achieving behavior change as the client is verbalizing the option the clinician does not want them to choose. Miller and Rollnick (2013) present motivational interviewing as a means to facilitate change via increasing a client's own change talk. The authors note that many well-intentioned professionals advise patients to make changes that are advantageous for the client; however, the act of giving advice is often not welcomed by clients and may not lead to positive change. Instead, patients are more likely to listen to their own reasons for making a change, making the facilitation of patient change talk an ideal method for successful intervention (Miller & Rollnick, 2013).

MI has the advantage in that primary care providers (PCPs) can be easily trained in its use. Also, training PCPs in MI provides a significant advantage in integrated care settings in regard to effectiveness and efficiency. First, the use of MI by the PCP would not take significantly more time than the normal time allotted for the appointment. Second, using MI would make the appointment more likely to create behavior change. Third, it would create another step in the stepped-care process, before having to refer to the behavioral health provider (BHP). However, given organizational limitations, training PCPs in MI may not be a viable option. Given this, it is recommended that all BCPs have experience in engaging in MI.

The use of brief MI interventions in a healthcare setting has been gathering significant empirical support. A meta-analysis of MI adaptations found support for the use of such interventions for improving diet and exercise (Burke, Arkowitz, & Menchola, 2003). Research has shown increased engagement in walking and reductions in cholesterol for overweight patients that were maintained at an 18-month follow-up (Hardcastle, Taylor, Bailey, Harley, & Haggar, 2013). Such changes have been found across a range of age groups, including meta-analytic support for changes in health behaviors of children (Gayes & Steele, 2014). Wong and Cheng (2013), for example, found that an MI intervention resulted in increased physical activity and improvements in caloric intake for children. Research examining the effectiveness of a telephone-based MI intervention for older adults found that posttreatment exercise levels and self-efficacy increased; however, a 6-month follow-up found that only increased self-efficacy was maintained. The researchers noted that this follow-up was conducted during the winter season, when barriers to exercise for the elderly may be higher than usual, indicating the need for addressing potential barriers to behavior change during the intervention process (Lilienthal, Pignol, Holm, & Vogeltanz-Holm, 2014).

In a study examining a stepped-care approach to treating obesity, participants assigned to a behavioral weight loss program enhanced with motivational interviewing lost more weight and engaged in more exercise than those who were assigned to a behavioral weight loss program alone (Carels et al., 2007). Indeed, MI is an ideal option for clinicians to consider implementing in stepped-care programs. For more information regarding the use of MI in healthcare settings, Rollnick, Miller, and Butler's (2008) *Motivational Interviewing in Healthcare: Helping Patients Change Behavior* provides further insight regarding its effective use.

Effective Goal Setting and Implementation

Developing goals provides an opportunity for increasing patient motivation, tracking progress, and increasing the likelihood of successful behavior change. However, ineffective goal setting has the potential to discourage patients and may lead to decreased motivation and self-efficacy. As such, evidence-based, behavioral principles should be used to ensure the goal setting process is completed in a manner that will enhance, rather than detract from, the treatment process. The use of realistic goal setting, shaping, monitoring, and an effective reward system will provide patients with a plan for behavior change that will maximize motivation and adherence rates (National Heart, Lung, and Blood Institute (NHLBI), n.d.). This subsection will briefly overview the use of said principles in the goal setting process.

First, emphasis should be placed on setting realistic goals. The use of reinforcement, monitoring, and other methods of improving adherence to goals cannot succeed if said goal is not achievable. To set achievable, positively oriented goals, healthcare providers should take a collaborative approach to goal identification with a focus on what behaviors should be performed rather than what behaviors should be avoided (NHLBI, n.d.). For example, telling patients not to eat sugary foods places emphasis on restrictions and does not offer information regarding what to do instead of consuming sugary foods. Instead, focusing on what patients should eat and what to do instead of eating sugary foods when experiencing a craving (e.g., chew gum, do something that will distract them from the craving, etc.) will lead to the creation of positively oriented goals that provide direction regarding the behaviors in which clients should engage.

In addition, creating achievable goals involves selecting appropriate goals for each patient. Setting a goal of running 3 miles, 5 days per week is not realistic for a patient currently living a sedentary lifestyle; therefore, prior to implementing a reward system, consideration of realistic goals should be made to increase the likelihood of meeting said goals (NHLBI, n.d.; Roberts, 2004). In the case of the aforementioned patient, while a clinician may intend for the patient to reach a fitness level that would allow them to run 3 miles, the initial goal could be more realistically set at walking 5 or 10 minutes, 4 days a week. Upon mastery of this level of activity, the shaping process can take place as the behavioral care provider works with the patient to increase engagement in health-promoting behaviors.

The shaping process is a behavioral intervention that involves reinforcing a smaller, more basic beginning point, followed by reinforcing subsequent increases in complexity or effort until the desired outcome is achieved (NHLBI, n.d.). For weight loss, the shaping process can be used to improve both diet and engagement in physical activity. An example of this would be the collaborative creation of a weekly meal plan that begins with a few, simple changes (e.g., using mustard instead of mayonnaise and trading one soda per day for a glass of water) and the selection of a reward for adhering to the plan. Over the course of a few weeks, each plan can be become progressively healthier such that no week led to a drastic change in eating habits. In time, the shaping process will lead to the desired outcome, a healthy lifestyle, in a manner that is less overwhelming and more likely to lead to a successful outcome (NHLBI, n.d.; CDC, 2015a, 2015b, 2015c, 2015d).

During the shaping process, the successful use of principles of reinforcement and/or punishment will greatly improve patient outcomes. Simply put, reinforcers lead to an increase in the reinforced behavior, while punishers lead to decreases in the punished behavior. Therefore, the use of reinforcers to increase engagement in health behavior as well as the use of punishers to decrease poor adherence to goals will lead to more desirable outcomes. Research supports the use of a rewards system as a more effective means to achieve weight loss (NHLBI, n.d.; Mahoney, Moura, & Wade, 1973). It is important to note that what works as an effective reinforcer or punisher for some may not be an effective strategy for others. Consideration of what rewards and negative outcomes will be effective for use may take time to identify for some patients. Verbal praise may be highly reinforcing for some patients and ineffective for others; therefore, collaborative creation of a rewards system is ideal. For example, client A may want to watch a movie in theaters and could use this as a reinforcer for following their weekly plan, but client B may not enjoy movies and would be better reinforced by a reward such as spending time with a friend or buying a new article of clothing. Another client may choose to use a punisher, such as giving a friend an envelope of money that will be donated to a cause that goes against the patient's values if the patient continues to engage in poor health habits. The collaborative approach to creating a reward system will ensure that patients feel involved in the process and that the rewards set in place are ideal for the individual.

Treatment outcomes can also be enhanced through self-monitoring (NHLBI, n.d.; Burke, Wang, & Sevick, 2012) Self-monitoring provides a means for patients to track their progress, see improvements, and provides clinicians with valuable information regarding goal adherence. The detection of patterns on logs can assist in the detection of environmental triggers and other barriers to healthy living that can then be addressed in treatment. To illustrate this point, if a clinician were to see a patient log with a sugary snack listed each day around 4 p.m., this information could stimulate a conversation regarding a stressful coworker that arrives each day around 4 p.m. In this particular case, teaching the client stress management techniques could assist in preventing the consumption of late afternoon sugary snacks. Self-monitoring provides insight about adherence as well as allowing clients to track their progress visually.

Because indirect factors may contribute to weight loss success, clinicians should also explore additional barriers to behavior change. Addressing sleep hygiene as well as effective stress management lead to improved outcomes for patients due to improving decision-making (AHA, 2016). Sleep loss is associated with increased self-reported hunger after a single night (Schmid, Hallschmid, Jauch-Chara, Born, & Schultes, 2008). For patients who are already trying to reduce caloric intake, increased hunger due to poor sleep leads to additional barriers to success. In addition, learning methods to reduce stress leads to improvements in goal compliance as higher levels of stress are associated with greater impulsivity (ADA, 2013). Undoubtedly, treatment of obesity requires a multifaceted approach that addresses the wide range of barriers to weight loss success.

What Doesn't Work

While rapid weight loss may be desirable to those seeking their ideal body weight, research indicates that rapid weight loss is often regained, whereas a slow, steady pace of weight reduction (1–2 pounds weekly) is more likely to lead to long-term maintenance of weight loss (CDC, 2015c). A survey of popular dieting strategies indicated that some popular diets may be hazardous to patient's health and lead to a relapse in weight loss after approximately 3–5 years (Miller, 1999). As such, highly restrictive diets and drastic lifestyle changes are shown to be far less effective than a slow shaping process. Rather, steady improvements that teach maintainable habits to incorporate into one's lifestyle which can be realistically maintained leads to improved long-term outcomes (CDC, 2015c). This may be due to learning healthy, realistic eating and exercising habits, an important aspect of long-term behavior change that is not present in drastic weight loss regimens, where a return to previous habits after weight loss is achieved will lead to a regaining of the lost weight.

Shifts from a sedentary or otherwise unhealthy lifestyle often involve the discontinuation of certain activities detrimental to patients' health. However, phrasing goals in a manner that emphasizes what behaviors patients should stop engaging in rather than what behaviors patients should engage in does not promote effective behavior change (NHLBI, n.d.; Charlton, Sobel, & Sobel, 2016). This approach is ineffective for several reasons. One such reason is that goals stating "I will not…" fail to involve engagement in a behavior and instead focus on a non-behavior, something they will not do. In addition, the goal is focused on the negative behavior rather than the desired behavior, thus placing emphasis on what has been done wrong previously rather than what can be done now. Recommendations regarding what should be avoided also fail to provide realistic options for replacing the undesirable behaviors. As such, goal setting should involve framing goals in a way that emphasizes the desirable, health behaviors rather than undesirable behaviors.

When to Refer to External Specialty Care

A stepped-care approach to the treatment of obesity ensures that clients receive the least invasive treatment possible to achieve a reduction in body fat. For those who do not respond to the treatment options available (see Stepped Care section for details), specialty referrals should be considered. To make appropriate referrals, healthcare providers should be aware of causes of obesity that are more appropriately treated in specialty care. In addition, knowledge regarding which specialty care providers are ideal based on the patient's needs is essential for appropriate referrals. While a bariatric specialist, a healthcare professional with specialized training in obesity, may be the forerunner for a specialty referral, if patient weight gain is an indirect result of a mental health issue that would be more appropriately treated in a mental health setting, a referral to a mental health provider is ideal (American Psychological Association, 2016). However, if lack of responsiveness to treatment is due to other factors, such as an inactive thyroid, the gland responsible for controlling metabolic functioning in the body, referral to a mental health professional would not provide the treatment modality necessary for achieving weight loss (Mullur, Liu, & Brent, 2014). As such, healthcare providers should be aware of not only when referrals are necessary but also which specialty providers are best suited to provide treatment for the patient.

The Role of the Primary Care Provider and Staff

Within the healthcare system, each professional interacting with the patient has the potential to play a positive role in the treatment process. Training in the basic principles used for motivational interviewing can equip healthcare professionals with the skills needed to respond to clients in a manner that promotes positive change during each step of their treatment process (Miller & Rollnick, 2013). Primary care physicians (PCPs) and nurses play multiple important roles when treating obesity. The medical team serves as the initial point of contact with the healthcare setting and usually assesses and tracks measures such as weight and blood test results (e.g., cholesterol and triglycerides). They are also the first point of contact where patients receive education about healthy living and diet and identify patients that could further be assisted by behavioral health interventions. Finally, the medical team determines if further referral to specialists beyond the primary care setting is needed to address issues a patient may be experiencing.

Outcome Assessment and Quality Improvement

Tracking treatment outcomes for obesity is multifaceted due to the array of health benefits associated with reductions in excess body fat; therefore, tracking outcomes can be best achieved through tracking multiple factors. Blood pressure and blood sugar, for example, have been found to improve over time as patients achieve even moderate weight loss (CDC, 2015c). Because a single outcome measure, such as BMI score, fails to capture the full array of health improvements available for patients with obesity, the addition of other measures is more likely to capture a complete picture of health improvements and further emphasizes the importance of the associated risk factors rather than body size (Miller, 1999). Presently, the use of multiple outcome measures (e.g., physical activity levels, cholesterol, blood pressure, weight, dietary changes, etc.) for research related to weight loss is common (Burke et al., 2003; Hardcastle et al., 2013). In addition to using outcome measures to track the changes made by individual patients, tracking patient progress and organizing outcomes in an easily accessible manner allows clinicians to use patient outcomes to inform and improve treatment for future clients (Bobbit, Cate, Beardslet, Azocar, & McCulloch, 2012). Such data can be submitted for publication, thereby assisting other professionals in their endeavor to provide the most effective treatment available. The use of patient outcomes to inform treatment and improve the treatment of future patients will ensure the highest quality treatment available is discovered and disseminated for use in all hospital settings. While the treatment of obesity may be a multifaceted process, a range of options are available to assist patients as they work toward living a healthier lifestyle.

References

American Diabetes Association. (2013). *Managing stress and diabetes*. Retrieved from http://www.diabetes.org/living-with-diabetes/parents-and-kids/everyday-life/managing-stress-and-diabetes.html

American Heart Association. (2016). *Understanding the American obesity epidemic*. Retrieved from http://www.heart.org/HEARTORG/HealthyLiving/WeightManagement/Obesity/Understanding-the-American-Obesity-Epidemic_UCM_461650_Article.jsp#. V1SsIZErK00

American Psychological Association. (2016). *Mind/body health: Obesity*. Retrieved from http://www.apa.org/helpcenter/obesity.aspx

Barnes, R. D., White, M. A., Martino, S., & Grilo, C. M. (2014). A randomized controlled trial comparing scalable weight loss treatments in primary care. *Obesity, 22*, 2508–2516.

Bobbit, B. L., Cate, R. A., Beardslet, S. D., Azocar, F., & McCulloch, J. (2012). Quality improvement and outcomes in the future of professional psychology: Opportunities and challenges. *Professional Psychology: Research and Practice, 43*(6), 551–559. https://doi.org/10.1037/a0028899

Burke, B. L., Arkowitz, H., & Menchola, M. (2003). The efficacy of motivational interviewing: A meta-analysis of controlled clinical trials. *Journal of Consulting and Clinical Psychology, 71*(5), 843–861. https://doi.org/10.1037/0022-006X.71.5.843

Burke, L.E., Wang, J., & Sevick, M.A. (2012). Self-monitoring in weight loss: A systematic review of the literature. *Journal of the Academy of Nutrition and Dietetics,111*(1), 92-102. doi: https://doi.org/10.1016/j.jada.2010.10.008

Carels, R. A., Wott, C. B., Young, K. M., Gumble, A., Darby, L. A., Oehlhof, M. W., … Koball, A. (2009). Successful weight loss with self-help: a stepped-care approach. *Journal of Behavioral Medicine, 32*(6), 503–509. https://doi.org/10.1007/s10865-009-9221-8

Carels, R. A., Young, K. M., Hinman, N., Gumble, A., Koball, A., Oehlhof, M. W., & Darby, L. (2012). Stepped-care in obesity treatment: matching treatment intensity to participant performance. *Eating Behaviors, 13*(2), 112–118. https://doi.org/10.1016/j.eatbeh.2012.01.002

Centers for Disease Control and Prevention. (2012). *Defining adult overweight and obesity*. Retrieved from http://www.cdc.gov/obesity/adult/defining.html

Centers for Disease Control and Prevention. (2015a). *Prevalence of overweight, obesity and extreme obesity among adults: United States, trends 1960-62 through 2005-2006*. Retrieved from http://www.cdc.gov/nchs/data/hestat/overweight/overweight_adult.htm

Centers for Disease Control and Prevention. (2015b). *Obesity facts*. Retrieved from http://www.cdc.gov/obesity/data/adult.html

Centers for Disease Control and Prevention. (2015c). *Losing weight*. Retrieved from http://www.cdc.gov/healthyweight/losing_weight/

Centers for Disease Control and Prevention. (2015d). *Losing weight: Getting started*. Retrieved from http://www.cdc.gov/healthyweight/losing_weight/getting_started.html

Charlton, S., Sobel, K., & Sobel, S. (2016). *Psychology: The science of who we are* (Vol. 1, 2nd ed.). Southlake, TX: Fountain Head Press.

Gayes, L. A., & Steele, R. G. (2014). A meta-analysis of motivational interviewing interventions for pediatric health behavior change. *Journal of Consulting and Clinical Psychology, 82*(3), 521–535. https://doi.org/10.1037/a0035917

Gormally, J., & Rardin, D. (1981). Weight loss and maintenance and changes in diet and exercise for behavioral counseling and nutrition education. *Journal of Counseling Psychology, 28*(4), 295–304. https://doi.org/10.1037/0022-0167.28.4.295

Hardcastle, S. J., Taylor, A. H., Bailey, M. P., Harley, R. A., & Haggar, M. S. (2013). Effectiveness of a motivational interviewing intervention on weight loss, physical activity and cardiovascular disease risk factors: A randomised controlled trial with a 12-month post-intervention follow-up. *The International Journal of Behavioral Nutrition and Physical Activity, 10*, 40. https://doi.org/10.1186/1479-5868-10-40

Jakicic, J. M., Tate, D. F., Lang, W., Davis, K. K., Polzien, K., Rickman, A. D., ... Finkelstein, E. A. (2012). Effect of a stepped-care intervention approach on weight loss in adults: A randomized clinical trial. *JAMA: Journal Of The American Medical Association, 307*(24), 2617–2626. doi:10.1001/jama.2012.6866

Lilienthal, K. R., Pignol, A. E., Holm, J. E., & Vogeltanz-Holm, N. (2014). Telephone-based motivational interviewing to promote physical activity and stage of change progression in older adults. *Journal of Aging and Physical Activity, 22*(4), 527–535. https://doi.org/10.1123/JAPA.2013-0056

Mahoney, M. J., Moura, N. G., & Wade, T. C. (1973). Relative efficacy of self-reward, self-punishment, and self-monitoring techniques for weight loss. *Journal of Consulting And Clinical Psychology, 40*(3), 404–407. https://doi.org/10.1037/h0034565

Marek, R. J., Heinberg, L. J., Lavery, M., Merrell Rish, J., & Ashton, K. (2016). A review of psychological assessment instruments for use in bariatric surgery evaluations. *Psychological Assessment, 28*(9), 1142–1157. https://doi.org/10.1037/pas0000286

Miller, W. C. (1999). How effective are traditional dietary and exercise interventions for weight loss? *Medicine and Science in Sports and Exercise, 31*(8), 1129–1134. Retrieved from http://www.ncbi.nlm.nih.gov/pubmed/10449014

Miller, W. R., & Rollnick, S. (2013). *Motivational interviewing: Helping people change*. New York: The Guilford Press.

Mitchell, N., Catenacci, V., Wyatt, H. R., & Hill, J. O. (2011). Obesity: Overview of an epidemic. *Psychiatric Clinics of North America, 33*(4), 717–732. https://doi.org/10.1016/j.psc.2011.08.005

Mullur, R., Liu, Y., & Brent, G. A. (2014). Thyroid hormone regulation of metabolism. *Physiological Reviews, 94*(2), 355–382. https://doi.org/10.1152/physrev.00030.2013

National Heart, Lung, and Blood Institute. (2012). *What are the health risks of overweight and obesity?* Retrieved from https://www.nhlbi.nih.gov/health/health-topics/topics/obe/risks

National Heart, Lung, and Blood Institute. (n.d.). *Guide to behavior change*. Retrieved from http://www.nhlbi.nih.gov/health/educational/lose_wt/behavior.htm

National Health Service. (2014). *Type 2 diabetes-Complications*. Retrieved from http://www.nhs.uk/Conditions/Diabetes-type2/Pages/Complications.aspx

Roberts, S. S. (2004). Defining success. Realistic goals are key to staying motivated about weight loss. *Diabetes Forecast, 57*(4), 52.

Rollnick, S., Miller, W. R., & Butler, C. C. (2008). *Motivational interviewing in healthcare: Helping patients change behavior*. New York: The Guilford Press.

Schmid, S. M., Hallschmid, M., Jauch-Chara, K., Born, J., & Schultes, B. (2008). A single night of sleep deprivation increases ghrelin levels and feelings of hunger in normal-weight healthy men. *Journal of Sleep Research, 17*(3), 331–334. https://doi.org/10.1111/j.1365-2869.2008.00662.x

Wong, E. Y., & Cheng, M. H. (2013). Effects of motivational interviewing to promote weight loss in obese children. *Journal of Clinical Nursing, 22*(17-18), 2519–2530. https://doi.org/10.1111/jocn.12098

25 Obsessive-Compulsive Disorder

M. Todd Sewell, Nicholas D. Wignall, and Bradford C. Richards

General Caution

Obsessive-compulsive disorder (OCD) is a serious mental illness and frequently leads to psychiatric disability. In addition, individuals struggling with OCD often have other comorbid anxiety-related disorders (Camuri et al., 2014). The treatment of OCD requires experienced mental health professionals with extensive training. There is no empirical evidence that the successful treatment of OCD has ever occurred within integrated health-care settings that typically restrict the number of sessions and session time with patients. One potentially poor outcome of trying to treat OCD within these limitations is that a compromised treatment occurs with marginal symptom reduction that effectively inoculates patients from an empirically supported treatment in the future when relapse occurs. Anecdotally, as a clinician, it is worrisome that this would leave patients discouraged about the treatment and less likely to engage in therapy in the future, especially in more severe presentations in which treatment adherence is less likely to begin with (Mancebo, Pinto, Rasmussen, & Eisen, 2008). One of the primary reasons that briefer treatments of OCD is contraindicated is that OCD is maintained by covert surreptitious safety cognitions that can continue to persist and evolve for years, often requiring years of treatment to extinguish (Jakubovski et al., 2013). It is strongly recommended that integrated health-care settings refer patients with OCD to an experienced mental health professional for treatment.

Definition/Description

OCD is characterized by intrusive and distress-provoking thoughts that are unreasonable and excessive. In addition to obsessive thoughts, mental or behavioral compulsions like counting, handwashing, and repeated checking behaviors are primary symptoms of OCD. Compulsions can appear related or unrelated to the obsessions and are usually performed with the intent of neutralizing the anxiety created by the obsessive thought pattern. Individuals with this disorder may not be able to discern whether their obsessive thoughts are reasonable or unreasonable. The obsessions and compulsions are often time consuming, have a negative impact on daily functioning, and cause a great deal of distress as the anxiety caused by the obsessions and the time devoted to performing compulsive acts can be significant (American Psychiatric Association, 2013).

M.T. Sewell, Ph.D. (✉) • N.D. Wignall, Ph.D.
B.C. Richards, Ph.D., A.B.P.P.
Cognitive Behavioral Institute of Albuquerque, Albuquerque, NM, USA
e-mail: ts@cogtherapy.com; nw@cogtherapy.com; br@cogtherapy.com

A. Maragakis, W.T. O'Donohue (eds.), *Principle-Based Stepped Care and Brief Psychotherapy for Integrated Care Settings*, https://doi.org/10.1007/978-3-319-70539-2_25

OCD is a common mental health disorder. It is estimated that the prevalence rate of OCD is between 3 and 5% of the population (Fineberg et al., 2013). Because the symptoms of OCD can be significant and potentially limit an individual's ability to perform activities of daily living, the economic impact of this disorder is significant. Many individuals who suffer from OCD also struggle with depression and other anxiety-related disorders. Research has also shown that less than half of individuals who struggle with OCD symptoms seek treatment for OCD (Veldhuis et al., 2012).

There are very few robust theories about the causes of OCD. Behavioral theories based on empirically tested and supported treatments suggest that fear is paired with obsessional topics in a classical conditioning process and then relief of these experiences is negatively reinforced through an operantly conditioned process of performing rituals to relieve distress (Dollard & Miller, 1950). Through repetition and reinforcement, the strength of the compulsions is strengthened. Other research has suggested OCD has similar familial rates to that of other anxiety-based disorders, and genetic factors may play a role in the transmission of OCD. One study compiling concordance rates for monozygotic twin research suggests these concordance rates are around 50% (Browne, Gair, Scharf, & Grice, 2014), suggesting a strong biological pathway for the development of OCD. Neurological causes of OCD have also been explored using neuroimaging and suggest individuals with OCD show significantly high activity within the frontal cortex as well as subcortical structures (Nakao, Okada, & Kanba, 2014). In addition, impairments in the caudate nucleus have been proposed as possible causes for OCD. The impairment inhibits the downregulation of output to the thalamus resulting in overactivity, and consequently, worry is not regulated adequately for individuals with OCD (Baxter et al., 1992). This theory has found support in more recent studies suggesting the caudate nucleus plays an important role in the dysregulation of mental processes (Hansen, Hasselbalch, Law, & Bolwig, 2002).

Because OCD does share some similarities with other disorders, such as generalized anxiety disorder and specific phobia disorder, in which abnormal or distressing thoughts are common symptoms, it is important to note the differences between OCD and other disorders. Assessment or screening within an integrated health-care setting would require someone with some basic training in screening and diagnosing mental health disorders to recognize the unique presentation of OCD and ensure a timely response to the patient's needs. The repetitive and perseverative behaviors of OCD are discriminating features of this disorder and distinguish it from other anxiety-related disorders. Even though the obsessions and accompanying compulsions can be unusual or irrational, their repetitive and perseverative behaviors distinguish them from other delusional disorders. OCD does not share symptoms present in other psychotic disorders like auditory or visual hallucinations. The presence of obsessions and compulsions differentiates OCD from a delusional disorder. The object of the anxiety is not specific to certain stimuli, responded to with strong avoidance or extreme focus on weight or food intake as is the case with specific phobia and eating disorders (APA, 2013).

Presentation in Medical Care Settings

Individuals who present to an integrated health-care setting with OCD may report concerns about anxiety or stress and may discuss their difficulty meeting the demands of their day-to-day routines due to obsessions and/or compulsions. Patients with OCD may have difficulty seeing medical professionals, going to medical settings, and taking medications due in part to fears or concerns about contamination or germs; they may also present to medical settings with possible skin problems that may be the result of excessive handwashing or cleaning rituals (APA, 2013). Complaints about lack of sleep, checking practices that are excessive and time consuming, washing rituals to address germs or contamination that lead to open sores or blisters, and difficulty completing tasks due to mental rituals like counting or word repetition may be reported to medical professionals to explain a current state of anxiety. The rituals will often be disconnected or unrelated to the worry or obsession; this incongruence should be a sign to include a behavioral specialist within an integrated care setting in the assessment of the patient. They may also complain about hygiene issues and/or be referred by individuals who have grown concerned for their physical and mental health. One study suggests that cardiologists and dermatologists were the health-care providers most commonly seen by patients with OCD (Kennedy & Schwab, 1997). Unlike other anxiety disorders in which gastrointestinal complaints are common, one study suggests that there is no evidence to suggest that patients with OCD will present with these issues (Kuiper, Batelaan, van Oppen, Hendriks, & van Balkom, 2013). Patients with OCD may seek medication to relieve the intense distress they experience as their obsessions and compulsions negatively impact their lives.

Screening and Assessment

In addition to the medical and health-related concerns mentioned in the previous section, providers can screen patients informally for OCD symptoms by noting and attending to their patients' verbal reports of anxiety that appears to be coupled with obsessive thoughts that are associated with or cause the individual to experience distress. In addition, it is important to screen patients who present with distress caused by extreme behavioral rituals they feel compelled to perform, take a significant amount of time, or impact the patient's ability to function normally. For example, a patient who presents with anxiety/worry related to fears of contracting a disease from public bathrooms, who states they drive home from work to use the bathroom, and has contracted urinary tract infections as a result of not relieving themselves displays obsessive thoughts and extreme behavioral compulsions indicative of OCD. Or an individual who reports significant anxiety and washes their hands for an excessive amount of time when they do use a public bathroom would warrant a screening for OCD. This patient exhibits significant anxiety and obsessional thoughts; their behavior impacts their job functioning, as well as compulsive handwashing that is excessive, and should be assessed further for OCD symptoms. Obsessive thought patterns and/or compulsive behavioral rituals are key indicators that should trigger a screening for OCD. Patient reports of anxiety or worry should trigger a screen for anxiety-related disorders.

How to Further Assess If a Screen Is Positive

The assessment of OCD within an integrated care setting is a vital part of ensuring patient needs that are identified quickly so that treatment and symptom relief can begin. The following assessments are either self-report or brief in nature and may lend themselves well to an integrated care setting.

The Yale-Brown Obsessive Compulsive Scale (Y-BOCS) (Goodman et al., 1989a, 1989b) is a clinician-administered, semi-structured interview, measuring the presence of 40 obsessions and 29 compulsions. It also includes a scale to measure the severity of symptoms. Items are rated on a 4-point scale (0–4; 0 = none, 4 = extreme), yielding two subscale scores (obsessions, compulsions) and a total score ranging from 0 to 40 (25 or more is moderately severe, 30 or more is considered severe, 35 is very severe) (Goodman et al., 1989a, 1989b).

Another quality self-report measure is the Florida Obsessive-Compulsive Inventory (FOCI) (Storch et al., 2007). This measure screens for the symptoms of OCD and provides a measure of symptom severity on endorsed items. The symptom scale is based on ten obsessions and ten compulsions taken from the Y-BOCS (Goodman et al., 1989a, 1989b). For an integrated care setting, this measure may be simpler to implement. The range for the symptom checklist is 0–20 with higher scores indicating a greater number of symptoms. Once a symptom is endorsed, individuals are directed to rate the severity of the symptom. The severity scale range is 0–25. Higher scores denote greater severity of the symptoms. The properties of the FOCI have been empirically tested in two studies (Aldea, Rahman, & Storch, 2009; Storch et al., 2007). Both studies suggest that the FOCI is an adequate OCD symptom screening device and provides clinicians with important data about the severity of endorsed symptoms. The severity of symptoms would be important in an integrated care setting as more severe cases would warrant a more significant intervention plan.

An additional self-report screening that has shown positive psychometric performance is the Obsessive Compulsive Inventory-Revised (Foa et al., 2002). This is an 18-item measure that assesses the distress experienced from obsession and compulsions. The items are ranked on a 4-point scale from "not at all" to "extremely." Higher scores indicate higher symptom severity. In addition to the total distress score, this measure provides subscales for neutralizing, checking, obsessing, hoarding, washing, and ordering (Foa et al., 2002).

Evidenced-Based Stepped Treatment Options

First-Line Treatments

This section will discuss various treatment modalities and techniques in the treatment of OCD, as well as formats for their delivery such as individual and group. We focus on cognitive behavioral therapy (CBT) as it has the most empirical support but also review second-line and adjunctive options such as bibliotherapy, e-health/teletherapy, and psychodynamic therapy.

CBT utilizing psychoeducation about the nature of OCD and exposure with response prevention (ERP) is widely considered the gold standard and first-line treatment for OCD as it has been shown to be effective (Abramowitz, 1997; Ougrin, 2011) and either equivalent or superior to pharmacotherapy (Belotto-Silva et al., 2012; Foa et al., 2005; Roshanaei-Moghaddam et al., 2011). A standard technique in most forms of CBT, ERP is based in behavioral theory and teaches the patient to expose themselves to intense manifestations of the feared/obsessive stimuli while simultaneously abstaining from any form of compulsive behavior, self-soothing, or avoidance, i.e., "safety behaviors." In the context of OCD, this typically takes the form of inducing a patient's feared obsessions via imaginal or in vivo exposure. For example, such an induction could consist of thinking about the possibility of catching a feared disease and what the outcomes might be, or deliberately touching a contaminated object for a period of time. Once the obsessional pattern has been provoked, the patient is prevented from engaging in their preferred ritual or compulsion as a means of lowering their anxiety. With repeated trials, patients learn (A) that their anxiety and discomfort will habituate and diminish on its own, independent of any action on their part, (B) the feared outcome that they anticipated will not come to pass despite having taken no action to prevent it, and (C) the feared outcome may come to pass, and the patient learns he/she can manage the risk. Because the obsessions are no longer negatively reinforced via the anxiety relief of the rituals or compulsions, they begin to diminish in both frequency and intensity via the operant extinction process.

CBT utilizing ERP is advantageous in several respects. First, it has a long history of documented effectiveness as mentioned above, with documented durable therapeutic effects up to 5 years posttreatment (McKay et al., 2015; Whittal, Robichaud, Thordarson, & McLean, 2008). Second, the hierarchical design of graded exposure means that, although the technique itself is challenging for patients, it can be administered gradually so as not to overwhelm the patient initially. Third, evidence suggests that many of the skills learned as a part of this approach are generalizable and may increase effectiveness of treatment for comorbid conditions such as depression (Abramowitz, Franklin, Street, Kozak, & Foa, 2000). Fourth, there is some evidence that this approach can be administered in diverse therapeutic settings with comparable effectiveness, including group (Jónsson, Hougaard, & Bennedsen,

2011), telephone (Lovell et al., 2006), and online (Andersson et al., 2012).

While highly effective, CBT utilizing ERP often requires significant investments of time, energy, and financial resources which some patients may not be willing or able to commit to. Minimum treatment duration, for example, is often in the range of 10–12 weeks, while the content of sessions with ERP is by definition challenging as it involves deliberate and repeated exposure to feared stimuli. Interestingly, while sometimes thought to produce higher dropout rates due to the challenging nature of the intervention, a recent meta-analysis suggested that ERP has dropout rates similar to other approaches for OCD (Ong, Clyde, Bluett, Levin, & Twohig, 2016).

Pharmacotherapy for OCD is also considered a first-line treatment and has been shown to be effective using specific FDA-approved selective serotonin reuptake inhibitors (SSRIs), including fluoxetine (Bergeron et al., 2002), fluvoxamine (Ackerman & Greenland, 2002), paroxetine (Hollander et al., 2003), and sertraline (Ninan et al., 2006). Escitalopram and citalopram, however, have not been FDA approved for the treatment of OCD. Additionally, CBT (using ERP) combined with pharmacotherapy is also considered first-line for OCD and has been demonstrated superior to medication alone (Foa, Franklin, & Moser, 2002; Simpson et al., 2004) but not CBT alone (van Oppen, van Balkom, de Haan, & van Dyck, 2005).

Second-Line Treatments

Various forms of CBT that do not emphasize behavioral techniques are often considered second-line psychological treatments. Cognitive therapy (CT) which emphasizes the identification and modification of maladaptive thoughts and beliefs has been shown to be effective in OCD (Ougrin, 2011; Rosa-Alcázar, Sánchez-Meca, Gómez-Conesa, & Marín-Martínez, 2008) and can be particularly helpful for manifestations of OCD where in vivo exposure is not feasible for some reasons (e.g., contamination with dangerous substances) (Krochmalik, Jones, Menzies, & Kirkby, 2004). Additionally, modular CT (Wilhelm et al., 2009) and CT aimed at obsessional doubt have been shown effective (O'Connor et al., 2005). Some limited data also suggests possible effectiveness for metacognitive therapy (Moritz, Jelinek, Hauschildt, & Naber, 2010; van der Heiden, van Rossen, Dekker, Damstra, & Deen, 2016), acceptance, and commitment therapy (ACT) (Twohig et al., 2010).

Motivational interviewing (MI) is a potential adjunctive treatment option for OCD. MI is designed to allow the patient an opportunity to explore their ambivalence about their disorder, as well as the costs and benefits for seeking treatment or not seeking treatment. Often this process aids patients in building motivation to make changes (Prochaska & DiClemente, 1982). As such, MI may be useful in either initially encouraging patients to begin treatment or to persist in their treatment despite challenges. The time-intensive nature of ERP may prohibit integrated care settings from implementing the treatment of OCD. Often the number of sessions allotted to patients in integrated health-care settings is limited, and the time constraints of those sessions would not be conducive to many protocols of ERP. Those sessions may be used to implement MI in order to move the client closer to a decision to seek or fully participate in a gold standard treatment like ERP or address a lack of commitment in medication and other treatment adherence issues.

Finally, while research suggests that therapist-assisted exposure is more effective than self-exposure (Rosa-Alcázar et al., 2008), there is some evidence to suggest that bibliotherapy can be an effective strategy for improving OCD symptoms compared to no treatment (Moritz et al., 2010; Moritz & Jelinek, 2011).

While clomipramine has a significant evidence base to support its effectiveness in treating OCD (Bisserbe, Lane, & Flament, 1997), it is generally considered second-line due to its increased side effect profile that includes primarily anticholinergic effects such as dry mouth, hypotension, sedation, and weight gain and safety concerns such as cardiac arrhythmias, seizures, and heightened overdose potential compared to SSRIs (Katzman et al., 2014).

Not Recommended

There is little support for the use of psychodynamic or stress management therapies in the treatment of OCD (Ponniah, Iliana, & Hollon, 2013). The following pharmacotherapies have not demonstrated effectiveness and are therefore not recommended in the treatment of OCD: clonazepam (Hollander, Kaplan, & Stahl, 2003), clonidine (Hewlett, Vinogradov, & Agras, 1992), desipramine (Hoehn-Saric et al., 2000), bupropion (Vulink, Denys, & Westenberg, 2005), and naltrexone (Amiaz, Fostick, Gershon, & Zohar, 2008). Additionally, adjunctive use of clonazepam (Crockett, Churchill, & Davidson, 2004), buspirone (Jenike, Baer, & Buttolph, 1991), or lithium (McDougle, Price, Goodman, Charney, & Heninger, 1991) is not recommended due to a lack of empirically supported evidence.

When and Why to Refer to Specialist

Treating OCD can be extremely challenging. The disorder's primary symptoms are excessive anxiety and compulsions that are functionally impairing. These presentations and the compulsions patients engage in can be extremely upsetting and stress inducing for the therapist as well. In accordance with APA guidelines, only individuals who have had adequate training or have adequate supervision should treat patients with OCD. Because exposure and response prevention is considered the frontline treatment for OCD (Öst, Havnen, Hansen, & Kvale, 2015) patients with OCD should be referred to mental health professionals who are trained to treat this disorder.

Even if there are mental health professionals on an integrated health-care treatment team trained to treat OCD, other limitations may warrant a referral to a specialist for therapy. Many integrated health-care settings have limitations for the number of sessions and session times offered to a patient, for example, five sessions at 20–30 min per session. Studies have shown that the amelioration of OCD symptoms is correlated to the number of sessions provided (Fisher & Wells, 2005). The dose-response nature of treatment is an important issue to assess within an integrated health-care setting as a treatment team considers the appropriate setting for clinical treatment. If an integrated health-care setting places limits on the number of sessions available for patients or if session times are limited in a way in which therapeutic treatment cannot be delivered, then a referral to a specialist is warranted. In sum, any integrated health-care setting that attempts to treat moderate to severe OCD should have adequately trained behavioral health professionals and the needed resources of adequate sessions and time for each session. It is strongly recommended that patients within an integrated health-care setting with OCD be referred to mental health professionals who have extensive training in empirically supported treatments.

Role of Primary Care Provider/Medical Team

The role of a primary care provider (PCP) and treatment teams who treat individuals with OCD can be extremely important and beneficial. The PCP can manage and prescribe important medical interventions as a supported first-line treatment or as a combined treatment with CBT for individuals who need an increased level of treatment. The PCP can also play a crucial role working with possible behavioral therapy providers to coordinate general care or to address specific symptoms. PCPs can remind patients about the benefits of treatment adherence and help manage medication needs reported by the patient and behavioral health providers.

Behavioral treatment providers can address both medication and therapy adherence issues with patients and the treatment team, provide feedback about symptoms addressed by medications, and provide information about therapeutic goals and the mechanisms of change for specific therapies. If behavioral treatment providers do not have the sufficient training, supervision, or resources to treat OCD, they can act as liaisons with specialists and coordinate care with the PCP and the referred specialist. As therapy progresses and the patient's symptoms improve, tapering medication could be one possible consideration for the behavioral health liaison. Behavioral health workers on an integrated treatment team could discuss therapeutic advantages of empirically supported treatments and discuss the specific symptoms that are likely to be addressed during therapy and which symptoms may benefit from medical interventions (Hazlett-Stevens, 2009). Treatment teams can function to remind patients to complete therapy homework, engage and attend therapy, and assess patient progress.

How to Assess Impact on Care/ Quality Improvement Processes

Many of the assessment measures previously covered in this chapter could be used to assess a patient's progress throughout treatment for OCD symptoms. Obvious measures of a successful integrated health-care setting assess the setting's ability to provide quality care and efficiency in the time required to identify, assess, and place patients in an effective treatment plan. Specifically in the case of OCD, assessment of an integrated care setting would require analysis of team's ability to identify possible symptoms of OCD and accurately measure the severity of the symptoms. In addition, efficiency in treatment delivery would also be an important measure of service quality. Only if adequate treatment can be offered within an integrated health-care setting, i.e., no restrictions on session time, number of sessions, and mental health professionals with extensive training for treatment delivery, treatment should begin in a timely fashion. If adequate treatment cannot be offered with the integrated health-care setting, then a timely referral to a specialist should be completed. Assessing progress throughout treatment as measured by symptom reduction is an excellent way to assess community referrals as well as treatment offered by behavioral health providers on the integrated team. Many of the assessment measures discussed in this chapter would be adequate for the assessment of OCD symptoms throughout treatment. Referred specialists may also share symptom assessments through coordinated care plans and patient feedback/consumer satisfaction efforts.

If MI is used to prepare clients to enter treatment, the Stages of Change Questionnaire (SOCQ) offers an excellent opportunity to assess the impact of the integrated care team in building motivation for future psychotherapy or for any number of positive health changes (McConnaughy, Prochaska, & Velicer, 1983). The SOCQ is a 32-item measure that assesses the patient's level of motivation for change. In the event that an integrated care setting does not have the appropriate resources to treat a patient with OCD and would need to refer treatment to an outside specialist, then the integrated care setting becomes a prime setting for working with patients to build motivation to engage in therapy with a specialist. MI has been shown to be effective in integrated health-care settings (Lakerveld et al., 2013).

References

Abramowitz, J. S. (1997). Effectiveness of psychological and pharmacological treatments for obsessive-compulsive disorder: A quantitative review. *Journal of Consulting and Clinical Psychology*, *65*(1), 44–52. https://doi.org/10.1037/0022-006X.65.1.44

Abramowitz, J. S., Franklin, M. E., Street, G. P., Kozak, M. J., & Foa, E. B. (2000). Effects of comorbid depression on response to treatment for obsessive-compulsive disorder. *Behavior Therapy*, *31*(3), 517–528. https://doi.org/10.1016/S0005-7894(00)80028-3

Ackerman, D., & Greenland, S. (2002). Multivariate meta-analysis of controlled drug studies for obsessive-compulsive disorder. *Journal of Clinical Psychopharmacology*, *22*(3), 309–317. https://doi.org/10.1097/00004714-200206000-00012

Aldea, M. A., Rahman, O., & Storch, E. A. (2009). The psychometric properties of the Florida Obsessive Compulsive Inventory: Examination in a non-clinical sample. *Individual Differences Research*, *7*(4), 228–238.

American Psychiatric Association. (2013). *Diagnostic and statistical manual of mental disorders* (5th ed.). Arlington, VA: American Psychiatric Publishing.

Amiaz, R., Fostick, L., Gershon, A., & Zohar, J. (2008). Naltrexone augmentation in OCD: A double-blind placebo-controlled cross-over study. *European Neuropsychopharmacology*, *18*(6), 455–461. https://doi.org/10.1016/j.euroneuro.2008.01.006

Andersson, E., Enander, J., Andrén, P., Hedman, E., Ljótsson, B., Hursti, T., … Rück, C. (2012). Internet-based cognitive behaviour therapy for obsessive–compulsive disorder: A randomized controlled trial. *Psychological Medicine*, *42*(10), 2193–2203. https://doi.org/10.1017/S0033291712000244

Belotto-Silva, C., Diniz, J. B., Malavazzi, D. M., Valério, C., Fossaluza, V., Borcato, S., … Shavitt, R. G. (2012). Group cognitive-behavioral therapy versus selective serotonin reuptake inhibitors for obsessive-compulsive disorder: A practical clinical trial. *Journal of Anxiety Disorders*, *26*(1), 25–31. https://doi.org/10.1016/j.janxdis.2011.08.008

Bergeron, R., Ravindran, A. V., Chaput, Y., Goldner, E., Swinson, R., Van Ameringen, M. A., … Hadrava, V. (2002). Sertraline and fluoxetine treatment of obsessive-compulsive disorder: Results of a double-blind, 6-month treatment study. *Journal of Clinical Psychopharmacology*, *22*(2), 148–154. https://doi.org/10.1097/00004714-200204000-00007

Bisserbe, J., Lane, R., & Flament, M. (1997). A double-blind comparison of sertraline and clomipramine in outpatients with obsessive-compulsive disorder. *European Psychiatry*, *12*(2), 82–93. https://doi.org/10.1016/S0924-9338(97)89646-0

Browne, H. A., Gair, S. L., Scharf, J. M., & Grice, D. E. (2014). Genetics of obsessive-compulsive disorder and related disorders. *Psychiatric Clinics of North America*, *37*(3), 319–335. https://doi.org/10.1016/j.psc.2014.06.002

Camuri, G., Oldani, L., Dell'Osso, B., Benatti, B., Lietti, L., Palazzo, C., & Altamura, A. C. (2014). Prevalence and disability of comorbid social phobia and obsessive–compulsive disorder in patients with panic disorder and generalized anxiety disorder. *International Journal of Psychiatry in Clinical Practice*, *18*(4), 248–254. https://doi.org/10.3109/13651501.2014.959972

Crockett, B. A., Churchill, E., & Davidson, J. R. (2004). A double-blind combination study of clonazepam with sertraline in obsessive-compulsive disorder. *Annals of Clinical Psychiatry*, *16*, 127–132.

Dollard, J., & Miller, N. E. (1950). *Personality and psychotherapy; an analysis in terms of learning, thinking, and culture*. New York, NY: McGraw-Hill.

Fineberg, N. A., Hengartner, M. P., Bergbaum, C. E., Gale, T. M., Gamma, A., Ajdacic-Gross, V., … Angst, J. (2013). A prospective population-based cohort study of the prevalence, incidence and impact of obsessive-compulsive symptomatology. *International Journal of Psychiatry in Clinical Practice*, *17*(3), 170–178. https://doi.org/10.3109/13651501.2012.755206

Fisher, P. L., & Wells, A. (2005). How effective are cognitive and behavioral treatments for obsessive-compulsive disorder? A clinical significance analysis. *Behaviour Research and Therapy*, *43*(12), 1543–1558. https://doi.org/10.1016/j.brat.2004.11.007

Foa, E. B., Franklin, M. E., & Moser, J. (2002). Context in the clinic: How well do cognitive-behavioral therapies and medications work in combination? *Biological Psychiatry*, *52*(10), 989–997. https://doi.org/10.1016/S0006-3223(02)01552-4

Foa, E. B., Huppert, J. D., Leiberg, S., Langner, R., Kichic, R., Hajcak, G., & Salkovskis, P. M. (2002). The obsessive-compulsive inventory: Development and validation of a short version. *Psychological Assessment*, *14*(4), 485–496. https://doi.org/10.1037/1040-3590.14.4.485

Foa, E. B., Liebowitz, M. R., Kozak, M. J., Davies, S., Campeas, R., Franklin, M. E., … Tu, X. (2005). Randomized, placebo-controlled trial of exposure and ritual prevention, clomipramine, and their combination in the treatment of obsessive-compulsive disorder. *The American Journal of Psychiatry*, *162*(1), 151–161. https://doi.org/10.1176/appi.ajp.162.1.151

Goodman, W. K., Price, L. H., Rasmussen, S. A., Mazure, C., Delgado, P., Heninger, G. R., & Charney, D. S. (1989a). The Yale-brown obsessive compulsive scale: II. Validity. *Archives of General Psychiatry*, *46*(11), 1012–1016. https://doi.org/10.1001/archpsyc.1989.01810110054008

Goodman, W. K., Price, L. H., Rasmussen, S. A., Mazure, C., Fleischmann, R. L., Hill, C. L., … Charney, D. S. (1989b). The Yale-brown obsessive compulsive scale: I. Development, use, and reliability. *Archives of General Psychiatry*, *46*(11), 1006–1011. https://doi.org/10.1001/archpsyc.1989.01810110048007

Hansen, E. S., Hasselbalch, S., Law, I., & Bolwig, T. G. (2002). The caudate nucleus in obsessive—Compulsive disorder. Reduced metabolism following treatment with paroxetine: A PET study. *The International Journal of Neuropsychopharmacology*, *5*(1), 1–10. https://doi.org/10.1017/S1461145701002681

Hazlett-Stevens, H. (2009). Assessment and treatment of anxiety in primary care. In L. C. James, W. T. O.'. Donohue, & L. C. James (Eds.), *The primary care toolkit: Practical resources for the integrated behavioral care provider* (pp. 169–182). New York, NY: Springer.

Hewlett, W. A., Vinogradov, S., & Agras, W. S. (1992). Clomipramine, clonazepam, and clonidine treatment of obsessive-compulsive disorder. *Journal of Clinical Psychopharmacology*, *12*(6), 420–430. https://doi.org/10.1097/00004714-199212000-00008

Hoehn-Saric, R., Ninan, P., Black, D. W., Stahl, S., Greist, J. H., Lydiard, B., … Harrison, W. (2000). Multicenter double-blind comparison of sertraline and desipramine for concurrent obsessive-compulsive and major depressive disorders. *Archives of General Psychiatry*, *57*(1), 76–82. https://doi.org/10.1001/archpsyc.57.1.76

Hollander, E., Allen, A., Steiner, M., Wheadon, D. E., Oakes, R., & Burnham, D. B. (2003). Acute and long-term treatment and prevention of relapse of obsessive-compulsive disorder with paroxetine. *The Journal of Clinical Psychiatry, 64*(9), 1113–1121. https://doi.org/10.4088/JCP.v64n0919

Hollander, E., Kaplan, A., & Stahl, S. M. (2003). A double-blind, placebo-controlled trial of clonazepam in obsessive-compulsive disorder. *World Journal of Biological Psychiatry, 4*, 30–34.

Jakubovski, E., Diniz, J. B., Valerio, C., Fossaluza, V., Belotto-Silva, C., Gorenstein, C., … Shavitt, R. G. (2013). Clinical predictors of long-term outcome in obsessive-compulsive disorder. *Depression and Anxiety, 30*(8), 763–772. https://doi.org/10.1002/da.22013

Jenike, M. A., Baer, L., & Buttolph, L. (1991). Buspirone augmentation of fluoxetine in patients with obsessive compulsive disorder. *The Journal of Clinical Psychiatry, 52*(1), 13–14.

Jónsson, H., Hougaard, E., & Bennedsen, B. E. (2011). Randomized comparative study of group versus individual cognitive behavioural therapy for obsessive compulsive disorder. *Acta Psychiatrica Scandinavica, 123*(5), 387–397. https://doi.org/10.1111/j.1600-0447.2010.01613.x

Katzman, M. A., Bleau, P., Blier, P., Chokka, P., Kjernisted, K., Van Ameringen, M., & the Canadian Anxiety Guidelines Initiative Group on behalf of the Anxiety Disorders Association of Canada/Association Canadienne des troubles anxieux and McGill University. (2014). Canadian clinical practice guidelines for the management of anxiety, posttraumatic stress and obsessive-compulsive disorders. *BMC Psychiatry, 14*(Suppl 1), S1. https://doi.org/10.1186/1471-244X-14-S1-S1

Kennedy, B. L., & Schwab, J. J. (1997). Utilization of medical specialists by anxiety disorder patients. *Psychosomatics: Journal of Consultation And Liaison Psychiatry, 38*(2), 109–112. https://doi.org/10.1016/S0033-3182(97)71478-6

Krochmalik, A., Jones, M. K., Menzies, R. G., & Kirkby, K. (2004). The superiority of danger ideation reduction therapy (DIRT) over exposure and response prevention (ERP) in treating compulsive washing. *Behaviour Change, 21*(4), 251–268. https://doi.org/10.1375/bech.21.4.251.66103

Kuiper, E. A., Batelaan, N. M., van Oppen, P., Hendriks, G., & van Balkom, A. J. (2013). Gastro-intestinal conditions in patients with obsessive compulsive disorder. *Journal of Obsessive-Compulsive and Related Disorders, 2*(4), 437–438. https://doi.org/10.1016/j.jocrd.2013.10.004

Lakerveld, J., Bot, S. D., Chinapaw, M. J., van Tulder, M. W., Kostense, P. J., Dekker, J. M., & Nijpels, G. (2013). Motivational interviewing and problem solving treatment to reduce type 2 diabetes and cardiovascular disease risk in real life: A randomized controlled trial. *The International Journal of Behavioral Nutrition and Physical Activity, 10*.

Lewis R. Baxter, (1992). Caudate Glucose Metabolic Rate Changes With Both Drug and Behavior Therapy for Obsessive-Compulsive Disorder. *Archives of General Psychiatry, 49*(9), 681 https://doi:10.1001/archpsyc.1992.01820090009002

Lovell, K., Cox, D., Haddock, G., Jones, C., Raines, D., Garvey, R., … Hadley, S. (2006). Telephone administered cognitive behaviour therapy for treatment of obsessive compulsive disorder: Randomised controlled non-inferiority trial. *BMJ: British Medical Journal, 333*(7574), 883. https://doi.org/10.1136/bmj.38940.355602.80

Mancebo M.C., Pinto A., Rasmussen S.A., Eisen J.L. (2008) Development of the treatment adherence survey–Patient version (TAS-P) for OCD. *Journal of Anxiety Disorders*. *22*(1), 32–43. DOI: 10.1016/j.janxdis.2007.01.009

McConnaughy, E. A., Prochaska, J. O., & Velicer, W. F. (1983). Stages of change in psychotherapy: Measurement and sample profiles. *Psychotherapy: Theory, Research & Practice, 20*(3), 368–375. https://doi.org/10.1037/h0090198

McDougle, C. J., Price, L. H., Goodman, W. K., Charney, D. S., & Heninger, G. R. (1991). A controlled trial of lithium augmentation in fluvoxamine-refractory obsessive-compulsive disorder: Lack of efficacy. *Journal of Clinical Psychopharmacology, 11*(3), 175–184. https://doi.org/10.1097/00004714-199106000-00005

McKay, D., Sookman, D., Neziroglu, F., Wilhelm, S., Stein, D. J., Kyrios, M., … Veale, D. (2015). Efficacy of cognitive-behavioral therapy for obsessive–compulsive disorder. *Psychiatry Research, 227*(1), 104–113. https://doi.org/10.1016/j.psychres.2015.02.004

Moritz, S., & Jelinek, L. (2011). Further evidence for the efficacy of association splitting as a self-help technique for reducing obsessive thoughts. *Depression and Anxiety, 28*(7), 574–581. https://doi.org/10.1002/da.20843

Moritz, S., Jelinek, L., Hauschildt, M., & Naber, D. (2010). How to treat the untreated: Effectiveness of a self-help metacognitive training program (myMCT) for obsessive-compulsive disorder. *Dialogues in Clinical Neuroscience, 12*(2), 209–220.

Nakao, T., Okada, K., & Kanba, S. (2014). Neurobiological model of obsessive–compulsive disorder: Evidence from recent neuropsychological and neuroimaging findings. *Psychiatry and Clinical Neurosciences, 68*(8), 587–605. https://doi.org/10.1111/pcn.12195

Ninan, P. T., Koran, L. M., Kiev, A., Davidson, J. T., Rasmussen, S. A., Zajecka, J. M., … Austin, C. (2006). High-dose sertraline strategy for nonresponders to acute treatment for obsessive-compulsive disorder: A multicenter double-blind trial. *The Journal of Clinical Psychiatry, 67*(1), 15–22. https://doi.org/10.4088/JCP.v67n0103

O'Connor, K. P., Aardema, F., Bouthillier, D., Fournier, S., Guay, S., Robillard, S., … Pitre, D. (2005). Evaluation of an inference-based approach to treating obsessive-compulsive disorder. *Cognitive Behaviour Therapy, 34*(3), 148–163. https://doi.org/10.1080/16506070510041211

Ong, C. W., Clyde, J. W., Bluett, E. J., Levin, M. E., & Twohig, M. P. (2016). Dropout rates in exposure with response prevention for obsessive-compulsive disorder: What do the data really say? *Journal of*

Anxiety Disorders, 40, 8–17. https://doi.org/10.1016/j.janxdis.2016.03.006

Öst, L., Havnen, A., Hansen, B., & Kvale, G. (2015). Cognitive behavioral treatments of obsessive–compulsive disorder. A systematic review and meta-analysis of studies published 1993–2014. *Clinical Psychology Review, 40*, 156–169. https://doi.org/10.1016/j.cpr.2015.06.003

Ougrin, D. (2011). Efficacy of exposure versus cognitive therapy in anxiety disorders: Systematic review and meta-analysis. *BMC Psychiatry, 11*.

Ponniah, K., Iliana, M., & Hollon, S. D. (2013). An update on the efficacy of psychological therapies in the treatment of obsessive-compulsive disorder in adults. *Journal of Obsessive-Compulsive and Related Disorders, 2*(2), 207–218.

Prochaska, J. O., & DiClemente, C. C. (1982). Transtheoretical therapy: Toward a more integrative model of change. *Psychotherapy: Theory Research and Practice, 19*, 276–288.

Rosa-Alcázar, A. I., Sánchez-Meca, J., Gómez-Conesa, A., & Marín-Martínez, F. (2008). Psychological treatment of obsessive-compulsive disorder: A meta-analysis. *Clinical Psychology Review, 28*(8), 1310–1325. https://doi.org/10.1016/j.cpr.2008.07.001

Roshanaei-Moghaddam, B., Pauly, M. C., Atkins, D. C., Baldwin, S. A., Stein, M. B., & Roy-Byrne, P. (2011). Relative effects of CBT and pharmacotherapy in depression versus anxiety: Is medication somewhat better for depression, and CBT somewhat better for anxiety? *Depression and Anxiety, 28*(7), 560–567. https://doi.org/10.1002/da.20829

Simpson, H. B., Liebowitz, M. R., Foa, E. B., Kozak, M. J., Schmidt, A. B., Rowan, V., … Campeas, R. (2004). Post-treatment effects of exposure therapy and clomipramine in obsessive-compulsive disorder. *Depression and Anxiety, 19*(4), 225–233. https://doi.org/10.1002/da.20003

Storch, E. A., Bagner, D., Merlo, L. J., Shapira, N. A., Geffken, G. R., Murphy, T. K., & Goodman, W. K. (2007). Florida obsessive-compulsive inventory: Development, reliability, and validity. *Journal of Clinical Psychology, 63*(9), 851–859. https://doi.org/10.1002/jclp.20382

Twohig, M. P., Hayes, S. C., Plumb, J. C., Pruitt, L. D., Collins, A. B., Hazlett-Stevens, H., & Woidneck, M. R. (2010). A randomized clinical trial of acceptance and commitment therapy versus progressive relaxation training for obsessive-compulsive disorder. *Journal of Consulting and Clinical Psychology, 78*(5), 705–716. https://doi.org/10.1037/a0020508

van der Heiden, C., van Rossen, K., Dekker, A., Damstra, M., & Deen, M. (2016). Metacognitive therapy for obsessive–compulsive disorder: A pilot study. *Journal of Obsessive-Compulsive and Related Disorders, 9*, 24–29. https://doi.org/10.1016/j.jocrd.2016.02.002

van Oppen, P., van Balkom, A. J., de Haan, E., & van Dyck, R. (2005). Cognitive therapy and exposure in vivo alone and in combination with fluvoxamine in obsessive-compulsive disorder: A 5-year follow-up. *Journal of Clinical Psychiatry, 66*, 1415–1422.

Veldhuis, J., Dieleman, J. P., Wohlfarth, T., Storosum, J. G., van Den Brink, W., Sturkenboom, M. M., & Denys, D. (2012). Incidence and prevalence of 'diagnosed OCD' in a primary care, treatment seeking, population. *International Journal of Psychiatry in Clinical Practice, 16*(2), 85–92. https://doi.org/10.3109/13651501.2011.617454

Vulink, N. C., Denys, D., & Westenberg, H. M. (2005). Bupropion for patients with obsessive-compulsive disorder: An open-label, fixed-dose study. *The Journal of Clinical Psychiatry, 66*(2), 228–230. https://doi.org/10.4088/JCP.v66n0211

Whittal, M. L., Robichaud, M., Thordarson, D. S., & McLean, P. D. (2008). Group and individual treatment of obsessive-compulsive disorder using cognitive therapy and exposure plus response prevention: A 2-year follow-up of two randomized trials. *Journal of Consulting and Clinical Psychology, 76*(6), 1003–1014. https://doi.org/10.1037/a0013076

Wilhelm, S., Steketee, G., Fama, J. M., Buhlmann, U., Teachman, B. A., & Golan, E. (2009). Modular cognitive therapy for obsessive-compulsive disorder: A wait-list controlled trial. *Journal of Cognitive Psychotherapy, 23*(4), 294–305. https://doi.org/10.1891/0889-8391.23.4.294

Oppositional Defiant Disorder (ODD)

26

Brittany M. Hayden and Brittany R. Patterson

Oppositional Defiant Disorder

What Is Oppositional Defiant Disorder?

Oppositional defiant disorder (ODD) is one of the most commonly occurring disorders in young children (Maughan, Rowe, Messer, Goodman, & Meltzer, 2004). According to the American Psychiatric Association's (APA) *Diagnostic and Statistical Manual of Mental Disorders*, Fifth Edition (DSM-5; 2013), ODD is included in the disruptive, impulse-control, and conduct disorders and is characterized by a pattern of irritable, argumentative, and vindictive behavior lasting at least 6 months, as evidenced by at least four of the following symptoms: loss of temper, being touchy or easily annoyed, being angry and resentful, arguing with authority figures, actively defying or refusing to comply with adults' rules and/or authority figures, deliberately annoying others, blaming others for their mistakes, or being spiteful or vindictive at least twice within the past 6 months. In addition, these symptoms must be demonstrated during interactions with at least one individual who is not a sibling (i.e., parent, teachers, authority figures, etc.). Children and adolescents with ODD may display negativity, rebelliousness, as well as antagonistic, and stubborn, and challenging behaviors. These behaviors are often difficult for parents, caregivers, teachers to manage.

It may be obvious that most of these behaviors are, on occasion, developmentally appropriate for most children and adolescents. As such, the frequency and intensity of these behaviors, as well as the overall impact on functioning and distress levels, should be considered to determine whether a behavior is symptomatic of ODD or is expected given the child/adolescent's developmental stage. To meet diagnostic criteria for ODD, children who are under 5 years old must demonstrate the aforementioned symptoms on most days for at least 6 months (APA, 2013), as some behavioral issues are typical for children of this developmental stage. Children and adolescents diagnosed with ODD exhibit behavioral disturbances that are significant enough to affect the social, academic, occupational, or other areas of functioning and/or cause distress in social contexts.

As mentioned previously, ODD is one of the most common mental health disorders seen among children. Current prevalence rates of ODD

B.M. Hayden, Ph.D. (✉)
Outpatient Behavioral Health Department, Sarah A. Reed Children's Center, Erie, PA, USA
e-mail: bhayden@sarahreed.org

B.R. Patterson, Ph.D.
Department of Psychiatry, Center for School Mental Health, University of Maryland School of Medicine, Baltimore, MD, USA
e-mail: bparham@som.umaryland.edu

A. Maragakis, W.T. O'Donohue (eds.), *Principle-Based Stepped Care and Brief Psychotherapy for Integrated Care Settings*, https://doi.org/10.1007/978-3-319-70539-2_26

in children and adolescents are around 3% of the population (APA, 2013; Canino, Polanczyk, Bauermeister, Rohde, & Frick, 2010), while other estimates indicate the disorder occurs in 1–16% of the population (Loeber, Burke, Lahey, Winters, & Zera, 2000). ODD occurs more often in boys during childhood, though gender differences in prevalence rates are not consistently found during adolescence (Loeber et al., 2000). There is growing research that suggests ODD symptoms manifest differently in boys and girls. For example, boys may display externalizing, antisocial behaviors such as being argumentative with adults, while girls with ODD are more likely to exhibit uncooperative or lying behaviors and less overt behaviors (Steiner & Remsing, 2007); regardless, these disruptive behaviors have a negative impact on the child's successful functioning. ODD symptoms are most likely to appear during the preschool or early school-age years, though, more rarely, it is possible for these behavioral disturbances to appear during adolescence.

Differential diagnosis and common co-occurring mental health conditions. ODD shares some common symptoms with conduct disorder (CD), attention-deficit/hyperactivity disorder (ADHD), mood disorders (i.e., depressive and bipolar disorders), disruptive mood dysregulation disorder (DMDD), intermittent explosive disorder (IED), and anxiety disorders. Compared to CD, ODD symptoms are less severe and do not include the violation of the rights of others such as destruction of property, physical aggression, or cruelty to animals, which may be seen in CD. In addition, ODD includes irritability and anger, whereas the diagnostic criteria in CD do not include emotional symptoms. It should be noted that ODD might precede CD if symptoms are not adequately addressed. Similarly, the severe aggressive behaviors observed in IED are not characteristic of individuals with ODD (Connor, 2002). ADHD and ODD are frequently diagnosed together, with comorbidity rates up to 60–70% in community and clinically referred samples (Steinhausen & Nøvik, 2006; Wilens, 2002). Through thorough screening and assessment, the mood symptoms seen with ODD (i.e., anger) should be differentiated from mood symptoms associated with depressive and mood disorders to aid in differential diagnosis and inform treatment recommendations; in addition, the chronic negative affect and temper tantrums are significantly more severe with DMDD compared to ODD. If criteria are met for DMDD, ODD is not diagnosed (even if all criteria for ODD are met; APA, 2013). Connor (2002) notes that children with anxiety or mood disorders may develop ODD symptoms in response to environmental and family stressors. When diagnosing ODD it is important to determine whether there may be any intellectual, learning, and/or language impairments that may be the root cause of oppositional behaviors, such as in an intellectual disability or language disorder (APA, 2013).

What causes ODD? While there is no clear cause of ODD, epidemiological studies have found a number of risk factors that increase the likelihood that an individual will develop the disorder. Awareness of risk factors that predispose children to ODD is essential in early detection and intervention. Experts believe that a combination of genetic, biological, social, psychological, and environmental factors plays a role in the development of ODD. A child's temperament or natural disposition may be a contributing factor to the development of the disorder as well. For example, a child who is highly emotionally reactive to perceived stressors or has difficulties with emotional regulation may be more likely to receive a diagnosis of ODD (Connor, 2002). An additional contributing factor includes neurological impairments, particularly those that affect the parts of the brain that manage impulse control, reasoning, and judgment. Physiologically, lower heart rates, lower skin conductance reactivity, decreased basal cortisol reactivity, and abnormalities in the prefrontal cortex and amygdala have been found in children with disruptive behavior disorders (APA, 2013). Children and adolescents are also more susceptible to ODD if they have a parent diagnosed with ODD, attention-deficit/hyperactivity disorder (ADHD), conduct disorder (CD), or a mood disorder (e.g., bipolar disorder or depression; Burke, Loeber, & Birmaher, 2002). Children whose parents have substance abuse problems or who have otherwise experienced prenatal exposure to alcohol, drugs, and even tobacco are at an increased risk for more disruptive behaviors (Burke et al., 2002). Exposure to toxins in the environment and poor nutrition may also contribute to increased risk for ODD.

Social, psychological, and environmental factors are also important to consider in the development of ODD. Perhaps most importantly, parental factors play a critical role in whether a child is at an increased risk for the development of the disorder. For example, a poor attachment with one or both parents, an absent caregiver, abuse or neglect, poor parental supervision, family disruptions/instability (e.g., frequent moves, divorce, separations, family discord, etc.), and inconsistent and/or harsh discipline place a child at increased risk for disruptive behavior disorders. Children and adolescents who have difficulty forming and maintaining relationships or who struggle to recognize and process social cues may also be at risk for developing ODD (Burke et al., 2002). There is additional support which suggests that female adolescents may be more likely to receive a diagnosis of ODD if their parents suspect the use or sale of drugs in the neighborhoods in which they live (Russell et al., 2015).

Impact of ODD. Children with ODD display impairments in social, academic, or other areas of functioning, and the symptoms of ODD are associated with distress in the individual and/or his/her caregivers (e.g., a parent or teacher; APA, 2013). The negative effects of ODD can include high levels of parental stress, parental relationship stress, poor parent-child relationships, academic difficulties, school suspensions/expulsions, low self-esteem, increased risk for substance use, delinquency, a lack of effective communication skills, social skills deficits, negative peer interactions, lack of friendships, and increased risk for perpetration of bullying (Burke et al., 2002; Connor, 2002). More importantly, if left untreated, children and adolescents with ODD are at risk for the development of other mental health conditions, as noted above. Although most children with ODD do not go on to develop CD, research suggests that approximately one-third of children who have ODD will go on to develop the disorder. Of those who subsequently develop CD, 40% will likely develop antisocial personality disorder in adulthood (Loeber et al., 2000). Given the serious consequences if left untreated (e.g., delinquency, substance abuse, etc.; Hamilton & Armando, 2008), early identification and treatment of ODD are critical. The next section will explore helpful screening tools to aid professionals working with children and adolescents suspected of having ODD.

Effective Ways to Screen in the Primary Care Setting

Family physicians in primary care settings are typically the first lifeline for parents of children suspected of having ODD. That is, parents initially call upon their primary care physician for help when they are struggling to manage their child's behaviors. The physician often begins by gathering medical history information, as well as conducting a thorough physical examination. Physicians should also carefully explore the possibility that the child's defiant behaviors are caused by abuse or neglect or some other type of trauma. After ruling out any trauma history or medical or physical causes for the disturbance of conduct, a brief interview and use of easily accessible screening tools can be utilized to quickly screen for ODD. Evidence-based screening and assessment tools offer more specificity in differentiating symptoms and disorders and are more sensitive in detecting changes in symptomology throughout treatment/intervention (Hamilton & Armando, 2008). Professionals in integrated health-care settings have access to a number of reliable and valid screening tools to assess for ODD. Measures such as the NICHQ Vanderbilt Assessment Scale (Vanderbilt; Wolraich et al., 2003) is a brief screening to assess for ADHD, ODD, CD, as well as anxiety and depression symptoms. The Vanderbilt also has a built-in impact scale, which assesses the severity of symptoms and their impact on children's functioning in home, at school, and interpersonally. This measure is useful for monitoring symptoms and tracking behaviors over time. Tools that assess for overall impact on functioning, such as the Vanderbilt or the Impairment Rating Scale (IRS), are essential in determining whether behavioral issues are significant enough to warrant diagnosis/treatment. See Table 26.1 for a comprehensive, though not exhaustive, review on easily accessible and empirically validated screening tools.

How to Assess Further If a Screen Returns Positive

A positive screen for a disruptive behavior disorder, such as ODD, can inform the selection of additional assessments to provide more detailed information about specific areas of concern (parental stress levels, cognitive abilities, peer relationships, etc.), as well as aid in differential diagnosis and assessment of coexisting conditions. As noted in Table 26.1, most screening tools include forms which other caregivers (e.g., teachers or daycare workers) or the child/adolescent can complete, which will provide valuable information for behavioral health clinicians in the integrated care setting to assess symptoms across domains. Gathering information from multiple sources provides information regarding a broad range of domains (e.g., relationship with peers, parent-child/family dynamics, academic performance, organization, etc.) and may also provide information regarding child and family strengths. Furthermore, the information received from these sources can contribute to the assessment and identification of ODD.

Direct observations and interaction rating scales provide additional assessment data for the diagnosis of ODD. After the brief screening is conducted, the behavioral health provider can gather information via teachers and other caregivers using a number of assessment tools. The Sutter-Eyberg Student Behavior Inventory-Revised (SESBI-R; Eyberg & Pincus, 1999) or the Revised Edition of the School Observation Coding System (REDSOCS; Bagner, Boggs, & Eyberg, 2010) can gather information regarding behavioral issues directly from the child's teachers. The child's teacher can also provide additional valuable data for assessment purposes using an Antecedent-Behavior-Consequence (ABC) chart which assists in determining the antecedents and consequences of problematic behaviors. The ABC form is most often a

Table 26.1 Screening tools to identify ODD

Tools	Ages	Domains assessed	Forms	Author(s)
BPC	7–17	Internalizing, externalizing	Parent report Youth report	Chorpita et al. (2010)
CADBI	3–18	Oppositionality, hyperactivity, impulsivity	Parent report Teacher report	Burns, Taylor, and Rusby (2001)
DBD-RS	6–17	ADHD, CD, ODD	Parent report Teacher report	Pelham, Gnagy, Greenslade, and Milich (1992)
IRS		Narrative description of overall impairment	Parent report Teacher report	Fabiano et al. (2006)
NICHQ Vanderbilt	6–12	ADHD, CD, ODD	Parent report Teacher report	Wolraich et al. (2003)
PSC/Y-PSC	3–17	Cognitive, behavioral, emotional	Parent report Youth report (11–17)	Gardner et al. (1999) (17-item)
SDQ	3–17	Emotional, conduct problems, hyperactivity/inattention, peer relationships, prosocial behavior	Parent report Teacher report Youth report (11–17)	Goodman (1997)
SNAP-IV	3–17	ADHD, ODD	Parent report Teacher report	Swanson et al. (2001)

See references for complete names of measures

These measures and others can be found at: http://csmh.umaryland.edu/Resources/Resources-for-Clinicians/ or http://www.cappcny.org/home/clinical-rating-scales/

component of a functional behavioral assessment, which is typically conducted in school settings to identify the function of a behavior (e.g., to avoid non-preferred tasks, to gain social attention, etc.) and develop individualized behavioral intervention plans, such as a daily report card (Vannest, Davis, Davis, Mason, & Burke, 2010).

Observations of the parent-child dyad may determine what, if any, dynamics may be contributing to the child's ODD symptoms. For example, the Keys to Interactive Parenting Scale (KIPS; Comfort & Gordon, 2006) or the Dyadic Parent-Child Interaction Coding System (DPICS; Eyberg, Nelson, Ginn, Bhuiyan, & Boggs, 2013) could be utilized to provide objective data regarding such domains as caregiver responsiveness, limits and consequences, and parenting skills acquisition.

Given that ODD is often comorbid with ADHD, anxiety, and mood disorders, a comprehensive assessment by a mental health clinician can provide information for differential and comorbid diagnoses. Are oppositional behaviors better explained by poor impulse control and hyperactivity, as seen in ADHD? Are ODD symptoms a result of a child struggling to manage anxiety or depression? Structured and semi-structured diagnostic interviews, like the Diagnostic Interview Schedule for Children (DISC; Shaffer, Fisher, Lucas, Dulcan, & Schwab-Stone, 2000), and more comprehensive psychosocial assessments, such as the Behavior Assessment System for Children (BASC; Kamphaus, Reynolds, Hatcher, & Kim, 2004), provide valuable information regarding differential diagnosis. Structured interviews are more time intensive for the behavioral health provider to administer, but are typically easy to score and provide valuable diagnostic information. Measures, such as the BASC or CBRS, can be completed by patients, caregivers, and teachers outside of sessions, and with the purchase of a subscription, providers typically have unlimited-use scoring software. Treating other co-occurring disorders or difficulties often decreases ODD symptoms. Table 26.2. provides a review of diagnostic interviews or rating inventories, which provide more comprehensive and/or in-depth symptom information.

Depending on the results of the screening and assessment procedures, primary care physicians may work with the parent or caregiver to request that a psychoeducational evaluation be completed by the child's school district to determine whether behavioral and learning supports are required in the academic testing. There is a consensus among experts that learning disabilities and/or communication disorders commonly coexist with ODD (Steiner & Remsing, 2007) and addressing learning difficulties may alleviate behavioral problems associated with academic frustrations or cognitive deficits. An individualized education program may be particularly important if a child's emotional and/or behavioral problems are negatively impacting his/her ability to learn. Once thorough, evidence-based screening and assessment have indicated the presence of ODD, the behavioral health clinician within the integrated care setting can implement

Table 26.2. Assessment tools to identify ODD

Tools	Domains assessed	Forms	Author(s)
BASC-3	Adaptive and problem behaviors	Parent, teacher, and youth version	Kamphaus et al. (2004)
CBCL; CBCL-YSR	Internalizing (anxiety, depression) externalizing (ADHD, ODD, CD), social skills, adaptive behavior	Parent, teacher, and youth report	Achenbach (1991)
Conners CBRS	Oppositionality, cognitive problems/ inattention, hyperactivity, anxiety, social problems, psychosomatic problems	Parent, teacher, and youth report	Conners et al. (1997)
DBDSPI	ADHD, ODD, CD	Interview	Pelham et al. (1992)
DISC-IV	Assesses for over 30 DSM disorders	Interview	Shaffer et al. (2000)

See references for complete names of measures

and provide brief, effective interventions to assist children and families. Given limited time and other constraints, the provider in the integrated care setting can utilize the screening measures in Table 26.1, such as the Vanderbilt, the PSC, the SNAP-IV, or the SDQ, which are free, available online, and typically take just 10–15 min to complete. The tools are sound measures in not only identifying ODD symptoms but also tracking the impact/severity of symptoms throughout treatment.

Evidence-Based Stepped Care and Brief Psychotherapeutic Approaches

Integrated care is a collaborative approach to addressing the biopsychosocial needs of a patient using evidenced-based stepped care and brief psychotherapeutic approaches. Stepped care includes increasing health-care literacy, bibliotherapy, e-health (i.e., using information and technology to improve health care; Eysenbach, 2001), groups therapy, brief individual therapy, and medications. The time frame used by most integrated health-care settings to implement "brief" psychotherapeutic approaches is limited to three to five sessions around 20–30 min in length. As a result, long-term and intensive therapies are not feasible; however, interventions for ODD with both parents and child can substantially improve short- and long-term outcomes (Hamilton & Armando, 2008). After gathering and reviewing clinical information from multiple respondents across settings, the clinician can provide the appropriate clinic-based treatment depending on the individual client/family needs, as well as the child's age and developmental level. The clinician may also provide referrals to community resources for children and families with more significant needs.

Prevention and Health-Care Literacy

There is substantial evidence which shows that early intervention and school-based programming, such as Head Start, can prevent disruptive behaviors associated with ODD (Burke et al., 2002); however, physicians in integrated care settings can provide prevention information to parents/caregivers as well. For example, physicians can direct families to information regarding strategies for use within the home to prevent problem behaviors. Organizations such as the Mayo Clinic or the American Academy of Family Physicians offer informational guides for families concerning ODD. Integrated care professionals can provide access to these materials in their clinics or offer informational sessions in the clinic on parenting strategies (e.g., praise positive behaviors, model appropriate behavior, set limits, develop a consistent routine, set aside quality child-caregiver time, identifying consequences, information concerning the potential for negative behaviors to increase before they improve; www.mayoclinic.org). The Department of Health and Human Services provides a Health Literacy Online Guide (https://health.gov/healthliteracyonline), which provides standards and best practices for physicians and professionals who wish to provide useful information via the web. Additionally, this tool provides guidance on how to present information in a manner that will assist consumers who may have limited literacy skills or other obstacles to obtaining such information.

Bibliotherapy

Bibliotherapy is a stepped care strategy meaning, simply, therapy through books. There are a number of applicable books based on sound research to address oppositionality, defiance, and anger in children, and research suggests that a minimal intervention, such as bibliotherapy, may improve family functioning just as effectively as a brief intervention (Lavigne et al., 2008). Most books addressing ODD symptoms provide behavioral management strategies, while others teach children and their caregivers better emotion management skills. In their book, *Your Defiant Child: 8 Steps to Better Behavior*, Barkley and Benton (2013) provide a step-by-step guide for parents to correct problem behaviors and explain the functions of such behaviors, stressing consistency, and use of praise. The book provides charts, checklists, and other tools for parental use. There are also a number of children's books with the goal of teaching children to improve their self-regulation and make better choices. For a number of effective titles and topics, physicians can point families to author Julia Cook's works, who wrote such books as *That Rule Doesn't Apply to Me* about a boy who finds that rules keep getting in the way of his fun. The Clear Lake Children's Center website offers a comprehensive list of books on a variety of topics (see http://clearlakechildrenscenter.com/resources/bibliotherapy). See Table 26.3 for a list (by no means exhaustive) of books addressing behavioral issues in children.

Brief Therapeutic Approaches/ Programs

Treatments for ODD typically include a combination of parent training programs/family therapy, individual therapy, problem-solving skills training, and social skills training. Most of the programs described hereafter have built-in prevention programming and stepped care based on the needs of the child/family and the intensity of behavioral problems. Typically, parent training and school-based programs are utilized with preschool and school-age children displaying disruptive behaviors. Across all age groups, interventions targeting parents are one of the most effective in decreasing behavioral symptoms associated with ODD. The AACAP and the California Evidence-Based Clearinghouse (CEBC) provide comprehensive lists of the most effective and well-known parenting management and intervention programs.

The Positive Parenting Program (Triple P; Sanders, 1999) is a multilevel system of parent/family training to offer preventative, early intervention, and treatment applications. Level 2 of Triple P is a brief intervention (one to two, 20-min sessions) and is appropriate for use by physicians, health-care providers, daycares, or schools. Similarly, Level 3 of Triple P is a more targeted intervention (one to four sessions)

Table 26.3 Bibliotherapy for oppositional defiant disorder

Book name	Author(s)	Target audience	Publication information
Help Me Be Good series	Berry, J.	Children (ages 4–7)	Joy Berry Books
I Just Don't Like the Sound of No and others	Cook, J.	Children (K–6)	Boys Town Press
Mindful Discipline: A Loving Approach to Setting Limits & Raising an Emotionally Intelligent Child	Shapiro, S. & White, C.	Parent/caregiver and child	New Harbinger Publications
Raising an Emotionally Intelligent Child: The Heart of Parenting	Gottman, J. & Declaire, J.	Parent/caregiver	Fireside
The Defiant Child: A Parent's Guide to Oppositional Defiant Disorder	Riley, D.	Parent/caregiver	Taylor Trade Publishing
SOS: Help for Parents: A Practical Guide for Handling Common Everyday Behavior Problems	Clark, L.	Parent/caregiver	SOS Programs & Parents Press
The Explosive Child: A New Approach for Understanding and Parenting Easily Frustrated, Chronically Inflexible Children	Greene, R. W.	Parent/caregiver	HarperCollins Publishers
The Kazdin Method for Parenting the Defiant Child	Kazdin, A. E.	Parent/caregiver	Houghton Mifflin Harcourt
The Whole-Brain Child: 12 Revolutionary Strategies to Nurture Your Child's Developing Mind	Siegel, D. J. & Payne Bryson, T.	Parent/caregiver	Bantam Books
Your Defiant Child: 8 Steps to Better Behavior	Barkley, R. A. & Benton, C. M.	Parent/caregiver	The Guilford Press

providing advice, rehearsal, and self-evaluation, which can also be provided by clinicians in primary care settings (Sanders, 1999). Social skills training programs have also been used as prevention/intervention programs for preschool/school-age children. The *Incredible Years* (IY; Reid & Webster-Stratton, 2001) is one such intervention. IY and similar programs teach children how to relate more positively to others and provide instruction for parents regarding setting limits, establishing rules, building a strong parent/child bond, and ways to manage oppositional behaviors (Reid & Webster-Stratton, 2001). Within the integrated care setting, well visits with the primary care physician present as opportunities for provision of parenting tips to parents and to provide written materials, offer parenting groups, and show video demonstrations of ideal parenting, as is provided by the IY program.

Brief Parent Training (BPT; Kjøbli & Ogden, 2012) has also shown promise as a short-term intervention for parent training and is associated with decreased conduct problems and increased social competence in children. BPT teaches parents proper use of praise, setting appropriate boundaries, and problem-solving day-to-day challenges over the course of three to five sessions. Kolko and Perrin (2014) identify other brief, evidence-based approaches, including Primary-Care Parent-Child Interaction Therapy (group therapy format) and the Play Nicely Program (multimedia trainings), as effective tools in decreasing externalizing behavior problems. Hamilton and Armando (2008) note that collaborative problem-solving strategies are comparably as effective as parent training programs. Collaborative problem-solving tasks parents and children to use cognitive approaches to resolve conflicts among family members (Greene et al., 2004). As demonstrated here, there are several brief, but effective, programs that can be implemented or adapted for use in integrated care settings.

What Doesn't Work

While there is no easy solution to addressing the behaviors associated with ODD, there are a number of measures that have been found to be ineffective and may worsen symptom issues. In recent years, there has been publicity and media attention for addressing behavioral problems in children and adolescents through scare tactics, boot camps, or so-called "tough love" camps. These quick, one-stop interventions are not effective in the treatment of ODD in children or adolescents, rarely incorporate parent/family dynamics, and are potentially harmful to child and family functioning (Connor, 2002). Similarly, harsh and/or hostile parenting and discipline practices used to force children into compliance may result in the reinforcement of maladaptive or aggressive behaviors (Connor, 2002). The possible effects of an "authoritarian" parenting style on children, which is characterized by a high degree of control or demandingness and strict discipline, may include increased aggressive behavior, poor anger management, and increased risk for resentment toward authority figures (Baumrind, 1966). Although harsh parenting practices do not work for addressing ODD symptoms, ignoring behavioral problems is not a wise strategy either. As mentioned previously, children with ODD who are left untreated are at risk for developing CD or even antisocial personality disorder as adults (Connor, 2002). Additionally, the use of medication alone has not been found to be an effective treatment for ODD; however, medication prescribed as part of a comprehensive treatment plan may be necessary to treat the symptoms of coexisting mental health disorders (e.g., ADHD, anxiety, etc.). Many medications used to treat ADHD, anxiety, or mood disorders have been found to decrease behavioral problems associated with ODD, when these conditions coexist (Hamilton & Armando, 2008).

Given that the majority of children improve with the assistance of behavioral interventions and/or therapy, hoping behavioral problems will just go away is contraindicated and may make matters worse. Research has shown that children and adolescents respond best to interventions which reward positive behavior, teach and model prosocial behaviors, and provide skills training on emotion management (Connor, 2002).

When to Refer to Specialty Mental Health

After comprehensive screening and assessment, professionals in integrated care settings will have a clear picture of whether more intensive and long-term services are required. Given the frequent comorbidity of ODD and other mental health conditions (Burke et al., 2002), a psychiatric evaluation may be warranted to determine whether a child would benefit from psychotropic medications. As previously mentioned, research suggests that pharmacological interventions targeted at treating coexisting mental disorders (e.g., ADHD or anxiety) can simultaneously decrease the frequency and/or intensity of behavioral symptoms (Hamilton & Armando, 2008).

As discussed earlier, prevention and early identification/intervention with behavioral problems are essential with regard to ODD treatment; however, the severity of symptoms across multiple settings may warrant long-term and individualized approaches. If children with ODD and their caregivers do not respond to the aforementioned evidence-based stepped care or brief therapy treatments, more targeted interventions are necessary. Additionally, there are typically longstanding social and environmental factors which give rise to and maintain ODD symptoms. In such cases, more intensive treatments such as Parent Child Interaction Therapy (PCIT; Eyberg, Boggs, & Algina, 1995) may be indicated. PCIT is an evidence-based treatment created by Sheila Eyberg in the 1970s for families with children ages 2–7 diagnosed with disruptive behavior disorders. PCIT uses live parent coaching to improve and increase positive parent-child interactions. Other evidence-based treatments designed to treat children with ODD and other disruptive behavior disorders are Triple P (Sanders, 1999), *Helping the Noncompliant Child* (HNC; McMahon & Forehand, 2003), Parent Management Training-Oregon (PMTO; Forgatch & DeGarmo, 1999), or Multisystemic Therapy (MST; Henggeler et al., 1986). Depending on the unique needs of the child and family, primary care physicians may refer families to clinicians trained in specific modalities.

Given the social and environmental issues that give rise to ODD symptoms, it is likely that children diagnosed with ODD and their families may require supports that ecologically and systemically target the factors contributing to disruptive behavior (e.g., family therapy to address family discord, referral to children services organizations if child is at risk for out-of-home placement, substance abuse counseling for caregiver/parent, etc.).

The Role of the Primary Care Provider/Medical Team in Treatment

For the past several years, the World Health Organization (WHO) and several others (e.g., AACAP, AAP, NAMI, NIMH, SAMHSA) have called for an integration of mental health services and primary care provision in an effort to close the alarming treatment gap for untreated mental illnesses (WHO, 2008). Integrated services are a cost-effective and logical means to providing necessary treatments (WHO, 2008), and it is widely acknowledged that mental and physical health are inextricably interwoven; therefore, treating the child holistically is best practice and produces better health outcomes (Asarnow, Rozenman, Wiblin, & Zeltzer, 2015). In a large-scale study assessing the national trends of office-based provision of mental health-care treatment for children and adolescents, over 70% of children presenting to office-based physicians received a diagnosis of a disruptive behavior disorder, such as ODD (Olfson, Blanco, Wang, Laje, & Correll, 2014). Of these office-based clinicians, nearly 68% were pediatric/family medicine physicians (Olfson et al., 2014). Given these trends, it is evident that primary care providers are playing an integral role in the identification, assessment, treatment, and monitoring of ODD and other mental disorders.

Using the previously mentioned tools and resources, primary care physicians can rule out any medical issues and efficiently and accurately assess for mental disorders. Once the provider diagnoses ODD, the primary care team can provide brief, solution-focused interventions and necessary resources for the child and family. Physicians can also explore pharmacological interventions, where appropriate, including education and discussions regarding potential side effects and limitations of various medications. Children and youth with ODD often exhibit symptoms in more than one setting (e.g., home and school, home and community, etc.); therefore, primary care physicians may provide (and receive) consultation and collaboration with other relevant important providers and caregivers (e.g., parents, teachers, therapists, etc.). One of the many benefits of integrated care is the ability to work collaboratively with a multidisciplinary team. There are opportunities for physician to screen for ODD and make a referral to the psychologist or psychiatrist on staff or other community resources, while the nurses are able to provide brief interventions or group classes on parenting strategies with the family/families in the clinic. Perhaps the most impactful role of the primary care provider is that of providing continuous, longitudinal care and monitoring of the overall healthy development of the child. Family physicians often have long-term contact with their patients and are in a unique position of providing ongoing support and monitoring of behavioral progress and functioning (Shi, 2012). There is also potential for primary care physicians to provide the family with referrals to more comprehensive/intensive assessment and evaluation, community resources, and specialty mental health treatment at any stage of the child's development.

Given the increased acknowledgement of integrated health care as best practice (WHO, 2008), primary care will continue to be increasingly important in the treatment of ODD and other mental health conditions. Primary care providers can offer easy access to brief, behaviorally focused parent training, psychoeducation, pharmacological interventions (given the presence of comorbid mental health conditions), consultation and collaborative care with other providers, progress monitoring, and referrals to more intensive and long-term family and individual psychotherapy.

How to Assess Impact on Primary Care/Quality Improvement Processes

Preventative efforts and strategies are important to moderating the risk factors associated with both mental and physical health problems. In the case of mental disorders, such as ODD, universal screenings at well visits throughout childhood and early intervention may prevent and/or reduce the likelihood of an ODD diagnosis (Burke et al., 2002), moderate the negative impact of mental health issues on a child's psychosocial functioning, and reduce the significant economic and environmental costs behavioral disorders have on communities/society (National Research Council; NRC & Institute of Medicine, 2009). The NRC and Institute of Medicine (2009) suggest that early intervention efforts (including early identification of risk factors) to prevent mental, emotional, and behavioral disorders are showing promising results. There is also research suggesting that screening pregnant women and new mothers for depression symptoms or substance abuse and providing treatment, where appropriate, can reduce the risk that their children will develop a mental illness (Bazelon Center for Mental Health Law, 2009a, 2009b). There are several global/universal screening tools which are easily accessible, have demonstrated sufficient reliability and validity, and have been successfully utilized in primary care settings in the identification of emotional and behavioral symptoms/disorders, such as the Pediatric Symptoms Checklist (PSC; Gardner et al., 1999), the Strengths and Difficulties Questionnaire (SDQ; Goodman, 1997), or the Early Childhood Screening Assessment (Gleason, Zeanah, & Dickstein, 2010). Concerns noted in these general psychosocial measures can prompt further screening with the tools identified in the screening and assessment section of this chapter. Furthermore, pediatricians and other behavioral health clinicians can assess treatment effectiveness through ongoing progress monitoring of ODD symptoms. Specifically, many of the screening tools identified above, such as the Vanderbilt, SNAP-IV-C, CADBI, or DBD-RS can be used to monitor and track progress.

In addition to regular behavioral health screenings, primary care physicians can, and should, provide education to parents regarding the nurturance of healthy social/emotional and cognitive development, in addition to information promoting the physical health of their children (Dosman & Andrews, 2012). Guidance and coaching in the primary care setting during well visits or immunization appointments regarding important developmental milestones such as strong parent-child attachments, healthy sleep habits, prosocial behaviors, self-discipline/self-regulation, and problem-solving skills can promote optimal developmental outcomes and reduce the likelihood that a child will develop ODD (Dosman & Andrews, 2012).

While it is clear that global assessment and universal screenings within the primary care setting are important, there is evidence that primary care providers report a lack of confidence with regard to their training and ability to address children's emotional and behavioral issues (Cunningham, 2009). Ongoing efforts to improve the quality of integrated care should address the barriers to providing mental health screenings and treatment in the primary care setting (e.g., lack of time, unavailability of mental health providers for referrals, increasing mandates, etc.; Cunningham, 2009; Weitzman, et al., 2015).

The support for the provision of behavioral health care in the primary care setting is strong, and the successful integration of services continues to be a dynamic process. There are a number of resources for primary care providers to address the quality improvement of integrated care and to offer strategies and tools to overcome barriers in service provision. The Bazelon Center for Mental Health Law (2009a, 2009b) identified the following strategies for quality assurance in integrated care and can be applied to the treatment of ODD within the integrated care setting: (a) use of evidence-based practices, (b) person-centered care, (c) measurement of improvement and outcomes, and (d) expanding the use of technology. The use of evidence-based practices in the assessment and treatment of ODD, with an emphasis on individualized treatment and care, is key.

The successful treatment of ODD can be accomplished by providing referrals to necessary resources and supports and offering guidance/coaching to help parents/caregivers make positive changes in their parenting approaches. Progress monitoring on an individual (patient/family) and aggregate basis (all patients receiving ODD-focused interventions) to determine treatment effectiveness is another useful strategy for quality improvement. Finally, the use of technology can assist in more efficient screening and assessment for ODD symptoms as well as improve collaboration among providers (e.g., coordination of care through teleconferencing, better electronic records, etc.; The Bazelon Center for Mental Health Law, 2009a, 2009b). Integrated care settings service the needs of children with ODD and their families to reduce problematic symptoms, increase access to necessary services, enhance the quality of care, and lower overall/long-term health-care costs.

References

American Psychiatric Association. (2013). *Diagnostic and statistical manual of mental disorders* (5th ed.). Arlington, VA: American Psychiatric Publishing.

Achenbach, T. M. (1991). *Manual for the child behavior checklist/4-18 and 1991 profile* (p. 288). Burlington, VT: Department of Psychiatry, University of Vermont.

Asarnow, J. R., Rozenman, M., Wiblin, J., & Zeltzer, L. (2015). Integrated medical-behavioral care compared with usual primary care for child and adolescent behavioral health: A meta-analysis. *JAMA Pediatrics, 169*(10), 929–937. https://doi.org/10.1001/jamapediatrics.2015.1141

Bagner, D. M., Boggs, S. R., & Eyberg, S. M. (2010). Evidence-based school behavior assessment of externalizing behavior in young children. *Education and Treatment of Children, 33*, 65–83.

Barkley, R. A., & Benton, C. M. (2013). *Your defiant child: 8 steps to better behavior* (2nd ed.). New York: The Guilford Press.

Baumrind, D. (1966). Effects of authoritative parental control on child behavior. *Child Development, 37*(4), 887–907.

Bazelon Center for Mental Health Law. (2009a). *Integration of mental health in quality-assurance policies (A healthcare reform issue brief)*. Washington, DC: Author.

Bazelon Center for Mental Health Law. (2009b). *Primary care providers' role in mental health (a healthcare reform issue brief)*. Washington, DC: Author.

Berry, J. (2010). *Help me be good: Disobeying*. New York: Joy Berry Books.

Burke, J. D., Loeber, R., & Birmaher, B. (2002). Oppositional defiant and conduct disorder: A review of the past 10 years, part II. *Journal of the American Academy of Child and Adolescent Psychiatry, 41*, 1275–1293.

Burns, G. L., Taylor, T. K., & Rusby, J. C. (2001). *Child and adolescent disruptive behavior inventory 2.3: Parent Version*. Pullman, WA: Washington State University, Department of Psychology.

Canino, G., Polanczyk, G., Bauermeister, J. J., Rohde, L. A., & Frick, P. J. (2010). Does the prevalence of CD and ODD vary across cultures? *Social Psychiatry and Psychiatric Epidemiology, 45*, 695–704. https://doi.org/10.1007/s00127-010-0242-y

Chorpita, B. F., Reise, S., Weisz, J. R., Grubbs, K., Becker, K. D., & Krull, J. L. (2010). Evaluation of the brief problem checklist: Child and caregiver interviews to measure clinical progress. *Journal of Consulting and Clinical Psychology, 78*(4), 526.

Clark, L. (2005). *SOS help for parents: A practical guide for handling common everyday behavior problems* (3rd ed.). Bowling Green, KY: SOS Programs & Parents Press.

Cook, J. (2011). *I just don't like the sound of NO!* Boys Town, NE: Boys Town Press.

Comfort, M., & Gordon, P. R. (2006). The Keys to Interactive Parenting Scale (KIPS): A practical observational assessment of parenting behavior. *NHSA Dialog, 9*(1), 22–48.

Connor, D. F. (2002). *Aggression and antisocial behavior in children and adolescents: Research and treatment*. New York: Guilford Press.

Conners, C. K., Wells, K. C., Parker, J. D., Sitarenios, G., Diamond, J. M., & Powell, J. W. (1997). A new self-report scale for assessment of adolescent psychopathology: Factor structure, reliability, validity, and diagnostic sensitivity. *Journal of Abnormal Child Psychology, 25*, 487–497.

Cunningham, P. J. (2009). Beyond parity: Primary care physicians perspectives on access to mental health care. *Health Affairs, 28*(3), w490–w501. https://doi.org/10.1377/hlthaff.28.3.w490

Dosman, C., & Andrews, D. (2012). Anticipatory guidance for cognitive and social-emotional development: Birth to five years. *Paediatric Child Health, 17*(2), 75–80.

Eyberg, S. M., Boggs, S. R., & Algina, J. (1995). Parent-child interaction therapy: A psychosocial model for the treatment of young children with conduct problem behavior and their families. *Psychopharmacology Bulletin, 31*, 83–91.

Eyberg, S. M., Nelson, M. M., Ginn, N. C., Bhuiyan, N., & Boggs, S. R. (2013). *Dyadic parent-child interaction coding system: Comprehensive manual for research and training* (4th ed.). Gainesville, FL: PCIT International.

Eyberg, S. M., & Pincus, D. (1999). *Eyberg child behavior inventory and sutter-eyberg behavior inventory-revised: Professional manual*. Odessa, FL: Psychological Assessment Resources.

Eysenbach, G. (2001). What is e-health? *Journal of Medical Internet Research, 3*(2), e20.

Fabiano, G. A., Pelham, W. E., Jr., Waschbusch, D. A., Gnagy, E. M., Lahey, B. B., Chronis, A. M., … Burrows-MacLean, L. (2006). A practical measure of impairment: Psychometric properties of the impairment rating scale in samples of children with attention deficit hyperactivity disorder and two school-based samples. *Journal of Clinical Child and Adolescent Psychology, 35*(3), 369–385.

Forgatch, M. S., & DeGarmo, D. (1999). Parenting through change: An effective parenting training program for single mothers. *Journal of Consulting and Clinical Psychology, 67*, 711–724.

Gardner, W., Murphy, J. M., Childs, G., Kelleher, K., Pagano, M. E., Jellinek, M. S., … Chiapetta, L. (1999). The PSC-17: A brief pediatric symptom checklist with psychosocial problem subscales. A report from PROS and ASPN. *Ambulatory Child Health, 5*, 225–236.

Gleason, M. M., Zeanah, C. H., & Dickstein, S. (2010). Recognizing young children in need of mental health assessment: Development and preliminary validity of the early childhood screening assessment. *Infant*

Mental Health Journal, 31(3), 335–357. https://doi.org/10.1002/imhj.20259

Goodman, R. (1997). The strengths and difficulties questionnaire: A research note. *Journal of Child Psychology and Psychiatry, 38*, 581–586.

Gottman, J., & Declaire, J. (1997). *Raising an emotionally intelligent child: The heart of parenting*. New York: Fireside.

Greene, R. W. (2014). *The explosive child: A new approach for understanding and parenting easily frustrated, chronically inflexible children*. New York: HarperCollins Publishers.

Greene, R. W., Ablon, J. S., Goring, J. C., Raezer-Blakely, L., Markey, J., Monuteaux, M. C., … Rabbitt, S. (2004). Effectiveness of collaborative problem solving in affectively dysregulated children with oppositional-defiant disorder: Initial findings. *Journal of Consulting and Clinical Psychology, 72*(6), 1157–1164. https://doi.org/10.1037/0022-006x.72.6.1157

Hamilton, S. S., & Armando, J. (2008). Oppositional defiant disorder. *American Family Physician, 78*(7), 861–866.

Henggeler, S. W., Rodick, J. D., Borduin, C. M., Hanson, C. L., Watson, S. M., & Urey, J. R. (1986). Multisystemic treatment of juvenile offenders: Effects on adolescent behavior and family interactions. *Developmental Psychology, 22*, 132–141.

Kamphaus, R. W., Reynolds, C. R., Hatcher, N. M., & Kim, S. (2004). Treatment planning and evaluation with the Behavior Assessment System for Children (BASC). In M. E. Maruish (Ed.), *The use of psychological testing for treatment planning and outcomes assessment, Instruments for children and adolescents* (Vol. 2, 3rd ed.). Mahwah, NJ: Lawrence Erlbaum.

Kazdin, A. E. (2008). *The Kazdin method for parenting the defiant child*. New York: Houghton Mifflin Harcourt Publishing Company.

Kjøbli, J., & Ogden, T. (2012). A randomized effectiveness trial of brief parent training in primary care settings. *Prevention Science, 13*(6), 616–626. https://doi.org/10.1007/s11121-012-0289-y

Kolko, D. J., & Perrin, E. C. (2014). The integration of behavioral health interventions in children's health care: Services, sciences, and suggestions. *Journal of Clinical Child and Adolescent Psychology, 43*(2), 216–228. https://doi.org/10.1080/15374416.2013.862804

Lavigne, J. V., LeBailly, S. A., Gouze, K. R., Cicchetti, C., Pochyly, J., Arend, R., … Binns, H. J. (2008). Treating oppositional defiant disorder in primary care: A comparison of three models. *Journal of Pediatric Psychology, 33*(5), 449–461. https://doi.org/10.1093/jpepsy/jsm074

Loeber, R., Burke, J. D., Lahey, B. B., Winters, A., & Zera, M. (2000). Oppositional defiant and conduct disorder: A review of the past 10 years, part I. *Journal of the American Academy of Child and Adolescent Psychiatry, 39*(12), 1468–1484. https://doi.org/10.1097/00004583-200012000-00007

Maughan, B., Rowe, R., Messer, J., Goodman, R., & Meltzer, J. (2004). Conduct disorder and oppositional defiant disorder in a national sample: Developmental etiology. *Journal of Child Psychology and Psychiatry, 45*(3), 609–621. https://doi.org/10.1111/j.1469.7610.2004.00250.x

McMahon, R., & Forehand, R. (2003). *Helping the noncompliant child: Family-based treatment for oppositional behavior* (2nd ed.). New York: Guilford Press.

National Research Council & Institute of Medicine. (2009). Preventing mental, emotional, and behavioral disorders among young people: Progress and possibilities. Committee on the prevention of mental disorders and substance abuse among children, youth, and young adults: Research advances and promising interventions. In M. E. O'Connell, T. Boat, & K. E. Warner (Eds.), *Board on children, youth, and families, division of behavioral and social sciences and education*. Washington, DC: The National Academies Press. Retrieved from https://www.ncbi.nlm.nih.gov/books/NBK32775/pdf/Bookshelf_NBK32775.pdf

Olfson, M., Blanco, C., Wang, S., Laje, G., & Correll, C. U. (2014). National trends in the mental health care of children and adolescents, and adults by office-based physicians. *JAMA Psychiatry, 71*(1), 81–90. https://doi.org/10.1001/jamapsychiatry.2013.3074

Oppositional defiant disorder (ODD). (n.d.). *Mayo Clinic*. Retrieved October 10, 2016, from http://www.mayoclinic.org/diseases-conditions/oppositional-defiant-disorder/basics/definition/con-20024559

Pelham, W. E., Gnagy, E. M., Greenslade, K. E., & Milich, R. (1992). Teacher ratings of DSM-III-R symptoms for the disruptive behavior disorders. *Journal of the American Academy of Child & Adolescent Psychiatry, 31*(2), 210–218.

Reid, M. J., & Webster-Stratton, C. (2001). The incredible years parent, teacher, and child intervention: Targeting multiple areas of risk for a young child with pervasive conduct problems using a flexible, manualized, treatment program. *Journal of Cognitive and Behavior Practice, 8*, 377–386.

Riley, D. A. (1997). *The defiant child: A parent's guide to oppositional defiant disorder*. Lanham, MD: Taylor Trade Publishing.

Russell, A. A., Johnson, C. L., Hammad, A., Ristau, K. I., Zawadzki, S., Villar, L. D. A., & Coker, K. L. (2015). Prenatal and neighborhood correlates of oppositional defiant disorder (ODD). *Child and Adolescent Social Work Journal, 32*, 375–381. https://doi.org/10.1007/s10560-015-0379-3

Sanders, M. R. (1999). Triple P-Positive Parenting Program: Towards an empirically validated multilevel parenting and family support strategy for the prevention of behavior and emotional problems in children. *Clinical Child and Family Psychology Review, 2*(2), 71–90. *Journal of the American Academy of Child and Adolescent Psychiatry, 39*(1), 28–38.

Shaffer, D., Fisher, P., Lucas, C. P., Dulcan, M. K., & Schwab-Stone, M. E. (2000). *NIMH Diagnostic Interview Schedule for Children Version IV (NIMH DISC-IV): Description, differences from previous versions, and reliability of some common diagnoses*.

Shapiro, S., & White, C. (2014). *Mindful discipline: A loving approach to setting limits and raising an emotionally intelligent child*. Oakland, CA: New Harbinger Publications, Inc..

Shi, L. (2012). The impact of primary care: A focused review. *Scientifica, 2012*, 1–22. https://doi.org/10.6064/2012/432892

Siegel, D. J., & Payne Bryson, T. (2011). *The whole-brain child: 12 revolutionary strategies to nurture your child's developing mind*. New York: Bantam Books.

Steiner, H., & Remsing, L. (2007). Practice parameter for the assessment and treatment of children and adolescents with oppositional defiant disorder. *Journal of the American Academy of Child and Adolescent Psychiatry, 46*(1), 126–141.

Steinhausen, H. C., & Nøvik, T. S. (2006). ADORE Study Group: Co-existing psychiatric problems in ADHD in the ADORE cohort. *European Child and Adolescent Psychiatry, 15*(1), i25–i29.

Swanson, J. M., Kraemer, H. C., Hinshaw, S. P., Arnold, L. E., Conners, C. K., Abikoff, H. B., … Wu, M. (2001). Clinical relevance of the primary findings of the MTA: Success rates based on sverity of ADHD and ODD symptoms at the end of treatment. *Journal of the American Academy of Child and Adolescent Psychiatry, 40*, 168–179.

Vannest, K. J., Davis, J. L., Davis, C. R., Mason, B. A., & Burke, M. D. (2010). Effective intervention for behavior with a daily behavior report care: A meta-analysis. *School Psychology Review, 39*(4), 654–672.

Weitzman, C., Wegner, L., & Section on Developmental and Behavioral Pediatrics, Committee on Psychosocial Aspects of Child and Family Health, Council on Early Childhood, & Society for Developmental and Behavioral Pediatrics. (2015). Promoting optimal development: Screening for behavioral and emotional problems. *Pediatrics, 135*(2), 384–395. https://doi.org/10.1542/peds.2014-3716

Wilens, T. E. (2002). Psychiatric comorbidity and functioning in clinically referred preschool children and school-age youths with ADHD. *Journal of the American Academy of Child and Adolescent Psychiatry, 41*(3), 262–268. https://doi.org/10.1097/00004583-2002030000-00005

Wolraich, M. L., Lambert, W., Doffing, M. A., Bickman, L., Simmons, T., & Worley, K. (2003). Psychometric properties of the Vanderbilt ADHD diagnostic parent rating scale in a referred population. *Journal of Pediatric Psychology, 28*(8), 559–568.

World Health Organization. (2008). *Integrating mental health into primary care: A global perspective*. Geneva, Switzerland: World Health Organization.

27 Panic Disorder and Agoraphobia

Ellen I. Koch and Michelle A. Fernando

Panic disorder (PD) is characterized by the presence of recurrent unexpected panic attacks and anxiety about their reoccurrence. Panic attacks can be defined as, "an abrupt surge of intense fear or intense discomfort that reaches a peak within minutes" (p. 208, APA, 2013). These involve a wide range of physiological symptoms, such as increased heart rate, shortness of breath, sweating, chest pain, gastrointestinal distress, dizziness, and numbness. The rapid onset of these symptoms is often accompanied by psychological distress, such as the feeling of "going crazy," losing control, or dying. In addition to panic attacks, a diagnosis of PD necessitates at least 1 month of anxiety or avoidance about future panic attacks. To cope with this fear, the individual may avoid activities that involve physiological arousal, with the belief that arousal will provoke a full panic episode. For example, the individual may avoid physical exercise because these activities often lead to accelerated heart rate, sweating, and shortness of breath, which may also be experienced during a panic attack. In general, PD is characterized by both recurrent panic attacks and a persistent fear or avoidance of future panic episodes.

For some individuals with PD, nocturnal panic attacks may also occur. Nocturnal panic attacks occur abruptly upon awakening from sleep, as if the individual has woken up with a panic attack. In general, nocturnal panic attacks occur during the first 1–3 h of sleep and last from 2 to 8 min (Craske & Rowe, 1997). Some evidence suggests that individuals with nocturnal panic attacks may experience a higher frequency of panic attacks than individuals that experience only diurnal panic attacks (Mahony & Ward, 2003). PD with nocturnal panic attacks often manifests with a different symptom profile, with greater respiratory distress, feelings of being choked or smothered, and fears of death compared to day-only panic attacks (Mahony & Ward, 2003; Sarísoy, Böke, Arík, & Şahin, 2008).

Agoraphobia

When diagnosing PD, it is also important to assess for agoraphobia symptoms. Agoraphobia is characterized by anxiety about being in public spaces, such as using public transportation, going to sporting events, going to the theater, being in a large public park, standing in line, or generally being outside of the home. Anxiety in these situations revolves around the fear that one may not be able to escape or get help if a panic attack occurs, possibly leading to public embarrassment or bodily harm (APA, 2013). To compensate for this

E.I. Koch (✉) • M.A. Fernando
Department of Psychology, Eastern Michigan University, Ypsilanti, MI, USA
e-mail: ellen.koch@emich.edu; mfernan3@emich.edu

A. Maragakis, W.T. O'Donohue (eds.), *Principle-Based Stepped Care and Brief Psychotherapy for Integrated Care Settings*, https://doi.org/10.1007/978-3-319-70539-2_27

anxiety, the individual may avoid public spaces, spend most of his or her time at home, or engage in safety signals or behaviors. For example, many individuals with agoraphobia carry water bottles, prescription medications, go places with a friend, or identify the location of the nearest hospital to ensure safety in the case of a panic attack (Craske & Barlow, 2014). Agoraphobia is identified mainly by an avoidance or fear of public situations in which panic attacks may occur and help will not be available.

Because PD involves recurrent and often unexpected panic attacks, it is not uncommon for agoraphobia to manifest as an extension of the avoidance/persistent worry seen in PD. About 50% of individuals with PD will develop agoraphobia within the course of their illness (Batelaan, De Graaf, Van Balkom, Vollebergh, & Beekman, 2007; Wittchen et al., 2008). Comorbid PD and agoraphobia is more common in females than males (Inoue, Kaiya, Hara, & Okazaki, 2016). Agoraphobia may increase the overall problem severity, as combined agoraphobia and PD is associated with higher levels of impairment (Wittchen et al., 2008), suicide risk (Inoue et al., 2016), cued panic attacks (Kessler et al., 2006), and longer course of illness (Kikuchi et al., 2005). Having both disorders is also associated with an increased rate of comorbidity with social anxiety disorder (SAD; Inoue et al., 2016) and other anxiety disorders, substance use, and major depressive disorder (MDD; Kessler et al., 2006). When diagnosing PD, it is important to assess for agoraphobia as having both PD and agoraphobia is associated with a more severe course of illness.

Prevalence and Comorbidity

PD is fairly common in the general population. About 23% of the population will experience at least one panic attack during their lifetime, although not all of these cases will meet the criteria for PD (Kessler et al., 2006). Lifetime prevalence rates for PD range from 3 to 4%, with 1.2% of the population diagnosed with PD at any given time (Chou, 2010; de Jonge et al., 2016). Within a US sample, rates of PD appear to be highest in European Americans (5.1%), followed by Hispanic/Latino Americans (4.1%), African-Americans (3.8%), and Asian-Americans (2.1%; Asnaani, Richey, Dimaite, Hinton, & Hofmann, 2010). In addition, PD is more prevalent in females than males (Kessler et al., 2012; Rogers et al., 1994). Many individuals with PD endorse a history of trauma, particularly sexual assault and childhood physical abuse (Leskin & Sheikh, 2002). Other risk factors for PD include living in urban areas, having a low income, parent psychiatric history, low education, being divorced or separated, and being unemployed (Batelaan et al., 2007; de Jonge et al., 2016). In general, PD is a relatively common disorder, primarily among females and individuals with a history of trauma.

There is a high rate of comorbidity in individuals with PD. Of those diagnosed, 83% of individuals with PD have at least one more comorbid psychiatric disorder (Kessler et al., 2006), commonly a mood or other anxiety disorder (Birchall, Brandon, & Taub, 2000). Comorbid MDD is found in 64% of individuals with PD (Sherbourne et al., 2010) and is associated with higher rates of suicidal ideation (Baldwin, 1998). Common comorbid anxiety disorders include SAD (30%), specific phobia (34%), generalized anxiety disorder (GAD; 18%), and obsessive-compulsive disorder (OCD; 4%). In addition, panic attacks and PD are common in individuals with bipolar disorder, although the relationship between these two disorders is still unclear (Freeman, Freeman, & McElroy, 2002; Goodwin & Hoven, 2002). Because of the increased risks and differences in treatment associated with these disorders, it is important to assess for comorbid psychiatric disorders when treating PD.

While PD is associated with a range of physiological symptoms during panic attacks, comorbid medical illnesses are also common. Individuals with PD tend to have higher rates of hypertension, gastritis, obesity, angina, ulcers, arthritis, and tachycardia (Chou, 2010). These health conditions often vary by gender; in males, angina is common, while in females, thyroid disease is prevalent (Rogers et al., 1994). Some researchers have hypothesized that the high rate of medical illness is caused by the strain that recurrent panic attacks and autonomic arousal puts on the body (Rogers et al., 1994), although the precise relationship between PD and medical illness is not yet known.

Onset and Course

The reported age of onset in PD varies between studies, although PD usually occurs before the age of 40 years. Wittchen et al. (2008) reported that a first episode of PD usually occurs in adolescence, between the ages of 16 and 19 years. Kessler et al. (2006) reported a later age of onset; for panic attacks, the mean age of onset was 23.6 years, and for PD, the mean age of onset was 22.9 years. Some reports have indicated mean ages of onset within the mid-thirties age range (de Jonge et al., 2016; Kikuchi et al., 2005). In general, a first episode PD can occur anywhere between adolescence and young adulthood.

After a PD diagnosis is given, the predicted course of the disorder is varied. Levels of anxiety tend to fluctuate over time, alternating between periods of high anxiety and frequent panic attacks and periods of relatively minimal anxiety. While symptoms may resolve over time, most individuals experience recurrent episodes of PD, and some will experience a chronic course without panic-free periods (Angst, 1998). Episodes of PD tend to be persistent, lasting anywhere from 35 weeks to greater than 12 months (Kessler et al., 2006; Kikuchi et al., 2005). The course of PD is intermittent, alternating between prolonged periods of high anxiety and low anxiety.

Individuals with PD often have a high level of impairment compared to other anxiety disorders (Sherbourne et al., 2010). This population often exhibits higher rates of disability, poorer physical and emotional functioning, less social involvement, and more days in bed compared to a typical population of primary care patients (Barsky, Delamater, & Orav, 1999; Sherbourne et al., 2010; Wittchen et al., 2008). Individuals with PD tend to endorse higher amounts of pain, which may prevent them from engaging in everyday physical activities and chores (Birchall et al., 2000). In general, individuals with PD have more negative views of their physical and mental health compared to non-PD individuals (Batelaan et al., 2007). Because PD is associated with a mix of physiological and psychological symptoms, individuals with PD endorse high levels of impairment in both general and mental health domains.

Medical Utilization

Individuals with PD often utilize a large amount of medical services (Barsky et al., 1999), possibly due to high somatization of symptoms (Simon & VonKorff, 1991) or increased prevalence of medical illness (Deacon, Lickel, & Abramowitz, 2008). Such individuals most commonly seek assessment and treatment in general or primary care settings (Kessler et al., 2006), meaning that PD is likely to be first identified and diagnosed within primary care. Identification and differential diagnosis may be challenging; in a study by Rees, Richards, and Smith (1998), only 45% of physicians correctly identified anxiety or panic as the cause of the patient's symptoms. Individuals with PD frequently use other specialty settings as well, including psychiatry/psychology, cardiology, gastroenterology, neurology, and pulmonology (Deacon et al., 2008; Rees et al., 1998). It is also not uncommon for individuals to present to emergency medicine after the onset of a panic attack, often complaining of chest pain or other physiological distress. Over 20% of individuals presenting to emergency departments meet diagnostic criteria for PD, and the rates are higher for those seeking an evaluation for chest pain in outpatient cardiology clinics (Huffman & Pollack, 2003). Individuals reporting chest pain are more likely to have PD if they do not have coronary artery disease, are female, younger, experience atypical chest pain, and have high self-reported anxiety (Huffman & Pollack, 2003). Taken together, frequent utilization of general medicine, specialty medicine, hospitalization, and emergency services results in high costs both to the individual and to the medical system (Rees et al., 1998). PD must be identified and treated adequately to reduce unnecessary medical utilization.

Screening Options in Integrated Care

Several brief measures are available to assess PD within a primary care setting. Many of the screening measures available are subscales or portions of lengthier validated assessment measures such as the Primary Care Evaluation of Mental Disorders (PRIME-MD).

Table 27.1 outlines the commonly used brief screeners, many of which have been validated in primary care settings. The Patient Health Questionnaire screeners for the PRIME-MD are publically available (www.phqscreeners.com) as are the Overall Anxiety Severity and Impairment Scale (OASIS) and the Panic Disorder Severity Scale-Self-Report Form (PDSS-SR).

Table 27.1 Panic disorder and anxiety screening measures

Measure	Diagnosis	Number of items (cutoff score)	Citation
Anxiety and Depression Detector (ADD)	PD, PTSD, social phobia, GAD, and depression	5	Means-Christensen, Sherbourne, Roy-Byrne, Craske, and Stein (2006)
Autonomic Nervous System Questionnaire (ANS)	PD	2 (any endorsed) + 3 follow-up questions (5)	Stein et al. (1999)
Beck Anxiety Inventory-Primary Care (BAI-PC)	PD, GAD, or both	7 (5)	Beck, Steer, Ball, Ciervo, and Kabat (1997)
Brief Panic Disorder Screen (BPDS)	PD	4 (11)	Apfeldorf, Shear, Leon, and Portera (1994)
Composite International Diagnostic Interview Screening Scale, Panic Disorder (CIDI-SC PD)	PD	15	Kessler et al. (2013)
Hospital Anxiety and Depression Scale (HADS), anxiety subscale	Anxiety	7 (10)	Zigmond and Snaith (1983)
Mental Health Index-5 (MHI-5) from the SF-36 mental health subscale	PD or MDD	5 (23 or less)	Berwick et al. (1991) and Stewart, Hays, and Ware (1988)
Overall Anxiety Severity and Impairment Scale (OASIS)	Anxiety severity and impairment	5 (8)	Norman, Cissell, Means-Christensen, and Stein (2006)
Panic Disorder Severity Scale—Self-Report (PDSS-SR)	PD	7 (8)	Houck, Spiegel, Shear, and Rucci (2002) and Shear et al. (1997)
PRIME-MD 1. Brief Patient Health Questionnaire (BPHQ)—panic module	PD	4 (4)	Spitzer et al. (1994)
2. Patient Health Questionnaire (PHQ)—panic module	PD	5	
3. Patient Questionnaire (panic and GAD components)	PD or GAD	3 (any endorsed)	
Symptom Checklist-90 (SCL-90) subscales	PD Agoraphobia	9 (10) 6 (2)	Hunter et al. (2005)
Symptom- Driven Diagnostic System for Primary Care (SDDS-PC)	PD	3 (any endorsed)	Broadhead et al. (1995)

Note. *SF-36* Medical Outcomes Study Short Form Health Survey (SF-36), *PRIME-MD* Primary Care Evaluation of Mental Disorders, *PD* panic disorder, *GAD* generalized anxiety disorder, *PTSD* post-traumatic stress disorder, and *MDD* major depressive disorder

In terms of a single screening item, Means-Christensen, Arnau, Tonidandel, Bramson, and Meagher (2005) suggested from the MHI-5, a positive response to the item, "in the past four weeks have you been 'a very nervous person'," should signal an evaluation for PD. Additionally, Löwe et al. (2003) suggested using, "In the last four weeks, have you had a panic attack—suddenly feeling fear or panic?." Although these single-item screeners are quick, the high rate of false positives will require additional clinician or physician time to determine if the individual actually meets diagnostic criteria for PD. Additionally, utilizing the BPDS with African-American patients should be done with caution given a concern with high rates of false positives (Johnson et al., 2007).

Along with the very brief screener for PD, the full SDDS-PC covers several diagnoses including alcohol abuse and dependence, GAD, MDD, OCD, and suicidal ideation (Broadhead et al., 1995). This brief 16-item questionnaire assesses several conditions likely to be comorbid with PD and may provide a more comprehensive screening option for some primary care settings.

Although several brief screening options are available to detect PD or anxiety, these could be followed by more comprehensive assessment if desired. However, given that individuals with PD present for treatment in many settings including primary care, emergency departments, and outpatient clinics, broad screening options could help detect those who are likely to benefit from stepped care interventions. Additionally, given the high medical costs (Rees et al., 1998; Roy-Byrne et al., 1999) and the lack of effective, evidence-based treatment offered to many individuals with PD in primary care settings (Marcks, Weisberg, & Keller, 2009; Roy-Byrne et al., 1999), effective screening and treatment selection are essential.

Evidence-Based Care and Brief Psychotherapeutic Approaches

PD with and without agoraphobia is common in primary care settings, and extensive research consistently demonstrates the value of cognitive behavioral treatments (CBT), but unfortunately fewer than half of patients receive high-quality medication or CBT within 6 months prior to their referral (Stein et al., 2011). The two primary CBT options with extensive empirical support include panic control treatment (PCT; Barlow & Craske, 2007a, 2007b) and cognitive therapy (CT; Clark, 1994). PCT includes psychoeducation, breathing retraining, cognitive restructuring, in vivo exposure, interoceptive exposure to bodily sensations, and relapse prevention. CT emphasizes cognitive restructuring and correcting catastrophic misinterpretations of the physical symptoms of PD. Primary care interventions for PD and agoraphobia rely heavily on these treatment approaches.

Psychoeducation

Typical treatment for PD includes a psychoeducation component covering the potential causes for PD (e.g., anxiety sensitivity), the sympathetic and parasympathetic nervous system response (fight or flight) to potential threats, and the contribution of anxious thoughts. Additionally, psychoeducation includes a description and rationale for treatment. In covering information about PD, it is particularly helpful to tie the explanation to symptoms the individual is experiencing but also to cover common reactions since the patient may not realize some symptoms relate to panic attacks (e.g., intestinal distress) or may be less comfortable sharing potentially embarrassing physical symptoms. Finally, psychoeducation should include correcting any misinformation the patient has about the anxiety process or effective treatment options.

Although psychoeducation alone is rarely sufficient in the stepped care model, Baillie and Rapee (2004) found that 1/3 of their sample did not require the next step of care (self-help workbook). The psychoeducational booklet alone resulted in no longer experiencing panic attacks or significant agoraphobic avoidance at 6 weeks for this subset of participants.

Psychoeducation can be an essential component for fostering treatment motivation and normalizing experiences. For individuals with mild symptoms or who only very recently began experiencing panic attacks, it may be beneficial. However, it is only the first option in the stepped care model and most individuals will require more intensive treatment.

Self-Help/Bibliotherapy

Evidence for using bibliotherapy without any therapist contact is limited and generally not suggested. However, a review by Carlbring, Westling, and Andersson (2000) identified three empirically validated self-help books including *Mastery of Your Anxiety and Panic, Workbook and Therapist Guide* (4th Ed.; Barlow & Craske, 2007a, 2007b), *Coping with Panic: A Drug-Free Approach to Dealing with Anxiety Attacks* (Clum, 1990), and *Living with Fear: Understanding and Coping with Anxiety* (2nd Ed.; Marks, 2005). Utilizing the *Coping with Panic* book, two studies found between-group effect sizes of 1.5, and one study had a 0.5 effect size after treatment and 0.8 at 2-month follow-up (Carlbring et al., 2000). Another study utilized *Mastery of Your Anxiety and Panic* and demonstrated within-group effect sizes of 1.1 at posttest and 1.0 at 6-month follow-up with no difference between therapist-directed and self-directed treatments (Carlbring et al., 2000).

The American Psychological Association, Division 12: Society of Clinical Psychology, provides resources related to PD on their website (www.div12.org/psychological-treatments/disorders/panic-disorder/cognitive-behavioral-therapy-for-panic-disorder/). Specifically, the following self-help books are recommended (in addition to *Mastery of your Anxiety and Panic* listed above): *10 Simple Solutions to Panic: How to Overcome Panic Attacks, Calm Physical Symptoms, and Reclaim Your Life* (Anthony & McCabe, 2004), *Don't Panic: Taking Control of Anxiety Attacks* (3rd ed., Wilson, 2009), and *An End to Panic: Breakthrough Techniques for Overcoming Panic Disorder* (2nd ed., Zuercher-White, 1998).

Although some self-help books are based on empirically validated treatments for PD, studies find fully self-administered treatment to be less effective than interventions with some therapist contact. Specifically, Power, Sharp, Swanson, and Simpson (2000) utilized the same treatment manual for three conditions and found bibliotherapy to be less effective than guided self-help or brief CBT interventions, in terms of statistical and clinical significance, at posttest and 6-month follow-up. The bibliotherapy condition resulted in 34.5% of participants being panic-free compared to 54.9% for guided self-help and 72.4% for brief CBT (Power et al., 2000). Additionally, Newman, Erickson, Przeworski, and Dzus (2003) found that fully self-administered treatments for PD were not better than self-monitoring or waitlist. However, interventions involving predominantly self-help (with at least minimal therapist contact) based on in vivo exposure procedures were significantly better than no treatment and consistent with treatments involving greater therapist contact (Newman et al., 2003). Finally, Lewis, Pearce, and Bisson (2012) indicated self-help options without any professional contact were not as efficacious as therapist-administered treatments, but guided self-help options (ranging from 3 to 7 h of therapist time) were equally effective. A recent study utilized an unguided, transdiagnostic, Internet-based intervention for PD, GAD, and SAD. The intervention included coping with cognitions, mindfulness and relaxation, exposure, social relationships, and relapse prevention and required approval from a physician prior to accessing the program. Adding the Internet-based intervention to care as usual produced significant improvement at posttest and follow-up (Berger et al., 2017). Although the results of this study are promising, given that the unguided intervention was not compared to active treatment conditions, the results should be viewed cautiously. Therefore, guided self-help options are preferred over fully self-administered treatment.

Guided Self-Help

Many studies utilize a variety of self-help options with some therapist contact including bibliotherapy, Internet-, and computer-based interventions (including virtual reality) for PD. These interventions vary in the amount of therapist contact provided from minimal (i.e., email or brief phone calls only) to extensive. Four meta-analyses found computer-aided or Internet-guided self-help interventions significantly improved PD symptoms similar to those found in face-to-face CBT or primarily cognitive therapy at posttest and follow-up (Amstadter, Broman-Fulks, Zinzow, Ruggiero, & Cercone, 2009; Andrews, Cuijpers, Craske, McEvoy, & Titov, 2010; Cuijpers et al., 2009; Reger & Gahm, 2009). The guided self-help interventions did not produce higher rates of attrition than face-to-face CBT. Andrews et al. (2010) found good adherence to guided self-help and a treatment effect size of 0.83. Andersson, Bergström, Carlbring, and Lindefors (2005) indicated that guided self-help modalities are safe to implement. Although severity level of agoraphobia impacts effectiveness of face-to-face CBT, this is not a factor for guided self-help (Andersson, Carlbring, & Grimlund, 2008). Finally, Reger and Gahm (2009) included subclinical symptoms as well and still found guided self-help to be effective. In general, guided self-help may be an effective approach within a stepped care model.

Two empirically validated, Internet-based, guided self-help programs are publically available addressing PD and agoraphobia: CALM Tools for Living, http://www.calmtoolsforliving.org/, and FearFighter, http://fearfighter.cbtprogram.com/. CALM is a therapist-guided program addressing PD, PTSD, GAD, or SAD. CALM includes the following modules: self-monitoring, psychoeducation, fear hierarchy, breathing retraining, cognitive restructuring, in vivo exposure, interoceptive/image/memory exposure, and relapse prevention. Professionals can access the program based on number of users (cost ranging from $450 for 1–2 users to $300 for 21 or more users per year). CALM is equally effective for patients with or without comorbid depression (Campbell-Sills et al., 2012), reduces comorbid SAD (Craske et al., 2011), and effectively treats individuals not responding to medications (Campbell-Sills et al., 2016). FearFighter is a program covering PD, agoraphobia, and other phobias and can be purchased with or without clinician support provided within the program and can cut clinician contact time by 73% (Marks, Kenwright, McDonough, Whittaker, & Mataix-Cols, 2004). Both programs are acceptable to clinicians and patients (Craske et al., 2009; MacGregor, Hayward, Peck, & Wilkes, 2009). Another program, Panic Online, has been empirically validated; however, it is not publically available. Finally, the Society for Clinical Psychology recommends two smartphone applications (iCBT and Stop Panic & Anxiety Self-Help) to be used in conjunction with treatment.

Virtual reality exposure (VRE) is another intervention that could be utilized as guided self-help. VRE has been successfully utilized to address agoraphobic avoidance and found to be equally effective to in vivo exposure, but is easier to implement given the difficulty completing exposure in numerous and diverse settings, and results in lower attrition (Meyerbröker & Emmelkamp, 2010). Additionally, VRE can be effectively implemented via computer or head-mount and with at least moderate presence (Meyerbröker, Morina, Kerkhof, & Emmelkamp, 2011). Although VRE is regularly used with agoraphobia, a novel approach involved VRE for interoceptive exposure. Perez-Ara et al. (2010) compared VRE with audio and visual interoceptive sensations in typically avoided agoraphobia settings with traditional VRE for agoraphobia and interoceptive exposure. Both treatments were effective at posttest and maintained gains with some additional improvements at follow-up. This study suggests that VRE can be used as guided self-help to simulate both in vivo and interoceptive exposure.

Guided self-help was also effectively implemented by nonmental health professionals. Rollman et al. (2005) utilized case managers to conduct telephone-based collaborative care with a guided self-help manual. The case managers conducted a detailed mental health assessment, provided psychoeducation, assessed treatment preferences, monitored treatment response, and informed the physician of treatment preference and progress. The patients remained improved at 12-month follow-up, reduced anxiety and depression, and increased quality of life including missing fewer work days and remaining employed. These changes occurred while not increasing the number of primary care visits as compared to a treatment as usual group (Rollman et al., 2005).

Guided self-help interventions reduce therapist time (Bergstrom et al., 2010) and increase accessibility of treatment particularly for those with difficulty engaging in treatment due to agoraphobia, comorbid conditions, stigma, or distance barriers. Although support is needed in guided self-help, this support could be effectively provided by an administer instead of a therapist (Cuijpers et al., 2009). General practitioners without prior CBT knowledge have been effectively trained to implement the intervention (Heatley, Ricketts, & Forrest, 2005). In one study, most participants recovered within the first two steps (psychoeducation and guided self-help) with very little therapist involvement (Nordgreen et al., 2016). Guided self-help with minimal contact from a professional is efficacious and should be utilized in primary care settings either with or without more intensive CBT or group treatment.

Group Treatment

Group treatment offers another effective stepped care option that reduces therapist contact per patient. Schwartze et al. (2017) conducted a meta-analysis of group treatments for PD and found large effect sizes when compared to no treatment and no difference between group and individual CBT. The group intervention also produced large effects on depression and general anxiety. Following group treatment, 78% of participants were classified as panic-free compared to 71% for other treatments and 33% for no treatment control. Additionally, the attrition rate for group was 15% compared to 16% for other active treatments (Schwartze et al., 2017). Group treatment is also effective when administered intensively over a weekend or 2 weeks (Austin, Sumbundu, Lykke, & Oestrich, 2008; Teng et al., 2015) with the weekend treatment also reducing PTSD, anxiety, and depression (Teng et al., 2015). Although group treatment is clearly effective, 95% of wait-list participants selected individual over group (Sharp, Power, & Swanson, 2004).

One recent study looked at factors contributing to attrition from group treatment. Bélanger et al. (2017) indicated higher attrition prior to exposure for patients with high expectations and prior treatment and during exposure for those with comorbid depression and children. Older participants were more likely to complete treatment. Being aware of potential characteristics contributing to attrition could allow clinicians to monitor progress and provide additional support to particular participants if needed.

Empirically validated CBT procedures can be effectively implemented in a group format within a stepped care model while attending to attrition risk factors. Participants also benefit from reducing symptoms of comorbid conditions and learning from other group members. Given this, group treatment can be effectively implemented within the primary care setting for individuals with PD with and without agoraphobia.

Brief Treatment

Within the stepped care model, the ability to have other professionals implement a portion of treatment reduces cost and time with the clinician. Additionally, these interventions typically involve a portion of an empirically validated treatment that is expected to produce some benefit for those that do not require more intensive intervention.

One portion of treatment for PD that could be implemented by other professionals is breathing retraining (i.e., diaphragmatic breathing); however, concerns regarding this technique should limit its use. Specifically, breathing retraining is likely to impact a minority of patients and runs the risk of suggesting the physiological sensations present during panic attacks should be avoided, which contradicts the purpose of interoceptive exposure and the treatment rationale for CBT (Taylor, 2001). Breathing retraining should only be used for those with problems related to hyperventilation or recurrent chest pain from chronic chest breathing at the beginning of treatment to reduce unwanted (but not dangerous) sensations and be discontinued once interoceptive exposure starts (Taylor, 2001). For those patients where breathing retraining is indicated, this could be taught in a single session by professional staff.

Professional staff could also be trained to complete cognitive restructuring in one visit. Specifically, the support staff could gather information about the estimated number of panic attacks experienced by the individual (calculated based on average number per week × 52 × years) and the feared consequences (e.g., dying, going crazy, losing control, fainting, having heart attack, etc.) and write this information down for the patient. Once the feared consequences are listed, the patient is asked to indicate how many times each of these feared consequences have occurred and the number is listed by each fear. The staff person could then provide information about the average number of panic attacks experienced by other patients and the numbers of times that each of the same feared consequences occurred and record this information on the same sheet. Finally, the patient is asked for any other evidence to indicate that the feared consequences are not likely to occur (e.g., medical tests ruling out cardiac problems, have not fainted so far, able to walk up flights of stairs so heart seems fine, etc.) and these are listed at the bottom of the page. The patient is asked to review this counter evidence to their feared consequences frequently. This could be completed fairly quickly within the primary care setting.

Along with other professionals completing a portion of treatment, clinicians have successfully implemented brief and very brief treatment for PD with effects similar to longer treatment options. Specifically, five to six sessions or an intensive 2-day option was as effective as longer CBT treatment and required much less therapist contact (Otto et al., 2012). One additional study utilized novice therapists to effectively implement brief CBT for PD. The intervention involved six sessions of CBT followed by six brief phone calls implemented by midlevel behavior health specialists without prior experience with CBT (Roy-Byrne, Craske, et al., 2005).

Non-clinicians can be effectively trained to implement empirically validated treatments, and clinicians can successfully utilize brief interventions for PD. However, which portions of the treatment should be completed by various levels of care remains unclear. CBT for PD with or without agoraphobia involves several aspects including cognitive restructuring, interoceptive exposure, and in vivo exposure with different approaches emphasizing the cognitive or the behavioral components with equal success. The ability to distinguish significant treatment components likely to be effective with a particular individual could provide guidance for brief interventions in primary care settings outside of the full treatment package. Once essential components are identified, it could be determined who would be best to implement each portion in the most cost-effective manner.

Longer Treatment

Individuals who do not fully respond to earlier levels of stepped care should receive a full course of CBT for PD with or without agoraphobia. One study found stepped care to be equal to immediate face-to-face treatment but had higher attrition (Nordgreen et al., 2016). Another study found 12 sessions of CBT was significantly better than only 6 sessions (Kenardy et al., 2003). Additionally, studies have found six or more sessions of CBT effectively helped individuals not responding to medication (Campbell-Sills et al., 2016; Rodrigues et al., 2011), and CBT alone outperformed the combination of CBT and medication (Campbell-Sills et al., 2016). A higher dose of CBT is needed for some individuals, particularly those non-responsive to previous treatment or those at higher risk for attrition.

Several meta-analysis and review studies have demonstrated the superiority of CBT for PD with and without agoraphobia in primary care settings. Westen and Morrison (2001) indicated that a substantial number of PD patients improve and remain improved over time with CBT more so than those with GAD and MDD. CBT is more effective than pharmacotherapy alone and has less attrition and refusal (Butler, Chapman, Forman, & Beck, 2006; Roshanaei-Moghaddam et al., 2011; Swift, Greenberg, Tompkins, & Parkin, 2017). In terms of the combination of CBT and medications, some studies find CBT alone to be more effective particularly at follow-up (Butler et al., 2006), and some find the combination to be superior to either treatment alone (Furukawa, Watanabe, & Churchill, 2006). Although only two studies met inclusion criteria, Watanabe, Churchill, and Furukawa (2007) indicated that combining CBT with benzodiazepines was helpful in the acute phase, but not for follow-up. Comparing cognitive versus behaviorally focused therapies, Furukawa et al. (2006) and Ougrin (2011) found both approaches to be equally effective at follow-up, while Mitte (2005) indicated the two were equal in terms of anxiety, but cognitive therapy was more successful with comorbid depression and resulted in lower attrition. Alternatively, exposure (both interoceptive and in vivo) and breathing retraining/anxiety management were more effective than cognitive therapy and in vivo exposure provided the greatest benefit for both PD and agoraphobia (Sánchez-Meca, Rosa-Alcázar, Marín-Martínez, & Gómez-Conesa, 2010). CBT also improved quality of life in general (Mitte, 2005) and over Internet-based intervention (Hofmann, Wu, & Boettcher, 2014). Finally, CBT for PD effectively reduces comorbid depression and general anxiety (Cuijpers, Cristea, Weitz, Gentili, & Berking, 2016; Cuijpers, Gentili, et al., 2016) with reductions in depression similar to those achieved with depression treatment.

CBT for PD with and without agoraphobia is well established and exceeds pharmacology alone but is also effective when implemented with medications particularly during the acute phase of treatment. Additionally, CBT should be continued or reinstated when medication is discontinued (Otto, Smits, & Reese, 2004). Both cognitive and behavioral interventions are equally effective, but cognitive therapy is more effective if comorbid depression is present (Mitte, 2005). CBT not only reduces the symptoms of PD and agoraphobia, it also increases the quality of life (Mitte, 2005) and reduces symptoms of depression and general anxiety (Cuijpers, Cristea, et al., 2016; Cuijpers, Gentili, et al., 2016). When given an option, many patients select CBT over medications (Roy-Byrne et al., 2010). Administering a greater number of high-quality CBT elements is associated with to more patient satisfaction (Stein et al., 2011). Therefore, CBT (either with or without medication in the acute phase) is the first-line treatment for PD with or without agoraphobia in primary care settings.

Other Treatment Options

Other treatment options for PD, or related conditions, have promising results, but additional research is needed to verify efficacy. Specifically, limited research supports interventions related to prevention and those utilized for non-cardiac chest pain as well as those focused on lifestyle changes, exercise alone, or transdiagnostic approaches. A study with individuals who experienced at least one panic attack in the past year, but did not meet diagnostic criteria for PD, were offered one 5-hour workshop covering CBT for PD and monthly calls for 6 months. Those in the intervention were less likely to develop PD, more improved with panic attacks, and less likely to avoid social situations compared to a waitlist (Gardenswartz & Craske, 2001). Interventions designed for non-cardiac chest pain within an emergency department include either a one (2-hour) session CBT panic management vs. seven session CBT (Lessard et al., 2012) or six sessions of cognitive therapy (Van Beek et al., 2013). All three options were effective, but individuals with more severe PD benefitted from the longer treatment (Lessard et al., 2012).

Lambert, Harvey, and Poland (2007) conducted a lifestyle-based, ten-session intervention over 16 weeks with occupational therapy focused on fluid intake; diet; exercise; caffeine, alcohol and nicotine use; negotiating positive lifestyle changes; and monitoring and reviewing impact of changes. Although the intervention reduced anxiety initially, the effect did not remain significantly different than treatment as usual at 10 months. Despite this, 67.7% of participants were panic-free at follow-up (compared to 48.5% for the control group) and maintained their lifestyle habits. Another study looked at exercise and found effects but also had very high attrition (31%) that was similar to rates for medications (Asmundson et al., 2013). Finally, one study found Acceptance and Commitment Therapy (ACT) to be efficacious compared to CBT for various anxiety disorders with 42% of the sample meeting diagnostic criteria for PD with or without agoraphobia (Arch et al., 2012). Although more research is needed, transdiagnostic and prevention approaches in particular seem promising as do interventions targeting non-cardiac chest pain.

What Does Not Work

Although nonsignificant studies are rarely published, Shear, Houck, Greeno, and Masters (2001) demonstrated that one condition (emotion-focused treatment) produced results similar to placebo even after 3 months of active treatment and 6 months of follow-up maintenance. The intervention addressed emotional reactions and current life problems utilizing reflective listening and supportive therapy. Both CBT and medication were significantly more effective compared to this treatment.

Another issue that potentially impacts treatment efficacy is the acute disease model that has been the focus of medical care. Such an approach does not allow time for education or follow-up care, both of which are important in treatment for PD and managing chronic diseases (Roy-Byrne, Wagner, & Schraufnagel, 2005). The ability to shift from historical care to more modern disease management and even prevention is likely to significantly impact treatments for PD in primary care settings.

Considering treatment preferences is important in the success of an intervention. Providing information about treatment options and the potential risks and benefits of each will be valuable for patients prior to selecting the best course of action. Along with implementing the preferred treatment approach ideally, it is important to increase homework compliance. Homework fosters generalization and assists with efficient treatment progress particularly for CBT.

In relation to exposure-based procedures, it is thought that anxiety control or safety behaviors reduce anxiety in the short term but increase or maintain anxiety in the long run (Helbig-Lang et al., 2014). However, Parrish, Radomsky, and Dugas (2008) conducted a review and indicated that anxiety control strategies are not always detrimental to exposure or need to be completely eliminated. Even though such behaviors can facilitate approach, it is important to distinguish the function of the behavior for the individual, particularly if the safety behaviors are serving as active coping compared to attempts to prevent feared catastrophes. Specifically, such behaviors are less counterproductive when they promote increased self-efficacy, do not require significant attention, lead to approach behavior and integration of new information, and do not promote misattributions of safety. Therefore the anxiety control or safety behaviors need to be classified as helpful or disruptive based on function and not form (Parrish et al., 2008). Although efficacious treatment is available for PD, some issues to consider include not using emotion-focused treatment, focusing on chronic disease management and prevention, following patient's treatment preference and facilitating homework compliance, reviewing function of any coping or safety behaviors, and knowing when to refer for specialty mental health.

When to Refer to Specialty Mental Health

Individuals who do not adequately respond to a sufficient dose and quality of CBT should be referred to specialty mental health. Additionally, individuals experiencing significant comorbidity or impairment of functioning would be good candidates for specialty care. Some individuals who do not respond to levels of stepped care may benefit from a longer or more intense trial of CBT or a combination of CBT and medications. If these options are not available within the primary care setting, referral to a specialist in anxiety disorders is warranted, particularly given that higher rates of high-quality medications or CBT are available from mental health providers in specialty care (Stein et al., 2011).

Role of Primary Medical Provider in Treatment

Given that many primary care patients are either not appropriately diagnosed or do not receive high-quality intervention (Roy-Byrne, Wagner, et al., 2005), the primary care physician can facilitate better screening and selection of stepped care interventions. The potential financial costs of under and misdiagnosis are significant given the high medical usage of individuals with PD (Barsky et al., 1999; Roy-Byrne, Wagner, et al., 2005). Medical providers should routinely screen for PD, MDD, and GAD given the prevalence of these conditions within the primary care setting. Specifically, about 4% of primary care patients will have PD, and the rates jump to 20–50% for those with cardiac or gastrointestinal presentations (Roy-Byrne, Wagner, et al., 2005). Additionally, positive screening should be followed with more detailed assessment as well as stepped care interventions. Given that CBT is effective for many disorders as well as subclinical conditions, the benefit of connecting patients with stepped care approaches is essential even if the exact diagnosis is unclear. Many of the effective CBT interventions were tested on several of the anxiety disorders, making a precise diagnosis less essential. Additionally, CBT significantly reduces comorbid anxiety disorders and depression in the context of treatment for PD (Haug et al., 2015). Therefore, increasing screening and treatment selection for individuals in primary care could potentially significantly decrease costs. Finally, treating PD early allows for briefer interventions before inflexible avoidance behaviors significantly negatively impact functioning (Haug et al., 2015). Fortunately given the high rate of medical usage, individuals with PD tend to present for treatment much earlier than other anxiety disorders allowing for early identification and treatment.

Assessing Impact on Care and Quality Improvement

Chen and Tsai (2016) identified potential risk factors contributing to treatment resistance. These included characteristics of PD, personal demographic factors, psychiatric and medical comorbidities, and psychosocial factors (see Chen & Tsai, 2016 for more details). Given the potential contribution of these risk factors for treatment resistance, their recommendation included the use of combined CBT and medication. Although this recommendation costs more than other stepped care treatment options, this intervention may be necessary for individuals who do not improve with stand-alone CBT treatment.

A few studies have specifically looked at the costs of stepped care interventions in relation to the expenses from high service utilization. Specifically, CBT for PD costs 1/3 less than medication treatment and leads to less utilization after treatment (Hunsley, 2003). When total medical costs are considered, CBT interventions save money and significantly increase anxiety-free days with moderate, incremental ambulatory costs (Joesch et al., 2012; Katon et al., 2006). CBT for both PD and GAD in stepped care is cost-effective while reducing work absences and increasing quality of life compared to care as usual (Goorden et al., 2014).

In terms of improving treatment quality, motivational interviewing techniques may increase treatment preference or motivation for change (Roy-Byrne, Wagner, et al., 2005). Determining the patient's current stage of change could highlight the most appropriate intervention for that individual initially. Additionally, identifying potential treatment barriers and conducting problem-solving to address issues will lead to greater treatment success (Roy-Byrne, Wagner, et al., 2005).

A significant amount of research demonstrates the efficacy of both the stepped care model in general and use of CBT techniques specifically for PD with and without agoraphobia in primary care settings. Interventions within primary care produce effects consistent with treatment from mental health specialists. Nonmental health workers can be effectively trained to implement portions of CBT, which would increase access to services and reducing overall cost of treatment implementation. Given the prevalent nature of PD and high service utilization, effective treatment options are essential and should be implemented as quickly as possible.

References

American Psychiatric Association. (2013). *Diagnostic and statistical manual of mental disorders* (5th ed.). Washington, DC: Author.

Amstadter, A. B., Broman-Fulks, J., Zinzow, H., Ruggiero, K. J., & Cercone, J. (2009). Internet-based interventions for traumatic stress-related mental health problems: A review and suggestion for future research. *Clinical Psychology Review*, *29*(5), 410–420. https://doi.org/10.1016/j.cpr.2009.04.001

Andersson, G., Bergström, J., Carlbring, P., & Lindefors, N. (2005). The use of the internet in the treatment of anxiety disorders. *Current Opinion in Psychiatry*, *18*(1), 73–77.

Andersson, G., Carlbring, P., & Grimlund, A. (2008). Predicting treatment outcome in internet versus face to face treatment of panic disorder. *Computers in Human Behavior*, *24*(5), 1790–1801. https://doi.org/10.1016/j.chb.2008.02.003

Andrews, G., Cuijpers, P., Craske, M. G., McEvoy, P., & Titov, N. (2010). Computer therapy for the anxiety and depressive disorders is effective, acceptable and practical health care: A meta-analysis. *PLoS One*, *5*(10), e13196. https://doi.org/10.1371/journal.pone.0013196

Angst, J. (1998). Panic disorder: History and epidemiology. *European Psychiatry*, *13*(Suppl. 2), 51s–55s. https://doi.org/10.1016/S0924-9338(98)80014-X

Anthony, M. M., & McCabe, R. E. (2004). *10 simple solutions to panic: How to overcome panic attacks, calm physical symptoms, and reclaim your life*. Oakland, CA: New Harbinger Publications, Inc..

Apfeldorf, W. J., Shear, M. K., Leon, A. C., & Portera, L. (1994). A brief screen for panic disorder. *Journal of Anxiety Disorders*, *8*(1), 71–78. https://doi.org/10.1016/0887-6185(94)90024-8

Arch, J. J., Eifert, G. H., Davies, C., Vilardaga, J. C. P., Rose, R. D., & Craske, M. G. (2012). Randomized clinical trial of cognitive behavioral therapy (CBT) versus acceptance and commitment therapy (ACT) for mixed anxiety disorders. *Journal of Consulting and Clinical Psychology*, *80*(5), 750–765. https://doi.org/10.1037/a0028310

Asmundson, G. J. G., Fetzner, M. G., Deboer, L. B., Powers, M. B., Otto, M. W., & Smits, J. A. J. (2013). Let's get physical: A contemporary review of the anxiolytic effects of exercise for anxiety and its disorders. *Depression and Anxiety*, *30*(4), 362–373. https://doi.org/10.1002/da.22043

Asnaani, A., Richey, J. A., Dimaite, R., Hinton, D. E., & Hofmann, S. G. (2010). A cross-ethnic comparison of lifetime prevalence rates of anxiety disorders. *The Journal of Nervous and Mental Disease*, *198*(8), 551–555. https://doi.org/10.1097/NMD.0b013e3181ea169f

Austin, S. F., Sumbundu, A. D., Lykke, J., & Oestrich, I. H. (2008). Treating panic symptoms within everyday clinical settings: The feasibility of a group cognitive behavioural intervention. *Nordic Journal of Psychiatry*, *62*(4), 287–293. https://doi.org/10.1080/08039480801984016

Baillie, A. J., & Rapee, R. M. (2004). Predicting who benefits from psychoeducation and self help for panic attacks. *Behaviour Research and Therapy*, *42*(5), 513–527. https://doi.org/10.1016/S0005-7967(03)00157-8

Baldwin, D. S. (1998). Depression and panic: Comorbidity. *European Psychiatry*, *13*(Suppl. 2). https://doi.org/10.1016/S0924-9338(98)80016-3

Barlow, D. H., & Craske, M. G. (2007a). *Mastery of your anxiety and panic, Therapist guide* (4th ed.). New York, NY: Oxford University Press.

Barlow, D. H., & Craske, M. G. (2007b). *Mastery of your anxiety and panic, Workbook* (4th ed.). New York, NY: Oxford University Press.

Barsky, A. J., Delamater, B. A., & Orav, J. E. (1999). Panic disorder patients and their medical care. *Psychosomatics*, *40*(1), 50–56.

Batelaan, N., De Graaf, R., Van Balkom, A., Vollebergh, W., & Beekman, A. (2007). Thresholds for health and thresholds for illness: Panic disorder versus subthreshold panic disorder. *Psychological Medicine*, *37*(2), 247–256. https://doi.org/10.1017/S0033291706009007

Beck, A. T., Steer, R. A., Ball, R., Ciervo, C. A., & Kabat, M. (1997). Use of the beck anxiety and depression inventories for primary care with medical outpatients. *Assessment*, *4*(3), 211–219. https://doi.org/10.1177/107319119700400301

Bélanger, C., Courchesne, C., Leduc, A. G., Dugal, C., El-Baalbaki, G., Marchand, A., … Perreault, M. (2017). Predictors of dropout from cognitive-behavioral group treatment for panic disorder with agoraphobia: An exploratory study. *Behavior Modification*, *41*(1), 113–140. https://doi.org/10.1177/0145445516656614

Berger, T., Urech, A., Krieger, T., Stolz, T., Schulz, A., Vincent, A., … Meyer, B. (2017). Effects of a transdiagnostic unguided internet intervention ("velibra") for anxiety disorders in primary care: Results of a randomized controlled trial. *Psychological Medicine, 47*(1), 67–80. https://doi.org/10.1017/S0033291716002270

Bergstrom, J., Andersson, G., Ljotsson, B., Ruck, C., Andreewitch, S., Karlsson, A., … Lindefors, N. (2010). Internet-versus group-administered cognitive behaviour therapy for panic disorder in a psychiatric setting: A randomised trial. *BMC Psychiatry, 10*, 54. https://doi.org/10.1186/1471-244X-10-54

Berwick, D. M., Murphy, J. M., Goldman, P. A., Ware, J. E. J., Barsky, A. J., & Weinstein, M. C. (1991). Performance of a five-item mental health screening test. *Medical Care, 29*(2), 169–176.

Birchall, H., Brandon, S., & Taub, N. (2000). Panic in a general practice population: Prevalence, psychiatric comorbidity and associated disability. *Social Psychiatry and Psychiatric Epidemiology, 35*(6), 235–241. https://doi.org/10.1007/s001270050233

Broadhead, W. E., Leon, A. C., Weissman, M. M., Barrett, J. E., Blacklow, R. S., Gilbert, T. T., … Higgins, E. S. (1995). Development and validation of the SDDS-PC screen for multiple mental disorders in primary care. *Archives of Family Medicine, 4*, 211–219.

Butler, A. C., Chapman, J. E., Forman, E. M., & Beck, A. T. (2006). The empirical status of cognitive-behavioral therapy: A review of meta-analyses. *Clinical Psychology Review, 26*(1), 17–31. https://doi.org/10.1016/j.cpr.2005.07.003

Campbell-Sills, L., Roy-Byrne, P. P., Craske, M. G., Bystritsky, A., Sullivan, G., & Stein, M. B. (2016). Improving outcomes for patients with medication-resistant anxiety: Effects of collaborative care with cognitive behavioral therapy. *Depression and Anxiety, 33*(12), 1099–1106. https://doi.org/10.1002/da.22574

Campbell-Sills, L., Sherbourne, C. D., Roy-Byrne, P., Craske, M. G., Sullivan, G., Bystritsky, A., … Stein, M. B. (2012). Effects of co-occurring depression on treatment for anxiety disorders: Analysis of outcomes from a large primary care effectiveness trial. *Journal of Clinical Psychiatry, 73*(12), 1509–1516. https://doi.org/10.4088/JCP.12m07955

Carlbring, P., Westling, B. E., & Andersson, G. (2000). A review of published self-help books for panic disorder. *Scandinavian Journal of Behaviour Therapy, 29*(June), 5–13. https://doi.org/10.1080/028457100439827

Chen, M. H., & Tsai, S. J. (2016). Treatment-resistant panic disorder: Clinical significance, concept and management. *Progress in Neuro-Psychopharmacology and Biological Psychiatry, 70*, 219–226. https://doi.org/10.1016/j.pnpbp.2016.02.001

Chou, K.-L. (2010). Panic disorder in older adults: Evidence from the national epidemiologic survey on alcohol and related conditions. *International Journal of Geriatric Psychiatry, 25*(8), 822–832. https://doi.org/10.1002/gps.2424

Clark, D. M. (1994). Cognitive therapy for panic disorder. In B. E. Wolfe & J. D. Maser (Eds.), *Treatment of panic disorder: A consensus development conference* (pp. 121–132). Arlington, VA: American Psychiatric Association.

Clum, G. A. (1990). *Coping with panic: A drug-free approach to dealing with anxiety attacks*. Pacific Grove, CA: Brooks/Cole Publishing.

Craske, M., & Barlow, D. H. (2014). Panic disorder and agoraphobia. In D. H. Barlow (Ed.), *Clinical handbook of psychological disorders* (pp. 1–61). New York, NY: The Guilford Press.

Craske, M. G., Rose, R. D., Lang, A., Welch, S. S., Campbell-Sills, L., Sullivan, G., … Roy-Byrne, P. P. (2009). Computer-assisted delivery of cognitive behavioral therapy for anxiety disorders in primary-care settings. *Depression and Anxiety, 26*(3), 235–242. https://doi.org/10.1002/da.20542

Craske, M. G., & Rowe, M. K. (1997). Nocturnal panic. *Clinical Psychology: Science and Practice, 4*(2), 153–174.

Craske, M. G., Stein, M. B., Sullivan, G., Sherbourne, C., Bystritsky, A., Rose, R. D., … Roy-Byrne, P. (2011). Disorder-specific impact of coordinated anxiety learning and management treatment for anxiety disorders in primary care. *Archives of General Psychiatry, 68*(4), 378. https://doi.org/10.1001/archgenpsychiatry.2011.25

Cuijpers, P., Cristea, I. A., Weitz, E., Gentili, C., & Berking, M. (2016). The effects of cognitive and behavioural therapies for anxiety disorders on depression: A meta-analysis. *Psychological Medicine, 46*(16), 3451–3462. https://doi.org/10.1017/S0033291716002348

Cuijpers, P., Gentili, C., Banos, R. M., Garcia-Campayo, J., Botella, C., & Cristea, I. A. (2016). Relative effects of cognitive and behavioral therapies on generalized anxiety disorder, social anxiety disorder and panic disorder: A meta-analysis. *Journal of Anxiety Disorders, 43*, 79–89. https://doi.org/10.1016/j.janxdis.2016.09.003

Cuijpers, P., Marks, I. M., van Straten, A., Cavanagh, K., Gega, L., & Andersson, G. (2009). Computer-aided psychotherapy for anxiety disorders: A meta-analytic review. *Cognitive Behaviour Therapy, 38*(2), 66–82. https://doi.org/10.1080/16506070802694776

de Jonge, P., Roest, A. M., Lim, C. C. W., Florescu, S. E., Bromet, E. J., Stein, D. J., … Scott, K. M. (2016). Cross-national epidemiology of panic disorder and panic attacks in the world mental health surveys. *Depression and Anxiety, 33*, 1–23. https://doi.org/10.1002/da.22572

Deacon, B., Lickel, J., & Abramowitz, J. S. (2008). Medical utilization across the anxiety disorders. *Journal of Anxiety Disorders, 22*(2), 344–350. https://doi.org/10.1016/j.janxdis.2007.03.004

Freeman, M. P., Freeman, S. A., & McElroy, S. L. (2002). The comorbidity of bipolar and anxiety disorders: Prevalence, psychobiology, and treatment issues. *Journal of Affective Disorders, 68*(1), 1–23. https://doi.org/10.1016/S0165-0327(00)00299-8

Furukawa, T. A., Watanabe, N., & Churchill, R. A. (2006). Psychotherapy plus antidepressant for panic disorder with or without agoraphobia: Systematic review. *British Journal of Psychiatry, 188*, 305–312.

Gardenswartz, C. A., & Craske, M. G. (2001). Prevention of panic disorder. *Behavior Therapy*, *32*(4), 725–737. https://doi.org/10.1016/S0005-7894(01)80017-4

Goodwin, R. D., & Hoven, C. W. (2002). Bipolar-panic comorbidity in the general population: Prevalence and associated morbidity. *Journal of Affective Disorders*, *70*(1), 27–33. https://doi.org/10.1016/S0165-0327(01)00398-6

Goorden, M., Muntingh, A., van Marwijk, H., Spinhoven, P., Adèr, H., van Balkom, A., … Hakkaart-van Roijen, L. (2014). Cost utility analysis of a collaborative stepped care intervention for panic and generalized anxiety disorders in primary care. *Journal of Psychosomatic Research*, *77*(1), 57–63. https://doi.org/10.1016/j.jpsychores.2014.04.005

Haug, T., Nordgreen, T., Öst, L.-G., Kvale, G., Tangen, T., Andersson, G., … Havik, O. E. (2015). Stepped care versus face-to-face cognitive behavior therapy for panic disorder and social anxiety disorder: Predictors and moderators of outcome. *Behaviour Research and Therapy*, *71*, 76–89. https://doi.org/10.1016/j.brat.2015.06.002

Heatley, C., Ricketts, T., & Forrest, J. (2005). Training general practitioners in cognitive behavioural therapy for panic disorder: Randomized-controlled trial. *Journal of Mental Health*, *14*(1), 73–82. https://doi.org/10.1080/09638230500047877

Helbig-Lang, S., Richter, J., Lang, T., Gerlach, A. L., Fehm, L., Alpers, G. W., … Wittchen, H.-U. (2014). The role of safety behaviors in exposure-based treatment for panic disorder and agoraphobia: Associations to symptom severity, treatment course, and outcome. *Journal of Anxiety Disorders*, *28*(8), 836–844. https://doi.org/10.1016/j.janxdis.2014.09.010

Hofmann, S. G., Wu, J. Q., & Boettcher, H. (2014). Effect of cognitive-behavioral therapy for anxiety disorders on quality of life: A meta-analysis. *Journal of Consulting and Clinical Psychology*, *82*(3), 375–391. https://doi.org/10.1037/a0035491

Houck, P. R., Spiegel, D. A., Shear, M. K., & Rucci, P. (2002). Reliability of the self-report version of the panic disorder severity scale. *Depression and Anxiety*, *15*(4), 183–185. https://doi.org/10.1002/da.10049

Huffman, J. C., & Pollack, M. H. (2003). Predicting panic disorder among patients with chest pain: An analysis of the literature. *Psychosomatics*, *44*(3), 222–236. https://doi.org/10.1176/appi.psy.44.3.222

Hunsley, J. (2003). Cost-effectiveness and medical cost-offset considerations in psychological service provision. *Canadian Psychology*, *44*(1), 61–73.

Hunter, E. E., Penick, E. C., Powell, B. J., Othmer, E., Nickel, E. J., & Desouza, C. (2005). Development of scales to screen for eight common psychiatric disorders. *The Journal of Nervous and Mental Disease*, *193*(2), 131–135. https://doi.org/10.1097/01.nmd.0000152786.61048.a1

Inoue, K., Kaiya, H., Hara, N., & Okazaki, Y. (2016). A discussion of various aspects of panic disorder depending on presence or absence of agoraphobia. *Comprehensive Psychiatry*, *69*, 132–135. https://doi.org/10.1016/j.comppsych.2016.05.014

Joesch, J. M., Sherbourne, C. D., Sullivan, G., Stein, M. B., Craske, M. G., & Roy-Byrne, P. (2012). Incremental benefits and cost of coordinated anxiety learning and management for anxiety treatment in primary care. *Psychological Medicine*, *42*(9), 1937–1948. https://doi.org/10.1017/S0033291711002893

Johnson, M. R., Hartzema, A. G., Mills, T. L., De Leon, J. M., Yang, M., Frueh, C., & Santos, A. (2007). Ethnic differences in the reliability and validity of a panic disorder screen. *Ethnicity & Health*, *12*(3), 283–296. https://doi.org/10.1080/13557850701235069

Katon, W., Russo, J., Sherbourne, C., Stein, M. B., Craske, M., Fan, M.-Y., & Roy-Byrne, P. (2006). Incremental cost-effectiveness of a collaborative care intervention for panic disorder. *Psychological Medicine*, *36*(3), 353–363. https://doi.org/10.1017/S0033291705006896

Kenardy, J. A., Dow, M. G. T., Johnston, D. W., Newman, M. G., Thomson, A., & Taylor, C. B. (2003). A comparison of delivery methods of cognitive-behavioral therapy for panic disorder: An international multicenter trial. *Journal of Consulting and Clinical Psychology*, *71*(6), 1068–1075. https://doi.org/10.1037/0022-006X.71.6.1068

Kessler, R. C., Avenevoli, S., McLaughlin, K. A., Green, J. G., Lakoma, M. D., Petukhova, M., … Merikangas, K. R. (2012). Lifetime co-morbidity of DSM-IV disorders in the US National Comorbidity Survey Replication Adolescent Supplement (NCS-A). *Psychological Medicine*, *42*, 1997–2010. https://doi.org/10.1002/mpr.357

Kessler, R. C., Calabrese, J. R., Farley, P. A., Gruber, M. J., Jewell, M. A., Katon, W., … Wittchen, H.-U. (2013). Composite international diagnostic interview screening scales for DSM-IV anxiety and mood disorders. *Psychological Medicine*, *43*(8), 1625–1637. https://doi.org/10.1017/S0033291712002334

Kessler, R. C., Chiu, W. T., Jin, R., Ruscio, A. M., Shear, K., & Walters, E. E. (2006). The epidemiology of panic attacks, panic disorder, and agoraphobia in the National Comorbidity Survey Replication. *Archives of General Psychiatry*, *63*(4), 415–424. https://doi.org/10.1001/archpsyc.63.4.415

Kikuchi, M., Komuro, R., Oka, H., Kidani, T., Hanaoka, A., & Koshino, Y. (2005). Panic disorder with and without agoraphobia: Comorbidity within a half-year of the onset of panic disorder. *Psychiatry and Clinical Neurosciences*, *59*(6), 639–643. https://doi.org/10.1111/j.1440-1819.2005.01430.x

Lambert, R. A., Harvey, I., & Poland, F. (2007). A pragmatic, unblinded randomised controlled trial comparing an occupational therapy-led lifestyle approach and routine GP care for panic disorder treatment in primary care. *Journal of Affective Disorders*, *99*(1–3), 63–71. https://doi.org/10.1016/j.jad.2006.08.026

Leskin, G. A., & Sheikh, J. I. (2002). Lifetime trauma history and panic disorder: Findings from the National Comorbidity Survey. *Journal of Anxiety Disorders, 16*(6), 599–603. https://doi.org/10.1016/S0887-6185(02)00125-1

Lessard, M.-J., Marchand, A., Pelland, M.-È., Belleville, G., Vadeboncoeur, A., Chauny, J.-M., … Lavoie, K. L. (2012). Comparing two brief psychological interventions to usual care in panic disorder patients presenting to the emergency department with chest pain. *Behavioural and Cognitive Psychotherapy, 40*(2), 129–147. https://doi.org/10.1017/S1352465811000506

Lewis, C., Pearce, J., & Bisson, J. I. (2012). Efficacy, cost-effectiveness and acceptability of self-help interventions for anxiety disorders: Systematic review. *British Journal of Psychiatry, 200*(1), 15–21. https://doi.org/10.1192/bjp.bp.110.084756

Löwe, B., Gräfe, K., Zipfel, S., Spitzer, R. L., Herrmann-Lingen, C., Witte, S., & Herzog, W. (2003). Detecting panic disorder in medical and psychosomatic outpatients: Comparative validation of the hospital anxiety and depression scale, the patient health questionnaire, a screening question, and physicians' diagnosis. *Journal of Psychosomatic Research, 55*(6), 515–519. https://doi.org/10.1016/S0022-3999(03)00072-2

MacGregor, A. D., Hayward, L., Peck, D. F., & Wilkes, P. (2009). Empirically grounded clinical interventions clients' and referrers' perceptions of computer-guided CBT (FearFighter). *Behavioural and Cognitive Psychotherapy, 37*(1), 1. https://doi.org/10.1017/S135246580800492X

Mahony, J. F. O., & Ward, B. G. (2003). Differences between those who panic by day and those who also panic by night. *Journal of Behavior Therapy and Experimental Psychiatry, 34*, 239–249. https://doi.org/10.1016/j.jbtep.2003.10.001

Marcks, B., Weisberg, R., & Keller, M. (2009). Psychiatric treatment received by primary care patients with panic disorder with and without agoraphobia. *Psychiatric Services, 60*(6), 823–830. https://doi.org/10.1176/appi.ps.60.6.823

Marks, I. M. (2005). *Living with fear: Understanding and coping with anxiety* (2nd ed.). New York, NY: McGraw-Hill Publishing Company.

Marks, I. M., Kenwright, M., McDonough, M., Whittaker, M., & Mataix-Cols, D. (2004). Saving clinicians' time by delegating routine aspects of therapy to a computer: A randomized controlled trial in phobia/panic disorder. *Psychological Medicine, 34*(1), 9–17. https://doi.org/10.1017/S003329170300878X

Means-Christensen, A. J., Arnau, R. C., Tonidandel, A. M., Bramson, R., & Meagher, M. W. (2005). An efficient method of identifying major depression and panic disorder in primary care. *Journal of Behavioral Medicine, 28*(6), 565–572. https://doi.org/10.1007/s10865-005-9023-6

Means-Christensen, A. J., Sherbourne, C. D., Roy-Byrne, P. P., Craske, M. G., & Stein, M. B. (2006). Using five questions to screen for five common mental disorders in primary care: Diagnostic accuracy of the anxiety and depression detector. *General Hospital Psychiatry, 28*(2), 108–118. https://doi.org/10.1016/j.genhosppsych.2005.08.010

Meyerbröker, K., & Emmelkamp, P. M. G. (2010). Virtual reality exposure therapy in anxiety disorders: A systematic review of process-and-outcome studies. *Depression and Anxiety, 27*(10), 933–944. https://doi.org/10.1002/da.20734

Meyerbröker, K., Morina, N., Kerkhof, G., & Emmelkamp, P. M. G. (2011). Virtual reality exposure treatment of agoraphobia: A comparison of computer automatic virtual environment and head-mounted display. *Annual Review of CyberTherapy and Telemedicine, 9*(1), 41–45. https://doi.org/10.3233/978-1-60750-766-6-51

Mitte, K. (2005). A meta-analysis of the efficacy of psycho- and pharmacotherapy in panic disorder with and without agoraphobia. *Journal of Affective Disorders, 88*(1), 27–45. https://doi.org/10.1016/j.jad.2005.05.003

Newman, M. G., Erickson, T., Przeworski, A., & Dzus, E. (2003). Self-help and minimal-contact therapies for anxiety disorders: Is human contact necessary for therapeutic efficacy? *Journal of Clinical Psychology, 59*(3), 251–274. https://doi.org/10.1002/jclp.10128

Nordgreen, T., Haug, T., Öst, L.-G., Andersson, G., Carlbring, P., Kvale, G., … Havik, O. E. (2016). Stepped care versus direct face-to-face cognitive behavior therapy for social anxiety disorder and panic disorder: A randomized effectiveness trial. *Behavior Therapy, 47*(2), 166–183. https://doi.org/10.1016/j.beth.2015.10.004

Norman, S. B., Cissell, S. H., Means-Christensen, A. J., & Stein, M. B. (2006). Development and validation of an overall anxiety severity and impairment scale (OASIS). *Depression and Anxiety, 23*, 245–249. https://doi.org/10.1002/da.20182

Otto, M. W., Smits, J. A. J., & Reese, H. E. (2004). Cognitive-behavioral therapy for the treatment of anxiety disorders. *Journal of Clinical Psychiatry, 65*(Suppl. 5), 34–41. Retrieved from http://www.scopus.com/inward/record.url?eid=2-s2.0-3843137540&partnerID=40&md5=ec83ac52323ff89fdb30f2d3ab6d066e

Otto, M. W., Tolin, D. F., Nations, K. R., Utschig, A. C., Rothbaum, B. O., Hofmann, S. G., & Smits, J. A. J. (2012). Five sessions and counting: Considering ultra-brief treatment for panic disorder. *Depression and Anxiety, 29*(6), 465–470. https://doi.org/10.1002/da.21910

Ougrin, D. (2011). Efficacy of exposure versus cognitive therapy in anxiety disorders: Systematic review and meta-analysis. *BMC Psychiatry, 11*(1), 200. https://doi.org/10.1186/1471-244X-11-200

Parrish, C. L., Radomsky, A. S., & Dugas, M. J. (2008). Anxiety-control strategies: Is there room for neutralization in successful exposure treatment? *Clinical Psychology Review, 28*(8), 1400–1412. https://doi.org/10.1016/j.cpr.2008.07.007

Perez-Ara, M. A., Quero, S., Botella, C., Banos, R., Andreu-Mateu, S., Garcia-Palacios, A., & Breton-Lopez, J. (2010). Virtual reality interoceptive exposure for the treatment of panic disorder and agoraphobia. *Annual Review of CyberTherapy and Telemedicine, 8*, 61–64.

Power, K. G., Sharp, D. M., Swanson, V., & Simpson, R. J. (2000). Therapist contact in cognitive behaviour therapy for panic disorder and agoraphobia in primary care. *Clinical Psychology and Psychotherapy, 7*, 37–46.

Rees, C. S., Richards, J. C., & Smith, L. M. (1998). Medical utilisation and costs in panic disorder: A comparison with social phobia. *Journal of Anxiety Disorders, 12*(5), 421–435.

Reger, M. A., & Gahm, G. A. (2009). A meta-analysis of the effects of internet- and computer-based cognitive-behavioral treatments for anxiety. *Journal of Clinical Psychology, 65*(1), 53–75. https://doi.org/10.1002/jclp

Rodrigues, H., Figueira, I., Gonçalves, R., Mendlowicz, M., Macedo, T., & Ventura, P. (2011). CBT for pharmacotherapy non-remitters-a systematic review of a next-step strategy. *Journal of Affective Disorders, 129*(1–3), 219–228. https://doi.org/10.1016/j.jad.2010.08.025

Rogers, M. P., White, K., Warshaw, M. G., Yonkers, K. A., Rodriguez-Villa, F., Chang, G., & Keller, M. B. (1994). Prevalence of medical illness in patients with anxiety disorders. *International Journal of Psychiatry in Medicine, 24*(1), 83–96. https://doi.org/10.2190/TXM9-EVX8-Q4WT-G03J

Rollman, B. L., Belnap, B. H., Mazumdar, S., Houck, P. R., Zhu, F., Gardner, W., … Shear, M. K. (2005). A randomized trial to improve the quality of treatment for panic and generalized anxiety disorders in primary care. *Archives of General Psychiatry, 62*(12), 1332–1341. https://doi.org/10.1001/archpsyc.62.12.1332

Roshanaei-Moghaddam, B., Pauly, M. C., Atkins, D. C., Baldwin, S. A., Stein, M. B., & Roy-Byrne, P. (2011). Relative effects of CBT and pharmacotherapy in depression versus anxiety: Is medication somewhat better for depression, and CBT somewhat better for anxiety? *Depression and Anxiety, 28*(7), 560–567. https://doi.org/10.1002/da.20829

Roy-Byrne, P., Craske, M. G., Sullivan, G., Rose, R. D., Edlund, M. J., Lang, A. J., … Stein, M. B. (2010). Delivery of evidence-based treatment for multiple anxiety disorders in primary care. *JAMA, 303*(19), 1921. https://doi.org/10.1001/jama.2010.608

Roy-Byrne, P. P., Craske, M. G., Stein, M. B., Sullivan, G., Bystritsky, A., Katon, W., … Sherbourne, C. D. (2005). A randomized effectiveness trial of cognitive-behavioral therapy and medication for primary care panic disorder. *Archives of General Psychiatry, 62*(3), 290–298. https://doi.org/10.1001/archpsyc.62.3.290

Roy-Byrne, P. P., Stein, M. B., Russo, J., Mercier, E., Thomas, R., McQuaid, J., … Sherbourne, C. D. (1999). Panic disorder in the primary care setting: Comorbidity, disability, service utilization, and treatment. *Journal of Clinical Psychiatry, 60*, 492–499.

Roy-Byrne, P. P., Wagner, A. W., & Schraufnagel, T. J. (2005). Understanding and treating panic disorder in the primary care setting. *The Journal of Clinical Psychiatry, 66*(Suppl 4), 16–22. Retrieved from http://www.ncbi.nlm.nih.gov/pubmed/15842183

Sánchez-Meca, J., Rosa-Alcázar, A. I., Marín-Martínez, F., & Gómez-Conesa, A. (2010). Psychological treatment of panic disorder with or without agoraphobia: A meta-analysis. *Clinical Psychology Review, 30*(1), 37–50. https://doi.org/10.1016/j.cpr.2009.08.011

Sarísoy, G., Böke, Ö., Arík, A. C., & Şahin, A. R. (2008). Panic disorder with nocturnal panic attacks: Symptoms and comorbidities. *European Psychiatry, 23*(3), 195–200. https://doi.org/10.1016/j.eurpsy.2007.08.003

Schwartze, D., Barkowski, S., Strauss, B., Burlingame, G. M., Barth, J., & Rosendahl, J. (2017). Efficacy of group psychotherapy for panic disorder: Meta-analysis of randomized, controlled trials. *Group Dynamics: Theory, Research, and Practice, 21*(2), 77–93. https://doi.org/10.1037/gdn0000064

Sharp, D. M., Power, K. G., & Swanson, V. (2004). A comparison of the efficacy and acceptability of group versus individual cognitive behaviour therapy in the treatment of panic disorder and agoraphobia in primary care. *Clinical Psychology and Psychotherapy, 11*, 73–82.

Shear, K. M., Brown, T. A., Barlow, D. H., Money, R., Sholomskas, D. E., Woods, S. W., … Papp, L. A. (1997). Multicenter collaborative panic disorder severity scale. *American Journal of Psychiatry, 154*(11), 1571–1575. https://doi.org/10.1176/ajp.154.11.1571

Shear, M. K., Houck, P., Greeno, C., & Masters, S. (2001). Emotion-focused psychotherapy for patients with panic disorder. *The American Journal of Psychiatry, 158*(12), 1993–1998. https://doi.org/10.1176/appi.ajp.158.12.1993

Sherbourne, C. D., Sullivan, G., Craske, M. G., Roy-Byrne, P., Golinelli, D., Rose, R. D., … Stein, M. B. (2010). Functioning and disability levels in primary care out-patients with one or more anxiety disorders. *Psychological Medicine, 40*(12), 2059–2068. https://doi.org/10.1017/S0033291710000176

Simon, G. E., & VonKorff, M. (1991). Somatization and psychiatric disorder in the NIMH epidemiologic catchment area study. *American Journal of Psychiatry, 148*(11), 1494.

Spitzer, R. L., Williams, J. B. W., Kroenke, K., Linzer, M., Verloin, F., Hahn, S. R., … Johnson, J. G. (1994). Utility of a new procedure for diagnosing mental disorders in primary care: The PRIME-MD 1000 study. *Journal of the American Medical Association, 272*(22), 1749–1756. https://doi.org/10.1001/jama.1994.03520220043029

Stein, M. B., Roy-Byrne, P. P., Craske, M. G., Campbell-Sills, L., Lang, A. J., Golinelli, D., … Sherbourne, C. D. (2011). Quality of and patient satisfaction with primary health care for anxiety disorders. *Journal of Clinical Psychiatry*, *72*(7), 970–976. https://doi.org/10.4088/JCP.09m05626blu

Stein, M. B., Roy-Byrne, P. P., Mcquaid, J. R., Laffaye, C., Russo, J., Mccahill, M. E., … Sherbourne, C. D. (1999). Development of a brief diagnostic screen for panic disorder in primary care. *Psychosomatic Medicine*, *61*(3), 359–364.

Stewart, A. L., Hays, R. D., & Ware, J. E. (1988). The MOS short-form general health survey: Reliability and validity in a patient population. *Medical Care*, *26*(7), 724–735. Retrieved from www.jstor.org/stable/37654

Swift, J. K., Greenberg, R. P., Tompkins, K. A., & Parkin, S. R. (2017). Treatment refusal and premature termination in psychotherapy, pharmacotherapy, and their combination: A meta-analysis of head-to-head comparisons. *Psychotherapy*, *54*(1), 47–57. https://doi.org/10.1037/pst0000104

Taylor, S. (2001). Breathing retraining in the treatment of panic disorder: Efficacy, caveats and indications. *Scandinavian Journal of Behaviour Therapy*, *30*(2), 49–56. https://doi.org/10.1080/02845710118895

Teng, E. J., Barrera, T. L., Hiatt, E. L., Chaison, A. D., Dunn, N. J., Petersen, N. J., & Stanley, M. A. (2015). Intensive weekend group treatment for panic disorder and its impact on co-occurring PTSD: A pilot study. *Journal of Anxiety Disorders*, *33*, 1–7. https://doi.org/10.1016/j.janxdis.2015.04.002

Van Beek, M. H. C. T., Oude Voshaar, R. C., Beek, A. M., Van Zijderveld, G. A., Visser, S., Speckens, A. E. M., … Van Balkom, A. J. L. M. (2013). A brief cognitive-behavioral intervention for treating depression and panic disorder in patients with noncardiac chest pain: A 24-week randomized controlled trial. *Depression and Anxiety*, *30*(7), 670–678. https://doi.org/10.1002/da.22106

Watanabe, N., Churchill, R., & Furukawa, T. A. (2007). Combination of psychotherapy and benzodiazepines versus either therapy alone for panic disorder: A systematic review. *BMC Psychiatry*, *7*(1), 18. https://doi.org/10.1186/1471-244X-7-18

Westen, D., & Morrison, K. (2001). A multidimensional meta-analysis of treatments for depression, panic, and generalized anxiety disorder: An empirical examination of the status of empirically supported therapies. *Journal of Consulting and Clinical Psychology*, *69*(6), 875–899. https://doi.org/10.1037/0022-006X.69.6.875

Wilson, R. (2009). *Don't panic: Taking control of anxiety attacks* (3rd ed.). New York, NY: HarperCollins Publishers.

Wittchen, H.-U., Nocon, A., Beesdo, K., Pine, D. S., Hofler, M., Lieb, R., & Gloster, A. T. (2008). Agoraphobia and panic. *Psychotherapy and Psychosomatics*, *77*, 147–157. https://doi.org/10.1159/000116608

Zigmond, A. S., & Snaith, R. P. (1983). The hospital anxiety and depression scale. *Acta Psychiatrica Scandinavica*, *67*(6), 361–370. https://doi.org/10.1111/j.1600-0447.1983.tb09716.x

Zuercher-White, E. (1998). *An end to panic: Breakthrough techniques for overcoming panic disorder* (2nd ed.). Oakland, CA: New Harbinger Publications..

Paraphilias: Problematic Sexual Interests

28

Daniel S. Bromberg

In the fifth edition of the American Psychiatric Association's *Diagnostic and Statistical Manual of Mental Disorders* (DSM-5; American Psychiatric Association, 2013), a problematic sexual interest, or paraphilia, is defined as "...any intense and persistent sexual interest other than sexual interest in genital stimulation or preparatory fondling with phenotypically normal, physically mature, consenting human partners" (p. 685). In cases in which intense and persistent sexual interests may not be present (e.g., very old or medically ill), "the term *paraphilia* may be defined as any sexual interest greater than or equal to normophilic (that is, normal) sexual interests" (p. 685).

There are eight paraphilic disorders listed in the DSM-5: voyeuristic disorder (spying on others engaging in private activities); exhibitionistic disorder (exposing one's genitals); frotteuristic disorder (touching or rubbing against a nonconsenting individual); sexual masochism disorder (undergoing humiliation, bondage, or suffering), sexual sadism disorder (inflicting humiliation, bondage, or suffering); pedophilic disorder (sexual attraction to prepubescent children); fetishistic disorder (using nonliving objects or having a highly specific focus on nongenital body parts) and; transvestic disorder (engaging in sexually arousing cross-dressing). However, it is noted that "the eight listed disorders do not exhaust the list of possible paraphilic disorders. Many dozens of distinct paraphilias have been identified and named, and almost any of them could, by virtue of its negative consequences for the individual or for others, rise to the level of a paraphilic disorder" (p. 685). Moreover, "A paraphilia is a necessary but not a sufficient condition for having a paraphilic disorder, and a paraphilia by itself does not necessarily justify or require clinical intervention" (p. 686). For example, if an individual engages in cross-dressing and is unconcerned about his behavior, there is no clear rationale for treatment. In contrast, acting on a sexual arousal pattern such as pedophilia would necessarily constitute a criminal offense, would likely result in harm to another individual, and, therefore, warrants clinical intervention.

Readers may notice numerous problems with DSM-5 conceptualizations of paraphilias and paraphilic disorders. Three such criticisms seem both compelling and relevant for the present discussion. First, there is no clear rationale for inclusion of the eight paraphilias listed in the DSM-5 and for the exclusion of the assortment of other paraphilias that are not listed. For example, inclusion of several "chronophilias" (Seto, 2016) or age/maturity categories other than arousal to young, sexually mature adults seems warranted because of the significant social and legal

D.S. Bromberg
Special Psychological Services, L.L.C., Bloomfield, NJ, USA
e-mail: danielbromberg@aol.com

A. Maragakis, W.T. O'Donohue (eds.), *Principle-Based Stepped Care and Brief Psychotherapy for Integrated Care Settings*, https://doi.org/10.1007/978-3-319-70539-2_28

consequences of acting on such arousal patterns. Two such chronophilias include nepiophilia (arousal to infants and toddlers) and hebephilia (arousal to pubescent children; Tanner Stages 2 and 3). However, these two "chronophilias" are not contained in the DSM-5 or in previous editions of the DSM.

Another criticism of DSM-5 conceptualizations of paraphilias and paraphilic disorders centers on the notion of "normophilic" sexuality. Those sexual interests considered to be normophilic (i.e., normal) depend on historical, political, and sociocultural factors, much more than on scientific evidence (Joyal, 2014). Until relatively recently, oral and anal sex, masturbation, and homosexuality were viewed as being symptoms or causes of mental disorders (Fedoroff, DiGioacchino, & Murphy, 2013). Such interests and behaviors are now accepted as being normative.

A third criticism pertains to *definitions* of paraphilias and paraphilic disorders. Some scholars have noted that the definitions employed may result in "unintentional paraphilias," or non-problematic sexual behaviors meeting diagnostic criteria for being paraphilic (e.g., Moser, 2016). For example, a man who prefers to achieve sexual arousal and orgasm by receiving oral sex from a consenting female peer rather than by having vaginal intercourse would seem to have a paraphilia because of the relative lack of interest in stimulating his partner's genitals. Similarly, if he prefers to achieve orgasm by having his consenting female partner stimulate his penis with her feet, that too constitutes a paraphilia. There is no clear scientific rationale why achieving orgasm by vaginal intercourse is "normal," but achieving orgasm by stimulation from the feet of one's partner should constitute a psychiatric disorder. Finally, having a preference to achieve orgasm with individuals who have tattoos, body piercings, or multicolored hair appears to meet diagnostic criteria for having a paraphilia because such characteristics are phenotypically nonnormative (Moser, 2016). O'Donohue (2016) provided an intriguing discussion of additional problems with paraphilias as a diagnostic category.

Screening for Paraphilias in Primary Care Settings

Although paraphilic disorders most commonly present in forensic and correctional settings, they are sometimes seen in general psychiatric (and medical) settings, as well. Presentation in general psychiatric and medical settings is most likely to occur when the paraphilia impairs sexual or relationship functioning with one's partner or spouse (Seto, Kingston, & Bourget, 2014). Moreover, males are more likely to present with paraphilias than are females (Bailey & Hsu, 2016; Dawson, Bannerman, & Lalumiere, 2016; Seto, 2016).[1]

Because sexual interests and behaviors are generally quite private, it is unlikely that a patient would volunteer information about paraphilic interests or behaviors during the course of a visit to a primary care practitioner. Therefore, such problems are likely to come to light only in response to direct inquiry or from the report of a third party such as a spouse. Certainly, direct inquiry is warranted if a patient presents with questions or concerns about sexual interests. Direct inquiry is also warranted for patients presenting with any of the following issues: difficulty becoming aroused while engaging in sexual behavior with one's partner and/or difficulty achieving orgasm; problematic or excessive use of internet pornography and; unexplained injuries to the genitalia or other parts of the body. It may also be useful to inquire about the extent to which the patient (and his or her partner) is concerned about this problem (or these problems) and if the patient or his partner find the problem(s) to be unusual, distasteful, or concerning. The practitioner might also consider asking the patient if law enforcement or child protective service authorities have ever questioned him about his sexual interests and behaviors. Affirmative responses to any of the foregoing questions, and/or the patient having injuries to the genitalia or other parts of the body with no plausible medical explanation,

[1] Because males are more likely to present with paraphilias than are females, I will use masculine pronouns throughout this chapter. However, statements made about men are applicable to women, as well.

suggests the need for further assessment. Under this last condition, the practitioner should also consider the possibility of the individual being a domestic violence victim. Practitioners should be mindful of mandated reporting requirements in their jurisdictions regarding suspected child or elder abuse.

There is a more general framework for circumstances under which further assessment is warranted. A thorough assessment is warranted when the patient's sexual interests and/or behaviors reach the following threshold: the sexual interest(s) would be illegal if acted upon and/or, the rights of others would be infringed if the sexual interest were acted upon and/or, the interest causes problems in social or sexual functioning. Such problems include impairment in work or school functioning and problems in relationships with one's spouse, partner, and/or children.

Research on characteristics of effective psychotherapists, including those who work with sex offenders, suggests the importance of the manner in which inquiry occurs. Practitioners who are warm, empathic, and nonjudgmental are likely to elicit important information about a patient's sexual interests and behaviors (e.g., Marshall & Marshall, 2015).

How to Further Assess If a Screen Returns Positive

Aside from the line of inquiry discussed previously in this chapter, there are no procedures to screen for paraphilias. Unlike many other clinical problems discussed in this book, further assessment of individuals with paraphilic interests is generally contraindicated in integrated care settings. There are two reasons underlying the recommendation to refrain from assessing further. First, specialized knowledge about, and experience in, assessing and managing problems of human sexuality is needed. Practitioners should be well-versed not only in information about human sexuality, but also about the complex legal and ethical issues regarding mandatory reporting requirements in one's jurisdiction. The content of a patient's disclosure may necessitate a referral to a state child protective service agency and/or to law enforcement authorities. The practitioner would then need to manage the difficult task of working therapeutically with one's patient after having notified authorities that the patient may pose a risk to the safety of others and/or after having disclosed commission of a criminal offense.

Second, such an assessment is a time-intensive process and requires specialized techniques. In most integrated care settings, it is impractical to conduct such assessments. Evaluations should consist of most of the following components: review of sexual history by way of interview and questionnaire; a mental status examination to assess for co-occurring disorders; psychophysiological testing of sexual arousal patterns; collateral information provided by current or former sexual partners and from files and; medical testing of hormone levels (Seto et al., 2014).

Evidence-Based Stepped Care and Brief Psychotherapeutic Approaches

Because treatment of individuals with paraphilic interests warrants specialized knowledge and experience, the brief psychotherapeutic approach of choice is psychoeducation. I suggest that practitioners address the following points with their patient:

- "Normal" human sexual interests and behaviors exist on an extremely broad continuum.
- Sexual interests and behaviors should be viewed as being concerning when the sexual interest(s) would be illegal if acted upon and/or, the rights of others would be infringed if the sexual interest were acted upon and/or, the interest causes problems in social or sexual functioning. The patient's sexual interests seem to fall into one or more of these categories. Therefore, specialized evaluation, and possibly treatment, is warranted.
- The practitioner should provide referrals to specialists or to an organization that can provide such referrals. State medical or

psychological associations are organizations that can often provide referrals to qualified specialists. Although there is no one hallmark of a qualified specialist, such practitioners generally devote most of their professional time to addressing problems with human sexuality, broadly defined. Specialists should also be experienced in some combination of the following assessment and intervention modalities: behavioral assessment and therapy; penile plethysmography; relapse prevention and/or; the Good Lives Model (of sex offender treatment). The clinician should offer to engage in ongoing communication with the specialty-level provider should the patient choose to give appropriate consent for exchange of information.

- Thank the patient for trusting you enough to bring this private and sensitive matter to your attention.

Few high-quality resources are available for laypersons seeking information about paraphilias and treatment options for paraphilic disorders. *The Sex Addiction Workbook* (Sbraga & O'Donohue, 2003) contains useful content. I am aware of two websites that provide accurate, albeit limited, information in this domain. These websites are https://www.ncbi.nlm.nih.gov and www.webmd.com.[2]

Safer Society Press located in Brandon, Vermont, has many relevant resources. Their books are primarily for professionals who deliver services to individuals whose sexual behaviors infringe on the rights of others. Although many of these publications are intended for a professional audience, others are intended for use by patients who are participating in treatment. Clinicians should consider the appropriateness of patient use of these materials in the absence of professional oversight before recommending them. Information about Safer Society Press publications is displayed on their website, www.safersociety.org.

The website of the Association for the Treatment of Sexual Abusers (ATSA) has limited information but contains links to other online resources. Their website is www.atsa.com.

Finally, there are resources appropriate only for mental health and medical professionals seeking further information about assessment and treatment of individuals with paraphilic interests. Beech and Harkins (2012) provided a useful summary of paraphilias listed in the DSM-IV-TR (not the DSM-5) and of evidence-based psychosocial and medical interventions for treatment of paraphilic disorders. Readers interested in learning more about assessment and treatment of these problems are encouraged to read Beech and Harkins's review. Assumpcao, Garcia, Garcia, Bradford, and Thibaut (2014) and Nair (2016) provide useful information about pharmacologic treatment of individuals with paraphilic interests.

What Does Not Work

There is an intuitively appealing notion that having "corrective" or "normative" sexual experiences, particularly ones culminating in orgasm, will result in a decrease or elimination of paraphilic interests. However, such an outcome is quite improbable. For example, extant research on pedophilia suggests the following:

> …pedophilia can be viewed as a sexual age orientation…regarding its age of onset, associations with sexual and romantic behavior, and stability over time….Changes in sexual arousal to children can be made using behavioral conditioning techniques, but follow-up studies have not shown evidence that this change generalizes outside the laboratory or persists over the longer-term…. Viewing pedophilia as a sexual orientation would suggest that treatment is more likely to be effective if it focuses on self-regulation skills (in order to effectively manage pedophilic urges, thoughts, etc.) than on trying to change sexual preferences. (Seto, 2012)

The preponderance of research on pedophilia and hebephilia is consistent with the foregoing

[2] However, readers should be aware that website information is subject to modification and cannot be assumed to be accurate in perpetuity. In addition, as of the date that this chapter was completed, changes taking place in the federal government suggest that information provided by federal agencies should also be viewed critically and checked for accuracy.

conclusion (e.g., Grundmann, Krupp, Scherner, Amelung, & Beier, 2016)[3] as is research regarding other paraphilias. Therefore, waiting for a paraphilic arousal pattern to disappear or self-correct is quite likely to be ineffective.

The Role of the Primary Care Provider/Medical Team in Treatment

The primary care provider and medical team can assume two roles in the treatment of individuals with paraphilic disorders. One important role is to reassure the patient that his concerns will be addressed in a professional and nonjudgmental manner. Communicating such a stance is likely to facilitate compliance with the clinician's recommendation for pursuing specialist-level assessment and treatment.

The second role is that of coordinator of mental health and medical services for the patient within a medical home. A medical home "strives to provide patient-centered, comprehensive, team-based, coordinated, accessible, and quality and safety-oriented health care delivery to individuals and families" (Kazak, Nash, Hiroto, & Kaslow, 2017). Thus, a primary care provider might coordinate services delivered to a single patient by professionals such as a behavior therapist, a psychiatrist, a urologist, and an endocrinologist. Such tracking might be particularly useful for the primarily medical bases of sexual functioning and for tracking all medications being prescribed. Tracking of medications is of particular importance to ensure that physicians are not inadvertently prescribing combinations of medications that might render the combination ineffective or harmful to the patient.

[3]However, it is important to note that there are many men with pedophilic and/or hebephilic interests who have never engaged in sexual behavior with a minor (Lasher & Stinson, 2016). Readers interested in learning more about "chronophilias" such as pedophilia and hebephilia are referred to Seto (2016) and Bailey and Hsu (2016) for cogent discussions of these topics.

Conclusion

A primary care provider may be the first professional to learn of a patient's paraphilic interests and behaviors. Therefore, (s)he is in an excellent position to determine if there is a need for a specialist-level comprehensive evaluation. Because of the need for specialized knowledge and experience to conduct such assessments, as well as the legal and ethical considerations inherent in doing so, a primary care provider should not attempt to conduct such an assessment. Instead, such a provider may serve in the important role of coordinating the patient's care with the assortment of other professionals with whom the patient may become involved.

References

American Psychiatric Association. (2013). *Diagnostic and statistical manual of mental disorders* (5th ed.). Arlington, VA: American Psychiatric Press.

Assumpcao, A. A., Garcia, F. D., Garcia, H. D., Bradford, J. M. W., & Thibaut, F. (2014). Pharmacologic treatment of paraphilias. *Psychiatric Clinics of North America, 37*, 173–181.

Bailey, J.M. & Hsu, K.J. (2016). Orienting basic research on chronophilias. *Archives of Sexual Behavior*, Advance online publication. https://doi: 10.1007/s10508-016-0885-1

Beech, A. R., & Harkins, L. (2012). DSM-IV paraphilia: Descriptions, demographics and treatment interventions. *Aggression and Violent Behavior, 17*, 527–539.

Dawson, S. J., Bannerman, B. A., & Lalumiere, M. L. (2016). Paraphilic interests: An examination of sex differences in a nonclinical sample. *Sexual Abuse: A Journal of Research and Treatment, 28*, 20–45.

Fedoroff, J. P., DiGioacchino, L., & Murphy, L. (2013). Problems with paraphilias in the DSM-5. *Current Psychiatry Reports, 15*, 363.

Grundmann, D., Krupp, J., Scherner, G., Amelung, T., & Beier, K. M. (2016). Stability of self-reported arousal to sexual fantasies involving children in a clinical sample of pedophiles and hebephiles. *Archives of Sexual Behavior, 45*, 1153–1162.

Joyal, C. C. (2014). How anomalous are paraphilic interests? *Archives of Sexual Behavior, 43*, 1241–1243.

Kazak, A. E., Nash, J. M., Hiroto, K., & Kaslow, N. J. (2017). Psychologists in patient-centered medical homes (PCMHs): Roles, evidence, opportunities, and challenges. *American Psychologist, 72*, 1–12.

Lasher, M. P., & Stinson, J. D. (2016). Adults with pedophilic interests in the United States: Current practices and suggestions for future policy and research. *Archives of Sexual Behavior*, Advance online publication. https://doi: 10.1007/s10508-016-0822-3

Marshall, W. L., & Marshall, L. E. (2015). Psychological treatment of the paraphilias: A review and an appraisal of effectiveness. *Current Psychiatry Reports*, *17*, 47.

Moser, C. (2016). DSM-5 and the paraphilic disorders: Conceptual issues. *Archives of Sexual Behavior*, *45*, 2181–2186.

Nair, M. (2016). Pharmacotherapy for sexual offenders. In A. Phenix & H. M. Hoberman (Eds.), *Sexual offending* (pp. 755–767). New York: Springer.

O'Donohue, W. (2016). Problems in the classification and diagnosis of the paraphilias: What is the evidence that the DSM warrants use? In D. R. Laws & W. O'Donohue (Eds.), *Treatment of sex offenders: Strengths and weaknesses in assessment and intervention*. New York: Springer.

Sbraga, T. P., & O'Donohue, W. T. (2003). *The sex addiction workbook*. Oakland, CA: New Harbinger.

Seto, M. C. (2012). Is pedophilia a sexual orientation? *Archives of Sexual Behavior*, *41*, 231–236.

Seto, M. C. (2016). The puzzle of male chronophilias. *Archives of Sexual Behavior*, Advance online publication. https://doi: 10.1007/s10508-016-0799-y

Seto, M. C., Kingston, D. A., & Bourget, D. (2014). Assessment of paraphilias. *Psychiatric Clinics of North America*, *37*, 149–161.

Pediatric Sleep Resistance

29

Michelle Byrd, Casiana Warfield, and Lauren Ostarello

Introduction

The developmental importance of sleep cannot be overstated from both physical and psychological perspectives. Not only can insufficient quantity or quality of sleep result in growth deficits and other negative physical health outcomes but can also mimic or exacerbate several behavioral concerns such as anxiety, learning disabilities, and/or attentional difficulties and has been shown to increase the incidence of accidents and injuries (Paruthi et al., 2016). Sleeplessness in teenagers has been associated with serious mood disorders and even higher rates of suicidal and parasuicidal behavior (Paruthi et al., 2016). Moreover, sleep problems create a behavioral ripple effect within the family system, often adversely affecting not only the identified child but also their parents and siblings. Surveys of both pediatric medical providers and parents suggest that upwards of 20% of young children experience clinically noteworthy difficulties falling or staying asleep on at least an intermittent basis (Davis et al., 2012; Owens, 2008). Despite the high prevalence of concern, however, sleep problems are often not adequately addressed in the primary care setting. Given that children are seen within primary care on a regular and frequent basis compared to adults both for well-child and sick visits, this is the ideal setting in which to assess for and intervene on sleep problems.

M. Byrd (✉) • C. Warfield • L. Ostarello
Eastern Michigan University, Ypsilanti, MI, USA
e-mail: mbyrd@emich.edu; lostarel@emich.edu

Defining Pediatric Sleep Problems

The American Academy of Sleep Medicine (Paruthi et al., 2016) recently revised their recommendations for optimal amount of sleep within a 24-h period, increasing the amount of time for several developmental categories. The current recommendations are:

- Ages 4–12 months: 12–16 h (including naps)
- Ages 1–2 years: 11–14 h (including naps)
- Ages 3–5 years: 10–13 h (including naps)
- Ages 6–12 years: 9–12 h
- Ages 13–18 years: 8–10 h

Any child who is getting less than the minimal recommended duration of sleep on a recurring basis is considered at risk for biopsychosocial sequelae and should be triaged in the primary care setting. The clinical presentation of pediatric sleep problems can range from common examples of poor sleep hygiene (e.g., inconsistent bedtime) to diagnosable sleep disorders. Interestingly, in a review of the literature, Honaker and Meltzer (2016) noted that parents report significantly more sleep concerns than do pediatricians,

A. Maragakis, W.T. O'Donohue (eds.), *Principle-Based Stepped Care and Brief Psychotherapy for Integrated Care Settings*, https://doi.org/10.1007/978-3-319-70539-2_29

indicating that there is a significant chasm between the phenomena itself and appropriate identification and treatment. Across studies, among both parents and primary care providers, the highest rates of concern are in children from birth to age 4, with higher prevalence of behaviorally based sleep disorders (e.g., sleep resistance or insomnia) than biologically based sleep disorders (e.g., night terrors, snoring/sleep apnea; Honaker & Meltzer, 2016). While sleep concerns among the youngest of children are legitimate developmentally, it is worrisome that adolescents are not perceived by parents or PCPs as having significant sleep concerns when some studies suggest that adolescent insomnia is at unprecedented levels globally (Gradisar, Gardner, & Dohnt, 2011).

The most prevalent sleep disturbance in children is behavioral insomnia of childhood which is characterized by either a delayed sleep onset of more than 20–30 min and/or nighttime awakenings that are either frequent and/or occurring for an extended time period requiring parental intervention to return to sleep (Morgenthaler et al., 2006). Childhood insomnia is typically associated with daytime symptoms such as sleepiness, irritability, and decreased focus. Topographically, delayed sleep onset manifests itself as bedtime resistance in the form of tantruming, repeatedly getting out of bed, crying and/or fussing excessively, and being highly oppositional at bedtime. Parents whose children are sleep resistant will sometimes describe bedtime as a "battleground" with their child and will go to great, and often unhealthy, lengths to avoid the drama and emotion dysregulation associated with refusal to go to sleep. For example, many parents will allow their child to sleep in their bed or conversely will begin sleeping with the child in the child's bed. It is not uncommon for bedtime resistance to spiral into a full-blown cycle of coercion (Patterson, 1982) where the parent and child mutually escalate the conflict through threats of punishment (e.g., "I'll lock the door and then you'll have to go to sleep!" "You can sleep outside for all I care!") typically resulting in parental acquiescence and mutual negative reinforcement when the child gets their way and the parent avoids further emotional turmoil and strife.

Nighttime awakenings may be thought of as a different form of sleep resistance characterized by the child initially falling asleep, presumably in their own bed, however, awakening during the night and either calling for their parent or getting out of their bed to seek out a parent to provide the comfort they need to be able to get back to sleep. For many families experiencing sleep resistance, children may be requiring parental intervention several times a week and sometimes several times in the same night. Moreover, it is not at all uncommon for a child to experience sleep resistance both at sleep onset and during nighttime awakening, causing a high level of sleep disturbance for the child themselves as well as their parent(s) and even potentially siblings who may either be disturbed by the behavior and kept awake or may even begin to model the behavior themselves.

Etiologically, sleep resistance can likely be best understood through both classical and operant conditioning paradigms. During infancy and young childhood, children associate particular setting events or stimuli with the experience of sleepiness and falling asleep. For example, it is common practice to rock a baby to sleep. However, as children grow beyond infancy, it is important that they expand their repertoire of events associated with sleep onset to be more developmentally appropriate and independent. Specifically, given that humans naturally wake up several times during a normal night's sleep, it is critical that young children develop self-soothing skills that they are fully capable of implementing on their own to fall asleep. If this expansion of stimuli does not occur, children will only associate the specific conditions their parents create (i.e., rocking, snuggling, singing, etc.) with sleep onset, rendering them unable to easily fall asleep without parental intervention. From the operant standpoint, when children demand their parents' attention or intervention to meet their classically conditioned needs for association and parents provide the desired attention, touch, etc., children are positively reinforced by the parental intervention and are more likely to engage in this behavior again in the future. From the parental perspective, when parents intervene in order to avoid oppositionality or emotion dysregulation (both leading to a longer sleep latency), they are negatively reinforced, making it more likely that they will engage in this behavior again in the future. Because most cases of childhood insomnia are learned through this behavioral paradigm, it follows that behavioral approaches are the gold standard in the treatment of sleep resistance and related problems. However, before an evidence-based approach can be implemented, the problem must first be detected.

Screening for Sleep Problems in Pediatric Primary Care

Given that approximately one quarter of children may be suffering from a sleep-related concern at any given time, it makes sense to screen for these concerns at every pediatric primary care visit. At the very least, children and adolescents should be screened at all well-child visits (typically occurring at least once per year) and, as immunization protocols are fulfilled and well-child visits become less frequent in older children and adolescents, at yearly sports physicals. If a child is not receiving a yearly checkup/physical, then sleep should be assessed at any available appointment, even if related to illness or injury.

To date, very few studies have examined screening practices for sleep problems in pediatric primary care. Across studies and methodologies, the majority of physicians report routinely screening for sleep problems in their child patients, while between 10 and 30% do not report screening at all (Faruqui, Khubchandani, Price, Bolyard, & Reddy, 2011; Owens, 2001). Parents report somewhat lower rates of screening, at about the 50% mark (National Sleep Foundation, 2004), and documentation of screening seems fairly uncommon (Chervin, Archbold, Panahi, & Pituch, 2001; Erichsen et al., 2012). Moreover, when physicians do report screening, they most commonly report only asking one question about sleep practices and often rely solely on parental report, rather than directly asking older children and adolescents (Owens, 2001). This single-reporter method is likely suboptimal for adequately and accurately detecting sleep problems.

Owens and Dalzell (2005) developed and tested a new sleep screening tool for pediatric primary care that meets both the demands of the setting and the need for more thorough assessment. The "BEARS" tool prompts questioning across critical sleep domains (*B*edtime issues, *E*xcessive daytime sleepiness, night *A*wakenings, *R*egularity and duration of sleep, and *S*noring) and was shown to exponentially increase screening practices (in the case of snoring by more than tenfold) and rates of detection of sleep problems and appropriate treatment recommendations. Although this instrument has only been tested in one study, it clearly shows promise and warrants additional research, ideally within an ongoing practice setting and with the inclusion of provider and parental acceptability ratings as indications of usability, as these key variables were not studied in the pilot testing. However, as this is currently the most comprehensive method available and has some limited data in support of its use, it is recommended for cautious implementation in the context of ongoing data collection and quality improvement procedures. If clinicians suspect a sleep problem based on screening but are seeking a more in-depth diagnostic tool, they might consider the Children's Sleep Habits Questionnaire (Owens, Spirito, & McGuinn, 2000); however, this instrument is likely too lengthy to be practical for routine use within the primary care setting. We would further recommend gathering data from both parents and children and adolescents themselves, beginning in elementary school, to improve accuracy of screening.

If there is any indication of sleep problems, at minimum clinicians should begin documenting these concerns in the medical record and having parents and children begin tracking relevant behavior using a sleep diary for a minimum of 2 weeks in order to discern a pattern across both weekdays and weekends (downloadable from the National Sleep Foundation: www.sleepfoundation.org/ or www.kidzzzsleep.com). Clinicians must decide whether the case requires additional assessment, immediate treatment (which could vary within a stepped care model from psychoeducation to self-help recommendations to referral for outpatient specialty behavioral healthcare), or monitoring with follow-up, depending on frequency and severity of symptoms, though no clear clinical guidelines on when to definitively intervene have been established. Clinically, it seems the case that physicians will initiate treatment when either parental tolerance for the sleep concerns or daytime sleepiness in the child has reached critical levels requiring attention. Importantly, any biological causes of sleep problems and/or biologically based diagnoses must be ruled out and adequately treated prior to engaging behavioral treatment for sleep concerns.

Evidence-Based Stepped Care and Brief Psychotherapeutic Approaches to Prevention and Intervention

As would be expected given the behavioral etiology of childhood insomnia, behavioral interventions have been demonstrated to be highly effective for the treatment of sleep resistance in infants and children. Specifically, behavioral treatment has been shown to alleviate problematic sleep behaviors in the child as well as improve intrapersonal and relational outcomes in caregivers (Mindell, Kuhn, Lewin, Meltzer, & Sadeh, 2006). However, in a review of the literature, it was noted that evidence-based treatment of sleep problems occurs at insufficient rates in primary care settings due to lack of physician training about pediatric sleep issues, time constraints, and low primary care provider confidence, despite the availability of interventions (Honaker & Meltzer, 2016).

As such, behavioral health specialists have several roles in integrated health settings when addressing this particular behavioral dysfunction including providing education about developmentally normative sleep behavior to primary care providers and caregivers, explaining the importance of sleep hygiene for other domains of well-being, and tailoring existing evidence-based interventions so they may be disseminated by PCPs efficiently and effectively (Honaker & Meltzer, 2016; Kuhn, 2014).

Interventions will be described below in the order that they would be likely to be implemented within a stepped care model, with the least intensive interventions presented first. In doing so, we will take care to highlight relevant research on and adaptations of these evidence-based practices within primary care.

Prevention/Early Intervention

Numerous studies have demonstrated the efficacy of the prevention of sleep dysfunction via providing psychoeducation concerning positive sleep routines to parents with infants or young children. In a stepped care model, psychoeducation may be provided at the population level to parents of newborn infants, to parents or children who are identified as at risk by the primary care provider, or when toddlers or preschool-aged children are showing early signs of sleep disturbance. Potential advantages of prevention or early intervention include reducing the suffering of children and parents by avoiding the development of sleep concerns, the potential for wider distribution of information if psychoeducation is provided via print or digital media, and low cost to the provider.

Primary components of establishing a healthy sleep routine that should be taught include knowledge of normal sleep cycles, timing feedings in infants to reduce and time-up nighttime awakenings to best suit parental sleep needs, fostering a consistent sleep schedule, developing bedtime routines that are soothing to the child and time-limited (less than 20 min), managing the caregivers' response to sleep resistance so as not to reinforce ineffective patterns, and putting the child to bed drowsy not asleep to encourage self-soothing (Kuhn, 2014). More details are provided on these principles of good sleep hygiene below.

Intervention

Establishing a positive bedtime routine. For children with significant bedtime oppositionality or resistance, it is common clinical practice to begin by establishing a positive bedtime routine that creates a new classical conditioning paradigm. Positive bedtime routines primarily involve caregivers creating a predetermined, consistent, and developmentally appropriate bedtime preceded by a period of quiet, child-preferred activities that end with the child being tucked in their bed drowsy but awake and alone with a transitional object such as a teddy bear or special blanket (Christophersen & Vanscoyoc, 2013; Mindell et al., 2006). Bedtime routines typically take less than 20 min and include activities such as putting on pajamas, brushing teeth, reading a story, saying prayers or meditating together, and snuggling/giving kisses goodnight. For some families it can be useful to write down these steps and post them in a relevant part of the house, such as the child's bedroom. Roughhousing or very active play is discouraged during the bedtime routine, as the goal is to calmly wind down before bed and provide comfort and attention to the child. In addition, the use of technology is not recommended because of the related cognitive stimulation. A positive bedtime is a critical building block of good sleep hygiene and is particularly important if parents and the child have been embroiled in conflict or coercion secondary to the bedtime resistance.

This intervention has great potential for use in the primary care setting because it is both easy and fast to explain to parents, as well as likely being intuitive to providers. Establishing a positive bedtime routine has been found to be satisfactory to caregivers and effective in reducing sleep resistance in a few studies; however, it has yet to be assessed empirically as a solitary intervention, and thus its efficacy or lack of independence of other strategies is uncertain (Mindell et al., 2006). Despite the need for additional empirical support, establishing positive routines is the most recommended sleep management strategy by pediatric primary care providers (83–95% of the time when problems were detected; Bruni et al., 2004; Mindell, Moline, Zendell, Brown, & Fry, 1994).

Daytime correction of sleep problems. Another method for reducing problematic sleep behavior is to use the daytime to manage bedtime behavior. First, it is critical to evaluate whether children are napping too much for their developmental level and/or too close to bedtime in such a manner as to give rise to resistance. Parents can use daytime opportunities to teach developmentally appropriate self-soothing skills during times of minor stress and/or boredom in order to get the young child used to being alone and calm, assuming that these behaviors will generalize to nighttime settings. By teaching the child self-quieting techniques during the day and ignoring unwanted behaviors at night, nighttime awakenings can be reduced and child's transition to bedtime improved (Christophersen & Vanscoyoc, 2013). Moreover, if the function of bedtime resistance seems to be attention rather than other drivers (e.g., anxiety), we would recommend that parents increase both the quality and quantity of time they are spending with their child during the day to meet their developmental needs for parental engagement during the appropriate time frame, rather than at bedtime. Finally, parents can use positive reinforcement strategies in the morning to reinforce compliance with the bedtime routine and staying in bed all night without requiring parental intervention. Some parents will choose to use an immediate tangible reinforcer, such as an edible, particularly for younger children, while others will employ a token economy, such as a sticker chart with achievable larger reinforcers, for elementary-aged children.

Daytime strategies can be taught in module form within the context of primary care, with the most challenging of these being teaching parents how to teach their children self-regulation and calming skills if they do not already have this skill. It would not be recommended to teach all of the daytime strategies within one brief intervention, as parents may become overwhelmed with trying to accomplish skill building at the same time as applying consistent reinforcement for compliant behaviors. However, clinicians might layer daytime strategies with nighttime strategies for optimal benefit. While these strategies are commonly used clinically in both traditional outpatient behavioral care and integrated primary care settings, there has not been research examining the efficacy of these techniques either used as a package or independently.

Relaxation. For children who have significant anxiety or an inability to calm themselves at bedtime, a related intervention involves facilitating the development of relaxation skills during the daytime to aid the child in coping with fears experienced at night. Relaxation skills may include diaphragmatic breathing, progressive muscle relaxation, learning, and repeating positive statements concerning one's ability to self-soothe. Children are then encouraged to utilize relaxation as part of their bedtime routine and, in particular, once their parents leave the bedroom. As with other skills, relaxation skill training and practice may be combined with reinforcement (Christophersen & Vanscoyoc, 2013). While relaxation has been empirically supported for use with children experiencing diagnostic levels of anxiety, it has not been well-studied for use in reducing sleep resistance (Gordon, King, Gullone, Muris, & Ollendick, 2001).

The bedtime pass. The bedtime pass is a brief intervention that lends itself well to the primary care environment, despite not having yet been tested in this forum. The bedtime pass intervention involves the caregivers making and giving the child a pass, physically represented by a small object such as a decorated note card or small stuffed animal, that the child may keep under their pillow and exchange once each night for a very brief (e.g., a few minutes) trip out of bed or the presence of a caregiver to engage in a preferred activity. For example, the child might use their pass to get a drink of water, another story, or five additional minutes of cuddling. After this pass is used, the caregivers follow an unmodified extinction protocol, specifically, ignoring the child's cries and returning the child to bed mechanically for the remainder of the night (see below; Christophersen & Vanscoyoc, 2013; Freeman, 2006; Kuhn, 2014). Clinically, many children have been observed to almost never use their bedtime pass, preferring to keep the option of using it later in the night but never needing to. In addition to being perceived as more acceptable by caregivers than pure extinction procedures, an additional advantage of this intervention is the reduced probability of the child exhibiting an extinction burst, or a temporary increase in frequency and/or intensity of unwanted behavior, as observed in other treatments, namely, unmodified and graduated extinction (Freeman, 2006).

Extinction paradigms. Once children are manifesting definitive sleep resistance resulting in notable daytime dysfunction, some level of extinction treatment is warranted. The strongest evidence in the extant literature is for extinction paradigms; however, these are also considered to be some of the most difficult to implement treatment strategies and should, therefore, be used only when other methods (described above) have failed within a stepped care model. As such, employing an extinction protocol may require multiple visits or potentially even referral to specialty outpatient behavioral healthcare for adequate support of the technique. Unfortunately, research has not yet been undertaken with regard to the feasibility of teaching these techniques within integrated care.

There is an excellent bibliotherapy resource for use in extinction for sleep resistance that may be used instead of or in addition to brief sessions. *Solve Your Child's Sleep Problems* is a classic self-help book by Dr. Richard Ferber (2006) first published decades ago that has been updated to be better suited for modern parents and to improve parent acceptability. Once criticized within the popular media for its seemingly harsh approach to "Ferberizing" the children of America, the latest edition takes a more measured approach that parents will likely find less daunting. Within a stepped care model, utilizing this book may be an excellent adjunct to professional behavioral care for parents who are very self-motivated. Unfortunately, there have been no studies to date examining the use of this modality in an integrated care setting.

Traditional, or unmodified, extinction paradigms for sleep resistance involve caregivers intentionally ignoring the child's unwanted behavior at bedtime and throughout the night (Christophersen & Vanscoyoc, 2013). As caregivers may find this approach unappealing or even distressing, it is important to caution caregivers that ignoring may first be met with increased frequency and/or intensity of the problem behavior such as crying, calling out to parents, and leaving the bed. It may be necessary to assure parents that this is temporary and that it is critical that they are consistent in ignoring so that the burst of behavior is not accidentally reinforced. Unmodified extinction has been investigated frequently, and in a review of behavioral treatments' efficacy in treating sleep resistance in infants and young children, ignoring demonstrated the strongest empirical support (Mindell et al., 2006). A more recent review of relevant articles found that unmodified extinction had the greatest effect on reducing unwanted behavior (i.e., night awakenings requiring parental involvement, bedtime disturbance) once these behaviors had risen to the level of daytime symptomology (Kuhn, 2014).

If parents are resistant to or demonstrate distress related to ignoring their child's cries at night, graduated extinction may be an efficacious intervention option (Kuhn, 2014). Graduated extinction involves allowing caregivers to check on the child at predetermined times during the night while lengthening the interval in which the parent ignores the child's cries over time, either over the course of a single night or a series of nights. In addition, parents are instructed to limit their checking behavior to mechanical, brief interactions with the child, to reduce the reinforcing nature of their behavior and breaking the operant conditioning paradigm which gave rise to the problematic behavior. The primary aim of graduated extinction is to facilitate the child's self-soothing skills so that they are able to fall asleep and back asleep without parental intervention. This technique may be more palatable to parents, and while it has slightly less empirical support than unmodified extinction or ignoring, the distinction is minimal and may be the result of less investigation of graduated extinction as compared to other extinction paradigms rather than a difference in efficacy (Mindell et al., 2006). Relatedly, while there is less empirical support, there is some evidence that a variation of extinction in which the caregiver remains in the room with the distressed child but does not physically respond to their requests, termed extinction with parental presence, may be a worthwhile intervention for sleep problems in children. However, this protocol instructs caregivers to progress to unmodified extinction practices eventually, and it is unclear how this shift in caregiver behavior may impact child response (Kuhn, 2014; Mindell et al., 2006).

Treatments Not Recommended

Despite the evidence for behavioral interventions to treat childhood insomnia, pharmacological treatment remains the most common intervention implemented in the primary care setting (Mindell et al., 1994) with over 80% of children presenting with a sleep disturbance being prescribed medication (Stojanovski, Rasu, Balkrishnan, & Nahata, 2007). While this may be an appropriate course of action for specific biologically based clinical phenomena, for the majority of children, this is not an optimal practice and may, in fact, be iatrogenic. Primary care providers may be inclined to treat pediatric sleep disturbance by prescribing sedative medications such as antihistamines, benzodiazepines, and chloral hydrate. However, research examining the outcomes of these interventions suggests that medications do not lead to long-term elimination of problematic behavior but rather postpone unwanted behavior until medications are discontinued. In addition, it is not clear what the long-term adverse effects of repeatedly medicating children with sedatives are. While it may be perceived as a simpler treatment to administer, parents may be reluctant to medicate their infants or young children and reasonably concerned about the long-term effects, wanted and unwanted, on the child's functioning (Kuhn & Weidinger, 2000). It is important to note that there are no FDA-approved medications to treat insomnia in children and concerns also within the medical community with regard to the safety of these drugs in developing children (Owens, Rosen, Mindell, & Kirchner, 2010).

In addition to noting the contraindications of medication management of sleep problems, it is also relevant to acknowledge the limitations of knowledge with regard to the application of behavioral principles. While behavioral treatments have been demonstrated to be efficacious in community pediatric populations, these interventions have not as of yet been well-tested in primary care. More importantly, they have not been as solidly supported in certain clinical pediatric samples including children with autism spectrum disorder, intellectual disabilities, or those who have experienced neglect (Kuhn, 2014). Further research in these populations is warranted in order to modify existing or develop novel interventions with similar efficacy. Therefore, clinicians should employ these techniques with caution when working with particularly vulnerable children.

The Role of the Primary Care Provider/Medical Team in Treatment

The two sections above outline evidence-based treatments for bedtime resistance as well as what does not work in reducing bedtime resistance. It is clear that behaviorally based interventions that shape parental behavior are the most effective in reducing child bedtime resistance (Mindell et al., 2006). Although bedtime resistance may not evolve into a clinical sleep disorder, primary care providers have a pivotal role in assessing for and treating sleep-related issues in their young patients. A study utilizing the Pediatric Sleep Survey (Owens, 2001) to assess general and specific sleep knowledge (e.g., clinical screening, diagnostic, and treatment practices) of pediatricians found that only 46% were confident in their ability to screen for sleep problems. Even more telling is that 34% reported confidence in their ability to assess, whereas only 25% were confident in their ability to treat sleep-related issues in children (Owens, 2001). These numbers are frightening given that pediatricians are the first line of defense in terms of recognizing, diagnosing, and treating or providing an appropriate referral for treatment of sleep-related issues in children.

It is also worth mentioning that the first study conducted in the United States surveying pediatricians on medication prescribing patterns for children with sleep resistance found that pediatricians reported prescribing both nonprescription and prescription medication for short-term situational use (e.g., travel, acute pain, acute stress) as well as more long-term chronic use (high-risk populations: children with neurologic impairment, developmental delays, psychiatric conditions, attention deficit hyperactivity disorder; Owens, Rosen, & Mindell, 2003). Perhaps more noteworthy is the fact that nearly 25% of pediatricians have prescribed medication to children with difficulty initiating sleep yet are otherwise healthy, despite the robust evidence in support of behavioral interventions. These providers even expressed reservations about appropriate medication options and nonexistent clinical guidelines in terms of medication treatment for children with sleep resistance.

It is clear that the lack of sufficient training for medical providers in how to clinically manage sleep has posed a system-wide problem. From a stepped care perspective, the role of the primary care provider in pediatric insomnia is primarily prevention. As stated above, it is critical to assess sleep patterns at least two time points: infant and early childhood well-child appointments and in adolescence. Pediatric primary care providers should be equipped with tools such as sleep logs for primary caregivers to complete in order to help better identify young children at risk for developing clinically disordered sleep. Handouts describing the importance of sleep in infancy and early childhood, the consequences of chronic sleep inadequacy, as well as strategies to improve children's bedtime routines should also be available in every patient room. Sleep logs and informational self-help materials could also be part of patient portals. Behavioral health professionals should be consulted when sleep issues develop despite prevention strategies implemented by the medical professional. With regard to intervention, some of the strategies described in this chapter may be well-delivered within the primary care environment; however, a referral to specialty outpatient behavioral services should be given when families are not benefitting from the level of care provided in the integrated setting or when more time or follow-up is needed related to the interventions being employed.

Impact on Care/Quality Improvement Processes

To evaluate the impact of assessing and treating bedtime resistance in a pediatric primary care setting, conducting a needs assessment will help develop a baseline of specific medical professionals' knowledge regarding this issue (Owens, 2001) given that it has been found that there is a gap in the knowledge and skills pediatric primary care professionals have in recognizing and appropriately targeting such sleep-related issues (Rosen & Zozula, 2001). Obtaining information regarding what pediatric medical professionals are already doing to screen for, evaluate, and treat sleep disorders will provide a starting point to address any gaps within a given system. Despite the fact that clinical sleep disorders are associated with morbidity, functional impairment, and a decreased quality of life, an insufficient amount of attention is given to sleep by pediatric medical professionals. Since chronic bedtime resistance and other sleep-related issues can manifest in a child's mood as well as through internalizing and externalizing behaviors, insufficient skills to recognize sleep disturbances could result in wrongly attributing these symptoms to psychiatric diagnoses such as ADHD (Mindell, Owens, & Carskadon, 1999). Such a system-wide gap in knowledge highlights the need for a pediatric sleep medicine curricula to be adapted into medical school, residency training, and as part of continuing education requirements (Owens, 2001).

Summary

Sleep is a critical indicator of both psychological and physical health in all people, but markedly so in developing children. When sleep becomes disrupted, a cascade of negative outcomes can quickly occur both for the individual child and for their family members. As such, it is of the utmost importance to create institutional tools and knowledge in both assessment and treatment to quickly triage and treat sleep problems when they occur in pediatric populations. Fortunately, as clinicians we have a wealth of tools that have been empirically proven in the outpatient behavioral health setting. However, we have a duty to test the portability and acceptability of these interventions within the primary care setting and make evidence-based modifications where appropriate.

References

Bruni, O., Violani, C., Luchetti, A., Miano, S., Verrillo, E., Di Brina, C., & Valente, D. (2004). The sleep knowledge of pediatricians and child neuropsychiatrists. *Sleep and Hypnosis*, *6*, 130–138.

Chervin, R. D., Archbold, K. H., Panahi, P., & Pituch, K. J. (2001). Sleep problems seldom addressed at two general pediatric clinics. *Pediatrics*, *107*(6), 1375–1380.

Christophersen, E. R., & Vanscoyoc, S. M. (2013). *Treatments that work with children: Empirically supported strategies for managing childhood problems*. Washington, DC: American Psychological Association.

Davis, D. W., Honaker, S. M., Jones, V. F., Williams, P. G., Stocker, F., & Martin, E. (2012). Identification and management of behavioral/mental health problems in primary care pediatrics: Perceived strengths, challenges, and new delivery models. *Clinical Pediatrics*, *51*(10), 978–982.

Erichsen, D., Godoy, C., Gränse, F., Axelsson, J., Rubin, D., & Gozal, D. (2012). Screening for sleep disorders in pediatric primary care: Are we there yet? *Clinical Pediatrics*, *51*(12), 1125–1129.

Faruqui, F., Khubchandani, J., Price, J. H., Bolyard, D., & Reddy, R. (2011). Sleep disorders in children: A national assessment of primary care pediatrician practices and perceptions. *Pediatrics*.

Ferber, R. (2006). *Solve your child's sleep problems*. New York, NY: Fireside.

Freeman, K. A. (2006). Treating bedtime resistance with the bedtime pass: A systematic replication and component analysis with 3-year-olds. *Journal of Applied Behavior Analysis*, *39*(4), 423–428.

Gordon, J., King, N. J., Gullone, E., Muris, P., & Ollendick, T. H. (2001). Treatment of children's nighttime fears: The need for a modern randomised controlled trial. *Clinical Psychology Review*, *27*(1), 98–113.

Gradisar, M., Gardner, G., & Dohnt, H. (2011). Recent worldwide sleep patterns and problems during adolescence: A review and meta-analysis of age, region, and sleep. *Sleep Medicine*, *12*(2), 110–118.

Honaker, S. M., & Meltzer, L. J. (2016). Sleep in pediatric primary care: A review of the literature. *Sleep Medicine Reviews*, *25*, 31–39.

Kuhn, B. R., & Weidinger, D. (2000). Interventions for infant and toddler sleep disturbance: A review. *Child & Family Behavior Therapy*, *22*(2), 33–50.

Kuhn, B. R. (2014). Practical strategies for managing behavioral sleep problems in young children. *Sleep Medicine Clinics*, *9*(2), 181–197.

Mindell, J. A., Moline, M. L., Zendell, S. M., Brown, L. W., & Fry, J. M. (1994). Pediatricians and sleep disorders: Training and practice. *Pediatrics*, *94*, 194–200.

Mindell, J. A., Owens, J. A., & Carskadon, M. A. (1999). Developmental features of sleep. *Child and Adolescent Psychiatric Clinics of North America*, *8*, 695–725.

Mindell, J. A., Kuhn, B., Lewin, D. S., Meltzer, L. J., & Sadeh, A. (2006). Behavioral treatment of bedtime problems and night wakings in infants and young children. *Sleep*, *29*(10), 1263–1276.

Morgenthaler, T. I., Owens, J., Alessi, C., Boehlecke, B., Brown, T. M., Coleman, J., Jr., … Swick, T. J. (2006). American Academy of Sleep Medicine. *Sleep*, *29*(10), 1277–1281.

National Sleep Foundation. (2004). Sleep in America Poll; Summary of Findings. Washington, D.C.

Owens, J. A., Spirito, A., & McGuinn, M. (2000). The Children's Sleep Habits Questionnaire (CSHQ): Psychometric properties of a survey instrument for school-aged children. *Sleep*, *23*, 1043–1051.

Owens, J. A. (2001). The practice of pediatric sleep medicine: Results of a community survey. *Pediatrics*, *108*(3), e51–e51.

Owens, J. A., Rosen, C. L., & Mindell, J. A. (2003). Medication use in the treatment of pediatric insomnia: Results of a survey of community-based pediatricians. *Pediatrics*, *111*(5), e628–e635.

Owens, J. A., & Dalzell, V. (2005). Use of the 'BEARS' sleep screening tool in a pediatric residents' continuity clinic: A pilot study. *Sleep Medicine*, *6*(1), 63–69.

Owens, J. (2008). Classification and epidemiology of childhood sleep disorders. *Primary Care*, *35*(3), 533e46.

Owens, J. A., Rosen, C. L., Mindell, J. A., & Kirchner, H. L. (2010). Use of pharmacotherapy for insomnia in child psychiatry practice: A national survey. *Sleep Medicine*, *11*(7), 692–700.

Paruthi, S., Brooks, L. J., D'Ambrosio, C., Hall, W. A., Kotagal, S., Lloyd, R. M., … Rosen, C. L. (2016). Recommended amount of sleep for pediatric populations: A consensus statement of the American Academy of Sleep Medicine. *Journal of Clinical Sleep Medicine*, *12*(6), 785.

Patterson, G. R. (1982). *Coercive family process* (Vol. 3). Castalia Publishing Company.

Stojanovski, S. D., Rasu, R. S., Balkrishnan, R., & Nahata, M. C. (2007). Trends in medication prescribing for pediatric sleep difficulties in US outpatient settings. *Sleep*, *30*(8), 1013–1017.

Rosen, R., & Zozula, R. (2001). Development of a brief, self-administered instrument for assessing sleep knowledge in medical education: The ASKME survey. *Sleep*, *24*, 227–233.

30 Posttraumatic Stress Disorder

David Austern, Jeffrey A. Cigrang, Sheila A. Rauch, and Ashley L. Evans

A Brief Description of the Disorder or Problem

After someone directly experiences, witnesses, or learns about a traumatic event, he or she may begin experiencing a variety of troubling cognitive, emotional, and physical symptoms. They may have intrusions of the event (e.g., nightmares), start avoiding reminders of the event, have unpleasant thoughts and feelings in relation to the event (e.g., self-blame), and could also have unpleasant physical symptoms in relation to the event (e.g., insomnia). While these symptoms are common in the aftermath of traumas, they typically subside after several weeks without the need for intervention. Posttraumatic stress disorder (PTSD) is a syndrome that can develop when the natural recovery process is thwarted.

D. Austern, Psy.D. (✉)
Veterans Affairs Maryland Healthcare System (VAMHCS), Baltimore, MD, USA

The Steven A. Cohen Military Family Clinic at NYU Langone Medical Center, New York, NY, USA
e-mail: david.austern@nyumc.org

J.A. Cigrang, Ph.D., A.B.P.P. • A.L. Evans, B.S.
Wright State University, Dayton, OH, USA
e-mail: Jeffrey.cigrang@wright.edu

S.A. Rauch, Ph.D., A.B.P.P.
Emory University School of Medicine and Atlanta VA Medical Center, Atlanta, GA, USA
e-mail: Sheila.a.m.rauch@emory.edu

PTSD is a common mental health problem in primary care populations, with prevalence estimates of approximately 12% in community-based (Stein, McQuaid, Pedrelli, Lenox, & McCahill, 2000) and Department of Veteran Affairs clinics (Magruder et al., 2005). Unfortunately, it is also quite burdensome; researchers have estimated the annual productivity loss resulting from PTSD may approximate $3 billion (Kessler, 2000). Veterans along with active duty military members may be especially vulnerable to developing PTSD and can experience unemployment, homelessness, and family disruption as a consequence of the disorder (Tanelian & Jaycox, 2008). Fortunately, there are a variety of treatment options for PTSD that include psychotherapy and medication management.

Research has established that trauma-focused psychotherapies (e.g., prolonged exposure, cognitive processing therapy) are efficacious in treating PTSD (Department of Veterans Affairs & Department of Defense, 2010; Institute of Medicine, 2014). However, people seeking help for PTSD symptoms can experience difficulty accessing these treatments, may drop out of treatment prematurely, or even find that the psychotherapy was not sufficiently helpful (Sloan, Marx, & Keane, 2011). Echoing these findings, a survey of returning veterans found that only one in four of those who met criteria for PTSD received minimally adequate treatment (Schell & Marshall,

A. Maragakis, W.T. O'Donohue (eds.), *Principle-Based Stepped Care and Brief Psychotherapy for Integrated Care Settings*, https://doi.org/10.1007/978-3-319-70539-2_30

2008). This is unfortunate because these evidence-based psychotherapies (EBPs) have been shown to reduce healthcare costs (Tuerk et al., 2013). Thus, untreated PTSD is a burdensome public health issue, and there is a growing need to improve the service delivery of psychological treatments.

One promising method of service delivery is stepped care. Patients are initially placed in the "least restrictive" treatment that is expected to offer them some benefit, while they maintain the option to be "stepped up" to a more intensive treatment if they are not benefitting. The stepped care service delivery model aims to increase efficiency by reserving more costly treatments (i.e., individual treatments requiring extensive therapist training and direct contact) for the patients most in need (Bower & Gilbody, 2005). However, applying stepped care principles to the service delivery of PTSD treatments is a relatively new endeavor.

The Veterans Affairs/Department of Defense practice guidelines (2010) propose a model of treating PTSD beginning with pharmacotherapy (e.g., prescribing antidepressants) and stepping patients up to psychotherapy and/or additional medication. This particular model presumes that patients are willing to engage in both forms of treatment, which may not be true. Military patients, for example, may have heightened concern toward medication's possible side effects, and this could create a significant barrier toward seeking treatment (Tanelian & Jaycox, 2008). In addition, many patients may not respond to medication or may experience side effects that prevent them reaching a therapeutic dose. Furthermore, there are inconclusive findings regarding the effectiveness of antidepressant medications for PTSD (Institute of Medicine, 2008). Recent meta-analyses support that trauma-focused psychotherapy should be a first-line treatment based on frequency and magnitude of response (Lee et al., 2016).

Within the Veterans Health Administration, PTSD treatment is commonly delivered inside specialty PTSD clinics (i.e., PTSD Clinical Teams) where providers often have specialized training and clinical expertise in treating PTSD. However, a study on service utilization found that returning veterans recently diagnosed with PTSD rarely completed treatment in the specialty clinics; results indicated that while 66% attended at least three PTSD clinic visits in the year following the positive PTSD screen, only 33% attended at least nine PTSD clinic visits in that same time frame. (Lu, Duckart, O'Malley, & Dobscha, 2011). The study's methodology makes it difficult to draw conclusions as to why more participants did not complete treatment in the study's time frame; although dropout is one theory, another possibility is that some participants benefitted and responded to treatment early. In fact, these authors questioned whether all veterans with PTSD require the same amount of treatment; perhaps more costly, intensive interventions could be reserved for those with more severe PTSD symptoms.

Perceived stigma about mental healthcare constitutes an additional barrier toward seeking treatment (Brown & Bruce, 2016; Hoge et al., 2004). Thus there may be an advantage to offering mental health services in primary care settings to decrease stigma associated with seeking treatment in the specialty mental health clinic (Pietrzak, Johnson, Goldstein, Malley, & Southwick, 2009). For example, the VHA provides a blended model of both colocated collaborative care (i.e., a mental health provider is embedded in a primary care clinic) and care management (i.e., a mental health provider is referred to patients from the primary care provider for telephone evaluation and triage of mental health problems) in order to most effectively meet veterans' mental health needs (Zeiss & Karlin, 2008). A recent study examined the effectiveness of a centrally assisted collaborative telecare (CACT) intervention among military service members; authors found that patients who received the intervention experienced significantly greater reductions in PTSD and depression symptoms over 12 months of follow-up compared to patients who received usual care (Engel et al., 2016). The purpose of this chapter is to summarize information on stepped care and brief behavioral treatments for PTSD in primary care settings in the service of optimizing assessment of and care for this challenging disorder.

Effective Ways to Screen for PTSD in the Primary Care Setting

Without effective screening tools in place, PTSD symptoms can be overlooked by primary care providers (Magruder et al., 2005). Although a variety of PTSD screeners specific to the primary care environment have been tested, the Primary Care Posttraumatic Stress Disorder Screen (PC-PTSD) and the PTSD Symptom Checklist (PCL) have received the most scientific evaluation specifically for primary care use.

The PC-PTSD was a four-item yes-no screener that assessed the four major symptom clusters of PTSD (reexperiencing, numbing, avoidance, and hyperarousal) the patient had experienced over the past month. Equal weight was given to all four items. Department of Veterans Affairs and Department of Defense guidelines for PTSD screening recommended a cutoff of three positive endorsements of symptoms when using the PC-PTSD (Department of Veterans Affairs & Department of Defense, 2010), while a cutoff of two positive symptoms had been recommended for the civilian population (Van Dam, Ehring, Vedel, & Emmelkamp, 2010). Due to the recent changes in PTSD diagnostic criteria implemented in the DSM-5, the PC-PTSD was updated to reflect these changes (PC-PTSD-5). The PC-PTSD-5 added a fifth item, which assesses for trauma-related blame and guilt. According to the DoD/VA, the PC-PTSD-5 is still undergoing validation (Primary Care PTSD Screen for DSM-5 (PC-PTSD-5)", n.d.). However, a cutoff score of 3 is recommended as consideration for a positive screen (Prins et al., 2016).

The PCL was originally a 17-item self-report measure based on DSM-IV criteria that asks patients to rate the severity of their trauma symptomatology on a 5-point severity scale (i.e., "not at all" to "extremely"). There were different versions of the PCL that were worded to be most relevant to certain populations. The PCL-M was designed for use with military populations and was recommended by VA/DoD Clinical Practice Guidelines when screening for PTSD in primary care settings (Peterson, Luethcke, Borah, Borah, & Young-McCaughan, 2011). In contrast, the language used on the PCL-C was tailored to screening for PTSD in civilian populations (Stein et al., 2000). The PCL-5 is the newest edition of the PCL, updated according to DSM-5 diagnostic criteria, and now contains 20 items. Similar to the PC-PTSD-5, research on the PCL-5 is continuing to grow; however, recommended cutoff scores currently fall within the 31–33 range for the most efficient in predicting a DSM-5 PTSD diagnosis (Bovin et al., 2015).

With both measures providing similar screening performance, the choice of which to use is largely up to the needs and preferences of the individual clinic. The PCL-5 is considered easy to administer and score but clearly requires more time to complete than the PC-PTSD-5. However, since the screener is only five items, there is the potential to miss out on valuable information that can be obtained by the lengthier PCL-5. If civilian primary care providers are unaccustomed to screening for PTSD, it may be helpful to begin by asking broadly about a patient's history of trauma exposure. One recent study found that rates of exposure to any trauma ranged from 66.38 to 83.66% of participants depending on their race and ethnicity; of these participants, 9.1% went on to develop PTSD (Roberts, Gilman, Breslau, Breslau, & Koenen, 2011). We recommend using the PC-PTSD-5 as a universal screener and then customizing the level of subsequent assessment based on the patient's clinical presentation and the available clinic resources.

How to Further Assess If a Screen Returns Positive

If the PC-PTSD-5 returns positive, further assessment of PTSD symptoms is recommended. However, the setting where one works will likely dictate the extent of additional assessment that is performed. This can range from administering the PCL-5 and querying about the patient's responses in an unstructured interview to administering structured PTSD assessments as part of a comprehensive battery of psychological measures. Given the fast-paced nature of the primary care environment, comprehensive psychological assessments are more likely to be performed in specialty mental healthcare settings (e.g., PTSD Clinical Teams). Even within those settings, it is often the case that varying levels of assessments are performed based on the referral question and the patient's presenting problems. The most comprehensive assessment batteries are reserved for patients who present with the most complexity. Therefore, stepped care principles applied to the assessment of PTSD are helpful in maximizing clinical resources.

For some patients it may be sufficient to administer the Life Events Checklist for DSM-5 (LEC-5), the PCL-5, and query their responses. The LEC-5 is an instrument used to assess traumatic exposure and help establish that a patient meets Criterion A for PTSD. Although the PC-PTSD-5 provides patients with examples of six potential traumatic events (i.e., serious accident or fire, physical or sexual assault or abuse, earthquake or flood, war, seeing someone be killed or seriously injured, having a loved one die through homicide or suicide), the LEC-5 lists 16 events plus provides patients with the option to add their own. Furthermore, the PC-PTSD-5 does not distinguish among the variety of ways a patient may "experience" a traumatic stressor, whereas the LEC-5 does. For example, it is important for providers to know whether a patient has directly experienced the trauma, whether they witnessed it happening to someone else, or whether they learned about it happening to a close friend or family member.

After a provider determines the patient meets Criterion A, they can help the patient establish which event is the "index trauma," usually the most distressing event and often the focus of treatment. Helpful questions for providers to ask may include "Which event is currently the most distressing to you?" "Which event are you having the most intrusions about?" "Which event would you *least* like to discuss?" and/or "Which event occurred first?"

Once the index trauma is established, patients can fill out the PCL-5 in relation to the index trauma. Patients should be encouraged to keep this particular event in mind as they respond to the items, given the potential for multiple events to lead to an overly general report of symptoms. Querying their responses to the PCL-5 will help determine whether they are providing an accurate report of symptoms or whether they may be interpreting item content idiosyncratically (e.g., patients often have difficulty discriminating between experiencing intrusive thoughts and their own rumination).

When querying a patient's PCL-5 responses is insufficient for a provider's purposes, it may be necessary to use the Clinician-Administered PTSD Scale for DSM-5 (CAPS-5), which is considered the "gold standard" in PTSD assessment. However, the CAPS-5 is unlikely to be administered in a primary care setting, and thus a referral to specialty mental health may be indicated in those instances.

Evidence-Based Stepped Care, Brief Psychotherapeutic Approaches, and Medications

There are no evidence-based guidelines for how behavioral health providers working in an integrated primary care clinic should treat PTSD (Possemato, 2011). Current Department of Veterans Affairs and Department of Defense guidelines for PTSD in primary care limit talk therapy options to supportive counseling (Department of Veterans Affairs & Department of Defense, 2010). However, the behavioral health provider interested in PTSD and primary care treatment is not without recourse. First, the remarkable growth in integrated care practice has resulted in publication of high-quality books authored by experienced clinicians (e.g., Hunter, Goodie, Dobmeyer, & Dorrance, 2009; Robinson & Reiter, 2007) that offer step-by-step guidance for using psychotherapy techniques adapted for the fast-paced environment of primary care. Though not specifically developed for PTSD, skills such as relaxation training, problem-solving, cognitive disputation, stimulus control, and sleep hygiene can provide some help to the patient in managing PTSD symptoms, while a referral for treatment to a specialty mental health provider is arranged. Second, several brief protocols for treating PTSD have been developed specifically for use in an integrated primary care environment (Cigrang et al., 2011, 2015; Corso et al., 2009; Harmon, Goldstein, Shiner, & Watts, 2014), though the current maturity of the science is limited to clinical case series and smaller pilot studies. Commonalities across these protocols are the short appointment durations (20–30 min) and limited number of appointments (2–4).

A primary distinction between the primary care protocols is whether treatment content includes a focus on the traumatic experience. Behavioral activation (BA) has been adapted for treatment of PTSD and used in an integrated primary care setting (Harmon et al., 2014). Originally developed for treatment of depression, BA helps patients identify and engage in activities that are potentially rewarding and consistent with their life goals. As applied to PTSD, the use of BA is viewed as a pragmatic way to target the avoidance symptoms of PTSD without specifically reviewing traumatic memories (Mulick, Landes, & Kanter, 2011). While working toward increased engagement with their environment, patients with PTSD may also encounter situations that are being avoided because of their association with traumatic memories.

Clinical case series with BA have shown good outcomes for BA with comorbid PTSD and depression (Jakupcak, Wagner, Paulson, Varra, & McFall, 2010; Mulick & Naugle, 2010; Nixon & Nearmy, 2011) and PTSD alone (Jakupcak et al., 2006) using protocols that are not consistent with integrated care (i.e., require 45–90-min weekly sessions over a 12–16-week period). When a brief version of BA was examined with 82 veterans in primary care using three, 20-min sessions, no changes were demonstrated from pre- to posttreatment in symptoms (Harmon et al., 2014). However, a majority (62%) of participants went on to specialty mental health treatment, suggesting that the intervention may have had a positive effect on referral follow-through compared to standard referral to specialty mental health (26%; Bohnert, Sripada, Mach, & McCarthy, 2015).

Primary care protocols for PTSD that have focused specifically on aspects of the traumatic experience have used written exposure as a key element. Corso and colleagues (Corso et al., 2009) examined two types of writing tasks in an integrated primary care clinic, but small sample size prevents any conclusions.

Over the past several years, there has been an ongoing effort by a Department of Defense and Department of Veteran Affairs' team to further develop and evaluate a brief exposure-based PTSD treatment for use by behavioral health providers working in integrated primary care (Cigrang et al., 2011, 2015). Prolonged Exposure for Primary Care (PE-PC) built on the writing exercises from Corso et al. (2009) and the PE protocol create a program that includes imaginal exposure through writing, processing through writing exercises, and in vivo exposure in detailed patient and provider manuals.

At the first 30-min PE-PC appointment, patients are provided a "Confronting Uncomfortable Memories" activity workbook to be completed at home and brought back for use in subsequent appointments. The workbook asks the patient to write a first-person, detailed narrative of the traumatic event associated with the greatest level of current distress and preoccupation, including recollection of personal thoughts, feelings, and physical reactions, and to answer emotional processing questions (e.g., "How has this event changed what you think about yourself?" and "How has this event changed how you think about others?"). Patients are instructed to write and then read the trauma narrative and their answers to the emotional processing questions for at least 30 min three times per week. During the second, third, and fourth appointments, patients are asked to read the narrative and their answers to the emotional processing questions out loud. The remainder of each 30-min appointment is devoted to trauma-associated emotional processing using a focused discussion of problematic beliefs and the emotions they evoke. At the end of the fourth appointment, the patient and provider review treatment progress and collaboratively decided whether to conclude treatment or to arrange a referral to specialty mental health services.

An open trial of PE-PC with active duty military service members has shown significant improvements in PTSD and depression symptoms based on both self-report and clinician interview measures. Treatment gains were maintained at 6- and 12-month follow-up assessments. The percentage of participants whose symptoms met diagnostic criteria for PTSD was reduced by nearly half (Cigrang et al., 2015). Thus, PE-PC holds great promise for behavioral health providers interested in a brief, manualized protocol for treating PTSD in integrated primary care. A randomized clinical trial was recently completed evaluating PE-PC compared to a minimal contact wait list condition, and the results are forthcoming. Readers interested in learning about the process for achieving competence in the use of PE-PC are encouraged to contact the second and third author.

In addition to brief psychotherapy, both sertraline and paroxetine have an FDA indication as effective for the treatment of PTSD (Department of Veterans Affairs & Department of Defense, 2010). Providers must consider patient preferences, current medications, and side effects when discussing medication as an option for PTSD treatment. For those who do not fully respond to medication, psychotherapeutic approaches may still be indicated to augment medication or function as stand-alone interventions. Readers who are considering medications are referred to the VA/DoD clinical guideline for PTSD that provides a more complete review of options for PTSD treatment and symptom management.

What Does Not Work

Use of evidence-based care by practitioners when treating PTSD is of the utmost importance. Unfortunately, there is an assortment of widely disseminated practices that lack sufficient research support to justify their use (e.g., cranial electrotherapy stimulation or CES devices) or may even be contraindicated after being exposed to scientific scrutiny. For example, many patients with PTSD are prescribed benzodiazepines (e.g., valium) despite evidence cautioning against their use. A recent meta-analysis (Guina, Rossetter, DeRhodes, Nahhas, & Welton, 2015) suggests that these drugs may be contraindicated for patients with PTSD. Particularly troubling for behavioral health providers is the finding that benzodiazepines may interfere with exposure-based psychological treatments like PE (Van Minnen, Arntz, & Keijsers, 2002). Thus, behavioral health providers should be mindful of a patient's medication regimen prior to initiating evidence-based behavioral treatment for PTSD in a primary care setting or before referring a patient to specialty mental health.

Another intervention that has seen widespread use is psychological debriefing – an umbrella term for a variety of technologies (e.g., Critical Incident Stress Debriefing) promoting brief emotional and psychological support after a trauma (e.g., meeting with people exposed to 9/11) to prevent the development of PTSD. Although well-intentioned, psychological debriefing has not yielded sufficient research support to justify its use. In contrast, a meta-analysis suggested that Critical Incident Stress Debriefing can actually have a detrimental effect on natural trauma recovery (van Emmerik, Kamphuis, Hulsbosch, & Emmelkamp, 2002). Behavioral health providers working in collaborative care settings should be mindful of these findings given that many hospitals unwittingly continue to employ psychological debriefing technologies (e.g., Critical Incident Stress Management Teams).

Providers benefit from having strong rationales for the treatments they recommend, especially when working with patients with PTSD who may have difficulty initially trusting providers. The stronger the scientific evidence that exists for the interventions we provide, the easier it is to recommend them. Although some interventions may be recommended within certain organizations, these interventions may nonetheless have questionable mechanisms of action (e.g., Eye Movement Desensitization and Reprocessing or EMDR). The purported mechanism of action (i.e., eye movements) of EMDR has largely been debunked in favor of a hypothesized exposure-based mechanism. Thus, it may be easier to explain to patients how exposure-based (i.e., PE) and cognitive-based (i.e., CPT) treatments work.

Providers may be tempted to use certain treatments that have some promising research support but are not yet considered well-established. For example, Acceptance and Commitment Therapy has been studied as an alternative PTSD treatment to PE/CPT over the past decade; however, the research is in its infancy with a recent RCT showing no benefit over present-centered therapy (Lang et al., 2016). When in doubt about whether a particular intervention would be effective, providers may benefit from seeking free consultation from the National Center for PTSD Consultation Program (http://www.ptsd.va.gov/professional/consult/).

When to Refer to External Specialty Mental Health

Behavioral health providers should be mindful of when a patient may benefit from a referral to a specialty mental health clinic or program for PTSD treatment. Examples include if the patient requires additional assessment, if the patient prefers to be treated there, if the patient may benefit from treatment options unavailable in primary care, if the patient has certain diagnostic features or comorbidities that require a higher level of care, or if the patient did not achieve remission from PTSD after behavioral health treatment was attempted in a primary care setting.

Some patients require assessment beyond what is feasible in a primary care setting, especially when there are concerns about symptom validity. The CAPS-5 is a structured interview that assesses for PTSD by providing standardized questions and probes about symptoms in relation to the index trauma; in contrast to self-report measures like the PCL-5, the provider uses their clinical judgment to make symptom severity ratings with the CAPS-5. In addition to assessing PTSD symptoms, the CAPS-5 queries subjective distress and functional impairment and allows providers to rate overall response validity. Ensuring symptom validity can be especially important when assessing PTSD with compensation-seeking patients. Research has shown that veterans, who may seek to become "service-connected" (i.e., when one receives financial compensation for a disability linked to their military service) for PTSD, may overreport or exaggerate their symptoms (Frueh et al., 2003). Such assessment batteries with multiple symptom validity measures (e.g., including an objective personality measure with validity scales) are most likely administered in specialty mental health settings.

Although some patients may feel stigmatized if they are referred to specialty PTSD clinics or programs, others may prefer to be treated in those environments. Eliciting patient preference regarding specialty mental health treatment is especially recommended to reduce combat mental health utilization disparities. A recent study found that Asian and African-Americans were less likely to receive referrals to specialty mental health clinics than White and Latino Americans (Meyer, Saw, Cho, & Fancher, 2015).

Some treatment offerings may only be available in specialty settings, such as a psychoeducational orientation group for patients new to PTSD treatment. A recent study examining veterans' satisfaction and treatment preferences who attended a PTSD Clinical Team 60-min orientation group found that veterans were highly satisfied with the group's ability to educate them about available treatment options (Schumm, Walter, Bartone, & Chard, 2015). This particular PCT offered six different PTSD treatments as well as medication management options, which may be too comprehensive a treatment package for a behavioral health provider working in a primary care setting.

Behavioral health providers may also consider a referral when patients present with co-occurring disorders (e.g., substance use disorders or SUD). A recent exploratory study of military veterans' treatment preferences found that the overwhelming majority preferred integrated PTSD and substance use treatment (Back et al., 2014). Seeking Safety (Najavits, 2002), an integrated PTSD/SUD treatment delivered across 25 sessions in a group format, may not be available or feasible in a primary care setting, and the evidence for efficacy for the treatment of PTSD is low (Berenz & Coffey, 2012). Occasionally, outpatient care may be insufficient to meet a patient's needs. Residential PTSD programs exist for patients who may have attempted EBPs in outpatient settings and were unsuccessful due to comorbidities (e.g., SUD) or psychosocial stressors. Additionally, it may be necessary to provide inpatient care to patients at risk of harming themselves; suicidal ideation and suicidal behavior have been found to be significantly associated with PTSD (Sareen, Houlahan, Cox, & Asmundson, 2005).

Finally, it may be indicated to refer patients for additional PTSD treatment if they do not respond or achieve remission after completing brief primary care-based treatments. For example, Cigrang et al. (2015) noted that a small minority of patients (2 of 24) requested to discontinue primary care-based PTSD treatment due to an increase in symptoms; both of these patients were offered a referral to specialty mental healthcare. The PE-PC protocol embodies the spirit of stepped care principles by emphasizing a collaborative decision between patient and provider regarding whether to refer patients to specialty mental healthcare.

The Role of the Primary Care Provider/Medical Team in Treatment

Behavioral health providers working in primary care settings are likely operating within the Primary Care Behavioral Health (PCBH) model (Robinson & Reiter, 2007), which is notably used in both VHA and military healthcare systems. In this model a behavioral health provider (e.g., psychologist) is embedded within a primary care clinic and works collaboratively with the medical team on behavioral health-related presenting problems of patients. The behavioral health provider may function in a variety of roles, including consultant, screener/assessor, and therapist. Clinical responsibility is typically maintained by the medical provider, with the behavioral health provider providing consultation and feedback regarding the patient's care. As such, this model is far more collaborative than other arrangements where patients may be referred from primary to specialty care and then clinical responsibility is transferred.

A recent study examined PCBH provider practices within two large healthcare settings, the VHA and the United States Air Force, and found that VHA behavioral health providers were more likely to regularly screen for PTSD than USAF providers (97% vs. 52%, respectively; Funderburk, Dobmeyer, Hunter, Walsh, & Maisto, 2013). Assuming that one's clinic and larger medical system is prepared to respond with help, it is important for providers to implement screening programs if there are not already ones in place. Furthermore, they should ensure that they are using DSM-5 consistent versions of the screening measures; it may be necessary to train support staff on how to orient patients to the screener if they are being administered the measures in a waiting room prior to meeting the PCBH provider. Consultation with primary care providers is also an important role for PCBH providers, although this may not occur with patients directly. Funderburk and colleagues noted that only 29–35% of VHA and USAF PCBH providers were regularly asked to join patient appointments by primary care providers; as such, providing important information (e.g., contraindications of benzodiazepines for PTSD patients) may need to take place at primary care staff meetings, which the majority of PCBH providers acknowledged attending. Ideally, the medical team will be receptive to the feedback and consultation offered by PCBH providers.

Some logistical considerations warrant mentioning when working with PTSD patients in primary care settings. Funderburk and colleagues found that the overwhelming majority of PCBH providers' offices were located within primary care clinics, and thus their patients used primary care waiting rooms. Patients with PTSD often have safety concerns and may be reluctant to sit with their backs to doors or other people. These concerns could be exacerbated by a hectic primary care environment. If feasible, it may be helpful to arrange the waiting area such that there is ample seating against the walls with at least some seats facing the door. Though reducing hypervigilance is a target of PTSD interventions, it is unrealistic to expect patients who are new to PTSD treatments to immediately stop scanning and tolerate the distress evoked by the situation. Similarly, to the extent possible, reducing levels of crowding in waiting areas will be helpful in creating a calmer environment for patients who are likely to avoid exposure to crowds. These environmental modifications may go a long way toward making patients feel comfortable enough to receive PTSD treatment in a primary care setting.

How to Assess Impact on Care/Quality Improvement Processes

There are numerous ways behavioral health providers working in primary care settings can assess the impact of their interventions. One important measure of an intervention's impact is whether it leads to symptom reduction and/or other improvements in subjective outcomes (e.g., enhanced quality of life) for patients. Depending on the setting, providers may want to measure symptoms on a weekly basis, or they may opt for measurement at fewer time points (e.g., pretreatment and posttreatment). Given the fast-paced nature of the primary care environment, administering the CAPS-5 at multiple time points is probably not feasible. However, the PCL-5 is well suited to function as a PTSD symptom outcome measure that can be easily administered on a weekly basis. Doing so allows the provider to make adjustments to the intervention if the patient's symptoms are not decreasing as expected. Although the collection of psychometric data on the PCL-5 is still an ongoing process, a recent study suggested that posttreatment scores at or below 24 likely represent clinically significant change for military members with PTSD (Wortmann et al., 2016).

Another important indicator of quality improvement is tracking outcomes related to attendance. Given how avoidance is one of the hallmark symptoms of PTSD, it is perhaps unsurprising that patients frequently have difficulties initiating and completing treatment. Monitoring patient attendance and noting whether they complete or drop out from treatment can be helpful in evaluating the tolerability of and satisfaction with the interventions being delivered. The PE-PC protocol was developed with these concerns in mind and seems to be well-tolerated (i.e., 71% of patients completed treatment) based on pilot study data (Cigrang et al., 2015). If providers are implementing a full PE or CPT protocol, they may consider patients who receive at least eight sessions as treatment completers based on Mott, Hundt, Sansgiry, Mignogna, and Cully's (2014) methodology; this is helpful in ascertaining whether patients are receiving an adequate dose of trauma-focused psychotherapy.

As previously discussed, evidence-based psychotherapies can reduce healthcare costs within a system, and a stepped care approach aims to maximize resources. Although it is beyond the scope of this chapter to provide a how-to guide in conducting health economic analyses, we can pinpoint several areas that may be fruitful targets for examination of cost-effectiveness. Does the intervention reduce the clinical burden on specialty PTSD care? The VHA has a mandate that all veterans must be scheduled for an initial appointment within 30 days or be compensated for a referral to a community provider. If even a small proportion of PTSD can be successfully treated in primary care, it may alleviate some of the need to provide community referrals, thus decreasing costs.

Another important question is how the receipt of the intervention impacts the overall healthcare spending on a particular patient. Ideally, patients receive the least restrictive, most cost-effective level of care necessary to benefit them and then do not receive additional, unnecessary mental healthcare. One may intuit that if a patient drops out of PTSD treatment, they will no longer be a financial burden on a healthcare system. However, Tuerk et al. (2013) found that veterans who dropped out of PE continued to use mental health services at a significantly higher rate than those veterans who completed PE. This finding underscores the importance of addressing dropout from PTSD treatments, as treatment completers may not require subsequent, costly mental health treatment.

As Bower and Gilbody (2005) note, a strong stepped care model of treatment is efficient and acceptable. It is clearly more efficient to treat patients over four brief sessions in primary care settings than immediately refer them to specialty PTSD clinics where they will receive 8–15 longer sessions of PE/CPT. This smaller dose of treatment may offer substantial relief to a significant proportion of the population of patients suffering from PTSD. Without primary care treatments, all patients suffering from PTSD would be referred to specialty care and quickly overwhelm their healthcare systems. Research suggests that the majority of patients find these brief interventions acceptable and some may even prefer them over specialty PTSD treatment due to perceived stigma. In sum, we encourage behavioral health providers working in primary care settings to consider adopting a stepped care model of treatment if feasible within their healthcare systems.

References

Back, S. E., Killeen, T. K., Teer, A. P., Hartwell, E. E., Federline, A., Beylotte, F., & Cox, E. (2014). Substance use disorders and PTSD: An exploratory study of treatment preferences among military veterans. *Addictive Behaviors, 39*(2), 369–373.

Berenz, E. C., & Coffey, S. F. (2012). Treatment of co-occurring posttraumatic stress disorder and substance use disorder. *Current Psychiatry Reports, 14*, 469–477.

Bohnert, K. M., Sripada, R. K., Mach, J., & McCarthy, J. F. (2015). Same-day Integrated Mental Health Care and PTSD diagnosis and treatment among VHA primary care patients with positive PTSD screens. *Psychiatric Services, 67*(1), 94–100.

Bovin, M. J., Marx, B. P., Weathers, F. W., Gallagher, M. W., Rodriguez, P., Schnurr, P. P., & Keane, T. M. (2015, December 14). Psychometric Properties of the PTSD Checklist for Diagnostic and Statistical Manual of Mental Disorders–Fifth Edition (PCL-5) in Veterans. *Psychological Assessment*. Advance online publication.

Bower, P., & Gilbody, S. (2005). Stepped care in psychological therapies: Access, effectiveness and efficiency. *The British Journal of Psychiatry, 186*(1), 11–17.

Brown, N. B., & Bruce, S. E. (2016). Stigma, career worry, and mental illness symptomatology: Factors influencing treatment-seeking for Operation Enduring Freedom and Operation Iraqi Freedom soldiers and veterans. *Psychological Trauma: Theory, Research, Practice, and Policy, 8*(3), 276–283.

Cigrang, J. A., Rauch, S. A. M., Avila, L. L., Bryan, C. J., Goode, J. L., Hryshko-Mullen, A., & Peterson, A. (2011). Treatment of active duty military with PTSD in primary care: Early findings. *Psychological Services, 8*(2), 104–113.

Cigrang, J. A., Rauch, S. A. M., Mintz, J., Brundige, A., Avila, L. L., Bryan, C. J., … the STRONG STAR Consortium. (2015). Treatment of active duty military with PTSD in primary care: A follow-up report. *Journal of Anxiety Disorders, 36*, 110–114.

Corso, K. A., Bryan, C. J., Morrow, C. E., Appolonio, K. K., Dodendorf, D. M., & Baker, M. T. (2009). Managing posttraumatic stress disorder symptoms in active duty military personnel in primary care settings. *Journal of Mental Health Counseling, 31*(2), 119–137.

The Management of Post-Traumatic Stress Working Group. (2010). *VA/DoD clinical practice guideline for Management of Post-Traumatic Stress*. Washington, DC: Department of Veterans Affairs, Department of Defense.

Engel, C. C., Jaycox, L. H., Freed, M. C., Bray, R. M., Brambilla, D., Zatzick, D., … Belsher, B. E. (2016). Centrally assisted collaborative telecare for posttraumatic stress disorder and depression among military personnel attending primary care: A randomized clinical trial. *JAMA Internal Medicine, 176*(7), 948–956.

Frueh, B. C., Elhai, J. D., Gold, P. B., Monnier, J., Magruder, K. M., Keane, T. M., et al. (2003). Disability compensation seeking among veterans evaluated for posttraumatic stress disorder. *Psychiatric Services, 54*, 84–91.

Funderburk, J. S., Dobmeyer, A. C., Hunter, C. L., Walsh, C. O., & Maisto, S. A. (2013). Provider practices in the primary care behavioral health (PCBH) model: An initial examination in the Veterans Health Administration and United States Air Force. *Families, Systems, & Health, 31*(4), 341.

Guina, J., Rossetter, S. R., DeRhodes, B. J., Nahhas, R. W., & Welton, R. S. (2015). Benzodiazepines for PTSD: A systematic review and meta-analysis. *Journal of Psychiatric Practice, 21*(4), 281–303.

Harmon, A. L., Goldstein, E. S. R., Shiner, B., & Watts, B. V. (2014). Preliminary findings for a brief posttraumatic stress intervention in primary mental health care. *Psychological Services, 11*, 295–299.

Hoge, C. W., Castro, C. A., Messer, S. C., McGurk, D., Cotting, D. I., & Koffman, R. L. (2004). Combat duty in Iraq and Afghanistan, mental health problems, and barriers to care. *New England Journal of Medicine, 351*(1), 13–22.

Hunter, C. L., Goodie, J. L., Oordt, M. S., & Dobmeyer, A. C. (2009). Behavioral health in primary care: A practitioner's handbook. Washington, DC: American Psychological Association.

Institute of Medicine (IOM). (2014). *Treatment for posttraumatic stress disorder in military and veteran populations: Final assessment*. Washington, DC: The National Academies Press.

Institute of Medicine (IOM). (2008). *Treatment of posttraumatic stress disorder: An assessment of the evidence*. Washington, DC: The National Academies Press.

Jakupcak, M., Robertsd, L. J., Martell, C., Mulick, P., Michael, S., Reed, R., … McFall, M. (2006). A pilot study of behavioral activation for veterans with posttraumatic stress disorder. *Journal of Traumatic Stress*, *19*, 387–391.

Jakupcak, M., Wagner, A., Paulson, A., Varra, A., & McFall, M. (2010). Behavioral activation as a primary care-based treatment for PTSD and depression among returning veterans. *Journal of Traumatic Stress*, *23*, 491–495.

Kessler, R. C. (2000). Posttraumatic stress disorder: The burden to the individual and to society. *The Journal of Clinical Psychiatry*, *61*(suppl 5), 4–12.

Lang, A. J., Schnurr, P. P., Jain, S., He, F., Walser, R. D., Bolton, E., Benedek, D. M., Norman, S. B., Sylvers, P., Flashman, L., Strauss, J., Raman, R., & Chard, K. M. (2016, June 20). Randomized controlled trial of acceptance and commitment therapy for distress and impairment in OEF/OIF/OND Veterans. *Psychological Trauma: Theory, Research, Practice, and Policy*. Advance online publication. https://doi.org/10.1037/tra0000127

Lee, D. J., Schnitzlein, C. W., Wolf, J. P., Vythilingam, M., Rasmusson, A. M., & Hoge, C. W. (2016). Psychotherapy versus pharmacotherapy for posttraumatic stress disorder: Systemic review and meta-analyses to determine first-line treatments. *Depression and Anxiety*, *33*, 792–806.

Lu, M. W., Duckart, J. P., O'Malley, J. P., & Dobscha, S. K. (2011). Correlates of utilization of PTSD specialty treatment among recently diagnosed veterans at the VA. *Psychiatric Services*, *62*, 943–949.

Magruder, K. M., Frueh, B. C., Knapp, R. G., Davis, L., Hamner, M. B., Martin, R. H., ... Arana, G. W. (2005). Prevalence of posttraumatic stress disorder in veterans affairs primary care clinics. *General Hospital Psychiatry*, *27*(3), 169–179.

Meyer, O. L., Saw, A., Cho, Y. I., & Fancher, T. L. (2015). Disparities in assessment, treatment, and recommendations for specialty mental health care: Patient reports of medical provider behavior. *Health Services Research*, *50*(3), 750–767.

Mott, J. M., Hundt, N. E., Sansgiry, S., Mignogna, J., & Cully, J. A. (2014). Changes in psychotherapy utilization among veterans with depression, anxiety, and PTSD. *Psychiatric Services*, *65*(1), 106–112.

Mulick, P.S. & Naugle, A.E. (2010). Behavioral activation in the treatment of comorbid posttraumatic stress disorder and major depressive disorder. International Journal of Behavioral Consultation and Therapy, 5(3&4), 330–350.

Mulick, P. S., Landes, S. J., & Kanter, J. W. (2011). Contextual behavior therapies in the treatment of PTSD: A review. *The International Journal of Consultation and Therapy*, *7*, 23–32.

Najavits, L. M. (2002). *Seeking safety: A treatment manual for PTSD and substance abuse*. New York: Guilford Press.

Nixon, R. D., & Nearmy, R. M. (2011). Treatment of comorbid posttraumatic stress disorder and major depressive disorder: A pilot study. Journal of Traumatic Stress, *24*, 451–455.

Peterson, A. L., Luethcke, C. A., Borah, E. V., Borah, A. M., & Young-McCaughan, S. (2011). Assessment and treatment of combat-related PTSD in returning war veterans. *Journal of Clinical Psychology in Medical Settings*, *18*(2), 164–175.

Pietrzak, R. H., Johnson, D. C., Goldstein, M. B., Malley, J. C., & Southwick, S. M. (2009). Perceived stigma and barriers to mental health care utilization among OEF-OIF veterans. *Psychiatric Services*, *60*, 1118–1122.

Possemato, K. (2011). The current state of intervention research for posttraumatic stress disorder within the primary care setting. *Journal of Clinical Psychology in Medical Settings*, *18*, 268–280.

Primary Care PTSD Screen for DSM-5 (PC-PTSD-5). (n.d.) Retrieved from https://www.ptsd.va.gov/professional/assessment/screens/pc-ptsd.asp.

Prins, A., Bovin, M. J., Smolenski, D. J., Marx, B. P., Kimerling, R., Jenkins-Guarnieri, M. A., ... Tiet, Q. Q. (2016). The primary care PTSD screen for DSM-5 (PC-PTSD-5): Development and evaluation within a veteran primary care sample. *Journal of General Internal Medicine*, 1–6.

PTSD Consultation Program. Retrieved from http://www.ptsd.va.gov/professional/consult/

Roberts, A. L., Gilman, S. E., Breslau, J., Breslau, N., & Koenen, K. C. (2011). Race/ethnic differences in exposure to traumatic events, development of posttraumatic stress disorder, and treatment-seeking for post-traumatic stress disorder in the United States. *Psychological Medicine*, *41*(01), 71–83.

Robinson, P. J., & Reiter, J. T. (2007). *Behavioral consultation and primary care*. New York: Springer.

Sareen, J., Houlahan, T., Cox, B. J., & Asmundson, G. J. (2005). Anxiety disorders associated with suicidal ideation and suicide attempts in the National Comorbidity Survey. *The Journal of Nervous and Mental Disease*, *193*(7), 450–454.

Schell, T. L., & Marshall, G. N. (2008). Survey of individuals previously deployed for OEF/OIF. In T. Tanelian & L. H. Jaycox (Eds.), *Invisible wounds of war: Psychological and cognitive injuries, their consequences, and services to assist recovery* (pp. 87–115). Santa Monica, CA: Rand Corporation.

Schumm, J. A., Walter, K. H., Bartone, A. S., & Chard, K. M. (2015). Veteran satisfaction and treatment preferences in response to a posttraumatic stress disorder specialty clinic orientation group. *Behaviour Research and Therapy*, *69*, 75–82.

Sloan, D. M., Marx, B. P., & Keane, T. M. (2011). Reducing the burden of mental illness in military veterans commentary on Kazdin and Blase (2011). *Perspectives on Psychological Science*, *6*(5), 503–506.

Stein, M. B., McQuaid, J. R., Pedrelli, P., Lenox, R., & McCahill, M. E. (2000). Posttraumatic stress disorder in the primary care medical setting. *General Hospital Psychiatry*, *22*(4), 261–269.

Tanelian, T., & Jaycox, L. (Eds.). (2008). *Invisible wounds of war: Psychological and cognitive injuries, their consequences, and services to assist recovery*. Santa Monica, CA: RAND Corporation.

Tuerk, P. W., Wangelin, B., Rauch, S. A., Dismuke, C. E., Yoder, M., Myrick, H., … Acierno, R. (2013). Health service utilization before and after evidence-based treatment for PTSD. *Psychological Services*, *10*(4), 401–409.

Van Dam, D., Ehring, T., Vedel, E., & Emmelkamp, P. M. (2010). Validation of the Primary Care Posttraumatic Stress Disorder screening questionnaire (PC-PTSD) in civilian substance use disorder patients. *Journal of Substance Abuse Treatment*, *39*(2), 105–113.

Van Emmerik, A. A., Kamphuis, J. H., Hulsbosch, A. M., & Emmelkamp, P. M. (2002). Single session debriefing after psychological trauma: A meta-analysis. *Lancet*, *360*, 766–771.

Van Minnen, A., Arntz, A., & Keijsers, G. P. J. (2002). Prolonged exposure in patients with chronic PTSD: Predictors of treatment outcome and dropout. *Behaviour Research and Therapy*, *40*(4), 439–457.

Wortmann, J. H., Jordan, A. H., Weathers, F. W., Resick, P. A., Dondanville, K. A., Hall-Clark, B., … Litz, B. T. (2016). Psychometric analysis of the PTSD Checklist-5 (PCL-5) among treatment-seeking military service members. *Psychological Assessment*. https://doi.org/10.1037/pas0000260

Zeiss, A. M., & Karlin, B. E. (2008). Integrating mental health and primary care services in the Department of Veterans Affairs health care system. *Journal of Clinical Psychology in Medical Settings*, *15*(1), 73–78.

31 Relationship Concerns

Tatiana D. Gray and James V. Cordova

Description of the Problem

Our personal relationships are intimately interwoven with nearly every aspect of our lives and, as such, are finally being recognized as a complete health system, on par with physical and emotional health (Cordova, 2013). More specifically, the quality of our intimate relationships is linked to physical health (e.g., Donoho, Crimmins, & Seeman, 2013; Kiecolt-Glaser & Newton, 2001; Whisman, Uebelacker, & Settles, 2010), emotional well-being (Gottman, & Levenson, 1992), mental health (Horwitz, White, & Howell-White, 1996; Whisman & Kaiser, 2008; Whisman, 2007), substance use and abuse (Rhule-Louie & McMahon, 2007), child outcomes (e.g., Cummings & Davies, 2002), and even mortality (Holt-Lunstad, Smith, & Layton, 2010). When our intimate relationships are healthy, nearly all aspects of our lives benefit; when our intimate relationships are distressed, nearly all aspects of our lives are made vulnerable to greater suffering. Therefore, reducing relationship distress and promoting healthy intimacy can prevent a range of psychological, behavioral, and physical disorders for the whole family.

T.D. Gray, Ph.D. • J.V. Cordova, Ph.D. (✉)
Department of Psychology, Clark University, Worcester, MA, USA
e-mail: jcordova@clarku.edu

Relationship distress comes with a considerable cost at both the individual and societal levels. Nearly half (40–50%) of first marriages in the USA end in divorce (Cherlin, 2010), and 20% of marriages are significantly distressed at any point in time (Beach, Arias, & O'Leary, 1986). In addition, researcher David Schramm recently estimated that divorces cost the US government $33.3 billion, *annually*, in direct and indirect expenses (Schramm, 2006). Given the high prevalence of relationship distress, the deleterious effects of that distress on individual and family well-being, and the resultant exorbitant cost to society, it is crucial that the field of relationship healthcare develop, empirically validate, and effectively disseminate brief and accessible professional care.

Unfortunately, there are multiple barriers for couples to attend traditional tertiary couple therapy, and we know from the literature that most couples never even consider seeking professional help for their relationships. Further, those who are willing to seek help primarily consult medical doctors (Veroff, 1981). This natural inclination for people to turn to their physicians for professional guidance can be capitalized on as an effective avenue for reaching quality relationship healthcare. In other words, when relationship interventions are brought into the world of primary care, doctors, nurses, and other medical personnel are able to act as a bridge between effective relationship therapies and couples in need.

A. Maragakis, W.T. O'Donohue (eds.), *Principle-Based Stepped Care and Brief Psychotherapy for Integrated Care Settings*, https://doi.org/10.1007/978-3-319-70539-2_31

In order to fit within an integrated care setting, relationship interventions need to meet several criteria. First, they need to be brief (typically between one and four sessions). Second, they need to be situated within the medical setting itself in order to facilitate a warm handoff from a doctor, nurse, or other medical staff to a behavioral health professional. This way, if a patient was meeting with their primary care doctor and brought up relationship concerns, their doctor would be able to literally walk them down the hall to a trained behavioral health specialist who could orient them to the relationship intervention and easily schedule a time for them to come in. Third, given the context and time limits, relationship interventions need to be action oriented in focus. Each of these components lowers traditional barriers to relationship help seeking and minimizes the stigma that is more often than not cemented to the notion of couple therapy.

Despite the advantages of utilizing integrated primary care settings to address relationship problems, very few behavioral health providers work with families or partners (Shepherd, 2014) and those that do tend to take a broad family systems/biopsychosocial approach (McDaniel & Le Roux, 2007) rather than implementing a brief evidence-based relationship protocol. This underutilization of brief couple-level protocols in integrated care is likely due to the fact that, until now, that type of empirically supported intervention did not exist. The remainder of this chapter will present the theory, structure, and protocol for the Marriage Checkup, which has been successfully adapted to primary care settings for military couples (Cigrang et al., 2016).

The Marriage Checkup (often referred to as the MC or relationship checkup/RC) fits perfectly within the integrated care setting for several reasons. First, the name itself (getting a relationship health *checkup*) immediately removes the connotations that come with tertiary couple therapy. It is made clear that the couples will meet with a behavioral health consultant for a brief assessment of their strengths and concerns within their relationship and be given personalized feedback with empirically guided options that they can choose what, if anything, to act upon. The MC is analogous to annual physical or mental health checkups and is another way for people to proactively take good care of their entire health. Next, the MC is both short term and brief (only three 30-min appointments). In addition, the MC is available and appropriate for any and all couples. Practically what this means is that any healthcare professional can refer a couple to receive a relationship checkup and all couples are eligible to receive a relationship checkup, regardless of their history, comorbid diagnoses, or severity of concerns. That being said, the checkup is meant to function as any other health checkup. For example, if you go to your primary care physician and you are generally healthy with very few concerns, your doctor may give you some general feedback (e.g., make sure you have a healthy diet and are getting regular exercise) and then schedule your annual checkup in another year and send you on your way. However, if you have a worrisome-looking mole, your doctor may examine it herself and then refer you to follow up with a specialist for further care. The MC consultant has a similar role, to look deeply at the relationship, assess strengths and concerns, offer suggestions and feedback where appropriate, and refer to a greater level of specialized care (e.g., long-term couple therapy) when it is indicated.

Effective Ways to Screen for the Problem

The first step in screening for relationship problems is to simply ask the patient how satisfied they are in their relationship and if they have any concerns. For example, "All things considered, on a scale from 1-10, how happy are you in your romantic relationship?" Many people will open up and express relationship stressors or concerns when given this opportunity. This type of question can be asked in person by medical staff or can be asked via the self-report mental health screen that a clinic might already give to patients.

How to Further Assess If the Screen Returns Positive

It is important to note that even if a person is not significantly distressed, medical staff can ask all patients if they would be interested in a relationship checkup. The checkup is not just for couples who are struggling but rather a proactive way to check the pulse of any relationship and help couples maintain a strong intimate connection. That being said, it may be particularly important to inform couples who report significant distress of the opportunity to participate in a relationship checkup.

If the couple would like to participate in a relationship checkup or talk about their relationship concerns in more depth, then the behavioral health consultant can administer the Couple Satisfaction Index (CSI; Funk & Rogge, 2007) in order to more thoroughly assess the patient's relationship functioning. There is a brief four-item version of this measure (readily available for clinical and research purposes at http://www.courses.rochester.edu/surveys/funk) ideal for medical settings. Once the patient completes the questionnaire, the physician or behavioral health consultant can quickly calculate the sum and then use the cut scores in order to determine his/her relationship distress level (scores range from 0 to 21, higher scores indicate higher levels of relationship satisfaction, and scores below 13.5 suggest notable relationship dissatisfaction).

Evidence-Based Stepped Care and Brief Psychotherapeutic Approaches

Overview of the Checkup Protocol

The MC is an assessment and feedback protocol that draws on therapeutic techniques from integrative behavioral couple therapy (IBCT; Jacobson & Christensen, 1996) and motivational interviewing (Miller & Rolnick, 2002). Ultimately the MC is designed to vitalize the intimate connection between partners by turning them compassionately toward one another and to activate them to take care of the health of their relationship. In order to fit within the integrated care model, the MC has been divided into three 30-min appointments. In the first appointment, the MC consultant reviews the couple's relationship history and primary strengths, appointment two is dedicated to discussing each partner's primary concern within the relationship, and, finally, the consultant reviews the information from the assessment and provides actionable feedback to the couple in appointment three.

General Guidelines

Given the brevity of the protocol, it is essential that behavioral health specialists capitalize on their time with the couple. This requires a delicate balance between building rapport quickly and diving right into the heart of the protocol (with little to no time for small talk or chitchat).

****Special Note:*** The MC protocol (available by paid subscription to Arammu: The Relationship Checkup) comes with clinical materials, including access to a healthcare platform with electronic questionnaires for the couple to complete prior to their checkup about their strengths and concerns as well as a program for automatically generating the couple's detailed feedback report. Without access to automation tools, clinicians will need to do a modified/abridged version of the checkup. It is recommended that all clinicians who use the checkup get training in the protocol by taking at least one relationship checkup workshop and utilizing *The Marriage Checkup Practitioner's Guide: Promoting Lifelong Relationship Health* (Cordova, 2013). **An upcoming workshop schedule can be found at www.arammu.org or workshops and can be arranged by contacting the authors at** James@arammu.org **or** Tatiana@arammu.org. **Training can be provided in person or via webinar.**

Assessment: Appointment One, Relationship History and Strengths

Appointment one begins with a brief orientation to the checkup by letting the couple know what to expect.

"Welcome to the relationship checkup. Overall, we will have three 30-minute appointments together. The first two appointments will be devoted to getting to know you and learn about your relationship strengths and concerns. Today I want to find out about your relationship history and your primary strengths as a couple. Next time we meet we will spend some time exploring any concerns that you might be having in your relationship. And then for our final meeting I will give you each a personalized feedback report and explore some options for maximizing your strengths, addressing your concerns, and continuing to take care of the health of your relationship."

Then MC consultant will then transition into a brief oral history interview (adapted from Gottman, 1994) by asking each partner about how they met. It is important to elicit each partner's unique version of their love story. It can be helpful to start with the partner who may be less talkative, often the male partner in opposite-sex relationships.

Question 1: *Why don't we start from the beginning…tell me how the two of you met and got together…what were your first impressions of each other? What initially attracted you to each other?*

Question 2: *Tell me about how you decided to commit to one another… of all the people in the world, what led you to decide that this was the person you wanted to be with?*

The intention of the OHI is twofold. First, the OHI is itself an assessment tool (Gottman, 1994). How partners talk about these early moments in their relationship appears to have some real predictive validity in terms of near-term and long-term relationship health. Relationship health appears to be particularly associated with husbands' expressions of fondness for their partners, and both partners expressed satisfaction with the relationship. In other words, in general, the most positive the emotional tone of the stories partners tell about how they met, fell in love, and decided to marry or commit to each other, the more robust their overall relationship health. The second intention of the OHI is to reorient the couple to the positive and endearing qualities that first attracted them to each other and to create a sweet, tender, and playful moment of intimacy between them in the session. The goal is to create a moment of intimate connection and to reestablish their focus on the positive foundation of the relationship.

After acknowledging, reflecting, and celebrating the sweet side of the couple's history and pulling out the key moments that laid the foundation for their relationship, the MC consultant will then move on to discussing each partner's primary strengths as a couple. If using the questionnaires, you will locate each partner's top three nominated relationship strengths and ask which one is the primary strength in the relationship. If the couple has not completed the questionnaires beforehand, the clinician asks about the strengths in the interview.

"There are many different aspects to our relationships, like our friendship, verbal affection, physical affection, parenting styles, communication, sexual intimacy, shared humor, and commitment to one another. Of those things, or if there is something else that stands out to you, what would you say is the primary strength in your relationship?"

Once the first partner has identified a strength, the therapist then proceeds with asking the following questions:

"Tell me about how you experience [primary strength, e.g., being affectionate toward each other on a daily basis] in your relationship."
"How does [primary strength, e.g., being affectionate toward each other on a daily basis] work to keep your relationship strong and healthy?"

After the first partner has discussed her primary strength, the MC consultant will turn to the other partner and repeat the same process.

As a strengths-based intervention, the intention of the strengths assessment within the MC is to draw out the areas in which the couple is functioning well and even thriving. The goal is to reorient the couple toward the things about each other and their relationship that attract them to each other and root their commitment to the relationship. Facilitating partners' celebration of and gratitude for what is best about them as a couple is meant to provide them with a strengths-based perspective from which to begin to consider and address their primary relationship concerns. It aims to provide a platform for the couple to celebrate the best and most satisfying aspects of their relationship and to instill a solid foundation from which to begin to address their concerns.

Ending the first meeting by assessing their strengths highlights for the couple the health-oriented nature of the checkup and asks them to reflect on these positive qualities between one meeting and the next. The couple is reassured, however, that they will have time to discuss their concerns in the next appointment.

Once the strengths assessment is complete, the MC consultant will thank the couple for coming in and schedule appointment two.

Assessment: Appointment Two, Concerns

At the start of appointment two, the MC consultant will briefly orient the couple to the time that they have together and move quickly into a discussion of each partner's primary concern in the relationship. Since the appointments are only 30 min, this allows for about 15 min to be devoted to each partner's concern. Similar to the strengths interview, if the couple has completed the questionnaires online, the clinician can use their top three concerns as a guide, if not the MC consultant can elicit the concerns in the interview.

> "We all have stuck-points and aspects of our relationship that we sometimes struggle with. Some of these might be how much time we get to spend together, how we communicate around conflict, handle finances, parent, and even individual issues that can impact the relationship. What would you say is your primary relationship concern at this time?"

Once the first partner has identified the concern, proceed with the therapeutic interview.

> "Can you tell me a little bit about that issue?"
> "How would you describe what the issue is and how it looks in your relationship?"

Therapeutic Techniques

The MC consultant will then use one of the three primary therapeutic techniques from IBCT: (1) uncovering soft emotions, (2) exploring understandable reasons, and (3) identifying relationship themes and patterns in order to elicit a more compassionate narrative of each partners' concern.

1. *Uncovering soft emotions*: The premise of uncovering soft emotions stems from the presumption that hard emotional expressions are complex emotion blends of both hard and soft emotions—often both hurt and anger. When we are hurt by our partners, we often lead with what we call hard emotions (i.e., anger, contempt, frustration, etc.), because it feels less vulnerable to do so. Couples often fall into the hard emotion trap when discussing their concerns. For example, "I feel like he is so flirtatious with other women, and he doesn't even consider how it makes me feel. It's infuriating." It is the therapist's job to use his or her own empathy to imagine what it might be like for that partner and dig beneath that anger in search of the softer more vulnerable emotion. Softer emotions are characterized as those that pull for a more compassionate and loving response from the partner (e.g., fear, loneliness, hurt, sadness, loss). In the case of our example, the MC consultant might respond by saying, "So there is something about the way that he interacts with other women that really scares you. It's not that you don't trust him, it's just that given your connection, that the thought of losing him or even just losing his attention to another woman for a few brief moments feels terrifying, because you don't even want to imagine not having him in your life in that way. And if he can be turned or enticed away from you by someone else, then your connection is threatened in a way that leaves you feeling really unsettled and unsafe. Is it anything like that?" This type of reflection is intended to connect the first partner with the deeper emotional roots of her concern, as well as allow for her partner to hear her concern in a new, less "hard" way, and hopefully, as a result, allow them both to understand one another with more compassion. The formulation is that it is easier to hear and empathize compassionately with

the pain minus the accusation. When both partners can experience that sense of being compassionately understood by each other around even an unsolvable problem, intimate connection can be reestablished and intimacy bridges can be built.

2. *Exploring understandable reasons*: We all have histories that have shaped the way we respond and behave in our lives, and clarifying these histories can help us to understand each other and ourselves more compassionately. The therapeutic technique of exploring understandable reasons consists of asking a series of questions that allow for the discovery of often very reasonable explanations and motives for why partners respond to one another, and issues within their relationship, in particular ways. For example, if one partner states that he is uncomfortable with the way in which his partner expresses anger toward him and argues with him in front of their children, the therapist could ask questions about the way that he learned about how to express anger growing up and how his relationship models (his parents) managed anger in the household. He might state that his parents never argued in front of them and in his entire childhood he never witnessed a harsh word exchanged between the two (perhaps classically conflict avoidant parents). It then becomes quite understandable why he would have a strong reaction to a more explicit and public display of disagreement. This increased understanding often allows for both partners to experience insight into why this particular issue has become a sticking point in their relationship.
3. *Identifying themes and relationship patterns*: The process of identifying themes and relationship patterns aims to bring the partners together around a shared concern and shift their perspective from blame to awareness. Thus, rather than seeing "the problem" as located within the bad behavior or poor character of the other, the couple is guided to see the problem as emerging from common and understandable differences between them that result in a shared pattern and mutual trap. For example, if the partners are concerned about how they handle finances in the household—one partner tends to be more fiscally conservative, whereas the other prefers to put their earnings toward vacations they can enjoy in the present moment—the MC consultant may point out that they have fallen into a spender/saver pattern. "Finances can be quite emotionally complicated for partners, and different people have different ways of responding to that complication. You can think of finances on a continuum, with spending on one end and saving on the other. Most people fall somewhere in the middle of this continuum, but may lean more towards one side than the other. Partners, who often start near each other on the continuum, can polarize over time as they respond to one another's money management styles. Say you get $100, one of you wants to put it in the bank and the other wants to go out for a nice dinner. If the person who wants to save it gets there first, then the other partner might be quicker to spend money on something nice the next time there is an opportunity. Then the person who prefers to save might try to cut back in other ways to make up for the spender's spending. The spending partner might then feel deprived and be more likely to look for other spending opportunities. You can see how couples can really polarize in this spot, and sort of pull one another off their own axes. Which is not to say either one of you is correct or incorrect, but just that you have this difference, and once we notice the patterns that we fall into, we have more space to respond to them gracefully."

For a more complete description of these techniques, see Jacobson and Christensen 1996 and Cordova 2014.

Feedback: Appointment Three, Review and Options

Before starting appointment three, the MC consultant would either use the computer program we have developed or Dr. Cordova's

Practitioner's Guide to the Marriage Checkup (2013) to create a feedback report for the couple. The feedback report consists of (a) a brief review of the couple's relationship history, (b) a review of their self-identified top strengths discussed in light of the current relationship health literature, (c) a review of their top areas of concern from the more intimacy productive perspective developed during Session 2, (d) a menu of options for each concern describing healthy ways of addressing their concerns as informed by the current relationship health literature, and (e) a space for brainstorming additional ways that the couple can actively take good and regular care of their relationship.

Within the feedback session, the clinician will review the couple's relationship history, spend some time reflecting on and celebrating their strengths, and emphasize the new compassionate narrative in response to their concerns. The review of the couples' history is, again, intended to remind them of the most positive aspects of their history together and, along with the review of their strengths, orients the couple toward what they value preserving and nurturing in their relationship. This sets a positive stage from which to present the newly developed intimacy productive narrative about their shared concerns, with the presumption that review and repetition helps to solidify their more compassionate understanding of each other. The MC consultant will then provide each partner with a menu of research-supported options (from the feedback report) for addressing their concerns, use motivational interviewing to capitalize on any available readiness for change, and collaboratively create a plan of action for the couple to continue to take regular active care of the health of their relationship.

What Does Not Work

We have some emerging evidence that the MC is efficacious as presented here within integrated healthcare systems (Cigrang et al., 2015, Cordova et al. *under review*), as well as strong randomized control trial evidence that the MC is efficacious in both clinical trial and private practice settings (Trillingsgaard, Fentz, Hawrilenko, & Cordova, 2016; Cordova et al., 2014). However, given the absence of other relationship health approaches that have been tested in this healthcare setting, it is not yet clear what else does and/or doesn't work in broad strokes.

In terms of clinical practice, it is clear that any intervention that cannot be conducted within the 30-min appointment standard within integrated behavioral healthcare will not work for the system. Therefore, focused clinical tools and automated processes appear to be a must for effectively integrating relationship healthcare into primary care.

Clinically, though 30 min may appear to be too short a period of time to conduct the emotionally rich work at the heart of the MC, it does not work to rush in a way that results in an emotionally superficial intervention. Our mantra when training new MC therapists has become "go deep, fast," and new therapists in training often remark on how surprised they are that the encounter can be so deeply meaningful to the couple in such a brief period of time.

Our sense is also that winging the MC untrained does not work. The effective implementation of the MC protocol requires training and at least an initial period of supervision. Working with couples is a complex work and a substantially different skill set from that required to do excellent individual work. Especially in such an abbreviated form, proper training is essential.

When to Refer

Since the relationship checkup is intended to do just that, *checkup* on the health of the relationship, it is expected that there will be instances in which a greater level of care is warranted. First, it is not uncommon for the couple to request a referral to a couple's therapist in order to continue the work that they started in the checkup. This is typically seen as a positive outcome, since the checkup may have served as a bridge to more specialized care that the couple may not have otherwise sought. Other concerns that may be illuminated through the checkup that call for a referral to a specialist include interpersonal violence, the aftereffects of an affair, significant substance use by one or both partners, and untreated mental health concerns such as depression or anxiety. One of the benefits of any kind of checkup is the opportunity to observe health issues that might not have been the obvious target of the checkup. For example, a standard eye exam can detect additional health issues from diabetes to cancer. The MC in integrated primary care is also a practical context in which to detect additional health issues such as substance abuse, untreated mental health issues, and childhood behavior problems, or even undiagnosed physical health issues of the other (potentially non-help-seeking) partner, that can then be referred back to the treating physician.

While the MC provides the most comprehensive checkup and thus most well-tailored set of options for couples to address their relationship health issues either on their own or through more extensive treatment, patients who are not interested in receiving a checkup can be provided with information about alternative resources. Perhaps the simplest alternative resource is bibliotherapy, although it has been our experience that this is an option pursued by a relatively select type of patient. The books we tend to recommend to couples include the following.

- *Reconcilable Difference* by Christensen, Doss, and Jacobson
- *The Marriage Checkup* by James Cordova
- *Fighting for your Marriage* by Markman and Stanley

Web-based resources are also available, and for these we recommend the following.

- Our Relationship: PREP online at www.our-relationship.com
- Couple CARE at www.couplecare.info

Patients might also be interested in relationship workshops that might be available in their area. A good resource for finding relationship skills workshops is available at www.prepinc.com.

The Role of Primary Care Provider/ Medical Team in Treatment

Primary care providers and the medical team are essential in terms of providing one of the easiest and most accessible and effective entry points for a relationship health checkup. It is essential to have provider buy-in to the importance of relationship health to a patient's overall health and understanding of the empirically supported effectiveness of the checkup in order to have a fully integrated and well-functioning relationship checkup within integrated primary care. Primary care providers and the medical team can help enormously in opening an easy pathway for patients to seek relationship healthcare by doing just a couple of simple things. One is allowing posting of educational posters about relationship health and the checkup in their exam rooms. The other is more actively assessing their patients' relationship health, even with just a one sentence query, like "In general, how satisfied are you with your relationship?"—much like the primary care provider might ask, "Have you been feeling down, depressed, or like life isn't worth living?" as a brief depression screen. If the patient then indicates relationship concerns, even mild relationship concerns, then a recommendation for a low-effort relationship health checkup can be made. Our sense is that a recommendation from their treating physician can go a very long way toward encouraging and normalizing relationship healthcare and educating patients about the importance of attending actively to relationship health.

Finally, and perhaps most importantly, medical providers can help facilitate the warm handoff to relationship checkup clinicians in order to decrease barriers for couples to follow up on the referral.

How to Assess Impact on Care/ Quality Improvement Processes

The research literature provides robust evidence that relationship health affects both mental and physical health, suggesting that assessing impact on care would involve assessing both for improvements in relationship health, via brief measures such as the CSI-4, and assessing for improvements in mental and physical health. Mental health might also be assessed actively through self-report questionnaires indicated by the patient's particular mental health history or through consultation with their mental health providers. Impact on physical health might be seen mostly on chronic conditions involving those inflammatory processes exacerbated by chronic stress and immune system functioning. One might expect to see fewer doctor visits as overall health improves. Paradoxically, for men, one might see a brief spike in doctor visits as increased relationship communication could facilitate partners' positive influence on necessary help seeking. Overall, impact on care assessment ideally involves a multifaceted approach attending to both relationship health directly and to the physical and mental health concomitants of relationship health.

References

Beach, S. R., Arias, I., & O'Leary, K. D. (1986). The relationship of marital satisfaction and social support to depressive symptomatology. *Journal of Psychopathology and Behavioral Assessment*, *8*(4), 305–316. https://doi.org/10.1007/BF00960728

Cherlin, A. J. (2010). Demographic trends in the United States: A review of research in the 2000s. *Journal of Marriage and Family*, *72*(3), 403–419. https://doi.org/10.1111/j.1741-3737.2010.00710.x

Cigrang, J. A., Cordova, J. V., Gray, T. D., Najera, E., Hawrilenko, M., Pinkley, C., Nielsen, M., Tatum, J., & Redd, K. (2016). The Marriage Checkup: Adapting and Implementing a Brief Relationship Intervention for Military Couples. Cognitive and Behavioral Practice. *23*(4), 561–570.

Cummings, M. E., & Davies, P. T. (2002). Effects of marital conflict on children: Recent advances and emerging themes in process-oriented research. *Journal of Child Psychology and Psychiatry*, *43*, 31–63. https://doi.org/10.1111/1469-7610.00003

Cordova, J. V. (2013). *The marriage checkup practitioner's guide: Promoting lifelong relationship health*. Washington, DC: American Psychological Association.

Cordova, J. V., Fleming, C. J., Morrill, M. I., Hawrilenko, M., Sollenberger, J. W., Harp, A. G., ... Wachs, K. (2014). The marriage checkup: A randomized controlled trial of annual relationship health checkups. *Journal of Consulting and Clinical Psychology*, *82*(4), 592–604.

Donoho, C. J., Crimmins, E. M., & Seeman, T. E. (2013). Marital quality, gender, and markers of inflammation in the MIDUS cohort. *Journal of Marriage and Family*, *75*, 127–141. https://doi.org/10.1111/j.1741-3737.2012.01023.x

Funk, J. L., & Rogge, R. D. (2007). Testing the ruler with item response theory: Increasing precision of measurement for relationship satisfaction with the couples satisfaction index. *Journal of Family Psychology*, *21*, 572–583.

Gottman, J. M., & Levenson, R. W. (1992). Marital processes predictive of later dissolution: Behavior, physiology, and health. *Journal of Personality and Social Psychology*, *63*, 221–233.

Gottman, J.M. (1994). What predicts divorce? The relationship between marital processes and marital outcomes. Hillsdale, NJ. Lawrence Erlbaum Associates.

Holt-Lunstad, J., Smith, T. B., & Layton, J. B. (2010). Social relationships and mortality risk: A meta-analytic review. *PLoS Medicine*, *7*(7), e1000316. https://doi.org/10.1371/journal.pmed.1000316

Horwitz, A. V., White, H. R., & Howell-White, S. (1996). Becoming married and mental health: A longitudinal study of a cohort of young adults. *Journal of Marriage and the Family*, *58*, 895–907.

Jacobson, N. S. & Christensen, A. (1996). Acceptance and change in couple therapy: A therapist's guide to transforming relationships. New York: Norton.

Kiecolt-Glaser, J. K., & Newton, T. L. (2001). Marriage and health: His and hers. *Psychological Bulletin*, *127*(4), 472–503. https://doi.org/10.1037/0033-2909.127.4.472

McDaniel, S. H., & Le Roux, P. (2007). An overview of primary care family psychology. *Journal of Clinical Psychology in Medical Settings*, *14*(1), 23–32.

Miller, W. R., & Rollnick, S. (2002). Motivational interviewing: Preparing people for change (2nd ed.). New York: Guilford Press.

Rhule-Louie, D. M., & McMahon, R. J. (2007). Problem behavior and romantic relationships: Assortative mating, behavior contagion, and desistance. *Clinical Child and Family Psychology Review*, *10*, 53–100.

Schramm, D. G. (2006). Individual and social costs of divorce in Utah. *Journal of Family and Economic Issues*, *27*(1), 133–151. https://doi.org/10.1007/s10834-005-9005-4

Shepherd, M. (2014). Do primary care psychological therapists 'think family'? Challenges and opportunities for couple and family therapy in the context of 'Improving Access to Psychological Therapies' (IAPT) services. *Journal of Family Therapy*, *36*, 39–61. https://doi.org/10.1111/j.1467-6427.2011.00559.x

Trillingsgaard, T., Fentz, H. N., Hawrilenko, M., & Cordova, J. V. (2016). A randomized controlled trial of the marriage checkup adapted for private practice. *Journal of Consulting and Clinical Psychology*. Advance online publication. https://doi.org/10.1037/ccp0000141

Veroff, J. B. (1981). The dynamics of help-seeking in men and women: A national survey study. *Psychiatry*, *44*, 189–200.

Whisman, M. A., & Kaiser, R. (2008). Marriage and relationship issues. In K. S. Dobson & D. J. A. Dozois (Eds.), *Risk factors in depression* (pp. 363–384). San Diego, CA: Academic. https://doi.org/10.1016/B978-0-08-045078-0.00016-2

Whisman, M. A. (2007). Marital distress and DSM-IV psychiatric disorders in a population-based national survey. *Journal of Abnormal Psychology, 116*(3), 638–643. https://doi.org/10.1037/0021-843X.116.3.638

Whisman, M. A., Uebelacker, L., & Settles, T. (2010). Marital distress and the metabolic syndrome: Linking social functioning with physical health. *Journal of Family Psychology, 24*, 367–370. https://doi.org/10.1037/a0019547

School Refusal Behavior

32

Heather Martens, J. Arthur Gillaspy Jr., and Stephen R. Gillaspy

A Brief Description of School Refusal Behavior

School refusal behavior (SRB), missing school due to truancy, school phobia, or anxiety, occurs in approximately 5–35% of students and often presents considerable challenges for educators, parents, and caregivers (Haight, Kearney, Hendron, & Schafer, 2011; Kearney, Lemos, & Silverman, 2004; Kearney, 2008b). Specifically, SRB is associated with school dropout, social dysfunction, low academic achievement, family conflict, poverty, employment difficulties, psychopathology, suicide attempts, and substance abuse. Not surprisingly, the majority students (56.7%) with SRB also have comorbid conditions such as anxiety disorders, mood disorders, enuresis, and posttraumatic stress disorder. A smaller percentage (4.2%) experience conduct disorder and attention deficit/hyperactivity disorder (Kearney, 2006).

School refusal behavior is usually understood in terms of operant conditioning or by the functional consequences of the SRB for the child or family. These functions include avoidance of school-based stimuli that promote negative affect, escape from social or evaluative situations, attention seeking, or obtain reinforcers outside of school (Kearney, 2008b; Kearney, Lemos, & Silverman, 2004; Wimmer, 2016). See Table 32.1 for a description of terms. Regardless of the function of the school refusal behavior, the powerful reinforcing effects of SRB often create a cycle that is difficult to break (Reid, 2006). The longer the child stays out of school, the more difficult it is to return to school. Parents and caregivers are often frustrated about SRB and will first seek assistance from a healthcare provider.

It is important for parents and healthcare providers to address the school refusal behavior as soon as possible. In most cases, SRB does not improve in the absence of treatment (Heyne, Sauter, Ollendick, Van Widenfelt, & Westenberg, 2014). Behavioral health providers (BHPs) in an integrated setting can play an important role in assessing of symptoms and risk factors, providing evidence-based psychological interventions, and when appropriate referring for more intensive treatment. This chapter will present a guide for BHPs in integrated care settings for the effective assessment and treatment of patients with SRB.

H. Martens (✉) • J.A. Gillaspy Jr., Ph.D.
University of Central Arkansas, Conway, AR, USA
e-mail: martensh@uca.edu

S.R. Gillaspy
The University of Oklahoma Health Sciences Center, Oklahoma City, OK, USA

A. Maragakis, W.T. O'Donohue (eds.), *Principle-Based Stepped Care and Brief Psychotherapy for Integrated Care Settings*, https://doi.org/10.1007/978-3-319-70539-2_32

Table 32.1 Types of absenteeism with explanation

Types of absenteeism	Parent knowledge	Reason for absence	SRB subtype
Typical absenteeism	Parent knowledge and legitimate absence	**Physical conditions**	
School refusal behavior	Parent knowledge, yet illegitimate absence	**Parent-motivated**	**School withdrawal** is a type of absence where a parent deliberately keeps a student home from school for financial purposes, to hide maltreatment, to prevent abduction from a noncustodial parent, to protect a student from a perceived school-based threat, to assist a parent with a mental health issue, or other reason
	Parent knowledge, yet illegitimate	**Student-motivated.** Usually involves anxiety about school. The reasons or functions for these absences can be avoidance of school due to student's negative affectivity, escape of aversive social or evaluative situations at school, or pursuing attention from significant others	**School refusal or extended school nonattendance** is a type of absence that is student-motivated refusal to attend school and/or difficulties remaining at school for the entire school day
	Lack of parent knowledge and illegitimate	**Student-motivated.** Absences may be linked to delinquency, academic problems, homelessness, and/or poverty	**Truancy** is a type of absence where a student obtains tangible reinforcers outside the school setting

Effective Ways to Screen for School Refusal in the Integrated Care Setting

Routine screening of school-aged children for behavioral health concerns is an important practice for medical and behavioral health providers. The American Academy of Pediatrics (AAP) recommends that all school-aged children receive mental health screening during well-child checks, as well as when indicated by clinical presentation, such as poor school performance, behavioral difficulties, or recurrent somatic complaints. Starting at age 5 and continuing throughout adolescence, engaging the child in a conversation about school is listed as a priority for well-child checks (Hagan, Shaw, & Duncan, 2008). Thus, well-child checks provide an ideal opportunity to identify SRB. This section will review screening methods for SRB that are appropriate for routine use in integrated care.

Specific screening for SRB is most likely when families report problematic absences and when students demonstrate one or more risk factors (Inglés, Gonzálvez-Maciá, García-Fernández, Vicent, & Martínez-Monteagudo, 2015; Wimmer, 2016):

- Anxiety/depression
- Abuse
- Pregnancy
- Physical complaints
- Homelessness
- Family conflict and/or drug/alcohol dependence
- Reports of feeling unsafe or unhappy at school
- Living in an impoverished neighborhood
- Lack of mental healthcare or social supports
- Asthma (the leading medical cause of school absenteeism)

Screening for SRB may also be triggered if parents report their child is frequently absent, absent on significant days, requesting to see the school nurse, requesting to call or go home, experiencing major family events, experiencing sleep difficulties, resisting getting out of bed, and/or reporting subjective health complaints and somatic symptoms (Havik, Bru, & Ertesvåg, 2014).

Several screening tools are available for screening for potential SRB. The Pediatric Symptom Checklist-17 (PSC-17; Gardner et al., 1999) is one of the most widely used screening tools in pediatric primary care. The PSC-17 assesses parent ratings of psychosocial symptoms along three dimensions, internalizing, externalizing, and attention for children 4–18 years old. Frequency of symptoms is rated on a Likert scale from 0 (*never*) to 2 (*often*). A positive screen is indicated by a total score of greater than 14, internalizing subscale greater than 4, externalizing subscale greater than 6, or attention subscale greater than 6. Positive screens do not diagnose a mental health disorder but rather signal the need for further evaluation to determine possible diagnosis. The PSC-17 is reported to have sound psychometric properties (Blucker et al., 2014). The PSC-17 can be accessed at https://brightfutures.aap.org/Bright%20Futures%20Documents/PSC-17%20Scoring%20Instructions.pdf.

How to Further Assess If a Screen Returns Positive

Although screening all patients for school absenteeism will increase the likelihood of identifying SRB, knowing the type or the function of SRB can help inform the appropriate intervention (Gregory & Purcell, 2014). Thus, further assessment may be needed to better understand the SRB and to develop appropriate treatment strategies. Ideally, a positive screen would trigger a protocol for a same-day follow-up assessment to determine the severity of the SRB, impact on family and school functioning, and factors maintaining the SRB. This brief assessment can be conducted by a primary care provider (PCP) or BHP and may involve further use of responses from the PCS-17 and the administration of more thorough measures such as the Screen for Child Anxiety Related Disorders (SCARED; Birmaher et al., 1999) or the School Refusal Assessment Scale-Revised (SRAS-R; Kearney, 2002).

The Screen for Child Anxiety Related Disorders (SCARED; Birmaher et al., 1999) consists of 41 items and 5 subscales that parallel the DSM-IV classification of anxiety disorders, panic disorder or significant somatic symptoms, generalized anxiety disorder, separation disorder, social anxiety disorder, and school avoidance. The SCARED has versions for both parents and children (8–18 years old). Respondents rate the frequency of symptoms on a Likert scale (0 = *not true or hardly ever true*, 1 = *somewhat true or sometimes true*, 2 = *very true or often true*). The SCARED demonstrates moderate parent-child agreement and good internal consistency, test-retest reliability, and discriminant validity. For SRB, the school avoidance subscale can be extremely helpful in identifying the role anxiety may play in SRB (Birmaher et al., 1999). The SCARED may be accessed at http://www.psychiatry.pitt.edu/sites/default/files/Documents/assessments/SCARED%20Child.pdf.

The School Refusal Assessment Scale-Revised (SRAS-R) is a quick method for measuring the relative strength of the four functions of the SRB—avoidance of school-based stimuli that promote negative student affect, escaping social or evaluative situations, pursuing attention from others, and obtaining tangible reinforcers outside the school setting. The parent and student versions of the scale each contain 24 items with 6 items devoted to each subscale. Healthcare professionals may use the scales to derive hypotheses about the function of the problem behavior in order to intervene with the family (Kearney, 2006). Scores from the SRAS-R have demonstrated excellent psychometric properties. In an investigation of concurrent validity, students who were diagnosed with separation, social, and generalized anxiety disorder were more likely to display an avoidance of school-based stimuli that provoked negative affect or escape from aversive social/evaluative situations rather than tangible reinforcement. Furthermore, students who were diagnosed with oppositional defiant and conduct disorder were more likely to display behaviors consistent with obtaining preferred items or activities outside of school. Parent-reported externalizing behaviors were higher for students who refused school for tangible, outside reinforcers (Kearney, 2002). A 2011 confirmatory factor analysis supported the four-factor model in a revision of the scale (Haight et al., 2011). The SRAS-R is included in *Helping school refusing children and their parents: A guide for school-based professionals* (Kearney, 2008a).

If using the SRAS-R is not preferred or possible, interviewing and observing may also be effective tools for understanding the function of the SRB. Helpful interview questions will aid a practitioner in understanding attendance history and patterns, comorbid conditions, instances of legitimate absences, family disruption, and a student's social and academic status. Furthermore, interview questions should identify specific school-related stimuli that provoke absenteeism, whether absence from the parent is the primary causative factor, and what tangible rewards the student receives during absence from school. The following questions are examples adapted from Kearney (2006):

- **When was the first time you purposefully avoided school? When did avoiding school become a common thing for you?** Ask to discern if SRBs are acute or chronic.
- **Do you feel sick before going to school?** Ask to determine if the following symptoms are present: diarrhea, fatigue, headache, stomachache, nausea, vomiting, palpitations, perspiration, pain, shaking, trembling, and sleep problems. Then, rule out medical conditions associated with symptoms.
- **If I were at your house on a morning before school, what would I see you doing?** Ask to determine types of behaviors and level of anxiety.
- **What do you not like about school?** Ask to understand why going to school is aversive and if the aversive condition is reasonable to avoid.
- **Would you be willing to attend school if your mom or dad went with you or if you got rewards for attending school?**
- **How do you feel when you wake up on the weekends?** Determine if somatic complaints and anxiety are present on weekends.

Evidence-Based Stepped Care and Brief Interventions

Interventions for SRB in an integrated setting usually involve a stepped care approach in which brief interventions are used first, followed by more intensive or specialty services. If the PCP suspects SRB at a well-child check or if the patient and family present with somatic complaints and school refusal, the PCP should first complete a full medical exam to rule out any physical problems. If there are no organic reasons for the symptoms, the PCP will further interview the patient and caregiver to determine factors associated with the SRB. At this point, the PCP may choose to provide research-based interventions such as reducing anxiety through relaxation techniques and breathing, gradually easing a child back into school, having the family engage in discussions about fears and challenging unreasonable thoughts, establishing morning routines, and establishing reinforcement systems for school attendance. In addition to these techniques, psychoeducational materials such as handouts, websites, or books may be offered to the family. An excellent overview of treating SRB in a primary care setting is provided by Kearney (2006), available at http://www.mdedge.com/jfponline/article/62306/dealing-school-refusal-behavior-primer-family-physicians.

Effective Treatments/Interventions for SRB

Generally, effective treatments/interventions for SRB involve the interruption of the reinforcing effects of absences. Additionally, interventions that involve school personnel, families, as well as children are most successful (Kearney, 2003). Younger children tend to have better outcomes compared to older children (Heyne et al., 2014). Brief cognitive behavioral interventions are the standard of care for SRB in the integrated care and school settings. Figure 32.1 illustrates how SRB may be conceptualized within a CBT framework. CBT interventions fall into four categories: child-based; parent-based; family-based; and school-based. These interventions are outlined in the following paragraphs.

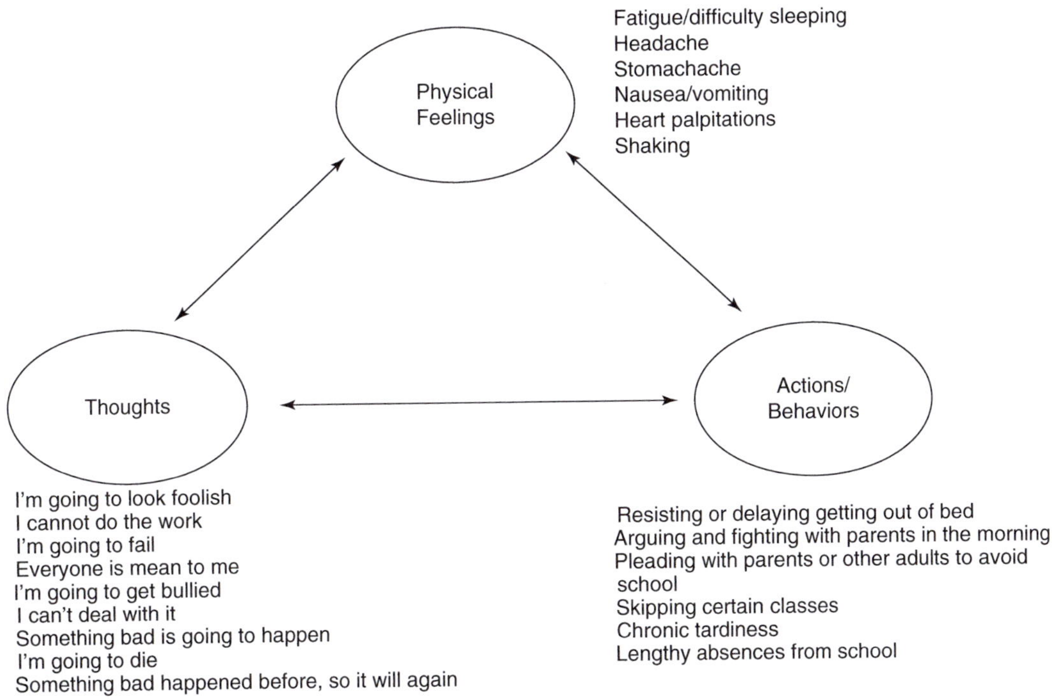

Fig. 32.1 Thoughts, feelings, and behaviors associated with SRB

Child-based. Child-based SRB treatments are cognitive behavioral in nature. Treatments for youth focus on reducing anxiety by teaching breathing retraining, relaxation techniques, and exposure-based techniques. Furthermore, youth are joined by the practitioner in creating a re-entry plan. For younger children, treatment should be adapted to include appropriate vocabulary and examples/illustrations of concepts that use familiar people, places, or things (Heyne et al., 2014). For example, a PCP or BHP might use Dora the Explorer or Scooby-Doo (who routinely follow clues to solve problems and mysteries) to illustrate the connections between thoughts, feelings, and behaviors and the utility of coping statements. Furthermore, small children will need more active support from their parents to overcome SRB whether the behavior is maintained by any of the four reasons or functions. For example, parents may need to prompt small children to identify thoughts and feelings during an emotional exchange. The course of treatment for children or youth, derived from CBT methods, would differ according to the function of the SRB.

Parent-based. Parent-based contingency management techniques are the standard for SRB. Techniques include modifying parental commands, providing attention-based consequences, and establishing morning and evening routines. A helpful publication for parents may be *Getting your child to say 'yes' to school: A guide for parents of youth with school refusal behavior* (Kearney, 2004). Helpful websites and web documents include:

- eMedicineHealth by WebMD http://www.emedicinehealth.com/school_refusal/article_em.htm
- National Association of School Psychologists: School Refusal search https://www.nasponline.org/search/search-results?keywords=school+refusal

Family-based. Family-based techniques may include contracting to increase incentives for school performance and decrease incentives for nonattendance, escorting students to school and class, and practicing with kids how to manage peer interactions. Additionally, the healthcare provider should discuss a referral for psychotropic medication when significant anxiety or depression is present.

School-based. School-based consultation is necessary for eliminating SRB. After identifying the function of the SRB, the school-based SRB antecedents in terms of CBT, and developing a re-entry plan, encourage the family and child to join in a consultative relationship with a school administrator and a teacher. Parents should be fully informed of what the healthcare provider intends to do in consultation as well as what information will be shared with the school prior to signing consent. In some cases, schools will require parents to sign the school district consent form prior to the beginning of consultation.

1. As soon as possible, contact the administrator in charge of attendance to inform of SRB. Inquire about supportive teachers to enlist in the plan.
2. Alternatively or in addition to contacting the administrator, ask the student to identify a supportive teacher. Students will likely have some idea of who will be receptive to helping with a re-entry plan.
3. Inform the teacher of SRB and function/s of SRB. An in-person meeting may not be possible. Using Skype™ or FaceTime is a reasonable alternative.
4. Outline the role of the teacher in the re-entry plan. In general, the teacher's role is to closely monitor attendance, inform parents of nonattendance, and encourage the student to return to school the following or same day.
5. Schedule regular follow-ups with the teacher to collect attendance data and address difficulties with the plan.

What Does Not Work

Although evidence-based treatments for SRB are readily available, healthcare providers need to ensure against interventions that are ineffective or may exacerbate the problem. These may include:

- Failing to assess risk factors when problematic school absenteeism is indicated during well checks
- Minimizing or ignoring SRB by forcing a quick return to school
- Writing excuses for children to stay home unless there is a medical cause that makes it necessary
- Using a SRB protocol that does not stress a collaborative team approach to SRB
- Creating a plan that includes immediate forced re-entry to school

When to Refer to External Providers and Specialty Mental Health

While it is the expectation that many patients with SRB will benefit from interventions in primary/integrated care setting, referral to specialty care offered in a traditional outpatient psychology clinic may be necessary. The decision to refer to external providers should be made in consultation with the treatment team after a thorough review of the medical record and assessment data and interview of the patient and family. These steps will assist in determining if the intervention can be provided in the primary/integrated care setting or if a referral for traditional psychological services is needed. Some indicators of the need for external referral include the following:

- When the SRB has been persistent or chronic
- When SRB does not improve with primary/integrated care-based treatment
- If the patient has comorbid conditions that negatively impact school and family functioning

Many families, however, may not be accepting of a referral outside the primary/integrated care practice or may want to try working with the behavioral health professional in the primary/integrated care setting before moving on to a higher level of care. Thus, it is important to set expectations with families about the level of treatment available in the primary/integrated care setting.

Roles of Team Members in the Integrated Care Team

To effectively address SRB in the integrated care setting, several systems-based processes must be in place. Appropriately trained BHPs working in integrated care settings should have the necessary skill set to assist in developing, implementing, and monitoring the outcomes of these systems-based processes. McDaniel and colleagues (2014) defined six competency areas for psychologists working in primary/integrated care: science, systems, professionalism, relationships, application, and education. They further identified within each competency area essential components or required elements as well as behavioral anchors for the essential components. Multiple competencies, numerous essential components, and specific behavioral anchors align with the role the behavioral health professional plays in the integrated care with regard to SRB.

First, the behavioral health professional would be involved in the development, implementation, and monitoring of the behavioral health screening process. This might include assisting with the selection of screening measures as well as determining processes for scoring and clinic flow. Because of the analytical skills of the psychologist working in an integrated setting, the BHP will typically lead efforts to compare screening results, to published prevalence rates, and will track rates across time.

The behavioral health professional may assist in developing and monitoring treatment algorithms, educating and training the PCP and staff on evidence-based interventions, and assisting in developing evidence-based handouts and resource lists. Additionally, the behavioral health professional may work to establish and maintain routine communication with school systems and personnel. Ensuring the healthcare system and school system collaborate is essential for effectively addressing SRB and evaluating treatment outcomes.

Lastly, the BHP will serve as a direct service provider and provide indirect care via clinical consultant. In cases where the PCP decides to intervene to address the SRB without directly involving the BHP, the BHP will provide consultation to the PCP. The BHP will provide direct care in brief (1–5 sessions) evidence-based interventions to address SRB. Additionally, the BHP may provide evidence-based treatment (traditional psychotherapy) to a subpopulation with comorbid mental health disorders.

The BHP operates as a collaborative member of the larger integrated care team, which typically involves integrated care providers (physicians, nurse practitioners, and physician assistants), nurses (RN and/or LPN), medical assistants (MA), and patient service representatives (PSR). All team members have a role to play in the effective assessment and treatment of patients with SRB. The process starts with the PSR who initially greets the patient at check-in. Part of the check-in process is to provide the patient/family with the appropriate paper work to complete prior to seeing the PCP. This paper work would include any screening measures, such as the PSC-17, SCARED, SRAS-R, or other screeners, the patient is scheduled to complete based on the patient's age and appointment type. The PSR collects the completed screeners and then provides the screeners to the MA. The MA is the professional who typically rooms the patient, performs and collects vital signs, and updates basic clinical information in preparation for the patient to see the PCP. As part of this preparation, the MA will score any screening measures. This scoring may be by hand or may involve entry into the electronic medical record. No matter the process, the MA scores the screens, so the PCP will be able to quickly review the results and discuss with the patient/family.

Nurses in integrated care are often involved in coordinating care planning and providing patient education. Therefore, nursing may collaborate with the BHP to ensure that screening measures are consistently followed and provide education and training to all clinic staff. Nursing may also provide the initial intervention for SRB by providing patients/families with patient education and additional resources. Lastly, nursing will be involved in the coordination of care ranging from coordination with the BHP and school personnel for patients treated within the integrated care setting to coordination and follow-up with outside referrals for ongoing psychotherapy for patients treated for SRB outside of the integrated care setting.

The PCP is responsible for the patient's overall care and responsible for ensuring the patient's treatment needs are appropriately addressed. In the integrated care process for effective assessment and treatment of patients with SRB, the PCP will be actively involved in the assessment process. The PCP will be involved in the treatment process, yet the level of involvement will vary depending on the level of severity, patient/family preference, and PCP level of confidence and competence.

How to Assess Impact on Care/Quality Improvement Process

Meaningful assessment of care and quality improvement involves monitoring patient outcomes related to SRB and the functioning of the integrated care team. SRB and any symptoms related to SRB should be tracked throughout the course of treatment through measures such as the SRAS-R or the PCS, as well as school attendance and functioning data from parents or school staff. Such tracking of outcomes provides important feedback to the treatment team about the impact of treatment and the need to adjust treatment if change is not occurring. In addition, monitoring the quality and fidelity of clinic protocols (e.g., screening for school problems with all pediatric patients during well checks, consistent use of assessments like the SRAS-R, warm handoff protocols to the BHP, etc.) will help ensure the overall success of the integrated care team. The following are examples for monitoring the quality and impact of screening and interventions for SRB:

- Assess administration rates for the PSC, SCARED, and SRAS-R.
- Assess administration rate of the SRAS-R when SRB was identified as a concern or was indicated on by SCARED.
- Assess documentation of discussion of school performance at well-child visits.
- Assess frequency of warm handoff to BHP when SRB was identified.
- Assess frequency of intervention plan when SRB was identified.
- Assess types of interventions for SRB provided: psychoeducation by PCP, brief intervention by PCP, brief interventions by BHP, and traditional psychotherapy.
- Assess frequency of communication with school when SRB was identified.
- Assess frequency of follow-up appointments with PCP or BHP after SRB was identified.
- Assess frequency of referrals for traditional outpatient therapy.
- Assess rates of re-administration of SCARED and SRAS-R when SRB was identified as a concern.
- Assess rates of returning to school and days missed from school.
- Assess child and caregiver quality of life.
- Assess caregiver satisfaction with intervention provided.
- Assess clinic staff familiarity and comfort with assessing and addressing SRB.

The list is not meant to be exhaustive but examples of aspects of care that might be periodically assessed. Additionally, the BHP working in an integrated setting will work collaboratively to routinely implement quality improvement projects, following the PDSA (plan-do-study-act) cycle to improve the process, care, and outcomes of the clinic population. Implementation of quality improvement projects provides the BHP an opportunity to provide leadership and utilize their competencies in science, systems, relationships, and application.

References

Birmaher, B., Brent, D., Chiappetta, L., Bridge, J., Monga, S., & Baugher, M. (1999). Psychometric properties of the Screen for Child Anxiety Related Emotional Disorders (SCARED): A replication study. *Journal of the American Academy of Child and Adolescent Psychiatry, 38*(10), 1230–1236.

Blucker, R. T., Jackson, D., Gillaspy, J. A., Hale, J., Wolraich, M., & Gillaspy, S. R. (2014). Pediatric Behavioral Health Screening in primary care: A preliminary analysis of the Pediatric Symptom Checklist-17 with functional impairment items. *Clinical Pediatrics, 53*(5), 449–455. https://doi.org/10.1177/0009922814527498

Gardner, W., Murphy, M., Childs, G., Kelleher, K., Pagano, M., Jellinek, M., … Sturner, R. (1999). The PSC-17: A brief pediatric symptom checklist including psychosocial problem subscales: A report from PROS and ASPN. *Ambulatory Child Health, 5*, 225–236.

Gregory, I. R., & Purcell, A. (2014). Extended school non-attenders' views: Developing best practice. *Educational Psychology in Practice, 30*, 37–50. https://doi.org/10.1080/02667363.2013.869489

Hagan, J. F., Shaw, J. S., & Duncan, P. M. (2008). *Bright futures: Guidelines for health supervision of infants, children, and adolescents* (3rd ed.). Elk Grove Village; IL: American Academy of Pediatrics.

Haight, C., Kearney, C. A., Hendron, M., & Schafer, R. (2011). Confirmatory analyses of the School Refusal Assessment Scale-Revised: Replication and extension to a truancy sample. *Journal of Psychopathology and Behavioral Assessment, 33*, 196–204. https://doi.org/10.1007/s10862-011-9218-9

Havik, T., Bru, E., & Ertesvåg, S. K. (2014). Parental perspectives of the role of school factors in school refusal. *Emotional and Behavioural Difficulties, 19*, 131–153. https://doi.org/10.1080/13632752.2013.816199

Heyne, D., Sauter, F. M., Ollendick, T. H., Van Widenfelt, B. M., & Westenberg, P. M. (2014). Developmentally sensitive cognitive behavioral therapy for adolescent school refusal: Rationale and case illustration. *Clinical Student and Family Psychology Review, 17*, 191–215. https://doi.org/10.1007/s10567-013-0160-0

Inglés, C. J., Gonzálvez-Maciá, C., García-Fernández, J. M., Vicent, M., & Martínez-Monteagudo, M. C. (2015). Current status of research on school refusal. *European Journal of Education and Psychology, 8*(1), 37–52. https://doi.org/10.1016/j.ejeps.2015.10.005

Kearney, C. A. (2002). Identifying the function of school refusal behavior: A revision of the School Refusal Assessment Scale. *Journal of Psychopathology and Behavioral Assessment, 24*, 235–245.

Kearney, C. A. (2003). Bridging the gap among professionals who address students with school absenteeism: Overview and suggestions for consensus. *Professional Psychology: Research and Practice, 34*(1), 57.

Kearney, C. A. (2006). Dealing with school refusal behavior: A primer for family physicians: Workable solutions for unhappy youth and frustrated parents. *The Journal of Family Practice, 55*, 685–692.

Kearney, C. A. (2004). *Getting your child to say "yes" to school: A guide for parents of youth with school refusal behavior*. New York, NY: Oxford University Press.

Kearney, C. A. (2008a). *Helping school refusing children and their parents: A guide for school based professionals*. New York, NY: Oxford University Press.

Kearney, C. A. (2008b). School absenteeism and school refusal behavior in student: A contemporary review. *Clinical Psychology Review, 28*(3), 451–471.

Kearney, C. A., Lemos, A., & Silverman, J. (2004). The functional assessment of school refusal behavior. *The Behavior Analyst Today, 5*(3), 275–283. https://doi.org/10.1037/h0100040

McDaniel, S. H., Grus, C. L., Cubic, B. A., Hunter, C. L., Kearney, L. K., Schuman, C. C., … Johnson, S. B. (2014). Competencies for psychology practice in primary care. *American Psychologist, 69*, 409–429.

Reid, K. (2006). The views of education social workers on the management of truancy and other forms of non-attendance. *Research in Education, 75*, 7540–7557.

Wimmer, M. B. (2016). Implementing evidence-based practices for school refusal and truancy. *Communiqué, 42*(4), 18–20.

33 Serious Mental Illness

Alexandros Maragakis and Michael Vriesman

Overview of Serious Mental Illness

The term serious mental illness (SMI) is commonly used in healthcare but lacks clear definition. This lack of clarity is due to SMI being used to describe multiple psychological issues, such as psychosis (Ruggeri, Leese, Thornicroft, Bisoffi, & Tansella, 2000), severe functional impairment (Federal Register Volume 58 No. 96, 1993), or as an umbrella term for diagnoses like schizophrenia, bipolar disorder, and major depressive disorder (De Hert et al., 2011). For the purposes of this chapter, we chose to refer to SMI as an umbrella term that captures a wide range of mental health disorders in order to provide a more inclusive perspective.

The prevalence rate of SMI is 4–6.8% among the global population (Kessler et al., 2009), and individuals with SMI are high utilizers of healthcare services. For example, a study that followed 437 patients with SMI over a 17-month period reported that the total additional costs to the healthcare system were $10.5 million in comparison to individuals without SMI (Mitton, Adair, McDougall, & Marcoux, 2005). Given this high utilization of healthcare services, it is imperative that healthcare providers and administrators understand the multifaceted (i.e., psychological, somatic, and social) issues individuals with SMI face.

Psychologically, individuals with SMI tend to experience more debilitating and persistent issues that lead to the manifestation of behaviors that can impact engagement with treatment. For example, individuals with SMI are more likely to be isolated, non-conformative, engage in bizarre (e.g., delusional beliefs, hallucinations) behavior, and experience some type of cognitive deficit (Young, Cohen, & Miotto, 2016). This constellation of psychological issues and behaviors results in individuals with SMI being less able to advocate for care and less likely to understand treatment plans.

Beyond psychological distress, individuals with SMI also face a disproportionate amount of preventable somatic conditions, which include cardiovascular disease, diabetes, hypertension, obesity, hyperlipidemia, and a reduction of 25 years in life expectancy (De Hert et al., 2011; Druss, Rosenheck, Desai, & Perlin, 2002; Kiraly & Gunning, 2008; Viron & Stern, 2010). These poorer health outcomes have been linked to sedentary lifestyle, poor diet, smoking, and the use of antipsychotic medications that are all highly prevalent in individuals with SMI. However, what is particularly problematic in regard to overall healthcare costs and quality of care is that individuals with SMI are less likely to access primary care and rely on more expensive emergency

A. Maragakis (✉) • M. Vriesman
Eastern Michigan University, Ypsilanti, MI, USA
e-mail: amaragak@emich.edu

A. Maragakis, W.T. O'Donohue (eds.), *Principle-Based Stepped Care and Brief Psychotherapy for Integrated Care Settings*, https://doi.org/10.1007/978-3-319-70539-2_33

care for somatic healthcare needs (Druss et al., 2002; Kiraly & Gunning, 2008). There have been several explanations for why this reliance on emergency care occurs. First, primary care providers (PCPs) have a difficult time interacting and engaging with individuals with SMI and report that individuals with SMI are beyond their scope of practice (Pastore, Griswold, Homish, & Wakins, 2013). This may lead PCPs to engage in "diagnostic overshadowing" when treating individuals with SMI and focus on the state of their mental health instead of their physical complaints (Jones, Howard, & Thornicroft, 2008). This results in PCPs being more likely to miss important somatic health concerns, which can lead to somatic issues not being appropriately treated (Graber et al., 2000). Second, individuals with SMI report that the primary care setting can be highly aversive (e.g., crowded, noisy) and feel that they have to exaggerate symptoms to be taken seriously and that they do not feel well-understood by their PCPs (Lester, Tritter, & Sorohan, 2005). Third, receiving care within the primary care context was a predictor of not receiving minimally adequate treatment for SMI (Wang, Demler, & Kessler, 2002). In combination, the current state of the primary care setting may create a difficult context for both PCPs and individuals with SMI (Maragakis, Siddharthan, RachBeisel, & Snipes, 2016).

Individuals with SMI also face unique resource issues. For example, individuals with SMI make up approximately 25–33% of the homeless population (Cortes et al., 2011) and are at a 10–20 times greater risk of homelessness than the general population (Susser et al., 1997). They also are likely to lack insurance, a vehicle, and general financial resources making it difficult for them to engage in treatment. These deficits can prevent these individuals from receiving evidence-based treatments for SMI as they are expensive and require consistent and long-term therapy. Furthermore, individuals with SMI face greater amounts of stigma, both in society and by healthcare professionals (Lawrence & Kisely, 2010). These resource issues become relevant in the context of receiving treatment in the primary care setting as individuals with SMI may miss medical appointments due to emergencies or unexpected appointments to address issues such as housing, insurance, and disability. Therefore, given that individuals with SMI have higher rates of social issues, it is imperative to not overlook them when providing care.

Individuals with SMI also experience unique difficulties as a result of medications used in their treatment, most common of which are antipsychotics. First-generation antipsychotics (also referred to as typical antipsychotics) have a wide range of side effects, including sexual and reproductive side effects, extrapyramidal side effects, and tardive dyskinesia (Glazer, 2000). Second-generation antipsychotics (also referred to as atypical antipsychotics) have improved upon first-generation antipsychotics by having a lower rate of sexual and reproductive side effects, extrapyramidal side effects, and tardive dyskinesia (Haro & Salvador-Carulla, 2006). However, second-generation antipsychotics also may cause metabolic syndrome which can lead to multiple somatic side effects, including hypertension, weight gain, and cardiovascular disease (Newcomer, 2007; Tschoner et al., 2007).

Finally, SMI is traditionally considered a lifetime issue. However, recent findings indicate that individuals with SMI can recover with appropriate treatment. Approximately 20% will make a complete recovery (exhibited by an absence of psychotic features), and another 40% of individuals make a social recovery (economic and residential independence with low social disruption). The key factors involved in these recoveries include satisfying relationships with clinicians and psychiatric medications, services at levels that are needed, and quality of care for medical conditions (Green et al., 2013). Therefore, proper detection, appropriate levels of care, as well as patient-centered approaches that promote patient-provider relationships are important factors to consider when delivering care for those with SMI in the primary care setting and have the potential of leading to greater outcomes than traditionally expected.

Ways to Screen in the Primary Care Setting

There have been several recommendations made to effectively screen for SMI in the primary care setting. The first involves using mental health screeners that have already been developed for the primary care setting, such as the Patient Health Questionnaire (PHQ-9 or GAD-7), to detect general mental health issues, because the disorders addressed in these screens may be highly correlated or directly related to certain SMI diagnoses (i.e., severe depression or bipolar disorder) (Minkoff & Parks, 2015). Second, the use of the Kessler Screening Scales (K6 or K10) (Kessler et al., 2010), which have been specifically created to discriminate cases of SMI, has been used internationally and by agencies like the World Health Organization. The K6 and K10 are consistent with the primary care setting in regard to length and ease of use and can be easily incorporated in a patient's previsit check before seeing the PCP (the K6 and K10 screens, as well as information on how they are scored are available at www.hcp.med.harvard.edu/ncs/k6_scales.php). Third, examining the individual's electronic health record can indicate SMI. Individuals with SMI often have a long treatment history and are likely to have previously received care. Finally, as discussed previously, behavioral symptoms of SMI are typically salient and noticeable (e.g., active delusions or hallucinations, manic behavior). If a patient engages any of these behaviors during the appointment, reports a history of these behaviors, or has a family member that is concerned due to these behaviors, then further assessment would be warranted.

How to Assess Further If a Screen Returns Positive

If a screen for SMI returns positive, there are several additional methods of assessing clinically relevant features that can impact treatment. First, individuals with SMI tend to have lower levels of independent and cognitive functioning (Young et al., 2016). Given this, assessing levels of independent functioning will determine the emphasis of treatment (see Evidence-Based Stepped Care section). The UCSD Performance-Based Skills Assessment (UPSA)-Brief is a brief measure that assesses an individual's communication and financial skills. It has been empirically validated, is a good predictor of residential independence, and is highly correlated with overall cognitive function and negative symptoms (Mausbach, Harvey, Goldman, Jeste, & Patterson, 2007). Furthermore, the UPSA-Brief is sensitive to changes due to treatment and can be used as an outcome measure (see Quality Improvement section).

Another key issue to assess for with this population is alcohol and substance abuse. Individuals with SMI are three to eight times more likely to abuse substances in comparison to the general population (Maisto, Carey, Carey, Gordon, & Gleason, 2000). The use of substances is particularly problematic in this population. For example, the use of substances has been linked to exacerbating positive symptoms, such as delusions and hallucinations, for those with schizophrenia (Wade, Harrigan, McGorry, Burgess, & Whelan, 2007). Therefore, assessing the presence, and the level, of substance and alcohol abuse is necessary to provide appropriate levels of care.

Measures, such as the AUDIT, which assesses for alcohol abuse, and DAST, which assesses for substance abuse, have been specifically designed to be used in the primary care setting. Both measures have been shown to adequately identify individuals that have abuse issues and provide clinical utility when used with the SMI population (Maisto et al., 2000) (see Substance Abuse chapter for further assessment methods).

Finally, an assessment of environmental factors and stressors is particularly important with this population. Therefore, assessing around issues, such as employment (or disability), housing, access to food, and access to other forms of healthcare, can provide valuable information in regard to what to focus on during treatment.

Evidence-Based Stepped Care

As discussed previously, providing adequate treatment to individuals with SMI can be difficult and typically beyond the scope of the primary care setting. Due to the difficulty providing treatment to individuals with SMI in the primary care setting, a stepped care model is suggested to assist in providing effective treatment and to meet the new demand of primary care integration. This method begins with the least invasive and lowest-cost treatment and allows for treatment to be intensified based on the needs of the individual. The following sections provide options for a stepped care model that can be used to treat a variety of issues.

It is important to note that the treatment of SMI is an ongoing and complex process that typically requires intensive mental health treatment (see When to Refer section). Therefore, given the limited time available to treat individuals, the primary goal when treating SMI within the primary care setting is to refer and get them connected with a case manager. However, given the time available when seeing individuals with SMI, it can also be useful to focus on smaller goals, such as improving diet and exercise routines, reducing smoking, or obtaining employment. By focusing on smaller goals, improvements in overall functioning may be actualized while the individual is being transitioned into long-term mental health treatment.

Psychoeducation

The use of psychoeducation with patients with serious mental illness has found to be effective, specifically for those with schizophrenia (Lukens & McFarlane, 2004). A review conducted in 2015 on the use of brief psychoeducation, including 20 studies with more than 2300 participants, indicated that brief psychoeducation reduced relapse rates and increased medication compliance, an important factor in the treatment in schizophrenia (Zhao, Sampson, Xia, & Jayaram, 2015). Brief psychoeducation consisted of less than ten sessions of didactic interventions discussing SMI from multiple dimensions, including familial, social, biological, and pharmacological perspectives. Individuals who participated in brief psychoeducation scored higher on mental state and social functioning scales. Multiple trials within this review showed that any form of psychoeducation produced more favorable short- to medium-term results than routine care. Additional reviews have also shown benefits in reduction in length of hospital stay as well as compliance with hospital readmissions (Xia, Merinder, & Belgamwar, 2011).

Family psychoeducation (FPE) has also been found to be effective in reducing hospital readmissions for individuals with schizophrenia. Research done by Baucom, Shoham, Mueser, Daiuto, and Stickle (1998) examined the efficacy of different FPE interventions. Their results indicated that readmission rates for individuals with SMI were lowered from 30 to 40% with routine treatment to 15% when FPE was included.

Useful materials for conducting family psychotherapy include:

- William McFarlane—Multifamily Groups in the Treatment of Severe Psychiatric Disorders (McFarlane, 2004). www.guilford.com/books/Multifamily-Groups-Treatment-Severe-Psychiatric-Disorders/William-McFarlane/9781593850951/reviews
- Family Psychoeducation Evidence-Based Practices (EBP) KIT (SAMHSA, 2009) http://store.samhsa.gov/product/Family-Psychoeducation-Evidence-Based-Practices-EBP-KIT/SMA09-4423

Online Interventions

Cognitive behavioral therapy for psychosis (CBTp) has been found to be an effective treatment for schizophrenia in that it reduces positive and negative symptoms and social anxiety and improves certain measures of functioning and mood (Wykes, Steel, Everitt, & Tarrier, 2008). However, CBTp is often difficult to access by individuals with SMI (Hazell, Hayward, Cavanagh, & Strauss, 2016). In response to this, a computerized version of CBTp has been developed called "Coping with Voices" (Gottlieb, Romeo, Penn, Mueser, & Chiko, 2013). A pilot study was conducted with 21 participants with schizophrenia spectrum disorder and auditory hallucinations. The 17 participants who experienced more than 50% of the program reported significant reductions in multiple measures, including the overall severity and perception of voices as an "outside entity" and intensity of "negative commentary," psychotic symptoms, and overall psychopathology. While additional research is needed, these results show the potential efficacy of using online CBT interventions for serious mental illness. While this is a promising intervention, it is current not available for public use.

Group Interventions

Multiple forms of group interventions have been found helpful for those with severe mental illness. However, given the limited time (15–20 min) allotted to patients, it is important to assess the number of patients needed to maintain productivity standards (approximated five to six patients) and whether or not this standard could be met before engaging in group processes.

Individuals with severe mental illness often have a deficit in social skills, and social skills groups have been shown to be effective at reducing these deficits (e.g., Chien et al., 2003; Kurtz & Mueser, 2008). Research has also been done showing the effectiveness of combining social skills groups and family psychoeducation. A study conducted by Valencia, Fresan, Juárez, Escamilla, and Saracco (2013) randomly assigned 119 people who were currently in outpatient and diagnosed with schizophrenia to either receive pharmacological treatment or participate in a social skills training group as well as family psychoeducation. The social skills training focused on areas where individuals were experiencing problems that interfered with their social functioning, including developing skills to manage social relations and problem-solving skills for better family relations. These trainings were conducted by the use of skill demonstrations by the trainers, role-playing, and constructive feedback. At a 6-month follow-up, they discovered that 91% of the individuals in the social skills group met criteria for symptomatic remission, while of those assigned to receive pharmacological treatment, only 66.7% met criteria. Additionally, 58.8% of individuals in the social skills group achieved functional improvement criteria, compared to only one individual receiving pharmacological treatment. Social skills training manuals, such as social skills training for schizophrenia (Bellack, Mueser, Gingerich, & Agresta, 2013), are low cost and provide very detailed instructions for clinicians that have never used them.

Groups can also be focused on lifestyle behaviors that are problematic for individuals with SMI. For example, smoking is a very common issue with individuals with SMI, with rates of smoking for those in psychiatric outpatient being over 60%, and even higher rates associated with more acute psychiatric illness (Vanable, Carey, Carey, & Maisto, 2003). However, it has been found that when provided with mental health treatment, individuals with severe mental illness are more likely to successfully quit smoking (Lê Cook et al., 2014). Therefore, engaging in groups that address some of these problematic behavioral issues commonly found in the SMI population could prove to be very beneficial in achieving the goal of functional improvement. (More information on specific smoking cessation interventions, as well as interventions for diet and substance abuse, can be found in their respective chapters in this book).

Individual Interventions

As there are currently no brief therapies for individuals with SMI that are appropriate for the primary care setting, providers should instead continue to focus on small achievable goals. This could best be served by providing referrals to social work interventions such as assisting the individual with acquiring disability, employment, living placement, and life skills. Life skills can include such things as self-care activities, household management, and finding employment. Mairs and Bradshaw (2004) created a manual and conducted a pilot study for a life skills intervention for people with a diagnosis of schizophrenia focusing on functional deficits and on the most important life skills for each individual. They discovered that participation led to a reduction in negative symptoms as well as overall general psychopathology.

What Doesn't Work

One of the primary treatments for individuals with SMI is CBTp (Hutton, Wood, Taylor, Irving, & Morrison, 2014). To effectively implement CBTp typically requires 16–20 individual therapy sessions over approximately 6 months. Given its length, more brief versions of CBTp have been examined and show comparable effect sizes to full CBTp (Hazell et al., 2016). However, even though it requires less than 16 sessions, brief CBTp still requires time-intensive individual therapy. Given this, engaging in CBTp or brief CBTp would be far beyond the scope of the primary care setting.

As discussed throughout this chapter, the primary care setting is not an adequate setting to treat the multifaceted issues faced by individuals with SMI. However, given the somatic health issues faced by SMI, the combination of mental health and primary care is desperately needed. The use of reverse integrated care (RIC) clinics, in which primary care is embedded within the mental health setting, has been suggested as an alternative that addresses many of the weaknesses faced when trying to deliver care in the primary care setting (Maragakis et al., 2016; Scharf et al., 2013). This model has been tested within the Department of Veteran Affairs, and the results have been promising. There has been evidence to suggest that this model of care has been effective at increasing the likelihood of individuals with SMI receiving alcohol misuse screenings and having good blood pressure control (Kilbourne et al., 2011b), as well as those on second-generation antipsychotics receiving cardiometabolic tests (Kilbourne, Lai, Bowersox, Pirraglia, & Bauer, 2011a). Given this, it can be argued that delivering care within the primary care setting itself "does not work" and ideally the integration of services ought to occur within the behavioral health setting.

When to Refer to External Mental Health

Due to the previously discussed difficulties of PCPs interacting with and treating individuals with SMI, referral of these individuals to a community mental health center should occur during the first appointment. To facilitate this transition, it is important that a clinic establishes rapport with a local community mental health center and try to create a service line that allows for clients to have immediate or expedited access to mental health services. Establishing interactive communication with a community mental health center and streamlining the transition would better ensure that individuals with SMI receive quality care (Foy et al., 2010). As the pharmacological treatment of SMI is beyond the scope of practice of PCPs, it is important to refer to a community mental health center that provides psychiatric services (Pastore et al., 2013).

It is important to note that referring out to mental health professionals for these interventions is often viewed by PCPs as a difficult and time-consuming process (Cunningham, 2009). Referral for behavioral treatment involves multiple steps, including problem identification, access to appropriate treatment resources, referral, referral acceptance, and treatment initiation, with failure in any of these steps resulting in the individual failing to receive treatment (Kessler, 2012). The success rates of referrals are also quite low, with only 33–50% of primary care patients referred for mental health services successfully completing the referral (Fisher, 1997). Community mental health centers also can suffer from long wait lists for appointments, which result in a lower rate of referral completion (Leung, Castan-Cameo, McGhee, Wong, & Johnston, 2003). Given these barriers, the primary focus of "individual intervention time" with the behavioral provider may be solely invested in the referral process and assisting the individual through the referral, such as assisting the individual in scheduling the appointment or filling out intake forms.

The Role of the Primary Care Team

Given the high prevalence of somatic health problems with individuals with SMI, the role of the primary care team is particularly important. However, as described earlier, there is commonly a "mismatch" between PCP and patient, which results in PCPs feeling that patients with SMI are beyond the scope of their care and patients feeling that their PCPs do not listen or address their concerns. Given this, it is an important intervention goal for the behavioral provider to discuss and support PCPs with any concerns or difficulties that they may be experiencing when treating an individual with SMI. This may require that PCPs receive training around how to effectively communicate treatment goals, medication regiments, and how to effectively handle the presence of positive symptoms during an appointment. It also may require that PCPs and behavioral providers have joint appointments in order to reduce any potential "mismatch" that might occur between patient and PCP and facilitate any concerns that either might be experiencing.

The medical team also has an important role of consistently monitoring somatic indicators, like BMI and HbA1c levels, for this population. Medications, like antipsychotics, can lead to metabolic syndrome, which results in rapid weight gain and diabetes. By appropriately tracking these indicators, potential side effects caused by antipsychotic medications can be reduced by early detection. Also, appropriate tracking may lead to new somatic diagnoses (e.g., type 2 diabetes), which would require for new medications to be prescribed.

Furthermore, it is important that medical providers be aware of potentially harmful medication interactions that would be unique to individuals with SMI. For example, angiotensin-converting enzyme (ACE) inhibitors are frontline treatments for hypertension. However, they decrease the elimination of lithium from the body. Therefore, individuals with SMI who are taking lithium as a mood stabilizer would be a greater risk for lithium toxicity if prescribed an ACE inhibitor.

Quality Improvement

Given that individuals with SMI face multifaceted issues discussed throughout this chapter (i.e., somatic, psychological, and social), there are multiple outcomes available to track for clinics and clinicians who wish to engage in quality improvement (QI). Given the wide range of outcomes available, the "optimal" QI approach will be highly dependent on the clinic's resources, the amount of individuals with SMI seen within the clinic, and the community resources within the area. Therefore, rather than recommend a specific QI plan, a description for possible outcomes and how to track them will be provided.

Since the primary goal of the primary care setting is to improve health outcomes, it is recommended that a QI initiative includes some monitoring of health improvement. Specifically, the monitoring of HbA1c levels and BMI is particularly important for this population due to the side effects of medications like antipsychotics. It is recommended that BMI is assessed every visit. For the purposes of QI, an example of a clinical goal is to ensure that BMI is at least stable or maintained when an individual has been prescribed an antipsychotic. If it increases more than X% (this is to be determined by the clinic), then contact must be made with the prescribing provider of the antipsychotic to inform them of the weight gain. The tracking of HbA1c should occur a minimum of every 6 months, with a goal of reducing HbA1c levels to 7. Again, if sudden changes to HbA1c levels occur, the prescribing provider of the antipsychotic should be informed. Clinics can decide to track multiple aspects, such as the percent of patients who actually received BMI and HbA1c checks during the recommended time period, percent of patients who are within recommended levels, and/or percent of prescribing providers contact if results are abnormal.

Psychological improvements in regard to symptom-specific issues faced by individuals with SMI that can be made during the course of treatment or overtime can be assessed through measures like the UPSA-Brief or other measures used during the assessment phase. Also, if a clinic decided to run groups on more general issues faced by individuals, such as smoking cessation or nutritional groups, pre-/post-assessments can be used to assess the effectiveness of these groups. Furthermore, if groups are available, an important QI metric could assess the number of people with SMI who have been referred to these groups (which should ideally be 100%) and the number of individuals who actually attend. This metric may provide information on potential barriers in regard to when the group is offered and may allow for the clinic to change services to better meet patient needs.

Finally, "social" improvements can also be tracked through QI. A particularly important metric to assess with this population is the percentage of individuals who follow through and are receiving care at a specialty mental health clinic. As discussed throughout this chapter, the level of care that is typically required for an individual with SMI is beyond the scope of the primary care setting. Therefore, receiving care at a mental health clinic is essential for this population to receive quality care. Assessing the number of completed referrals would allow the clinic and providers to react in multiple ways. For example, if the total percentage of completed referrals is low, then an assessment of potential barriers patients face when transitioning into specialty care is warranted. Further metrics of interest could involve percent of patients with health insurance, disability, employment, or other assistance programs. By engaging in QI across these domains, clinics and providers can make more informed treatment decisions and augment the treatment of individuals with SMI in the primary care setting.

References

Baucom, D. H., Shoham, V., Mueser, K. T., Daiuto, A. D., & Stickle, T. R. (1998). Empirically supported couple and family interventions for marital distress and adult mental health problems. *Journal of Consulting and Clinical Psychology*, *66*(1), 53–88. Retrieved from http://ezproxy.emich.edu/login?url=http://search.proquest.com/docview/614400143?accountid=10650.

Bellack, A. S., Mueser, K. T., Gingerich, S., & Agresta, J. (2013). *Social skills training for schizophrenia: A step-by-step guide*. New York: Guilford Publications.

Chien, H. C., Ku, C. H., Lu, R. B., Chu, H., Tao, Y. H., & Chou, K. R. (2003). Effects of social skills training on improving social skills of patients with schizophrenia. *Archives of Psychiatric Nursing*, *17*(5), 228–236.

Cortes, A., Leopold, J., Rothschild, L., Buron, L., Khadduri, J., & Culhane, D. (2011). *The 2010 annual homeless assessment report to congress*. Washington, DC: U.S. Department of Housing and Urban Development.

Cunningham, P. J. (2009). Beyond parity: Primary care physicians' perspectives on access to mental health care. *Health Affairs*, *28*(3), w490–w501.

De Hert, M., Cohen, D., Bobes, J., Cetkovich-Bakmas, M., Leucht, S., Ndetei, D., & Correll, C. (2011). Physical illness in patients with severe mental disorders. Barries to care, monitoring and treatment guidelines, plus recommendations at the system and individual level. *World Psychiatry*, *10*, 138–151.

Druss, B., Rosenheck, R., Desai, M., & Perlin, J. (2002). Quality of preventive medical care for patients with mental disorders. *Medical Care*, *40*, 129–136.

Fisher, L. (1997). Developing health care within the context of primary care. *Archives of Family Medicine*, *6*, 324–333.

Foy, R., Hempel, S., Rubenstein, L., Suttorp, M., Seelig, M., Shanman, R., & Shekelle, P. G. (2010). Meta-analysis: Effect of interactive communication between collaborating primary care physicians and specialists. *Annals of Internal Medicine*, *152*(4), 247–258.

Glazer, W. M. (2000). Extrapyramidal side effects, tardive dyskinesia, and the concept of atypicality. *The Journal of Clinical Psychiatry*, *61*, 16–21. Retrieved from http://ezproxy.emich.edu/login?url=http://search.proquest.com/docview/619494009?accountid=10650.

Gottlieb, J. D., Romeo, K. H., Penn, D. L., Mueser, K. T., & Chiko, B. P. (2013). Web-based cognitive–behavioral therapy for auditory hallucinations in persons with psychosis: A pilot study. *Schizophrenia Research*, *145*(1), 82–87.

Graber, M., Bergus, G., Dawson, J., Wood, G., Levy, B., & Levin, I. (2000). Effect of patient's psychiatric history on physicians' estimation of probability of disease. *Journal of General Internal Medicine*, *15*, 204–206.

Green, C., Perrin, N., Leo, M., Janoff, S., Yarborogh, B., & Paulson, R. (2013). Recovery in serious mental illness: Trajectories, characteristics and the role of mental health care in the STARS study. *Psychiatric Services, 64*(12), 1203–1210.

Haro, J. M., & Salvador-Carulla, L. (2006). The SOHO (Schizophrenia Outpatient Health Outcome) Study. *CNS Drugs, 20*(4), 293–301.

Hazell, C. M., Hayward, M., Cavanagh, K., & Strauss, C. (2016). A systematic review and meta-analysis of low intensity CBT for psychosis. *Clinical Psychology Review, 45*, 183–192. Retrieved from http://ezproxy.emich.edu/login?url=http://search.proquest.com/docview/1779462575?accountid=10650.

Hutton, P., Wood, L., Taylor, P. J., Irving, K., & Morrison, A. P. (2014). Cognitive behavioural therapy for psychosis: Rationale and protocol for a systematic review and meta-analysis. *Psychosis: Psychological, Social and Integrative Approaches, 6*(3), 220–230. Retrieved from http://ezproxy.emich.edu/login?url=http://search.proquest.com/docview/1560816250?accountid=10650.

Jones, S., Howard, L., & Thornicroft, G. (2008). Diagnostic overshadowing: Worse physical health care with people with mental illness. *Acta Psychiatrica Scandinavica, 118*, 169–171.

Kessler, R., Aguilar-Gaxiola, S., Alonso, J., Chatterji, S., Lee, S., Ormel, J., … Wang, P. (2009). The global burden of mental disorders: An update from the WHO World Mental Health (WMH) surveys. *Epidemiologia E Psichiatria Sociale, 18*, 23–33.

Kessler, R., Greif Green, J., Gruber, M., Sampson, N., Bromet, E., Cuitan, M., … Zaslavsky, A. (2010). Screening for serious mental illness in the general population with the K6 screening scale: Results from the WHO world mental health (WMH) survey initiative. *International Journal of Methods in Psychiatric Research, 19*, 4–22.

Kessler, R. (2012). Mental health care treatment initiation when mental health services are incorporated into primary care practice. *Journal of the American Board of Family Medicine, 25*(2), 255–259.

Kilbourne, A. M., Lai, Z., Bowersox, N., Pirraglia, P., & Bauer, M. S. (2011a). Does colocated care improve access to cardiometabolic screening for patients with serious mental illness? *General Hospital Psychiatry, 33*(6), 634–636.

Kilbourne, A. M., Pirraglia, P. A., Lai, Z., Bauer, M. S., Charns, M. P., Greenwald, D., … Yano, E. M. (2011b). Quality of general medical care among patients with serious mental illness: Does colocation of services matter? *Psychiatric Services, 62*(8), 922–928.

Kiraly, B., & Gunning, K. (2008). Primary care issues in patients with mental illness. *American Family Physician, 78*, 355–362.

Kurtz, M. M., & Mueser, K. T. (2008). A meta-analysis of controlled research on social skills training for schizophrenia. *Journal of Consulting and Clinical Psychology, 76*(3), 491–504. Retrieved from http://ezproxy.emich.edu/login?url=http://search.proquest.com/docview/614484214?accountid=10650.

Lawrence, D., & Kisely, S. (2010). Inequalities in healthcare provision for people with serious mental illness. *Journal of Psychopharmacology, 24*(11), 61–68.

Lê Cook, B., Wayne, G. F., Kafali, E. N., Liu, Z., Shu, C., & Flores, M. (2014). Trends in smoking among adults with mental illness and association between mental health treatment and smoking cessation. *JAMA, 311*(2), 172–182.

Lester, H., Tritter, J., & Sorohan, H. (2005). Patients' and health professionals' views on primary care for people with serious mental illness: Focus group study. *British Medical Journal, 330*, 1122.

Leung, G. M., Castan-Cameo, S., McGhee, S. M., Wong, I. O., & Johnston, J. M. (2003). Waiting time, doctor shopping, and nonattendance at specialist outpatient clinics: Case-control study of 6495 individuals in Hong Kong. *Medical Care, 41*(11), 1293–1300.

Lukens, E. P., & McFarlane, W. R. (2004). Psychoeducation as evidence-based practice: Considerations for practice, research, and policy. *Brief Treatment and Crisis Intervention, 4*(3), 205.

Mairs, H., & Bradshaw, T. (2004). Life skills training in schizophrenia. *British Journal of Occupational Therapy, 67*(5), 217–224.

Maisto, S., Carey, M., Carey, K., Gordon, C., & Gleason, J. (2000). Use of the AUDIT and the DAST-10 to identify alcohol and drug use disorder among adults with severe and persistent mental illness. *Psychological Assessment, 12*(2), 186–192.

Maragakis, A., Siddharthan, R., RachBeisel, J., & Snipes, C. (2016). Creating a 'reverse' integrated primary and mental healthcare clinical for those with serious mental illness. *Primary Health Care Research & Development, 17*, 421–427.

Mausbach, B., Harvey, P., Goldman, S., Jeste, D., & Patterson, T. (2007). Development of a brief scale of everyday functioning in persons with serious mental illness. *Schizophrenia Bulletin, 33*(6), 1364–1372.

McFarlane, W. R. (2004). *Multifamily groups in the treatment of severe psychiatric disorders*. New York: Guilford Press.

Minkoff, K., & Parks, J. (2015). Primary health-behavioral health integration for the population of individuals with serious mental illness. In W. O'Donohue & A. Maragakis (Eds.), *Integrated primary and behavioral care: Role in medical homes and chronic disease management* (pp. 171–200). New York: Springer.

Mitton, C. R., Adair, C. E., McDougall, G. M., & Marcoux, G. (2005). Continuity of care and health care costs among persons with severe mental illness. *Psychiatric Services, 56*(9), 1070–1076. Retrieved from http://ezproxy.emich.edu/login?url=http://search.proquest.com/docview/213081313?accountid=10650.

Newcomer, J. W. (2007). Metabolic considerations in the use of antipsychotic medications: A review of recent evidence. *The Journal of Clinical Psychiatry, 68*(suppl 1), 20–27.

Pastore, P., Griswold, K., Homish, G., & Wakins, R. (2013). Family practice enhancements for patients with severe mental illness. *Community Mental Health Journal, 49*, 172–177.

Ruggeri, M., Leese, M., Thornicroft, G., Bisoffi, G., & Tansella, M. (2000). Definition and prevalence of severe and persistent mental illness. *The British Journal of Psychiatry, 177*, 149–155. Retrieved from http://ezproxy.emich.edu/login?url=http://search.proquest.com/docview/619463803?accountid=10650.

Scharf, D., Eberhart, N., Schmidt, N., Vaughn, C., Dutta, T., Pincus, H., & Burnam, M. (2013). Integrating primary care into community behavioral health settings: Programs and early implementation experiences. *Psychiatric Services, 64*(7), 660–665.

Substance Abuse and Mental Health Services Administration (SAMHSA). (2009), *Family psychoeducation: How to use the evidence-based practices KITs.* HHS Pub. No. SMA-09-4422. Rockville, MD: Center for Mental Health Services, Substance Abuse and Mental Health Services Administration, U.S. Department of Health and Human Services. Retrieved November 30, 2016, from http://store.samhsa.gov/product/Family-Psychoeducation-Evidence-Based-Practices-EBP-KIT/SMA09-4423

Susser, E., Valencia, E., Conover, S., Felix, A., Tsai, W., & Wyatt, R. (1997). Preventing recurrent homelessness among mentally ill men: A "critical time" intervention after discharge from a shelter. *American Journal of Public Health, 87*(2), 256–262.

Tschoner, A., Engl, J., Laimer, M., Kaser, S., Rettenbacher, M., Fleischhacker, W. W., … Ebenbichler, C. F. (2007). Metabolic side effects of antipsychotic medication. *International Journal of Clinical Practice, 61*(8), 1356–1370.

Valencia, M., Fresan, A., Juárez, F., Escamilla, R., & Saracco, R. (2013). The beneficial effects of combining pharmacological and psychosocial treatment on remission and functional outcome in outpatients with schizophrenia. *Journal of Psychiatric Research, 47*(12), 1886–1892.

Vanable, P. A., Carey, M. P., Carey, K. B., & Maisto, S. A. (2003). Smoking among psychiatric outpatients: Relationship to substance use, diagnosis, and illness severity. *Psychology of Addictive Behaviors, 17*(4), 259.

Viron, M., & Stern, T. (2010). The impact of serious mental illness on health and healthcare. *Psychosomatics, 51*, 458–465.

Wade, D., Harrigan, S., McGorry, P., Burgess, P., & Whelan, G. (2007). Impact of severity of substance use disorder on symptomatic and functional outcome in young individuals with first-episode psychosis. *Journal of Clinical Psychiatry, 68*, 767–774.

Wang, P. S., Demler, O., & Kessler, R. C. (2002). Adequacy of treatment for serious mental illness in the United States. *American Journal of Public Health, 92*(1), 92–98.

Wykes, T., Steel, C., Everitt, B., & Tarrier, N. (2008). Cognitive behavior therapy for schizophrenia: Effect sizes, clinical models, and methodological rigor. *Schizophrenia Bulletin, 34*(3), 523–537.

Xia, J., Merinder, L. B., & Belgamwar, M. R. (2011). Psychoeducation for schizophrenia. *The Cochrane Library*.

Young, A., Cohen, A., & Miotto, K. (2016). Improving the quality of care for serious mental illness. In W. O'Donohoue & A. Maragakis (Eds.), *Quality improvement in behavioral health* (pp. 275–288). Cham, Switzerland: Springer International.

Zhao, S., Sampson, S., Xia, J., & Jayaram, M. B. (2015). Psychoeducation (brief) for people with serious mental illness. *The Cochrane Library*.

34 Sexual Abuse and PTSD in Children

Caroline Cummings and William T. O'Donohue

A Brief Description of the Disorder or Problem

Child sexual abuse is a type of a traumatic event that may involve "unwanted and inappropriate sexual solicitation of, or exposure to, a child by an older person; genital touching or fondling; or penetration in terms of oral, anal or vaginal intercourse or attempted intercourse" (Andrews, Corry, Slade, Issakidis, & Swanston, 2004). In a study using data collected from Child Protective Services, it was found that there were 60,956 reports of child sexual abuse investigated between October 2012 and September 2013 (U.S. Department of Health and Human Services, 2015). Another national survey found that 6.1% of children in the United States reported being a victim of child sexual abuse in the previous year (Finkelhor, Turner, Ormrod, Hamby & Kracke, 2009). A portion of these victims of child sexual abuse may later develop psychological issues, including posttraumatic stress disorder (PTSD).

When a child directly experiences, or witnesses or learns about traumatic events that a family member or friend endures, they are susceptible to developing PTSD (American Psychiatric Association, 2013). PTSD manifests as intrusive thoughts, distress, physiological reactivity, and avoidant behavior following the traumatic event(s). Diagnostic criteria for PTSD specifically includes "recurrent, involuntary, and intrusive distressing" memories and dream of the traumatic event, along with dissociative reactions (sometimes occurring in play), and psychological distress and physiological reactions in response to cues that assimilate aspects of the event (American Psychiatric Association, 2013). Additionally, there needs to be an avoidance of stimuli associated with the traumatic event, which may be indicated by avoidance of memories, thoughts, feelings, and external reminders. Professionals also find negative alterations in cognitions and mood of children with PTSD, as demonstrated by social withdrawal, reduction of positive emotional expression, and increased negative emotional states (American Psychiatric Association, 2013). Last, there are alterations in arousal and reactivity, as demonstrated by irritability, angry outbursts, hypervigilance, exaggerated startle response, concentration difficulties, sleep disturbances, or reckless behavior. If the symptoms last more than 1 month, they may be eligible for a PTSD diagnosis. However, this only occurs if their natural trauma recovery process is disrupted or they have few factors that promote resiliency (Bonanno & Mancini, 2008). In fact, a large percentage of individuals do not later develop PTSD following a traumatic event, and the prevalence rate of children with PTSD following a traumatic event is unclear. Data suggest that 60.6% of children between 0 and 17.2 children

C. Cummings (✉) • W.T. O'Donohue
Department of Clinical Psychology,
University of Nevada, Reno, NV, USA
e-mail: caroline.cummings@nevada.unr.edu

A. Maragakis, W.T. O'Donohue (eds.), *Principle-Based Stepped Care and Brief Psychotherapy for Integrated Care Settings*, https://doi.org/10.1007/978-3-319-70539-2_34

had experienced trauma within a 1-year period, yet only 5% of adolescents have met the criteria for PTSD in their lifetime (Finkelhor et al., 2009; Merikangas et al., 2010). For those who do develop PTSD, it can have detrimental effects on a child's development such as learning difficulties, hyperarousal, and problems with affect modulation. Thus, PTSD typically causes problems in the child's relationships and academic performance (Streeck-Fischer & Kolk, 2000).

Despite an alarming prevalence of child sexual abuse and PTSD and their documented negative effects on a victim's life, there is no empirically supported treatment that has been used in the primary care setting. A stepped care approach may provide an avenue for providers to engage in effective practices that may help those who seek mental health treatment in the primary care setting. There are significant advantages to implementing a stepped care model, which is an approach toward treatment that is intended to be less restrictive, self-correcting, and patient centered—involving shared decision-making. Additionally, stepped care aims to reduce the financial burden of healthcare, as well as provide more efficient treatment for patients. The provider first screens, then with a positive screen further assesses the patient, and then conjointly with the patient or patient's family decides which level of treatment they would most benefit from. The patient or guardian can then decline or opt out of the stepped care approach but should be provided with the correct decision tools and information to make an informed decision. Because people are more likely to present in a primary care setting with symptoms of abuse and mental health issues, a stepped care approach in primary care may increase the number of patients who will receive treatment, as well as efficiently use the provider's allotted time.

Effective Ways to Screen for PTSD in the Primary Care Setting

If a child presents with bruises or other visible injuries, the parent or child discloses child sexual abuse may have occurred, or if there is any suspicion by the primary care provider that the child may have been victimized, screening for PTSD is recommended. There are various screening tools for PTSD that are age-appropriate for use with child patients as well as their caregivers. Tools that directly screen for sexual abuse and PTSD and have the most psychometric support include the Clinician-Administered PTSD Scale for Children and Adolescents (CAPS-CA), PTSD Checklist-Civilian Version (PCL-C), Primary Care Posttraumatic Stress Disorder Screen (PC-PTSD), and Child PTSD Symptoms Scale (CPSS).

The CAPS-CA is a 30-item scale that screens for a diagnosis of PTSD in children 7 and above (Pynoos et al., 2015). A recent version was designed to use the Diagnostic and Statistical Manual of Mental Disorders Fifth Edition (DSM-5) criteria (CAPS-CA-5) and takes about 45–60 min to administer. The scale targets symptoms, distress, impairment, and relevant specifiers. It can be completed by the child, as it has picture response options and was constructed with age-appropriate language. Responses are on a 4-point scale, ranging from 0 (absent) to 4 (extreme/incapacitating). A positive screen is indicated by a rating of 2 (moderate/threshold) or higher on at least one symptom on both Criteria B and C, at least two symptoms on both D and E, as well as the disturbance lasting at least 1 month and causing clinically significant distress or functional impairment (criteria F and G). The CAPS scale is considered the gold standard of PTSD screening and is endorsed by the United States Department of Veteran Affairs, though it does take 30–45 min to administer, which may not be appropriate for all primary care settings. To obtain the scale, a request form may be accessed at http://www.ptsd.va.gov/professional/assessment/ncptsd-instrument-request-form.asp.

The PCL-C is a 17-item checklist that assesses the symptoms of PTSD in civilian populations. It was derived from the CAPS, and researchers found a high correlation between the two, providing some evidence for its ability to detect symptoms (Blanchard, Jones-Alexander, Buckley, & Forneris, 1996). An adapted version is available for the purpose of assessing symptoms in children during the previous month (PCL-C/PR). The checklist can be completed by either the child or, most often, the caregiver and typically takes 10 min to administer and score. Responses follow a 5-point scale ranging from "not at all" to "extremely." A positive screen is indicated by a suggested cutoff score of 30. Studies suggest an internal consistency of between 0.89 and 0.92 and test-retest reliability of 0.92 (Daviss et al., 2000; Ford et al., 1999). Additionally, Spanish versions are presently available for use. The PCL-C scale can be accessed at http://www.integration.samhsa.gov/clinical-practice/Abbreviated_PCL.pdf, and the PCL-C/PR can be obtained from the developer, Dr. Julian D. Ford, by emailing him at ford@psychiatry.uchc.edu.

The PC-PTSD is a screening tool that can be completed by the child or parent. The tool assesses whether the patient experienced a traumatic event that triggered various PTSD-like symptoms within the past month. A recent revised version, called PC-PTSD-5, includes PTSD diagnostic criteria from the DSM-5 and demonstrates promising results, with high diagnostic accuracy and sensitivity, efficiency, or specificity, depending on the cutoff score (Prins et al., 2016). The screen was revised to be five items, in contrast to the previous four-item design. It has a dichotomous response scale with options of yes or no. It is considered a positive screen if the patient responds "yes" to three or more items and should be followed by an interview. A PDF version of the scale can be accessed at http://www.ptsd.va.gov/professional/assessment/screens/pc-ptsd.asp.

The CPSS is a 26-item self-report form that looks at traumatic events, symptoms, and functioning to determine a possible PTSD diagnosis. Responses are scored on a 4-point Likert scale, ranging from 0 (not at all) to 3 (five or more times a week) and correspond with frequency of symptoms within the past month. An additional seven items are scored dichotomously (absent or present) and assess level of impairment. The CPSS should be completed by the child with adult assistance and takes about 15 min to administer and score. A score of 16 or above suggests at least a mild level of PTSD severity. Studies suggest a 0.89 internal consistency and 0.84 test-retest reliability for the tool (Foa, Johnson, Feeny, & Treadwell, 2001). A PDF version of the scale can be accessed at https://www.aacap.org/App_Themes/AACAP/docs/resource_centers/resources/misc/child_ptsd_symptom_scale.pdf.

Any of these screening tools and measurements can be efficiently incorporated into appointments considering the relatively small amount of time required to complete and score each. Consideration should be taken for individuals who may not speak English as their first language. In those cases, the Spanish version of the PCL-C is recommended. Additionally, depending on the child's developmental level, they may require assistance from their caregiver.

How to Further Assess If a Screen Is Positive

If results return a positive screen, further assessment is recommended. First, conducting a Structured Clinical Interview for DSM-5 Disorders-Civilian Version (SCID-5-CV) to ensure a correct diagnosis is an option although it is fairly time-consuming. This manual provides step-by-step guidelines for interviewing and assessing various mental disorders (First, Williams, Karg, & Spitzer, 2016). To gain more insight into how the symptoms manifest, talking with the caregiver(s) of the child is highly recommended. A conversation should include details of the trauma, as well as a discussion regarding how often the child presents with symptoms, symptom onset, in which contexts the symptoms are expressed, what alleviates and exacerbates symptoms, course of the symptoms, and their perception of the severity of the symptoms. Additionally, providers should ask the caregiver(s) if the child displays any other negative behaviors, either at home or at school. These behaviors can be tracked using the Child Behavior Checklist (Achenbach, 1991a; Achenbach & Rescorla, 2000). There are currently two versions, one designated for patients preschool age and the other for patients between 6 and 18 years of age. Parents score 100 and 118 problem behavior questions on a 3-point scale, ranging from "not true" to "very true". If possible, it is also recommended to provide the child's teacher with the Teacher's Report Form adaptation of the Child Behavior Checklist to actively document the child's behavior in a school context (Achenbach, 1991b). Each checklist is available online (http://www.aseba.org/preschool.html; http://www.aseba.org/schoolage.html) and can provide further insight into the nature of the problem.

Following assessment of the degree of symptoms, understanding the number of traumatic events the patient has endured is important. If they have experienced various instances of trauma, the behavior care provider (BCP) cannot realistically address all of those events in therapy. Understanding which specific traumatic event drives their symptoms and causes the most impairment can help guide the treatment plan. Ways to probe for this information may include asking "What event do you think of the most?," "What event can you best describe?," or "What event bothers you the most?." Additionally, noting what they reenact in play may help provide insight regarding what about the event is most distressing and intrusive.

Evidence-Based Stepped Care and Brief Psychotherapeutic Approaches

There currently are no empirically supported protocols for treating children presenting with PTSD in primary care. Typically, the children will need to be referred to specialty care only once the symptoms severely impact their functioning. In order to intervene early for the child's benefit and to ensure providers are efficiently able to provide services for as many children as possible, a stepped care approach is recommended. Stepped care follows a five-step model: watchful waiting, psychoeducation, bibliotherapy, group therapy, and finally individual therapy.

The first step, watchful waiting, follows the notion that some children will improve and recover naturally. Many patients have intrinsic strengths and mechanisms to recover from trauma, both physical and emotional. Resilience from trauma has been associated with no premorbid pathology, supportive parent or parents, instrumental-based coping, as well as perceived self-efficacy and behavioral flexibility (Pat-Horenczyk, Rabinowitz, Rice, & Tucker-Levin, 2009). Thus, not all children who experience trauma will later develop PTSD. For patients who do not meet diagnostic criteria for PTSD and/or who report experiencing trauma but do not return with a positive screen on the screening tools, it is acceptable to suggest they return if the symptoms develop, begin to worsen, or impair their functioning. Typically, it is suggested for patients to wait for at least a month before being moved to the next step, as symptoms may spontaneously remit and the patient will not be eligible for a PTSD diagnosis until a month following the trauma. In cases where the patient presents with symptoms of PTSD for less than a month, acute stress disorder would be the appropriate diagnosis.

The second step, psychoeducation, consists of the physician or BCP providing psychoeducational tools to provide both the parent and child with further understanding of the prognosis, treatment options, and other information about PTSD. These should be age-appropriate and can be found online through the Substance Abuse and Mental Health Services Administration (SAMHSA), National Institute of Mental Health (NIMH), Association for Behavioral and Cognitive Therapies (ABCT), or the United States Department of Veteran Affairs (https://www.samhsa.gov/capt/tools-learning-resources/coping-traumatic-events-resources; https://www.nimh.nih.gov/health/topics/post-traumatic-stress-disorder-ptsd/index.shtml; http://www.abct.org/Information/?m=mInformation&fa=fs_PTSD; http://www.ptsd.va.gov/professional/materials/fslist-handouts.asp). Each agency has websites with pamphlets discussing symptoms, risk factors, and treatment options. The purpose of providing these materials is to increase health literacy to correct misperceptions, normalize reactions, as well as provide positive steps that can help victims cope with the trauma. While there are no data demonstrating the efficacy of psychoeducation alone, when combined with trauma-focused cognitive behavioral therapy (TF-CBT) psychoeducation has been proven to be successful at reducing symptomatology (Scheeringa, Weems, Cohen, Amaya-Jackson, & Guthrie, 2011).

Following psychoeducation, bibliotherapy that utilizes Cognitive Behavioral Therapy (CBT) techniques has proven to be moderately effective in helping increase knowledge about PTSD, as well as help survivors develop coping skills. Bibliotherapy tools should be provided for both the child and caregiver and typically consist of books and/or workbooks that serve as a guide for moving forward and coping with symptoms. Suggested materials for children and caregivers are listed next.

For children, *Let's Talk About Taking Care of You: An Educational Book about Body Safety* and *Let's Talk About Taking Care of You: An Educational Book about Body Safety for Young Children* are two interactive workbooks for children in elementary school and between 2 and 6 years of age, respectively (Stauffer & Deblinger, 1990; Stauffer & Deblinger, 2004). The books provide the reader with emotional expression skills and education about body parts, appropriate and inappropriate touch, as well as personal safety skills.

For caregivers, *The PTSD Workbook: Simple, Effective Techniques for Overcoming Traumatic Stress Symptoms* provides evidence-based CBT techniques they can use, in order to help individuals cope with prior trauma (Williams & Poijula, 2016). Parents can read these and help convey appropriate ways of coping to their child, as well as familiarize them with the process of PTSD and how it manifests.

All of these books are under $20 and are available for purchase online. It is recommended to have a few copies readily accessible for patients who cannot access the Internet or cannot afford the products. Consideration should be taken regarding language preference for both the patient and caregiver, as they may differ. Additionally, developmental level should be considered for both the patient and caregiver when choosing the appropriate bibliotherapy material.

The next step in the model is group therapy. Group therapy is beneficial because it can utilize scarce resources efficiently if multiple clients are willing to participate. Additionally, interacting with other individuals with similar situations can help a child learn to normalize his or her reactions, learn more effective coping skills and can create a support network for the child. Group therapy would entail cognitive behavioral therapy for a group of children with symptoms of PTSD and their caregivers. The overall structure of the group would consist of understanding the maintaining factors of the symptoms, then proceed to building coping skills utilizing cognitive restructuring to reshape their maladaptive cognitions, as well as prolonged exposure. In order to further develop these skills outside of the group, homework may be assigned for each individual and discussed in the following sessions.

In the context of clinical trials, group therapy has shown to be effective in alleviating symptoms. One study compared the effects of CBT group therapy versus supportive counseling (Deblinger, Stauffer, & Steer, 2001). The study consisted of 44 maternal caregivers and their sexually abused children, all of whom received either group CBT or supportive counseling. Parents in the CBT group attended 11 sessions, in which topics covered were education, coping, communication, modeling, gradual exposure, and behavior management. Children in the CBT group attended 11 sessions, in which techniques used included interactive workbooks, role play, behavioral rehearsal, and joint parent-child exercises. Results demonstrated that children in the CBT group had significantly higher increases in knowledge and coping skills; thus, CBT group therapy for sexually abused children yields promising results. Additionally, the study demonstrated group therapy for caregivers may be beneficial, as demonstrated by a decrease in intrusive thoughts and negative emotional reactions. This is essential, as decreasing parental distress can help the child better adjust post-trauma (Cohen & Mannarino, 1996).

Lastly, individual therapy can be administered to children who would not or do not otherwise benefit from the other steps in the stepped care model. One study suggests two possible sub-steps:

parent-led, therapist-assisted trauma-focused cognitive behavioral therapy (TF-CBT) and/or therapist-led TF-CBT (Salloum et al., 2014).

Parent-led, therapist-assisted TF-CBT requires less time for the therapist to provide treatment and equips the parent with tools to help address the child's symptoms (Salloum et al., 2014). This approach consists of 3 face-to-face therapist meetings over 6 weeks, weekly 15 min phone support sessions, bibliotherapy (parent-child workbook), National Child Traumatic Stress Network psychoeducation, and a maintenance phase for 6 weeks. It is intended for the parent to utilize the bibliotherapy and psychoeducation tools during regular parent-child meetings, in order to help their child develop appropriate coping skills, as well as provide parents the opportunity to speak with a therapist semi-regularly for guidance and support. One major aspect of this step is exposure therapy, which begins with creating a hierarchy of anxiety-provoking situations, followed by the child drawing the incident, imagining it, then presenting the child with environmental cues (e.g., smells, sounds, locations) of the trauma. The provider would orient the parent and child to the steps of exposure therapy, but the parent would guide the exposure at home with the child. Details are outlined in the parent workbook, *Stepping Together*, and accompanying child workbook, *My Steps*. If the child successfully completes the therapy, the provider would then incorporate a relapse prevention plan into the session. This consists of assessing possible triggers following the termination of treatment and identifying appropriate and realistic guidelines for reacting (e.g., utilizing relaxation skills).

Limited research has examined parent-led, therapist-assisted TF-CBT. A pilot study using parent-led, therapist-assisted TF-CBT demonstrated that 5 out of 6 children responded to the treatment and did not require further treatment (Salloum et al., 2014). The study suggests this treatment may be effective in treating children following a traumatic experience.

Alternatively, if parent-led, therapist-assisted TF-CBT is not successful, the parent does not comply with the principles, or if the parent is the perpetrator of the trauma-related incident, the therapist would lead the sessions. This step entails the therapist leading trauma-focused CBT for nine sessions (Salloum et al., 2014). In each session, which is 90 min, the therapist introduces and practices relaxation and emotion regulation skills with the patients. Additionally, creating a hierarchy of anxiety-provoking events can help the provider build the gradual exposure aspect of treatment. Gradual exposure progresses from written to verbal retelling of the traumatic event(s) and concludes with in vivo exposure. Written exposure includes the child writing about the traumatic incident. If the child does not possess these skills, drawing may be substituted. Verbal exposure includes the child recalling the incident and verbally retelling it in detail. In vivo exposure includes bringing environmental cues into the treatment room. This may consist of sounds, smells, or locations that remind the patient of the traumatic event and initiate the stress response. The goal is for the child to use healthy coping skills (e.g., muscle relaxation, deep breathing). If these are successful, a relapse prevention plan is constructed, and the therapy is terminated. As this step takes 90 min a session, if this is not possible in the primary care setting, a child should be referred to a TF-CBT therapist.

TF-CBT following parent-led TF-CBT has only been studied with one child in a clinical trial, as the other five children responded to the parent-led TF-CBT aspect (Salloum et al., 2014). The child successfully completed the treatment. It is also important to note that traditional TF-CBT demonstrates significant improvements in children suffering from PTSD, as demonstrated by significant changes in "interpersonal trust, perceived credibility and shame" as well as substantial decreases in symptoms (Cohen, Deblinger, Mannarino, & Steer, 2004).

Research has demonstrated the efficacy of individual TF-CBT outside of the two-step model previously described. In a randomized controlled trial of 229 children between 8 and 14 years of age who were sexually abused, children who were assigned to the TF-CBT condition had improved significantly more than their counterparts who received child-centered therapy (Cohen et al., 2004). Improvements were indicated by less behavioral problems, depression, and PTSD symptoms, as well as decreased shame. Additionally, for parents who were assigned to TF-CBT, there was an increase in support of the child and a decrease in parental distress and depression related to the abuse. This is important to note, as parental support is a protective factor for children who experience trauma.

In order to assess and track the improvement of the child to determine whether the patient would benefit from therapist-led, TF-CBT, the researchers suggest using the clinical global impression-improvement scale to detect symptom improvement (Busner & Targum, 2007). The scale is used to compare the clinician's perceptions of the patient's condition at various points in treatment to the baseline. It is scored from 1 (very much improved since the initiation of treatment) to 7 (very much worse since the initiation of treatment), with higher scores indicating poorer progress.

What Does Not Work

It is important to provide evidence-based treatment, and, despite a plethora of treatment options available, there are various treatment options that are not suggested based upon a lack of empirical support. First, for adults suffering from PTSD, psychopharmacology is sometimes explored in conjunction with therapy; however, there is a lack of randomized controlled trials demonstrating its efficacy (Institute of Medicine (U.S.), 2008). Thus, there is a controversy surrounding whether or not children should be prescribed medication. In fact, there is very little empirical investigation and evidentiary support for psychopharmacology for children, unless the child has comorbid diagnoses (Cohen, Mannarino, Perel, & Staron, 2007). Additionally, studies that examine medication administration combined with psychotherapy do not demonstrate statistically differences in treatment outcomes when compared to therapy-only participants (Cohen et al., 2007). If psychiatric medications are prescribed, providers should be cognizant and acknowledge the importance of medication stability prior to starting treatment, as it can impact treatment outcomes. In regard to therapy, there is little recent empirical support for Thematic Apperception Test, Rorschach inkblot testing, and other psychotherapies (Lilienfeld, Wood, & Garb, 2000). Additionally, there have been no randomized controlled trials that support these forms of therapy.

When to Refer to External Specialty Mental Health

The previously proposed stepped care model, like any treatment, will not suffice as treatment for all individuals. First, not all children presenting with symptoms of PTSD in primary care should be prescribed a level in the stepped care model but instead immediately referred out to a specialty care behavioral health provider. An instance where the child should be referred to specialty care would be if, when the problem is initially presented, symptoms are causing high functional impairment, as demonstrated by significant impairment in more than one domain (i.e., school and home) or if the child reports suicidal ideation/attempts. Additionally, if the child progresses through all recommended levels of the stepped care model and does not appear to have improved, they should then be referred out to a specialty care provider to receive more intensive and long-term evidence-based care. Lastly, if the child presents with comorbid diagnoses, they should be referred to specialty care for extensive treatment that can address all diagnoses. As with any step in the process, if the patient insists on having a specialty care provider, they should be referred but still be informed of the provider's recommendation for which step best fits the patient's presentation.

In these instances, the preferred method of therapy would be evidence-based practice of CBT and exposure therapy. Randomized controlled trials demonstrate that CBT is the recommended choice of therapy for individuals presenting with PTSD, particularly for children with a sexual abuse trauma history (Cohen et al., 2004).

If the child presents with symptoms that are severe and/or has comorbid diagnoses, intensive individual therapy is highly recommended. This can be provided either by private or public sectors.

In intensive individual therapy, patients will go through a motivational interviewing process for the therapist to build rapport and identify the functionality issues the patient suffers from, as well as allow the patient to identify advantages and disadvantages of engaging in treatment. Following this, the therapist could walk the patient through the process of prolonged exposure, as this has proven to be effective in the treatment of PTSD specifically (Foa, Chrestman, & Gilboa-Schechtman, 2008). Parental involvement may be necessary depending on the child and their relationship with the parent.

Quality Improvement

The purpose of any treatment approach is to improve the quality of therapy clients are receiving, as demonstrated by better quality of life, cost efficiency, satisfaction, and various other measures. The first step is to ensure the services being provided are evidence-based. Staying updated on new advances in the field will ensure the best therapy is being provided. Secondly, quality of treatment can be measured using patient satisfaction surveys. Patient satisfaction is important because if these stakeholders are not satisfied, then they will not continue seeking treatment and/or may be reluctant to later engage in therapy. Patient satisfaction surveys can include asking patients whether they find the treatment time-effective and if they would recommend it to someone they know who suffers from PTSD.

Other ways to assess quality improvement opportunities include ensuring all appropriate individuals are screened and none are overlooked Further, examining treatment outcomes is essential to determining opportunities for quality improvement. This would entail looking at attrition rates, percentage of patients who show improvement of symptoms and function, and the magnitude of improvement. Comparing these results to alternative treatment options is imperative to assess whether the treatment is as effective, if not more. Additionally, re-administration of screening tools can be useful in determining the level of improvement in specific individuals. Screening tools typically indicate the frequency at which re-administration scores are valid. Lastly, a percentage of patients do not complete treatment. An important aspect of quality improvement is to look at the number of complete and incomplete referrals. Assessing for reasons why patients do not complete the referral process can help inform ways of addressing these concerns/barriers. Conversely, completed referrals may help inform specific problems with a stepped care approach, as they are more representative of the entire treatment process.

Conclusions

In sum, PTSD expression in children following sexual abuse is a problem that can be identified in primary care. Primary care providers and their teams have the opportunity to provide treatment for patients who present with mild to moderate symptoms. Screening patients for PTSD symptoms and implementing a stepped care approach may help. Given the potential benefits of implementing a stepped care model in the primary care setting, it is strongly suggested.

References

Achenbach, T. M. (1991a). *Manual for the child behavior checklist/4-18 and 1991 profile*. Burlington, VT: Department of Psychiatry, University of Vermont.

Achenbach, T. M. (1991b). *Manual for the Teacher's report form and 1991 profile*. Burlington, VT: University of Vermont, Department of Psychiatry.

Achenbach, T. M., & Rescorla, L. (2000). *Manual for the child behavior checklist: Preschool forms and profiles*. Burlington, VT: University of Vermont College of Medicine.

American Psychiatric Association. (2013). *Diagnostic and statistical manual of mental disorders (5th ed.)*. Arlington, VA: American Psychiatric Association.

Andrews, G., Corry, J., Slade, T., Issakidis, C., & Swanston, H. (2004). Child sexual abuse. In Ezzati, M. , Lopez, A. D., Rodgers, A., & Murray, C.J.L. (Eds.), *Comparative quantification of health risks: Global and regional burden of disease attributable to selected major risk factors*. Geneva, Switzerland: World Health Organization.

Blanchard, E. B., Jones-Alexander, J., Buckley, T. C., & Forneris, C. A. (1996). Psychometric properties of the PTSD checklist (PCL). *Behaviour Research and Therapy, 34*(8), 669–673.

Bonanno, G. A., & Mancini, A. D. (2008). The human capacity to thrive in the face of potential trauma. *Pediatrics, 121*(2), 369–375.

Busner, J., & Targum, S. D. (2007). The clinical global impressions scale: Applying a research tool in clinical practice. *Psychiatry (Edgmont), 4*(7), 28.

Cohen, J. A., Deblinger, E., Mannarino, A. P., & Steer, R. A. (2004). A multisite, randomized controlled trial for children with sexual abuse–related PTSD symptoms. *Journal of the American Academy of Child & Adolescent Psychiatry, 43*(4), 393–402.

Cohen, J. A., & Mannarino, A. P. (1996). Factors that mediate treatment outcome of sexually abused preschool children. *Journal of the American Academy of Child & Adolescent Psychiatry, 35*(10), 1402–1410.

Cohen, J. A., Mannarino, A. P., Perel, J. M., & Staron, V. (2007). A pilot randomized controlled trial of combined trauma-focused CBT and sertraline for childhood PTSD symptoms. *Journal of the American Academy of Child & Adolescent Psychiatry, 46*(7), 811–819.

Daviss, W. B., Mooney, D., Racusin, R., Ford, J. D., Fleischer, A., & McHugo, G. J. (2000). Predicting posttraumatic stress after hospitalization for pediatric injury. *Journal of the American Academy of Child & Adolescent Psychiatry, 39*(5), 576–583.

Deblinger, E., Stauffer, L. B., & Steer, R. A. (2001). Comparative efficacies of supportive and cognitive behavioral group therapies for young children who have been sexually abused and their nonoffending mothers. *Child Maltreatment, 6*(4), 332–343.

Finkelhor, D., Turner, H., Ormrod, R., Hamby, S., & Kracke, K. (2009). *Children's exposure to violence: A comprehensive national survey*. Washington, DC: United States Department of Justice, Office of Justice.

First, M. B., Williams, J. B., Karg, R. S., & Spitzer, R. L. (2016). *Structured clinical interview for DSM-5 disorders: SCID-5-CV clinician version*. Arlington, VA: American Psychiatric Association.

Foa, E. B., Chrestman, K. R., & Gilboa-Schechtman, E. (2008). *Prolonged exposure therapy for adolescents with PTSD emotional processing of traumatic experiences, therapist guide*. New York, NY: Oxford University Press.

Foa, E. B., Johnson, K. M., Feeny, N. C., & Treadwell, K. R. (2001). The child PTSD symptom scale: A preliminary examination of its psychometric properties. *Journal of Clinical Child Psychology, 30*(3), 376–384.

Ford, J. D., Racusin, R., Daviss, W. B., Ellis, C. G., Thomas, J., Rogers, K., … Sengupta, A. (1999). Trauma exposure among children with oppositional defiant disorder and attention deficit–hyperactivity disorder. *Journal of Consulting and Clinical Psychology, 67*(5), 786.

Institute of Medicine (U.S.). (2008). *Treatment of posttraumatic stress disorder: An assessment of the evidence*. Washington, DC: National Academies Press.

Lilienfeld, S. O., Wood, J. M., & Garb, H. N. (2000). The scientific status of projective techniques. *Psychological Science in the Public Interest, 1*(2), 27–66.

Merikangas, K. R., He, J. P., Burstein, M., Swanson, S. A., Avenevoli, S., Cui, L., … Swendsen, J. (2010). Lifetime prevalence of mental disorders in US adolescents: Results from the National Comorbidity Survey Replication–Adolescent Supplement (NCS-A). *Journal of the American Academy of Child & Adolescent Psychiatry, 49*(10), 980–989.

Pat-Horenczyk, R., Rabinowitz, R. G., Rice, A., & Tucker-Levin, A. (2009). The search for risk and protective factors in childhood PTSD. In D. Brom, R. Pat-Horenczyk, & J. D. Ford (Eds.), *Treating traumatized children risk, resilience and recovery*. New York, NY: Routledge/Taylor & Francis Group.

Prins, A., Bovin, M. J., Smolenski, D. J., Marx, B. P., Kimerling, R., Jenkins-Guarnieri, M. A., … Tiet, Q. Q. (2016). The primary care PTSD screen for DSM-5 (PC-PTSD-5): Development and evaluation within a veteran primary care sample. *Journal of General Internal Medicine, 31*(10), 1206–1211.

Pynoos, R. S., Weathers, F. W., Steinberg, A. M., Marx, B. P., Layne, C. M., Kaloupek, D. G., … Kriegler, J. A. (2015). *Clinician-Administered PTSD Scale for DSM-5 Child/Adolescent Version*. Scale available from the National Center for PTSD at www.ptsd.va.gov.

Salloum, A., Robst, J., Scheeringa, M. S., Cohen, J. A., Wang, W., Murphy, T. K., … Storch, E. A. (2014). Step one within stepped care trauma-focused cognitive behavioral therapy for young children: A pilot study. *Child Psychiatry & Human Development, 45*(1), 65–77.

Scheeringa, M. S., Weems, C. F., Cohen, J. A., Amaya-Jackson, L., & Guthrie, D. (2011). Trauma-focused cognitive-behavioral therapy for posttraumatic stress disorder in three through six year-old children: A randomized clinical trial. *Journal of Child Psychology and Psychiatry, 52*(8), 853–860.

Stauffer, L., & Deblinger, E. (1990). *Let's talk about taking care of you: An educational book about body safety*. Hatfield, PA: Hope for Families.

Stauffer, L. B., & Deblinger, E. (2004). *Let's talk about taking care of you: An educational book about body safety for young children*. Hatfield, PA: Hope for Families.

Streeck-Fischer, A., & Kolk, B. A. (2000). Down will come baby, cradle and all: Diagnostic and therapeutic implications of chronic trauma on child development. *Australian and New Zealand Journal of Psychiatry, 34*(6), 903–918.

United States Department of Health and Human Services. (2015). *Child maltreatment 2013*. Washington, DC: Administration on Children, Youth and Families, Administration for Children and Families.

Williams, M. B., & Poijula, S. (2016). *The PTSD workbook: Simple, effective techniques for overcoming traumatic stress symptoms*. Oakland, CA: New Harbinger Publications.

35 Sexual Dysfunction

Catalina Vechiu and William T. O'Donohue

Sexual dysfunction is a major health concern in the general population and is associated with impaired quality of life, diminished satisfaction with one's sexual life, and personal and/or relationship difficulties. A multifaceted interplay of psychological, somatic, emotional, and relational factors contributes to the development and maintenance of sexual dysfunction in both women and men. An overwhelming number of studies aimed at understanding the etiology of sexual dysfunction have led to the development of pharmaceutical and psychological interventions for the treatment of male sexual dysfunction. Unfortunately, sexual dysfunction is poorly understood and rarely recognized by providers despite the high prevalence of sexual dysfunction among women of all ages (Laumann, Paik, & Rosen, 1999).

Traditional models of sexual functioning assumed that both women and men experience a linear cycle of excitement, plateau, orgasm, and resolution (Kammerer-Doak & Rogers, 2008; Masters & Johnson, 1966). More contemporary models of sexual response more adequately capture the intricacies of the female sexual cycle, which is not linear but rather cyclical and includes both social and psychological features into female sexual functioning, such as physical and emotional satisfaction, sexual desire, and emotional intimacy (Basson, 2001). The differences between the sexual response of women and men contribute to variations in sexual function and dysfunction. A number of psychosocial approaches are available for the treatment of sexual dysfunction, although few have been empirically validated. The aim of this chapter is to provide behavioral healthcare professionals with the tools necessary to (1) screen and assess for sexual dysfunction, (2) provide brief empirically supported psychotherapeutic interventions, and (3) streamline the referral process to specialty mental healthcare.

C. Vechiu, M.A. (✉) • W.T. O'Donohue, Ph.D.
Department of Clinical Psychology, University of Nevada, Reno, NV, USA
e-mail: cvechiu@gmail.com

A Brief Description of the Disorders

In the *Diagnostic and Statistical Manual of Mental Disorders (DSM-5)*, sexual dysfunctions "are typically characterized by a clinically significant disturbance in a person's ability to respond sexually or to experience sexual pleasure" (American Psychiatric Association [APA], 2013, p. 423). For females, there are currently three sexual dysfunctions:

1. *Female sexual interest/arousal disorder*: New category that represents the combination of

A. Maragakis, W.T. O'Donohue (eds.), *Principle-Based Stepped Care and Brief Psychotherapy for Integrated Care Settings*, https://doi.org/10.1007/978-3-319-70539-2_35

sexual desire and arousal disorders diagnosed by the decrease or absence of three of the following: sexual activity, sexual interest, erotic thoughts or fantasies, initiation of sexual activity or responsiveness to a partner's attempts, sexual excitement, response to sexual cues, and genital and non-genital sensations during sexual activity (see chapter 21 this volume)

2. *Female orgasmic disorder*: Presence of one or both of the following: delay, infrequency, or absence of orgasm and/or reduced intensity of orgasm present 75–100% of the time
3. *Genito-pelvic pain/penetration disorder*: New category that represents the merging of dyspareunia and vaginismus and diagnosed by the persistence and recurrent occurrence of one or more of the following difficulties: vaginal penetration, marked vulvovaginal or pelvic pain during penetration or attempt at penetration, fear or anxiety about pain in anticipation of, during, or after penetration, and tightening or tensing of pelvic floor muscles during attempted penetration (APA, 2013)

For males, there are four sexual dysfunctions:

1. *Erectile disorder*: Difficulty in at least one of the following approximately 75–100% of the time: obtaining or maintaining an erection during sexual activity or decrease in erectile rigidity
2. *Male hypoactive sexual desire disorder*: Persistent and recurring deficient or absent desire for sexual activity or sexual, erotic thoughts or fantasies
3. *Premature ejaculation*: Persistent or recurrent pattern of ejaculation within 1 min following vaginal penetration approximately 75–100% of the time
4. *Delayed ejaculation*: The experience of delay, infrequency, or absence of ejaculation approximately 75–100% of the time (APA, 2013)

Prevalence of Sexual Dysfunction

Data from the 1992 National Health and Social Life Survey in the United States indicates that the national prevalence rates of sexual dysfunction are 43% of women and 31% of men experience (Laumann et al., 1999). For specific sexual dysfunctions, research indicate a current prevalence of 3% for dyspareunia (now genito-pelvic pain/penetration disorder), 6% for female sexual arousal disorder, 7–10% for female orgasmic disorder, 0–3% for male hypoactive sexual desire disorder, 0–5% for erectile disorder, and 4–5% for premature ejaculation (Simons & Carey, 2008). In a sample of women age 18–39, 18% of women reported experiencing pain during sexual intercourse, 27% of women reported an inability to achieve orgasm, and 32% reported an absence of sexual interest in the past 12 months (Laumann et al., 1999). For DSM-IV female sexual dysfunction disorders, estimates for female orgasmic disorder range from 4 to 7% in the general population to 5–42% in primary care settings; estimates for dyspareunia range from 3 to 18% in the general population to 3–46% in primary care settings; estimates for vaginismus (now genito-pelvic pain penetration disorder) range from 0.5 to 1% in the general population to up to 30% in primary care settings; and estimates for female sexual interest/arousal disorders range from 6 to 46% in the general population (APA, 2000; Frank, Mistretta, & Will, 2008; Simons & Carey, 2008).

Male sexual dysfunction has historically been more widely examined; however, the variability in prevalence rates is significant, possibly due to poor methodology and varying definitions. Existing data estimates that approximately 30% of adult men report at least one sexual dysfunction (Lewis et al., 2004). Although some studies report high rates of sexual dysfunction for older men, it is also common in younger men. For example, estimates of erectile dysfunction in the past 12 months range from 30% for individuals aged 18–29, 32% for those aged 30–39, 28% for those aged 40–49, 55% for those aged 50–59, and 20–40% for those aged 60–69 (Laumann et al., 1999). In the same study, 14% of men aged 18–29 reported low sexual interest compared to 17% of men aged 50–59 in the past year (Laumann et al., 1999). Despite variability in the rates of prevalence, it is evident that sexual dysfunction poses a significant challenge for a large portion of the general population. Given that prevalence rates are typically higher in primary care settings, it is important for providers to conduct a detailed and systematic evaluation during routine examinations.

Screening for Sexual Dysfunction in the Primary Care Setting

Because of the sensitive nature of sexual dysfunctions, it is often difficult for providers to evaluate, diagnose, and treat sexual dysfunction, especially for individuals who hold conventional or traditional beliefs regarding sex and sexuality. Other factors such as limited treatment options, lack of available referral choices, difficulty with diagnosis, provider or patient discomfort, and lack of knowledge regarding obtaining a comprehensive sexual history also limit a thorough evaluation of sexual dysfunction at first presentation (Bachmann, 2006; Clayton, 2003). It is important that the provider takes an active role in discussing sexual health difficulties, as most patients are hesitant to disclose their concerns and typically wait for the provider to initiate a discussion (Gott & Hinchliff, 2003). It is recommended that therapists working in a time-limited integrated care setting use the following three questions to initiate a conversation regarding the patient's sexual functioning:

1. Are you sexually active?
2. Are there any problems?
3. Do you have pain with intercourse? (Plouffe, 1985)

Although not comprehensive, if asked in a confident, neutral, and culturally sensitive manner can normalize discussions of sexual health and sexual dysfunction. If the patient indicates a positive answer to any of the three questions, the therapist can then further assess for any dissatisfaction or concern with the patient's sexual life by utilizing one of the following commonly used and empirically supported screening tools:

- Brief Sexual Symptom Checklist (BSSC; Hatzichristou et al., 2010). The BSSC is a four-item self-report questionnaire that assesses the type and duration of sexual problem experienced, the patient's satisfaction with sexual functioning, and the patient's willingness to address his or her concerns with the provider (Hatzichristou et al., 2010).
- Arizona Sexual Experiences Scale (ASEX; McGahuey et al., 2000). The ASEX is a five-item questionnaire that contains a male and female version and assesses sex drive, arousal, vaginal lubrication/penile erection, ability to reach an orgasm, and satisfaction from orgasm. Scores range from 5 to 30, with higher scores indicating more sexual dysfunction.
- The Female Sexual Distress Scale-Revised (FSDS-R; DeRogatis, Clayton, Lewis-D'Agostino, Wunderlich, & Fu, 2008). The FSDS-R is a 13-item questionnaire that assesses the presence of sexually related personal distress in women. A recommended cutoff score of ≥11 discriminates between women with FSD and no FSD.
- Brief Sexual Function Inventory for Urology (BSFI; O'Leary et al., 1995). The BSFI is an 11-item questionnaire that measures male sexuality across five domains: (1) sexual desire, (2) ejaculation, (3) erectile function, (4) perception of sexual problems, and (5) sexual satisfaction. The individual questions are examined for positive answers, which indicate difficulty in one of the five domains of sexual functioning.

How to Further Assess if a Screen Returns Positive

If a sexual concern is elicited, further assessment of functioning in the following domains should be conducted:

- *Sexual history*: Including sexual activity, practices, experiences, problems and satisfaction, sexually transmitted infections, reproductive, and menstrual and obstetric histories
- *Medical history*: Including the use of medications, alcohol, drugs, tobacco, as well as an evaluation of cardiovascular, diabetes, neurological, cancer, trauma, and surgical histories
- *Psychosexual history*: Including experiences of sexual trauma or abuse; personal, family, and cultural beliefs about sexuality; psychological and interpersonal factors; history of psychological distress; partner attitudes and beliefs; and patient's self-esteem and coping skills

However, a comprehensive assessment of a patient's psychosexual history is highly unlikely given the time-limited nature of the integrated care setting and is more likely to be conducted in specialty mental healthcare centers. Additionally, to date, no structured or semi-structured clinical interviews have been developed and empirically validated for sexual dysfunction, which adds a layer of complication to the assessment and diagnosis of sexual dysfunction disorders. As such, the ALLOW algorithm can be utilized to assess and manage sexual dysfunction.

The **ALLOW** (Ask, Legitimize, Limitations, Open, Work; Hatzichristou et al., 2004) method is a succinct and helpful guide that can be used to further inquire about sexual functioning, guide the conversation, and make a shared decision regarding treatment options (see Table 35.1 for a description; Murtagh, 2010). The **ALLOW** method provides a framework for therapists to further inquire about sexual activity and dysfunction while recognizing the therapists' own limitations in providing treatment for any elicited problems (Hatzichristou et al., 2004). Once the therapist reaches the third step (Limitations), he or she can provide a referral to specialty mental healthcare and rest assured that "the clinician has done it *all* for the patient" (Hatzichristou et al., 2004, p. 51).

Evidence-Based Stepped Care and Brief Psychotherapeutic Approaches

There are a number of treatment approaches for sexual dysfunction; however, research on the efficacy of such interventions is scarce, and evidence-based treatment guidelines for behavioral healthcare providers working in an integrated care setting have yet to be developed. Additionally, there are no brief psychotherapeutic approaches for sexual dysfunction, particularly because the most effective treatments include the patient's partner. However, there are promising interventions in the context of a stepped care model of treatment for sexual dysfunction. Evidence-based stepped care is a healthcare delivery system in which the intensity of treatment is organized in a hierarchy of intensity typically associated with cost. The emphasis on evidence-based within this model

Table 35.1 ALLOW method for the assessment of sexual dysfunctions

Level	Scope	Examples
Ask	Ask the patient about sexual functioning and activities	"How would you describe the problem(s)?" "How satisfied are you with your current sexual relationships?"
Legitimize	Normalize the clinical relevance of sexual health and the patient's experiences of sexual function or dysfunction	"Patients with [condition] often experience sexual difficulties. What has been your experience?" "Many patients find that they often experience changes in their sexual satisfaction/desire/interest. Is it okay if we discuss this?"
Limitations	Identify the limitations the clinician may have about the evaluation of sexual dysfunction	This step includes a self-evaluation (i.e., lack of knowledge, discomfort discussing issues with sexual functioning) by the clinician, and he/she may choose to refer out to specialty mental healthcare
Opening up the discussion	Further investigate the patient's problem	"Are there any sexual/nonsexual problems with your partner?" What emotions, life stressors, or physical health issues could contribute to this problem?"
Work together to develop a treatment plan	Identify an appropriate goal and treatment option through shared decision-making	"Some patients find it helpful to talk to someone who has experience in this area. Are you interested in getting more support for the issues we've discussed?" "There are a number of websites/books that some of my patients with similar concerns have found helpful. Are you interested in that information?"

indicates that the recommendations in each step have scientific support in the form of randomly controlled trials (RCT) that have examined their effectiveness, efficacy, feasibility, and patient satisfaction. Stepped care treatment models have been effectively implemented for the treatment of depression, and emerging research supports stepped care in the treatment of PTSD. Stepped care has been less examined in the sexual dysfunction literature; however, an evidence-based stepped care system has the potential to decrease costs and increase patient satisfaction.

Psychoeducation

Psychoeducation is a potential first-line treatment for sexual dysfunction, particularly because the few studies that have examined the effects of psychoeducation on sexual dysfunction have yielded positive results, with women reporting significant improvement across various domains of sexual dysfunction (i.e., arousal, desire, lubrication, orgasm, and satisfaction) after participating in a group psychoeducational intervention conducted by a women's health nurse practitioner (Smith, Beadle, & Shuster, 2008). At this level, the role of the provider is to provide accurate education about the diagnosis, physiological basis of sexual dysfunction, the variety of sexual expressions and responses, and dispelling common myths about optimal sexual functioning. Psychoeducation should also include information regarding the impact of the patient's lifestyle on his or her sexual functioning. For instance, reducing stress factors, exercising, and adopting a healthy diet by eliminating smoking, drinking, and illicit drug use may positively affect a patient's sexual functioning. Psychoeducation can be provided in multiple formats, including mobile apps, websites, and free resources that can be found online (see Appendix A for some of the most common psychoeducational resources).

Because psychoeducation is a flexible model, it can incorporate both information specific to sexual dysfunction and tools for managing it and other related problems (Lukens & McFarlane, 2004). As a result, behavioral healthcare professionals can provide psychoeducation in 20- or 30-min sessions, depending on the context in which they work. Providers can schedule a follow-up with patients to monitor their progress. If symptoms do not abate, patients can then be "stepped up" to the next level. Monitoring is an important component of any stepped care model of treatment and allows for timely and effective triage. However, clinically significant symptom reduction hinges on the severity of the patient's sexual dysfunction and any co-occurring issues.

Self-Help and Bibliotherapy

Patients who do not show improvement after receiving psychoeducation may need further treatment, and self-help can be a viable option. Many consumers now turn to various forms of self-help, and the number of self-help books has proliferated in the medical and psychological field. Research on the use of self-help in the treatment of sexual dysfunction has yielded mixed results, with some studies indicating that self-help can effectively treat sexual dysfunctions and others indicating that any gains made during the course of treatment are lost at follow-up (van Lankveld, 2009). Leusink and Aarts (2006) found that 81% of men who utilized online consultation reported improvement in erectile dysfunction. In another study, men who completed web-based CBT for erectile dysfunction reported increased sexual functioning and well-being and improved quality and satisfaction of their sexual relationship (McCabe, Price, Piterman, & Lording, 2008). Self-help and bibliotherapy increases the accessibility to treatments for sexual dysfunction and is an effective alternative for individuals with mild symptoms and can be used as a complementary tool for individuals who might benefit more from traditional therapy approaches (see Appendix B for some of the most popular self-help books).

What Does Not Work

Medical Interventions

There is an overwhelming amount of research on medical interventions for the treatment of erectile dysfunction, but a dearth for female sexual dysfunction or mixed sexual dysfunction in males. A review of existing medical options is beyond the scope of this chapter and can be found elsewhere (i.e., Allahdadi, Tostes, & Webb, 2009; Holmes, 2000; Kammerer-Doak & Rogers, 2008). Although medication may be effective in treating physiological symptoms, it may not alleviate the causes of sexual dysfunction. It has been well established that relationship factors, psychosocial stressors, and psychological distress such as anxiety and depression impact sexual functioning. These issues are better addressed by psychological interventions, are typically more cost-effective, and are not associated with negative side effects.

When to Refer to External Specialty Mental Health

Stepped care is inherently a collaborative model that facilitates shared decision-making. Patients may often benefit from more intensive treatments and decisions regarding referrals to specialty mental healthcare that should be made together with the patient. Referral may be made for a number of reasons:

1. The patient did not respond to psychoeducational or self-help interventions.
2. The patient prefers a more intensive intervention as a first-line treatment.
3. The patient has comorbidities that require specialty mental healthcare (i.e., psychosis, suicidality).
4. The patient requires additional comprehensive assessment.
5. The patient has strong traditional beliefs about sex and sexuality.

The behavioral healthcare provider can assess for these reasons in conjunction with assessment of symptomology. The screening tools mentioned in an earlier section can also be used as monitoring tools at each step of the intervention. If patients do not improve on the questionnaire chosen by the provider, a referral to specialty mental healthcare should be provided. Options for treatment include:

Sex Therapies

Although psychoeducation and self-help interventions are increasing in popularity, the treatment of choice is often sex therapy. The most commonly examined treatment approaches are those based on specialized sex therapy, which are derivatives of the Masters and Johnson (1970) intervention. This was an intensive treatment provided daily for approximately 2–3 weeks by a team of mixed-sex therapists with both the patient and his or her partner (Fruhauf, Gerger, Schmidt, Munder, & Barth, 2013). The focus of the intervention was on alleviating performance anxiety and increasing sexual pleasure. Other sex therapies include:

- Sexual skills training (SST) for female/male orgasmic disorder: Treatment comprised of nine steps focused on improving sexual skills through directed masturbation and other sensate-focused exercises. The partner assists in guiding the client's progress through the program (Farah, 2011).
- Systematic desensitization (SD) for genito-pelvic pain/penetration disorder: Focused on alleviating anxiety associated with intercourse and includes vaginal dilator training and pelvic floor muscle therapy (Fruhauf et al., 2013).
- Marital therapy: Focused on resolving issues with communication, listening to one's partner, understanding the feelings, thoughts, behaviors, and needs of one's partner, and trust can improve sexual satisfaction. Also includes the use of sensate focused and general body awareness exercises to increase intimacy (Fruhauf et al., 2013).
- Cognitive behavioral therapy (CBT): Includes sexual education and is focused on helping patients understand how dysfunctional beliefs

about the self or his/her partner's sexual needs can lead to sexual dysfunction and satisfaction (Fruhauf et al., 2013).

- Sex therapy (ST): Includes the standardized sex therapy proposed by Masters and Johnson (1970) and other modifications. It is based on the sexual response cycle and includes sexual education, couple exercises, and counseling (Masters & Johnson, 1970).
- Orgasm consistency training (OCT) for hypoactive sexual disorder: CBT-based treatment focused on mutual interdependence and rewards for orgasm through coital alignment, sensate-focused exercises, and directed masturbation (Hurlbert, White, Powell, & Apt, 1993).

The Role of the Primary Care Provider/Medical Team in Treatment

Research indicates that any illness, medical intervention, or treatment has the potential to affect a patient's sexual health. Therefore, sexuality falls within the realm of medical care, although which aspects are particularly relevant should rest with the patient (Taylor & Davis, 2006). Thus, the role of the physician and the medical team is to routinely screen and assess for sexual dysfunction in all of their patients. Once initial screening is conducted, primary care physicians can refer the patient to the behavioral healthcare provider for further assessment, streamlining the treatment process and providing continuity of care. One of the most critical components of integrated healthcare is collaboration and consultation with the treatment team. As such, the behavioral healthcare provided should consult with primary care providers regarding screening, assessment, etiology, and treatment options. This is particularly relevant with patients suffering from sexual dysfunction because of the potential comorbidities of medical illnesses and impact of medications on sexual functioning. Consultation and effective communication is vital during the screening and assessment phase because the primary care provider can order laboratory tests and make recommendations and indicate contraindications for treatment based on the patient's medical health history and current medical status.

Quality Improvement (QI) and Impact on Care

Assessing patient outcomes and satisfaction and conducting quality improvement on the care practitioners provide are increasingly complex. There is a necessity for QI, and healthcare systems across the USA are evaluating the likelihood of obtaining desired health outcomes while minimizing medical errors and patient dissatisfaction. It is important that the treatment team measure the quality and impact of the healthcare they provide in a systematic manner. This allows them to increase efficiency, determine if their procedures are scientifically based, if they are consistent with patient preferences, and if patients' concerns regarding their sexual health improve. QI often requires a paradigm shift at the systems level as well as the individual behavioral healthcare level. Hughes (2008) proposes 14 common factors of successful quality improvement efforts:

1. Leadership
2. Stakeholders
3. Multidisciplinary teams
4. Standardized care process
5. Evidence-based practice
6. Methodologically sound approach
7. Sufficient resources
8. Serve multiple purposes
9. Flexibility
10. Appropriate use of technology
11. Culture of safety and improvement
12. Consensus on the definition of the problem
13. Continuous assessment, monitoring, and communication of quality improvement efforts
14. Change takes time

Given the complexity of both healthcare and sexual dysfunction, assessing quality improvement likely requires the implementation of multiple quality tools that have been effectively adopted within medical settings. QI may be initially difficult in the assessment of treatment of sexual dysfunction because of the variability in its etiology as well as in the quality of available treatments. However, providers have the opportunity to implement QI at every step in the assessment process. For instance, QI can be conducted on the initial evaluation by appraising the following questions:

- How many patients are asked about their sexual health and satisfaction with sexual activity?
- What are the barriers to discussing sexuality?
- How many providers initiate the conversation?
- What are patient preferences regarding discussions of sexuality with their providers?
- How time-efficient are existing questionnaires that assess sexual health?
- Are there newer assessment tools available?

Behavioral healthcare providers can learn valuable information from including a standard QI questionnaire incorporating these questions and others into a patient's regular visit or follow-up visits. The process must start somewhere, and the point of change is one that must be determined by the healthcare team.

Conclusion

Sexual dysfunction is a complex and highly prevalent class of disorders with multiple etiologies, maintaining factors, and pathways to care are varied in both quality and quantity. A standardized management protocol or unified treatment plan for sexual dysfunction does not exist, which complicates how providers evaluate and treat sexual dysfunction. Additionally, several medical, interpersonal, biological, and psychological factors can affect an individual's sexual functioning and contribute to various forms of sexual dysfunction. Since sexual dysfunction is a multifactorial problem, treatment should be tailored to the individual. Although psychological and medical interventions for sexual dysfunctions are available, the field lacks evidence-based treatments. However, there are a number of steps that behavioral healthcare providers can take to begin the evaluation and assessment process of sexual dysfunction in males and females.

Initial evaluation should target all patients, regardless of symptom presentation, as the overwhelming majority of patients are uncomfortable discussing sexuality and often wait for their providers to initiate the conversation. Healthcare providers should be compassionate and flexible and create a comfortable atmosphere for the patient to disclose any concerns with their sexual health. If concerns are uncovered, assessment should include a comprehensive psychosocial and medical history, a physical exam, and in some instances, laboratory testing is also necessary. This chapter has provided suggestions and guidelines for the effective implementation of evaluation, assessment, and treatment of sexual dysfunction that may be the first step in enabling providers to increase their knowledge and practice of sexual dysfunction.

Appendix 1: Psychoeducational Resources for Sexual Dysfunction

- American College of Obstetrics and Gynecologists: Provides a free psychoeducational resource regarding women's sexual health (Also available in Spanish).
  http://www.acog.org/~/media/For%20Patients/faq072.pdf
- Mayo Clinic: Provides a free resource with information regarding female sexual dysfunction.
  http://www.mayoclinic.org/diseases-conditions/female-sexual-dysfunction/basics/definition/CON-20027721?p=1
- Hormone Health Network: Provides a free brochure with educational information regarding the therapeutic use of androgens for women who experience low sexual desire.
  http://www.hormone.org/sitecore%20modules/web/~/media/Hormone/Files/Patient%20Guides/Womens%20Health/PGAndrogensWoman%20523.pdf
- The Ohio State University Medical Center: Provides a free informational booklet regarding erectile dysfunction.
  https://patienteducation.osumc.edu/Documents/erectile-dysfunction-what.pdf

- Cleveland Clinic: Provides a website with information regarding the causes and treatments of erectile dysfunction. http://my.clevelandclinic.org/health/diseases_conditions/hic_Erectile_Dysfunction_Overview
- The Institute for Sexual Medicine: Provides a free informational resource regarding male hypoactive sexual desire disorder. https://sexualmed.org/known-issues/male-hypoactive-sexual-desire-disorder/

Appendix 2: Self-Help and Bibliotherapy Resources

- Heiman, J., LoPiccolo, J., & Palladini, D. (1988). *Becoming orgasmic: A sexual and personal growth program for women* (2nd ed.). New York: Simon & Schuster.
- Goldstein, A., & Brandon, M. (2009). *Reclaiming desire: 4 keys to finding your lost libido*. New York: Rodale Books.
- McCarthy, B.W., & Metz, M.E. (2004). *Coping with premature ejaculation: How to overcome PE, please your partner, and have great sex*. Oakland, CA: New Harbinger Publications.
- McCarthy, B.W., & Metz, M.E. (2004). *Coping with erectile dysfunction: How to regain confidence and enjoy great sex*. Oakland, CA: New Harbinger Publications.
- McCarthy, B.W., & McCarthy, W. (2003). *Rekindling desire: A step-by-step program to help low-sex and no-sex marriages*. New York: Taylor & Francis Group.
- Castleman, M. (2004). *Great sex: A man's guide to the secret principles of total-body sex*. New York: Rodale Books.

References

Allahdadi, K. J., Tostes, R. C. A., & Webb, R. C. (2009). Female sexual dysfunction: Therapeutic options and experimental challenges. *Cardiovascular & Hematological Agents in Medicinal Chemistry*, *7*(4), 260–269.

American Psychiatric Association. (2000). *Diagnostic and statistical manual of mental disorders* (4th ed., pp. 493–538). Washington, DC: American Psychiatric Association.

American Psychiatric Association. (2013). *DSM-5: Diagnostic and statistical manual for mental disorders* (5th ed.). Arlington, VA: American Psychiatric Press.

Bachmann, G. (2006). Female sexuality and sexual dysfunction: Are we stuck on the learning curve? *Journal of Sexual Medicine*, *3*(4), 639–645.

Basson, R. (2001). Are the complexities of women's sexual function reflected in the new consensus definitions of dysfunction? *Journal of Sex & Marital Therapy*, *27*, 105–112.

Clayton, A. H. (2003). Sexual function and dysfunction in women. *Psychiatric Clinics of North America*, *26*(3), 673–682.

DeRogatis, L., Clayton, A., Lewis-D'Agostino, D., Wunderlich, G., & Fu, Y. (2008). Validation of the female sexual distress scale-revised for assessing distress in women with hypoactive sexual desire disorder. *Journal of Sexual Medicine*, *5*(2), 357–364. https://doi.org/10.1111/j.1743-6109.2007.00672.x

Farah, L. K. (2011). The effects of sexual skills training on marital satisfaction. *Procedia-Social and Behavioral Sciences*, *30*, 2581–2585.

Frank, J. E., Mistretta, P., & Will, J. (2008). Diagnosis and treatment of female sexual dysfunction. *American Family Physician*, *77*(5), 635–642.

Fruhauf, S., Gerger, H., Schmidt, H. M., Munder, T., & Barth, J. (2013). Efficacy of psychological interventions for sexual dysfunction: A systematic review and meta-analysis. *Archives of Sexual Behavior*, *42*, 915–933. https://doi.org/10.1007/s10508-012-0062-0

Gott, M., & Hinchliff, S. (2003). How important is sex in later life? The views of older people. *Social Science and Medicine*, *56*(8), 1617–1628.

Hatzichristou, D., Rosen, R. C., Broderick, G., Clayton, A., Cuzin, B., Derogatis, L., … Seftel, A. (2004). Clinical evaluation and management strategy for sexual dysfunction in men and women. *Journal of Sexual Medicine*, *1*(1), 49–57.

Hatzichristou, D., Rosen, R. C., Derogatis, L. R., Low, W. Y., Meuleman, E. J., Sadovsky, R., & Symonds, T. (2010). Recommendations for the clinical evaluation of men and women with sexual dysfunction. *Journal of Sexual Medicine*, *7*(1), 337–348. https://doi.org/10.1111/j.1743-6109.2009.01619.x

Holmes, S. (2000). Treatment of male sexual dysfunction. *British Medical Bulletin*, *56*(3), 798–808.

Hughes, R. G. (2008). Tools and strategies for quality improvement and patient safety. In R. G. Hughes (Ed.), *Patient safety and quality: An evidence-based handbook for nurses*. Rockville, MD: Agency for Healthcare Research and Quality.

Hurlbert, D. F., White, L. C., Powell, R. D., & Apt, C. (1993). Orgasm consistency training in the treatment of women reporting hypoactive sexual desire: An outcome comparison of women-only groups and couples-only groups. *Journal of Behavior Therapy and Experimental Psychiatry*, *24*(1), 3–13.

Kammerer-Doak, D., & Rogers, R. G. (2008). Female sexual function and dysfunction. *Obstetrics and Gynecology Clinics of North America*, *35*, 169–183.

Laumann, E. O., Paik, A., & Rosen, R. (1999). Sexual dysfunction in the United States: Prevalence and predictors. *JAMA, 281*, 537–544.

Leusink, P. M., & Aarts, E. (2006). Treating erectile dysfunction through electronic consultation: A pilot study. *Journal of Sex and Marital Therapy, 32*, 401–407.

Lewis, R. W., Fugl-Meyer, K. S., Bosch, R., Fugl-Meyer, A. R., Laumann, E. O., Lizza, E., & Martin-Morales, A. (2004). Epidemiology/risk factors of sexual dysfunction. *The Journal of Sexual Medicine, 1*, 35–39.

Lukens, E. P., & McFarlane, W. R. (2004). Psychoeducation and evidence-based practice: Considerations for practice, research and policy. *Brief Treatment and Crisis Intervention, 4*(3), 205–225.

Masters, W. H., & Johnson, V. E. (1966). *Human sexual response*. Boston: Little, Brown & Co.

Masters, W. H., & Johnson, V. E. (1970). *Human sexual inadequacy*. New York: Bantam Books.

McCabe, M. P., Price, E., Piterman, L., & Lording, D. (2008). Evaluation of an Internet-based psychological intervention for the treatment of erectile dysfunction. *International Journal of Impotence Research, 20*, 324–330.

McGahuey, C. A., Gelenberg, A. J., Laukes, C. A., Moreno, F. A., Delgado, P. L., McKnight, K. M., & Manber, R. (2000). The Arizona Sexual Experience Scale (ASEX): Reliability and validity. *Journal of Sex & Marital Therapy, 26*(1), 25–40. https://doi.org/10.1080/009262300278623

Murtagh, J. (2010). Female sexual function, dysfunction, and pregnancy: Implications for practice. *Journal of Midwifery & Women's Health, 55*(5), 438–446. https://doi.org/10.1016/j.jmwh.2009.12.006.

O'Leary, M. P., Fowler, F. J., Lenderking, W. R., Barber, B., Sagnier, P. P., Guess, H. A., & Barry, M. J. (1995). A brief male sexual function inventory for urology. *Urology, 46*, 697–706.

Plouffe, L. (1985). Screening for sexual problems through a simple questionnaire. *American Journal of Obstetrics & Gynecology, 151*, 166–169.

Simons, J. S., & Carey, M. P. (2008). Prevalence of sexual dysfunctions: Results from a decade of research. *Archives of Sexual Behavior, 30*(2), 177–219.

Smith, W. J., Beadle, K., & Shuster, E. J. (2008). The impact of a group psychoeducational appointment on women with sexual dysfunction. *American Journal of Obstetrics and Gynecology, 198*(6), 687.e1–697.e7. https://doi.org/10.1016/j.ajog.2008.03.028

Taylor, B., & Davis, S. (2006). Using the extended PLISSIT model to address sexual healthcare needs. *Nursing Standard, 21*(11), 35–40.

van Lankveld, J. (2009). Self-help therapies for sexual dysfunction. *The Journal of Sex Research, 46*(2–3), 143–155. https://doi.org/10.1080/00224490902747776.

36 Sexual Pain Disorder

Rory Newlands and William T. O'Donohue

The assessment and treatment of sexual pain presents a daunting challenge and demands close collaboration between the behavioral health provider (BHP) and the medical treatment team. Some of the primary factors that contribute to the difficulty of assessing and treating sexual pain include confusion about what constitutes "sexual pain" (and what separates it from nonsexual pain, e.g., for those with ongoing pain in the area), the wide array of etiological factors that shape the course and presentation of the pain, and the paucity of empirically supported treatments (Binik et al., 2002; Van Lankveld et al., 2010). The purpose of this chapter is to serve as a guide for navigating assessment and treatment of sexual pain.

Sexual Pain or Genital Pain?

Historically, female sexual pain had been conceptualized as two discrete disorders: *dyspareunia*, which encompasses general genital and pelvic pain, and *vaginismus*, an involuntary and painful tightening or spasm of pelvic muscles (Binik et al., 2002). The DSM-5 integrated both disorders into genito-pelvic pain/penetration disorder, based on their high comorbidity (Wincze & Weisberg, 2015). The decision to classify female sexual pain as a sexual dysfunction in the DSM-5, rather than as a pain disorder, has been contentious among some mental health-care professionals. Much of the disagreement stems from the fact that sexual pain occurs in nonsexual contexts (e.g., gynecological exams, tampon insertion, etc.), suggesting that sexual pain may better be conceptualized as a chronic pain disorder than as a sexual dysfunction (Bergeron, Binik, Khalifé, Pagidas, & Glazer, 2001; Binik et al., 2002). Epidemiological research supporting this conclusion discovered that virgin adolescent girls who reported severe pain at first tampon insertion were more likely to develop sexual pain later in life (Landry & Bergeron, 2009). Furthermore, research has found that chronic pain disorders, such as migraine headaches, correlate with chronic sexual pain (Paterson, Davis, Khalifé, Amsel, & Binik, 2009) and that many urogenital and pelvic pain conditions (e.g., interstitial cystitis, loin pain/hematuria syndrome, vulvar vestibulitis syndrome, etc.) appear to be linked to inflammation (Van Lankveld et al., 2010). These findings, coupled with the lack of a general lack of treatment success, suggest that approaching sexual pain as a pain disorder that interferes with sex, rather than as a sexual dysfunction, may increase treatment options and success (Binik, 2005). However, this reframing is not intended to discount the role that psychological factors play in the development and maintenance of either sexual or nonsexual pain.

R. Newlands (✉) • W.T. O'Donohue
Department of Clinical Psychology, University of Nevada, Reno, NV, USA
e-mail: rorynewlands@gmail.com

A. Maragakis, W.T. O'Donohue (eds.), *Principle-Based Stepped Care and Brief Psychotherapy for Integrated Care Settings*, https://doi.org/10.1007/978-3-319-70539-2_36

Prevalence

Inferences regarding the prevalence of sexual pain are inconclusive, given the wide range of estimates (Wincze & Weisberg, 2015). Note: Although some men experience sexual pain, the necessary empirical and clinical literature is limited; thus, this chapter examines sexual pain in women only. For dyspareunia, estimates range from 3 to 43% and vary with sample demographics (clinical vs. nonclinical) and client age (Van Lankveld et al., 2010; Wincze & Weisberg, 2015). The prevalence of dyspareunia ranges from 3 to 46% in general practice settings and from 10 to 20% in gynecological clinics (Van Lankveld et al., 2010). For vaginismus, conclusions about prevalence remain elusive, as few studies have assessed the rate of affliction; existing research estimates rates between 1 and 6% (Van Lankveld et al., 2010). Rates of vaginismus are highest in cultures where women have few rights and arranged or forced marriages are normative (Amidu et al., 2010; Yasan & Gürgen, 2009), which highlights the importance of psychosocial factors. Despite the high prevalence of sexual pain in women, studies have found that only 60% of women experiencing sexual pain sought treatment and, of those women, only 60% received a diagnosis (Harlow, Wise, & Stewart, 2001).

Etiology

The causes for development of sexual pain remain as unclear as the definition of the disorder itself. Numerous physiological and biological conditions influence the experience of sexual pain including, but not limited to, pelvic inflammatory disease, endometriosis, interstitial cystitis, uterine fibroids, STIs, STDs, side effects of chemotherapy, IBS, prolapsed ovaries, congenital abnormalities, and vaginal septum (Fugl-Meyer et al., 2013; Kingsberg & Althof, 2009; Kingsberg & Knudson, 2011). Additionally, research has shown that women who experience sexual pain have decreased general touch and pain thresholds compared to controls (Van Lankveld et al., 2010). Although biological/physiological factors play an important role in the development of sexual pain, it is crucial that psychosocial factors are not discounted, as these factors may contribute significantly to the development and course of sexual pain (Wincze & Weisberg, 2015).

Childhood physical and sexual abuses are some of the most robust predictors of sexual pain development (Wincze & Weisberg, 2015). Fear or avoidance of sex may be a causal mechanism for sexual pain; sufferers are 4.1 times more likely to report experiencing severe childhood physical abuse and 6.5 times more likely to report severe childhood sexual abuse (Harlow & Stewart, 2005). Chronic pain patients show persistent patterns of catastrophizing pain, fear of pain, pain-related anxiety, and avoidance of pain-inducing activities (Crombez, Vlaeyen, Heuts, & Lysens, 1999; Vlaeyen, Kole-Snijders, Boeren, & Van Eek, 1995; Vlaeyen & Linton, 2000). Such findings contributed to the development of the *fear-avoidance model of chronic pain* (Leeuw et al., 2007), which posits that pain is maintained in a cyclical fashion, with individuals who are high in pain-related fear, anxiety, and catastrophizing paying greater attention to pain cues and displaying more worry about the pain and their ability to cope with the pain, which causes the individual to avoid pain-provoking activities as well as pain-related thoughts. This avoidance leads to relief, which reinforces the individual's avoidance and maintains their pain-related fear, anxiety, and catastrophizing. This fear-avoidance model can be applied to the conceptualization of sexual pain; research has found that women with sexual pain also have an increased sensitivity to pain cues (Payne, Binik, Amsel, & Khalifé, 2005), increased fear of pain (Peters et al., 2007), and greater catastrophizing around sexual pain (Pukall, Binik, Khalifé, Amsel, & Abbott, 2002).

Relationship satisfaction and dyadic adjustment have not been shown to play important roles in sexual pain as they do in other sexual dysfunctions, but the partner's response to the pain has been found to moderate the client's experience of pain (Wincze & Weisberg, 2015). Specifically, partner responses that encouraged adaptive coping predicted decreased pain intensity (Bergeron, Rosen, & Pukall, 2014; Rosen et al., 2014), while hostile/frustrated and overly attentive/concerned partner communication styles predicted increased pain intensity (Desrosiers et al., 2008). All of these factors (physiological/biological conditions, history of childhood abuse, fear avoidance, and relationship dynamics) contribute to the difficulty of assessing and treating sexual pain and solidify the importance of thorough assessment and close collaboration between medical experts and BHP.

Screening in a Primary Care Setting

The medical nature of sexual pain, in conjunction with the many possible comorbid or relevant medical and psychological conditions, warrants close collaboration between the BHP and the medical treatment team. A comprehensive medical exam is required to establish the presence of a contributing or causal medical condition (e.g., infection, scarring, malformations, etc.). Traditionally, to determine the presence of sexual pain, a cotton swab test was used during a gynecological exam (Basson et al., 2004). A recently developed device, the vulvalgesiometer, provides a more sophisticated way of detecting and measuring sexual pain. This device enables practitioners to distinguish between types of sexual pain (i.e., superficial vs. deep), can assist in quantifying the severity and location of pain, and can be used posttreatment to evaluate treatment success (Basson et al., 2004). Characteristics and location of the pain are the soundest predictors of its organicity (Meana, Binik, Khalifé, & Cohen, 1997). Additionally, the sensation (e.g., throbbing vs. burning vs. stabbing) and characteristics (reactive vs. spontaneous, dispersed vs. confined) of the pain provide insight into its nature (somatic, visceral, neuropathic); these insights, in turn, guide treatment decisions (Rosenbaum, 2005). Understanding where the pain occurs in the sexual response cycle (e.g., arousal vs. orgasm) and how the client deals with the pain also provides the practitioner with important treatment considerations (Rosenbaum, 2005). However, depending on the patient's presenting complaint, performing the medical exam first may not be optimal. Additionally, some patients may be reluctant or uncomfortable discussing sexual issues (Montgomery, 2008) and may only disclose detailed information when asked directly or if prompted by a questionnaire. See Table 36.1 for assessment questions if patients indicate

Table 36.1 Helpful assessment questions

Pain	Can you tell/show me where it hurts? (having an anatomical model can aid patients with limited anatomical knowledge.) How would you describe your pain? How long does the pain last? Does touching elsewhere in the genital/pelvic area hurt? Do you feel pain when riding a bike or wearing tight clothes?
Pain and penetration	When during intimacy does the pain occur? • When the opening of your vagina has contact • Once your vagina is partially penetrated • When you are fully penetrated • After some thrusting • After deep thrusting • After withdrawal • With your partner's ejaculation Do other forms of penetration hurt, such as inserting a tampon or finger? Do you find your body tensing up when your partner attempts to penetrate you? If so, what thoughts go through your mind?
Pelvic floor tension	Do you notice the feeling of your pelvic floor muscle tensing during sexual contact? Do you notice your pelvic floor muscle tensing in nonsexual situations?
Arousal	Are you excited when you attempt intercourse/sex? Does your vagina become sufficiently moist? Do you ever feel like you are losing vaginal moisture or drying up?
Consequences	What happens when you experience pain during sexual contact? (e.g., continue anyway, stop, try something else, etc.) Does the pain affect other aspects of your relationship? And if so, in what way?
Biomedical factors	When and how did the pain first occur? Have medical tests been performed? And if so, what was the conclusion? Have you received treatment? And if so, what kind?
Other pain	Do you suffer from any other types of chronic pain? (e.g., migraines, chronic back pain, etc.)

*Adapted from Basson et al. (2004)

sexual pain or consider using the self-report Female Sexual Functioning Index (FSFI; Rosen et al., 2000).

Even if relevant medical conditions are identified, evaluating psychosocial factors is still paramount, as these factors provide key information regarding treatment options. In some cases, medical treatment may not be possible, and psychological approaches offer the most promise, because they help patients and their partner cope with the pain and adapt their behaviors to minimize it (Wincze & Weisberg, 2015). All patients with sexual pain should be assessed for thoughts and behaviors around their pain (specifically fear, catastrophizing, and avoidance), psychological functioning, and relationship and sexual difficulties (Boyer, Goldfinger, Thibault-Gagnon, & Pukall, 2011). Given the high prevalence of physical and sexual abuse in this population, practitioners should also assess for psychological trauma (Harlow & Stewart, 2005). Haefner et al. (2005) created a treatment algorithm designed to help clinicians reach treatment decisions based on the client's presentation. With its concrete approach, this algorithm can be a useful tool, but many clinicians prefer individualized assessments due to the wide array of contributing and maintaining factors (Goldfinger & Pukall, 2011).

Further Assessment for Positive Screens

Given that sexual pain in women encompasses a complex interaction among physical, psychological, and social factors (Boyer et al., 2011), finding the right treatment can be challenging. Research shows that chronic pain patients and those suffering from sexual pain both demonstrate catastrophizing pain, fear of pain, pain-related anxiety, and avoidance of pain-inducing activities (Crombez et al., 1999; Payne et al., 2005; Peters et al., 2007; Pukall et al., 2002; Vlaeyen et al., 1995; Vlaeyen & Linton, 2000). For individuals experiencing sexual pain without comorbid sexual dysfunction, trauma history, or distorted/maladaptive ideas about sex, whose pain is not specific to sex or a certain sexual activity, treatment incorporating chronic pain protocols may offer promise (Payne et al., 2005). For patients endorsing one or more psychosocial factors, treatments employing cognitive behavioral therapy involving psycho-education, cognitive restructuring, and self-coping statements in conjunction with pain management strategies have shown positive results (Bergeron et al., 2014). Because of the cross-disciplinary complexity of women's sexual pain, thorough medical and psychosocial evaluations and a multidisciplinary treatment team are prerequisites for successful treatment. With evaluation results in hand and applying a stepped-care approach, practitioners can tailor treatments so that each client receives an appropriate balance of medical and psychological interventions, while patients needing extended psychotherapy and/or serious medical intervention can be directed to the appropriate referral.

Level One: psycho-education

Guided by the stepped-care framework (Bower & Gilbody, 2005), Level One treatments are optimal for highly motivated patients with simple presentations (i.e., few contributing and maintaining etiological factors). Once sexual pain is identified as the primary culprit, rather than as a side effect or vestige of another condition, practitioners should provide the patient with psycho-education. regarding their diagnosis, sexual anatomy and physiology, and "normal" sexual functioning. Practitioners should also provide education on the fear-avoidance model of chronic pain and the cyclical nature of pain and fear (Leeuw et al., 2007). Patients may also benefit from education on general health issues such as sleep hygiene, diet, substance abuse, and exercise and on the role these factors play in maintaining their pain. Given that research has linked sexual pain and neurogenic inflammation in females suffering from sexual pain (Basson et al., 2004), diet and exercise should definitely be addressed. Low-inflammation diets (i.e., high fat, reduced starch and sugar intake, increased fruit and vegetable intake) are recommended for those suffering from pain disorders (Seaman, 2002); additionally, diets high in ketogenic fats have been found to reduce pain and inflammation markers in animal studies (Ruskin, Kawamura, & Masino, 2009). Self-help books such as *Diet for a Pain-Free Life* (McIlwain & Bruce, 2006) can aid patients in making lifestyle changes relevant to their pain.

Level Two: Group Psychotherapy or Guided Self-Help

Given the multifaceted nature of sexual pain, many patients need treatments more intensive than Level One. In terms of group treatments, group cognitive behavioral therapy (GCBT) appears the most promising; however, more randomized control trials (RCTs) are needed (Landry, Bergeron, Dupuis, & Desrochers, 2008). Bergeron et al. (2001) designed and evaluated an 8–12-week 2-h GCBT treatment plan intended to reduce pain, fear of pain, and maladaptive affect and coping and to increase sexual activities. The treatment is composed of these eight elements: (1) psycho-education on sexual pain, sexual anatomy, the impact of sexual pain on desire and arousal, and the biopsychosocial view of pain, (2) calming skills (i.e., progressive muscle relaxation and diaphragmatic breathing), (3) Kegel exercises, (4) vaginal dilation, (5) focusing on sexual imagery as a distraction technique, (6) self-coping statements, (7) communication skills training, and (8) cognitive restructuring.

The noninvasive nature of GCBT, combined with its focus on reducing pain and the resultant psychological, social, and sexual consequences, makes it an appealing treatment option (Landry et al., 2008). However, more RCTs evaluating treatment efficacy of GCBT are needed. The GCBT program may also benefit from incorporating mindfulness and acceptance-based principles (Rosenbaum, 2013) as well as from expanding instruction about the fear-avoidance model of pain (Thomtén & Linton, 2013).

While few self-guided treatments exist for sexual pain, self-guided treatments for chronic pain have expanded in recent years, with e-health programs leading the way. In patients suffering from chronic pain, one e-health program, Chronic Pain Management Program (CPMP), demonstrated success in decreasing pain severity, catastrophizing, perceived disability, pain-related interference and emotional burden, pain-induced fear, anxiety, depression, and stress (Ruehlman, Karoly, & Enders, 2012). CPMP consists of four modules focusing on the following domains: thinking better (cognitive), doing more (behavioral), relating better (social), and feeling better (emotional regulation). Each module provides participants with psycho-education, interactive activities to teach skills and provide practice, self-monitoring, an exercise regimen, and relaxation skills. CPMP is available commercially and can be purchased at https://pain.goalistics.com. While e-health programs such as CPMP have not been evaluated for the treatment of sexual pain, the overlap between sexual pain and chronic pain (Bergeron et al., 2001; Binik et al., 2002) suggests that treatments such as Ruehlman et al.' (2012) program could be applied to this population; however, further research is needed.

Level Three: Brief Individual Psychotherapy

Sexual pain disorders lack empirically validated brief individual therapies (i.e., three to five sessions). Applying brief CBT augmented for the treatment of sexual pain is a possibility, given the success of prolonged CBT for the treatment of sexual pain (Landry et al., 2008; LoFrisco, 2011). Using the Bergeron et al. (2001) group CBT model as a template, individual therapy could take this form:

- Session (1) Psycho-education (i.e., sexual pain, sexual anatomy, the impact of sexual pain on desire and arousal, the fear-avoidance model of chronic pain, and the cyclical nature of pain and fear), skills training (i.e., progressive muscle relaxation, diaphragmatic breathing, Kegel exercises), and an introduction to cognitive restructuring.
  Homework: Thought records, pain diary, and skills practice.
- Session (2) Creating self-coping statements (e.g., "No pain no gain," "I'm stronger than my pain," "I choose to see this as a challenge," etc.) and continued focus on cognitive restructuring.

Homework: Thought record, pain diary, skills practice, and practice of self-coping statements.
- Session (3) Work on communication skills, assess/address cognitive distortions regarding relationship, body, or self, and continue with cognitive restructuring.
  Homework: Thought record, pain diary, skills practice, and practice of self-coping statements.
- Session (4) Introduction to vaginal dilation, psycho-education regarding focusing on sexual imagery as a distraction technique, continued communication skills training and cognitive restructuring.
  Homework: Thought record, pain diary, skills practice, vaginal dilation, practice of self-coping statements, and practice the use of sexual imagery as a distraction technique.
- Session (5) Review psycho-education from Session 1, cognitive restructuring, and wrap-up.

Research regarding the efficacy of brief CBT interventions for the treatment of sexual pain is needed, as the multifaceted and multidisciplinary nature of the disorder may require more intensive treatments. Unfortunately commercial treatment manuals are not available at this time.

What Does Not Work

Sex therapy may seem like the obvious treatment of choice for sexual pain disorders. While incorporating elements of sex therapy (such as sensate focus, graded exposure, involvement of the partner, etc.) can benefit the treatment of sexual pain (Masters & Johnson, 1970), using the original Masters and Johnson (1966) sex therapy manual is not recommended. One reason for not recommending the manual is that sex therapy has not been empirically validated as a treatment for sexual pain (Landry et al., 2008; LoFrisco, 2011). Another more practical reason is that sexual pain can occur in contexts outside of sexual contact (Bergeron et al., 2001; Binik et al., 2002), and traditional sex therapy fails to address many of the psychological and interpersonal factors relevant to sexual pain.

When to Refer Out: Level Four—Long-Term or Biomedical Interventions

Practitioners have a range of long-term or biomedical intervention options. One option, *vestibulectomy* (the surgical removal of the skin from the vaginal vestibule), has been shown to be significantly more effective than CBT or biofeedback in terms of reducing pain (Landry et al., 2008). However, vestibulectomy did not outperform CBT or biofeedback in terms of psychosexual functioning; additionally, the CBT group had a significantly lower attrition rate than those in the vestibulectomy group and higher patient satisfaction than those in the biofeedback group (Landry et al., 2008). Given its success, vestibulectomy may be an appealing treatment (Landry et al., 2008; LoFrisco, 2011). However, it is crucial that practitioners address all aspects of sexual pain (e.g., psychosocial components) as, for most patients, sexual pain encompasses more than just the physical (Wincze & Weisberg, 2015).

For patients who demonstrated resistance to lower-level treatments, and for those presenting with many contributing etiological factors, cognitive behavioral sex therapy and pain management coupled with physical therapy has been recommended as the treatment of choice (Bergeron & Lord, 2003). This multidisciplinary treatment approach addresses the biopsychosocial factors contributing to and maintaining sexual pain and demonstrates success rates comparable to other medical treatments (Landry et al., 2008). Traditional CBT (i.e., 10–12 sessions) for the treatment of sexual pain has garnered empirical support, with studies finding that participants reported less pain during intercourse, greater perceived pain control, and increased sexual satisfaction (Bergeron et al., 2001; Ter Kuile & Weijenborg, 2006). Biofeedback has also demonstrated treatment success (Landry et al., 2008; LoFrisco, 2011) and can be used in conjunction with CBT (Wincze & Weisberg, 2015).

The Role of the Primary Care Provider/Medical Team in Treatment

The nature of sexual pain requires close collaboration of a multidisciplinary team. The medical work-up provides valuable information regarding relevant etiological factors, which in turn dictates treatment decisions. The BHP should also be actively involved in the assessment process, given that the medical team may miss relevant etiological factors (e.g., trauma history, maladaptive beliefs about pain or sex, body image, etc.) (Basson et al., 2004). Some researchers have argued that the treatment of sexual pain would benefit from integrating psychotherapy and medical assessment/physical therapy, as the behaviors displayed during the gynecological assessment or physical therapy offer insight about treatment targets (Rosenbaum, 2005). It is important for health-care professionals to agree on a common lexicon; communication between team members can be strained by the fact that a variety of terms are used when discussing sexual pain (e.g., vulvodynia, vulvar vestibulitis, dyspareunia, genito-pelvic pain/penetration disorder, etc.).

Quality Improvement

When it comes to improving treatment efficiency and patient satisfaction, treatment of sexual pain disorders has much ground to cover. Understanding the nature of sexual pain is one of the greatest impediments in facing the treatment of this disorder (i.e., Is it a sexual dysfunction, or is it chronic pain that interferes with sex?). Research investigating the efficacy of chronic pain treatments adapted for sexual pain is needed. Additionally, understanding whether certain patient characteristics (e.g., patient beliefs about pain, beliefs about sex, cultural affiliation, religiosity, etc.) mediate or moderate treatment success requires greater attention, as these idiographic features could have profound treatment implications. Basic research and treatment guidelines are also lacking in the area of treatment of sexual pain in men (Goldfinger & Pukall, 2010). Luzzi and Law (2006), who have created a preliminary definition and classification system for sexual pain in men, recommend approaching this disorder much the same as sexual pain in women. However, more work in this area is needed. Additionally, anal sexual pain, or anodyspareunia, deserves further attention in men (Damon & Rosser, 2005).

Patient and practitioner discomfort addressing sex and sexual dysfunction presents another major impediment to the treatment of sexual pain. Health-care professionals must create an atmosphere in which patients feel comfortable and understood. Given that many health-care professionals have limited training in treating sexual health (Kingsberg & Rezaee, 2013), creating staff trainings at integrated care sites to promote open communication is recommended. Still, not all patients will be comfortable discussing sexual health (Montgomery, 2008). Self-report questionnaires, such as the Female Sexual Functioning Index (FSFI; Rosen et al., 2000), may provide practitioners insight into the patient's diagnosis and treatment options. Because sexual pain presents many conceptual and treatment-related challenges, increasing communication between researchers, practitioners, patients, and other disciplines is necessary.

References

Amidu, N., Owiredu, W. K., Woode, E., Addai-Mensah, O., Quaye, L., Alhassan, A., & Tagoe, E. A. (2010). Incidence of sexual dysfunction: A prospective survey in Ghanaian females. *Reproductive Biology and Endocrinology*, *8*(1), 106. https://doi.org/10.1186/1477-7827-8-106

Basson, R., Weijmar Shultz, W. C., Binik, Y. M., Brotto, L. A., Eschenbach, D. A., Laan, E., … Redmond, G. (2004). Women's sexual desire and arousal disorders and sexual pain. In *Sexual medicine: Sexual dysfunctions in men and women* (pp. 851–974). Paris, France: Health Publications.

Bergeron, S., Binik, Y. M., Khalifé, S., Pagidas, K., & Glazer, H. I. (2001). Vulvar vestibulitis syndrome: Reliability of diagnosis and evaluation of current diagnostic criteria. *Obstetrics & Gynecology*, *98*(1), 45–51. https://doi.org/10.1016/s0029-7844(01)01389-8

Bergeron, S., & Lord, M. (2003). The integration of pelvi-perineal re-education and cognitive-behavioural therapy in the multidisciplinary treatment of the sexual pain disorders. *Sexual and Relationship Therapy*, *18*(2), 135–141. https://doi.org/10.1080/1468199031000099406

Bergeron, S., Rosen, N. O., & Pukall, C. F. (2014). Genital pain in women and men: It can hurt more than your sex life. In Y. M. Binik & K. S. Hall (Eds.), *Principles and practice of sex therapy* (5th ed., pp. 159–176). New York, NY: Guildford Press.

Binik, Y. M. (2005). Should dyspareunia be retained as a sexual dysfunction in DSM-V? A painful classification decision. *Archives of Sexual Behavior*, *34*(1), 11–21. https://doi.org/10.1007/s10508-005-0998-4

Binik, Y. M., Reissing, E., Pukall, C., Flory, N., Payne, K. A., & Khalifé, S. (2002). The female sexual pain disorders: Genital pain or sexual dysfunction? *Archives of Sexual Behavior*, *31*(5), 425–429. https://doi.org/10.1023/A:1019892125163

Bower, P., & Gilbody, S. (2005). Stepped care in psychological therapies: Access, effectiveness and efficiency. *The British Journal of Psychiatry*, *186*(1), 11–17. https://doi.org/10.1192/bjp.186.1.11

Boyer, S. C., Goldfinger, C., Thibault-Gagnon, S., & Pukall, C. F. (2011). Management of female sexual pain disorders. In R. Balon (Ed.), *Sexual dysfunction: Beyond the brain-body connection* (Vol. 31, pp. 83–104). Basel: Karger. https://doi.org/10.1159/000328810

Crombez, G., Vlaeyen, J. W., Heuts, P. H., & Lysens, R. (1999). Pain-related fear is more disabling than pain itself: Evidence on the role of pain-related fear in chronic back pain disability. *Pain*, *80*(1), 329–339. https://doi.org/10.1016/s0304-3959(98)00229-2

Damon, W., & Rosser, B. R. (2005). Anodyspareunia in men who have sex with men. *Journal of Sex & Marital Therapy*, *31*(2), 129–141. https://doi.org/10.1080/00926230590477989

Desrosiers, M., Bergeron, S., Meana, M., Leclerc, B., Binik, Y. M., & Khalifé, S. (2008). Original research—Pain: Psychosexual characteristics of vestibulodynia couples: Partner solicitousness and hostility are associated with pain. *The Journal of Sexual Medicine*, *5*(2), 418–427. https://doi.org/10.1111/j.1743-6109.2007.00705.x

Fugl-Meyer, K. S., Bohm-Starke, N., Petersen, C. D., Fugl-Meyer, A., Parish, S., & Giraldi, A. (2013). Standard operating procedures for female genital sexual pain. *The Journal of Sexual Medicine*, *10*(1), 83–93. https://doi.org/10.1111/j.1743-6109.2012.02867.x

Goldfinger, C., & Pukall, C. F. (2011). Sexual pain disorders. In J. P. Mulhall, L. Incrocci, I. Goldstein, & R. Rosen (Eds.), *Cancer and sexual health* (pp. 163–182). New York, NY: Humana Press. ISBN: 978-1-60761-915-4.

Haefner, H. K., Collins, M. E., Davis, G. D., Edwards, L., Foster, D. C., Hartmann, E., … Wilkinson, E. J. (2005). The vulvodynia guideline. *Journal of Lower Genital Tract Disease*, *9*(1), 40–51. https://doi.org/10.1097/00128360-200501000-00009

Harlow, B. L., & Stewart, E. G. (2005). Adult-onset vulvodynia in relation to childhood violence victimization. *American Journal of Epidemiology*, *161*(9), 871–880. https://doi.org/10.1093/aje/kwi108

Harlow, B. L., Wise, L. A., & Stewart, E. G. (2001). Prevalence and predictors of chronic lower genital tract discomfort. *American Journal of Obstetrics and Gynecology*, *185*(3), 545–550. https://doi.org/10.1067/mob.2001.116748

Kingsberg, S. A., & Althof, S. E. (2009). Evaluation and treatment of female sexual disorders. *International Urogynecology Journal and Pelvic Floor Dysfunction*, *20*(S1), 33–43. https://doi.org/10.1007/s00192-009-0833-x

Kingsberg, S. A., & Knudson, G. (2011). Female sexual disorders: Assessment, diagnosis, and treatment. *CNS Spectrums*, *16*(02), 49–62. https://doi.org/10.1017/s109285291200017x

Kingsberg, S. A., & Rezaee, R. L. (2013). Hypoactive sexual desire in women. *Menopause*, *20*(12), 1284–1300. https://doi.org/10.1097/gme.0000000000000131

Landry, T., & Bergeron, S. (2009). How young does vulvo-vaginal pain begin? Prevalence and characteristics of dyspareunia in adolescents. *The Journal of Sexual Medicine*, *6*(4), 927–935. https://doi.org/10.1111/j.1743-6109.2008.01166.x

Landry, T., Bergeron, S., Dupuis, M., & Desrochers, G. (2008). The treatment of provoked vestibulodynia. *The Clinical Journal of Pain*, *24*(2), 155–171. https://doi.org/10.1097/ajp.0b013e31815aac4d

Leeuw, M., Goossens, M. E., Linton, S. J., Crombez, G., Boersma, K., & Vlaeyen, J. W. (2007). The fear-avoidance model of musculoskeletal pain: Current state of scientific evidence. *Journal of Behavioral Medicine*, *30*(1), 77–94. https://doi.org/10.1007/s10865-006-9085-0

Lofrisco, B. M. (2011). Female sexual pain disorders and cognitive behavioral therapy. *Journal of Sex Research*, *48*(6), 573–579. https://doi.org/10.1080/00224499.2010.540682

Luzzi, G. A., & Law, L. A. (2006). The male sexual pain syndromes. *International Journal of STD & AIDS*, *17*(11), 720–726. https://doi.org/10.1258/095646206778691220

Masters, W. H., & Johnson, V. E. (1966). *Human sexual response*. Boston, MA: Little, Brown and Company.

Masters, W. H., & Johnson, V. E. (1970). *Human sexual inadequacy*. Boston: Little, Brown.

McIlwain, H. H., & Bruce, D. F. (2006). *Diet for a pain-free life: A revolutionary plan to lose weight, stop pain, sleep better, and feel great in 21 days*. New York: Marlowe &.

Meana, M., Binik, Y. M., Khalifé, S., & Cohen, D. R. (1997). Biopsychosocial profile of women with dyspareunia. *Obstetrics & Gynecology, 90*(4), 583–589. https://doi.org/10.1016/s0029-7844(98)80136-1

Montgomery, K. A. (2008). Sexual desire disorders. *Psychiatry (Edgemont), 5*(6), 50–55.

Paterson, L. Q., Davis, S. N., Khalifé, S., Amsel, R., & Binik, Y. M. (2009). Persistent genital and pelvic pain after childbirth. *The Journal of Sexual Medicine, 6*(1), 215–221. https://doi.org/10.1111/j.1743-6109.2008.01063.x

Payne, K. A., Binik, Y. M., Amsel, R., & Khalifé, S. (2005). When sex hurts, anxiety and fear orient attention towards pain. *European Journal of Pain, 9*(4), 427–427. https://doi.org/10.1016/j.ejpain.2004.10.003

Peters, K. M., Killinger, K. A., Carrico, D. J., Ibrahim, I. A., Diokno, A. C., & Graziottin, A. (2007). Sexual function and sexual distress in women with interstitial cystitis: A case-control study. *Urology, 70*(3), 543–547. https://doi.org/10.1016/j.urology.2007.04.037

Pukall, C. F., Binik, Y. M., Khalifé, S., Amsel, R., & Abbott, F. V. (2002). Vestibular tactile and pain thresholds in women with vulvar vestibulitis syndrome. *Pain, 96*(1), 163–175. https://doi.org/10.1016/s0304-3959(01)00442-0

Rosen, C., Brown, J., Heiman, S., Leiblum, C., Meston, R., Shabsigh, D., … D'Agostino, R., Jr. (2000). The Female Sexual Function Index (FSFI): A multidimensional self-report instrument for the assessment of female sexual function. *Journal of Sex & Marital Therapy, 26*(2), 191–208. https://doi.org/10.1080/009262300278597

Rosen, N. O., Bergeron, S., Sadikaj, G., Glowacka, M., Delisle, I., & Baxter, M. (2014). Impact of male partner responses on sexual function in women with vulvodynia and their partners: A dyadic daily experience study. *Health Psychology, 33*(8), 823–831. https://doi.org/10.1037/a0034550

Rosenbaum, T. Y. (2005). Physiotherapy treatment of sexual pain disorders. *Journal of Sex & Marital Therapy, 31*(4), 329–340. https://doi.org/10.1080/00926230590950235

Rosenbaum, T. Y. (2013). An integrated mindfulness-based approach to the treatment of women with sexual pain and anxiety: Promoting autonomy and mind/body connection. *Sexual and Relationship Therapy, 28*(1–2), 20–28. https://doi.org/10.1080/14681994.2013.764981

Ruehlman, L. S., Karoly, P., & Enders, C. (2012). A randomized controlled evaluation of an online chronic pain self-management program. *Pain, 153*(2), 319–330. https://doi.org/10.1016/j.pain.2011.10.025

Ruskin, D. N., Kawamura, M., Jr., & Masino, S. A. (2009). Reduced pain and inflammation in juvenile and adult rats fed a ketogenic diet. *PLoS One, 4*(12), E8349. https://doi.org/10.1371/journal.pone.0008349

Seaman, D. R. (2002). The diet-induced proinflammatory state. *Journal of Manipulative and Physiological Therapeutics, 25*(3), 168–179. https://doi.org/10.1067/mmt.2002.122324

Ter Kuile, M. M., & Weijenborg, P. T. (2006). A cognitive-behavioral group program for women with vulvar vestibulitis syndrome (VVS): Factors associated with treatment success. *Journal of Sex & Marital Therapy, 32*(3), 199–213. https://doi.org/10.1080/00926230600575306

Thomtén, J., & Linton, S. J. (2013). A psychological view of sexual pain among women: Applying the fear-avoidance model. *Women's Health, 9*(3), 251–263. https://doi.org/10.2217/whe.13.19

Van Lankveld, J. J., Granot, M., Weijmar Shultz, W. C., Binik, Y. M., Wesselmann, U., Pukall, C. F., … Achtrari, C. (2010). Women's sexual pain disorders. *Journal of Sexual Medicine, 7*(1 pt 2), 615–631. https://doi.org/10.1111/j.1743-6109.2009.01631.x.

Vlaeyen, J. W., Kole-Snijders, A. M., Boeren, R. G., & Van Eek, H. (1995). Fear of movement/(re)injury in chronic low back pain and its relation to behavioral performance. *Pain, 62*(3), 363–372. https://doi.org/10.1016/0304-3959(94)00279-n

Vlaeyen, J. W., & Linton, S. J. (2000). Fear-avoidance and its consequences in chronic musculoskeletal pain: A state of the art. *Pain, 85*(3), 317–332. https://doi.org/10.1016/s0304-3959(99)00242-0

Wincze, J. P., & Weisberg, R. B. (2015). *Sexual dysfunction: A guide for assessment and treatment* (3rd ed.). New York, NY: Guildford Press. ISBN: 9781462520596.

Smoking Cessation

37

Brandon T. Sanford

Smoking Prevalence and Impact

Smoking prevalence is commonly defined as percentage of daily smokers in a population. Worldwide this rate is approximately 31.1% for men and 6.2% for women (Ng et al., 2014). Prevalence estimates in the United States are slightly lower for men at 22.2% and considerably higher for women at 17.9% (Dwyer-Lindgren et al., 2014). Dwyer-Lindgren et al. (2014) also observed regions in the southern United States and regions with higher Native American populations to have elevated prevalence rates. Smoking rates are higher in US veteran populations (Brown, 2010), lower socioeconomic status populations, and rural populations (Casetta et al., 2016; Nagelhout et al., 2012). Concerningly, prevalence rates for smoking have been observed to be higher in several vulnerable populations. For example, those with poorer mental health are over twice as likely to be smokers (Steinberg, Williams, & Li, 2015), and while smoking rates have been slowly decreasing both in the United States and worldwide, this is not true to those with poor mental health. Among youths with mental health or substance abuse problems, rates have been observed to be as high as 64.5% for those between the ages of 12 and 18 and 72.7% among those between the ages of 19 and 24 (Catchpole, McLeod, Brownlie, Allison, & Grewal, 2016). Those admitted for inpatient medical care are approximately 33% more likely to be smokers (Harrison, Preston, Bucur, & Fletcher, 2012). Likewise, those diagnosed with COPD are 48% more likely to be smokers than those who are not (Vozoris & Stanbrook, 2011). Finally, approximately 26.6% of women are smokers during their first month of pregnancy (Alshaarawy & Anthony, 2015). It should be noted that this is in line with the point prevalence rate for women between the ages of 12 and 44. This study reports 11.3% of women continue to smoke through the entirety of their pregnancy. In summary, smoking is a highly common problem which is especially likely to be confronted in an integrated care setting. Clinics which primarily serve low SES or Native American populations, are located in the southern United States, or who see a higher than average rate of individuals with poor mental health are especially likely to engage with smokers.

These prevalence data are important in the context of the deleterious effects of tobacco smoking. As will not likely come as a shock to readers of this text, smoking dramatically increases mortality. Smoking is the leading cause of preventable death in the United States (CDC,

B.T. Sanford
Department of Psychology, University of Nevada, Reno, Reno, NV, USA
e-mail: Brandon.Sanford0030@gmail.com

A. Maragakis, W.T. O'Donohue (eds.), *Principle-Based Stepped Care and Brief Psychotherapy for Integrated Care Settings*, https://doi.org/10.1007/978-3-319-70539-2_37

2002). In a large review which examined three cohorts spanning 50 years, researchers concluded: "The age-standardized relative risk for death from all causes among current smokers, as compared with those who had never smoked, increased across all three time periods, with a relative risk of 2.80 (95% CI, 2.72–2.88) for male smokers and 2.76 (95% CI, 2.69–2.84) for female smokers in the contemporary cohorts" (Thun et al., 2013). It is a well-established finding that individuals who smoke are 2.8–3 times as likely to die from any cause compared to non-smokers (Banks et al., 2015; Carter et al., 2015; Jha et al., 2013). Specifically, the rate of death from ischemic heart disease was 2.86 times higher for men and 2.5 times for women; these numbers increase to 3 times as likely in smokers between the ages of 55 and 74. In terms of raw figures, smoking-related deaths have been estimated to amount to more than 480,000 per year (Jamal et al., 2014). This report notes that smoking has been found to negatively impact nearly every organ and organ system in the body. Smokers are more likely to suffer from COPD, diabetes, heart disease, at least six different forms of cancer, and stroke (Rostron, Chang, & Pechacek, 2014). Smoking during pregnancy, which was noted to be at around 11% prevalence, has also been shown to increase the rates of infertility, spontaneous abortion, ectopic pregnancy, fetal growth restriction, preterm birth, perinatal/neonatal mortality, stillbirth, congenital malformations, SIDS, childhood respiratory problems, cancer, and early in life behavior and psychiatric problems (Cnattingius, 2004).

In addition to the above list of health problems, smoking accounts for a staggering degree of economic impact, which is measured as direct (i.e., healthcare expenditures resulting from smoking-related disease) or indirect (i.e., cost of secondhand smoking, cost to employers due to smokers' loss of productivity and absenteeism, smoking-related fires). Up to 18% of all healthcare expenditures in the Unites States are related to smoking (Ekpu & Brown, 2015). In total, smoking costs Americans up to 321 billion dollars per year, or 1.9% of the annual gross domestic product, in both health costs and loss of productivity.

Fortunately, the morbidity and mortality associated with smoking can be largely ameliorated following cessation. Those who quit smoking between the ages of 25 and 34 have nearly identical survival curves to those that have never smoked, which accounts for a life expectancy gain of approximately 10 years (Jha et al., 2013). Life expectancy gain is about 9 years for those who quit between the ages of 35 and 44, meaning excess risk of death from all causes is reduced by 90%. Those who quit between the ages of 45 and 54 reduce their excess risk by 66%. Similarly, every 10 years of smoking cessation is associated with a 16% decrease in the likelihood of being hospitalized for congestive heart failure, diabetes-related complications, COPD, or angina (Tran, Falster, Douglas, Blyth, & Jorm, 2015). The benefits of smoking cessation are not limited to the individuals themselves. Children's odds of smoking are reduced by 39% if their parents quit by the time they start 3rd grade (Bricker, Leroux, Andersen, Rajan, & Peterson, 2005). Similarly, for children who do start smoking, they are 39% more likely to quit if their parents quit late in their childhood (ages 8–17) and 53% more likely if their parents quit before they were age 8 (Bricker, Otten, Liu, & Peterson, 2009). As should be abundantly clear, the negative impacts of smoking are significant, both in terms of health and economics. The benefits of smoking cessation should also be readily apparent. Thus, smoking cessation programs represent an opportunity to make a large impact in an integrated healthcare setting intervening with a high volume of patients.

Screening

As is likely echoed throughout this text, effective integrated care for smoking cessation requires efficient and seamless screening and referral mechanisms. As such, using approaches already commonly recommended to primary care provider (PCP) is optimal. Perhaps the easiest of these screening approaches is to simply ask patients about their current smoking habits. Fortunately, there is a standardized protocol already widely used in medical settings which reinforces the importance of asking patients about smoking in the 5As approach (Fiore et al., 2000; Whitlock, Orleans, Pender, & Allan, 2002). The 5As are Ask, Advise, Assess, Assist, and Arrange. This strategy is compliant with the US Public Health Service evidence-based Treating Tobacco Use and Dependence: Clinical Practice Guidelines to reduce the effects of smoking which strongly recommend all patients be systematically screened for current tobacco use and their readiness to make a quit attempt (Fiore et al., 2000; Fiore et al., 2008). Here we will focus on the first two As before covering the remainder in later sections. Physicians have been estimated to come into contact with about 70% of all smokers each year (Davis, 1988; Zwar, Zwar, Richmond, Zwar, & Richmond, 2006). However, screening rates are consistently observed to be lower than desirable. Multiple studies have found outpatient physicians screening rates to range between 60 and 77% of patients (Jamal et al., 2012; Lawson, Flocke, & Casucci, 2009; Park et al., 2015). Behavioral health providers (BHP) cannot take it for granted that patients are currently being asked about their smoking habits. Furthermore, despite a growing body of evidence supporting the notion that a PCP's advice to quit smoking increases motivation to quit (Eckert & Junker, 2001; Fiore et al., 2008; Kreuter, Chheda, & Bull, 2000; Ossip-Klein et al., 2000), rates of completion for the Advise stage are similar to that of Ask (King, Dube, Babb, & McAfee, 2013; Park et al., 2015). Advice from PCPs should be clearly worded and unequivocal, strong/firm, and personalized.

Fortunately, several studies support the efficacy of brief training interventions to increase the rate of 5A completion (Chen et al., 2015; Payne et al., 2014; Sarna et al., 2014). These training programs emphasize tobacco dependence overview, the role of medical staff in smoking cessation, review of the 5As approach, and role-playing with simulated motivated and unmotivated patients. It is highly recommended that training occur prior to the implementation of an integrated care smoking cessation program. If possible, posters which clearly state the 5As will also aid in keeping the program salient for practitioners. In a recent comprehensive review of interventions designed to increase engagement in the 5As approach, Papadakis et al. (2010) found significant evidence for two strategies: implementation of checklists and prompts inside the electronic medical record (EMR) system. The Adult Screening Inventory (ASI; Maragakis & O'Donohue, in prep) represents a useful checklist as it briefly screens for a wide variety of behavioral health issues and can be quickly reviewed without the need for scoring. The ASI presents a total of 40 domains for which BHPs can provide intervention, for each item patients are simply asked to report whether it is "a concern" or "not a concern." Providers should be advised to have all patients complete the ASI and quickly review it during the course of care. For patients who mark smoking as a concern, this will serve as a cue to advise the patient to quit and continue with the 5As approach. Secondly, where possible, a pop-up window should display whenever the chart of a smoker is pulled up in an EMR system. A message such as "This patient is listed as a smoker, please Ask, Advise, Assess, Assist, and Arrange for follow-up with this patient" should be displayed to prompt the provider to act. Papadakis et al. (2010) found mixed results for auditing charts; however, this may be useful in ensuring all possible referrals are being made. Physicians should also be reminded that the current best-practice guidelines recommend all smokers be at minimum asked about their current smoking habit and be advised to quit (Fiore et al., 2008). A physician's recommendation to quit is associated with a 76% increased likelihood of quitting and requires minimal change in the workflow (Hartmann-Boyce, Stead, Cahill, & Lancaster, 2014). This should be the initial focus of integrated care smoking cessation programs as it ensures consistent referrals for those who may benefit from care.

How to Further Assess if a Screen Returns Positive

Once a patient has been screened and advised to quit smoking by their PCP, a warm handoff (WHO) should be initiated with the BHP who will assess and motivate readiness to attempt cessation due to the following reasons: (1) Rates of completion for the Assess step consistently drop by over 10% when compared to rates of completion for Ask and Advise, as low as 42.6% of patients (King et al., 2013; Park et al., 2015). This may be due to unwillingness on the part of the provider to engage in smoking cessation counseling, perceived lack of self-efficacy, or simply time constraints. Regardless of the reason, stepping in at this point represents an opportunity for the BHP to apply their expertise and allow for increased efficiency on the part of the PCP who is then free to move on to their next patient. (2) BHPs are able to go beyond the recommended forms of assessment which frequently are limited to "are you willing to attempt to quit at this time?" and apply evidence-based methods for increasing motivation to change. It is in the course of this WHO that Motivational Interviewing (MI; Miller & Rollnick, 2002) is recommended. While not a comprehensive system of psychotherapy, MI was developed to specifically address ambivalence toward change and facilitate willingness to engage in change behavior (Miller, 2012). While the breadth of evidence supporting MI is well beyond the scope of the present chapter, it is worth noting that two large (31 trials) meta-analyses have concluded that MI is effective for smoking cessation with those in the MI condition having a 45% increased chance of succeeding at abstinence (Heckman, Egleston, & Hofmann, 2010; Hettema & Hendricks, 2010). A more recent meta-analysis demonstrates the effectiveness of MI delivered in short (less than 20-min) sessions (Lindson-Hawley, Thompson, & Begh, 2015). MI has also been tested in combination with the 5As approach in primary care settings and has been shown to reduce nicotine use in patients compared to TAU (Ridner et al., 2014). Counselors employ the principles of expressing empathy, avoiding argument, managing resistance without confrontation, and supporting the individual's self-efficacy. Specifically, counseling techniques such as open-ended questions, reflective listening, summarizing, affirming, and eliciting client self-motivational statements are used. The goal of WHO is to utilize MI to engage with the patient and increase the amount of patient-generated change talk. Change talk includes patient-generated reasons to quit and statements expressing a desire or commitment to change. For example, a BHP might start with an open-ended question such as "what are your current concerns about smoking" while listening for any potential motivations for quitting such as general health, longevity, improved mobility, children, etc. This might be followed by employing readiness to change ruler such as "on a scale of 1-10, how important is it for you to quit smoking"; this is followed up by "why did you choose [#] instead of [lower-value]." This prompts the patient to give additional context for the importance of the change. If a patient is resistant to engage in change, a useful technique is to deploy discrepancies. For example, the BHP might ask "On the one hand you're coughing and are out breath, and on the other hand you are saying cigarettes are not causing you any problems. What do you think is causing your breathing difficulties?" (cf. Sobell & Sobell, 2011). This is intended to be asked in a curious, nonconfrontational manner, allowing the BHP to explore discrepancies without evoking defensiveness. It is important that the BHP respond to patient with reflective and normalizing statements to reinforce these responses and promote increases in change talk. The interested reader is advised to read *Motivational Interviewing in Health Care* (Rollnick, Miller, & Butler, 2007) and visit http://www.motivationalinterviewing.org/ for resources and a list of upcoming trainings. Once a patient is sufficiently motivated to engage in the treatment, the BHP can move to the Assist stage.

One domain in which MI is likely to be particularly useful is ameliorating fears of excessive weight gain following smoking abstinence. Concerns about weight gain have been shown to prevent attempts to quit (Brouwer & Pomerleau, 2000). Additionally, weight gain following cessation predicts relapse in white women, though this was found to be the inverse in Hispanic women (Mukhopadhyay & Wendel, 2011). The Clinical Practice Guidelines on treating tobacco use and dependence suggest warning patients about the likelihood of weight gain and quelling exaggerated fears of weight gain (Fiore et al., 2008). After an immediate period of weight gain following cessation (approximately 1 lb. per year more for those who quit compared to those who continually smoke over the first 5 years; Travier et al., 2012), former smokers tend to have weights similar to those who never smoked and tend to have similar weight gain trajectories (Flegal, 2012). Additionally, the benefits of smoking far outweigh the potential deleterious effects of weight gain, including cardiovascular benefits and increases in muscle mass and bone density (Clair et al., 2013; Rom, Reznick, Keidar, Karkabi, & Aizenbud, 2015). BHPs should also be prepared to counsel patients on diet and exercise in order to minimize the impact of smoking cessation on weight.

Evidence-Based Stepped Care and Brief Psychotherapeutic Approaches

Stepped care and brief psychotherapeutic interventions represent the Assist stage. In treatment-as-usual conditions, physician-supported assistance for smoking cessation and arranging for follow-up were associated with a 40% increase and 46% increase, respectively, in the odds of quitting (Park et al., 2015). However, here again we see compliance rates far below what best-practice guidelines recommend. Assistance is provided in the form of smoking cessation counseling to approximately 20–28% of patients who smoke (Bernstein, Yu, Post, Dziura, & Rigotti, 2013; Jamal et al., 2012; Nelson et al., 2015; Payne et al., 2012). With 73% of physicians failing to complete the 5As (Lawson et al., 2009), and only 17.5% having arranged follow-up (King et al., 2013). Upon referral, BHPs have a range of options in assisting patients in their attempts to smoke. Depending on the needs of their patients and the demands of their organization, BHPs may choose to refer patients to stepped-care interventions such as smartphone apps, quitlines, or nicotine replacement therapy and/or provide brief evidence-based counseling.

Stepped Care Interventions

Smartphone and Web-Based Interventions

Over 64% of American adults are smartphone owners, and over half of smartphone users have used their phone to look up information about a health condition in the past year (Smith, 2015). The advantages of using smartphone apps to aid in smoking cessation are readily apparent as they are widespread and readily available to be used by patients virtually whenever needed. In a recent review of mobile phone-based interventions, 12 trials were found to have sufficient randomization and follow-up data to be meaningfully evaluated, representing almost 12,000 participants (Whittaker, McRobbie, Bullen, Rodgers, & Gu, 2016). The authors found mobile phone-based interventions to be effective, resulting in a 67% increased rate of abstinence at follow-up. It should be noted that most trials included in this analysis were text message-based and did not take advantage of the complexity and custom-tailoring of interventions afforded by smartphone apps. A recent content analysis of smoking cessation apps available on the Android operating system found 225 to be currently available (Hoeppner et al., 2015). They found the majority of these apps to be free and well rated on the application store. However, despite the established benefits of tailoring interventions (Hawkins, Kreuter, Resnicow, Fishbein, & Dijkstra, 2008), only 10% of apps studied included this feature. The most commonly observed features pertaining to the Assist step were basic information about smoking and its health impacts; trackers for money saved, health benefits accrued after quitting, or cigarettes not smoked over a period of time; or simple distractor tasks. Fortunately, they found app quality to be strongly correlated with popularity (i.e., number of total downloads). This is important as the number of smoking cessation apps available to patients is expected to continue to grow rapidly, making it difficult for BHPs to be familiar with the wide range of options. As a general rule, the most popular options available tend to be free or low cost and best provide tailoring of the intervention based on input from patients.

Only one app will be discussed in detail here as it represents the best demonstrated efficacy across multiple trials. SmartQuit was designed based on content from two successful web-based trials (Bricker, Mann, Marek, Liu, & Peterson, 2010; Bricker, Wyszynski, Comstock, & Heffner, 2013). Broadly speaking, it seeks to (1) increase motivation to quit using personalized patient input regarding values; (2) develop a personalized quit plan identifying social support and providing information on FDA-approved nicotine replacement therapy; (3) promote acceptance, discussed later, as a coping strategy in the context of urges to smoke; (4) address shame and self-judgment in the context of lapses in smoking behavior; and (5) track urges and amount of time spent practicing exercises provided by the app. In a large ($n = 256$) trial, participants randomized to the SmartQuit condition were 62–88% more likely to quit than those who used the National Cancer Institute's QuitGuide app (Bricker et al., 2014). A feature-level analysis of the trial found that those who spent time viewing their personalized quit plan, and tracked their practice of acceptance in the context of urges, were most likely to succeed at cessation (Heffner, Vilardaga, Mercer, Kientz, & Bricker, 2015). A follow-up was conducted which examined a modified version of the app emphasizing the features found to be most predictive of cessation (Bricker et al., 2017). Compared to those in the initial trial, those receiving the modified version reported higher satisfaction, similar quit rates, and significantly higher reductions in smoking. The primary drawback to SmartQuit is the price, listed at $50 at the time of this writing after a free trial period. For those working with a primarily low SES population, this may be more than they are willing to spend; however BHPs may be able to justify the purchase by leveraging the current amount the patient is spending on cigarettes.

Finally, as noted above text messaging-based interventions have proved to be useful. BHPs may choose to integrate this into their programs by having staff provide patients (1) reminders of their chosen quit date, (2) referrals to information about smoking or nicotine replacement treatments, (3) encouragement regarding their quit attempts, (4) reminders to engage in skills practice, or (5) reminders to follow up with BHP. This is a relatively simple and low-cost way of boasting the efficacy of brief interventions.

Quitlines

Smoking cessation quitlines are telephone-based programs which provide services ranging from mailed materials and counseling to information and access regarding nicotine replacement therapy (North American Quitline Consortium, 2009). These services are often free for the patient. Similar to app-based interventions, quitlines offer access to the intervention at the patients' convenience. They also allow for counselors to proactively call patients to engage in follow-up and are often structured in such a way that effective evidence-based protocols can be delivered. A review and meta-analysis which encompassed eight trials and over 18,000 participants found that quitlines which included call-back counseling resulted in a 41% likelihood of cessation as follow-up when compared to either a single patient-initiated counseling session or mailed materials (Stead, Perera, & Lancaster, 2007). An up-to-date reference for the quitline services offered nationally and state by state can be found at http://map.naquitline.org/. BHPs are encouraged to review the services offered in their area so as to best advise and prepare patients to use quitlines.

Nicotine Replacement Therapy (NRT)

NRT can take the form of gum, patches, lozenges, inhalers, or nasal sprays which replace the nicotine in tobacco products. These products were widely available over the counter in 1996. The goal of NRT is to replace some of the nicotine from tobacco in order to reduce cravings to smoke and ameliorate withdrawal symptoms. In a meta-analysis which included data from 12 reviews, covering 105 trials, those using NRT were 84% more likely to be abstinent at follow-up (Cahill, Stevens, Perera, & Lancaster, 2013). Of note, NRT has been shown to significantly increase the rate of chest pain and heart palpitations; however, this is still a rare event with only 2.5% of participants reporting this effect. In sum, the benefits of increased rates of abstinence outweigh the potential cardiovascular risks, though more personalized intervention strategies accounting for individual differences in nicotine reactions may further inform their use (Samet, 2013).

Evidence-Based Principles for Brief Intervention

Counseling for tobacco cessation is unfortunately an under-researched domain. In the most recent Cochrane Review of tobacco addiction interventions, only 51 of 506 reported trials (10%) included face-to-face counseling (Hartmann-Boyce et al., 2014). This may in part be due to psychologists' tendency to ignore smoking cessation counseling in the course of standard clinical work (Lichtenstein, Zhu, & Tedeschi, 2010). Thus, it is perhaps unsurprising that this review found individual counseling to improve cessation rates by only 39%. However, group therapy was associated with nearly a twofold improvement in cessation rates as compared to self-help interventions. This is likely because group therapy is ideal for fostering social support and makes delivering evidence-based protocol more likely. It should also be noted that counseling has been demonstrated to be particularly effective for patients who are either pregnant or those who have received a diagnosis of depression (Hartmann-Boyce et al., 2014). Additionally, counseling interventions are typically equally effective in young adult populations (Suls et al., 2012). Troublingly, a recent meta-analysis of healthy behavior change interventions for low-income individuals found smaller intervention effects which fell to only an 11% increased chance of cessation at follow-up (Bull, Dombrowski, McCleary, & Johnston, 2014). Those working with low-income populations are strongly encouraged to include as many treatment components as possible to account for this effect. This is important as there is a demonstrated dose-response effect for behavioral interventions, at least up until the 30-min encounter mark (Fiore et al., 2008). Often BHPs will be in the role of conducting brief 10–30-min WHO encounters utilizing MI to facilitate engagement with the stepped care interventions. This will ensure the patient sets a quit date, tracks cigarette smoking or abstinence length, is given skills to practice, and is provided encouragement to quit. For patients who either refuse or are not able to access the aforementioned stepped care resources, similar materials can be accessed at https://www.SmokeFree.gov/ either by the patient or printed out by the BHP. In some cases, given the resources of the integrated healthcare center, three to five session counseling interventions may be conducted. If stepped care interventions are not utilized, BHP must ensure they cover the above mentioned domains. Individual/group counseling may be especially useful for patients who report high levels of stress. The link between perceived stress and smoking is well established (Carey, Kalra, Carey, Halperin, & Richards, 1993; Cohen & Lichtenstein, 1990; Kassel, Stroud, & Paronis, 2003). Individuals who report consistently high levels of stress are less likely to succeed in quit attempts, less likely to utilize skills, and more likely to relapse. Thus, targeting stress is critical during cessation counseling. Additionally, as most behavioral treatments for smoking cessation are designed to be between

7 and 12 weeks in length (Hitsman et al., 2013), we will illustrate two particularly useful principles to incorporate into counseling.

Acceptance

Experiential acceptance, defined as an individual's willingness to remain in contact with an aversive private experience, such as an urge to smoke, has been shown to mediate the effect of stress on smoking and smoking cessation (Farris et al., 2015; Garey, Farris, Schmidt, & Zvolensky, 2016). It has also been found to be associated with length of delay to relapse, with those who are intolerant of the distress caused by urges more likely to quickly relapse (Brown, Lejuez, Kahler, & Strong, 2002), as well as experience greater levels of withdrawal, more intense cravings, and more negative affect at the start of treatment (Farris, Zvolensky, & Schmidt, 2015). Treatments which specifically target willingness to experience psychological distress during attempts to quit smoke, such as intense urges, have been shown to be highly effective. An acceptance-based treatment has been shown to significantly outperform NRT with 35% abstinence rate vs. 15% abstinence rate at 1-year follow-up (Gifford et al., 2004). Acceptance was further shown to mediate changes in cessation rates. This has also been shown to be the case for quitline (Schuck, Otten, Kleinjan, Bricker, & Engels, 2014) and web-based interventions (Bricker et al., 2013). In sum, a meta-analyses which examined the five trials of acceptance-based treatment for smoking cessation found a medium-effect size advantage over competing active treatments (Lee, An, Levin, & Twohig, 2015). An example protocol with additional information about acceptance-based treatment for smoking cessation can be found at Brown et al. (2008). As it pertains to brief treatment, acceptance skills are likely to be taught by eliciting an urge to smoke and helping the patient to come into contact with the urge without attempting to distract or avoid. Additionally, a patient may be instructed to wait for 5 min after noticing an urge before smoking. This delay can then be extended until urges come and go without the patient smoking in response. It may also be useful to provide patients with handouts outlining accepting/willingness or distress tolerance skills to practice.

Mindfulness

Mindfulness in this context could be meaningfully considered to be another form of acceptance/willingness, but is specifically mentioned here in order to orient clinicians to its utility in fostering distress tolerance. Mindfulness interventions are most simply described as "paying attention in a particular way: on purpose, in the present moment, and nonjudgmentally" (Kabat-Zinn, 1994) and as "bringing one's complete attention to the present experience on a moment-to-moment basis" (Marlatt & Kristeller, 1999). Mindfulness interventions have been particularly effective as it pertains to lapse recovery (Brewer et al., 2011; Heppner et al., 2016; Vidrine et al., 2016). Specifically, mindfulness skills have proved useful in reducing cravings in response to smoking-related stimuli (Elwafi, Witkiewitz, Mallik, Thornhill, & Brewer, 2013; Westbrook et al., 2013) and reducing affective volatility during cessation attempts (Adams et al., 2014). In practice, BHPs may practice mindfulness interventions during encounters with patients or provide them with materials, links to recorded exercises online, or texts on the subject. There are a wide variety of freely available mindfulness exercises available on the Internet and video hosting websites, making it ideal for lower SES patients.

What Does Not Work

The most recent Cochrane Review on tobacco addiction treatments lists a number of interventions which result in either no increased probability of cessation or worse outcomes than treatment as usual (Hartmann-Boyce et al., 2014). Those interventions listed as largely inert include partner-based interventions, carbon monoxide measurement in primary care settings, spirometry in primary care settings, naltrexone (a medication primarily prescribed to treat opioid and alcohol abuse), and selective serotonin reuptake inhibitors (SSRIs). Additionally, their review revealed the following to decrease chances of abstinence versus comparison: buspirone (a medication typically prescribed to treat generalized anxiety) is associated with a 24% lower chance of cessation when compared to placebo, and similarly St. John's wort is associated with a 19% lower chance of cessation. Programs should be designed to avoid these strategies, and training with medical staff should specifically review the two contraindicated psychoactive substances.

When to Refer to External Specialty Mental Health

Although 100% of patients should be asked about smoking and advised to quit, there are times when treatment should be referred to community mental health resources. The patient characteristics mentioned here will likely be echoed throughout this text, and as a general rule, patients with symptomology more severe than can be safely treated in three to five 30-min sessions should be referred out. As it pertains to smoking, there are three groups which are especially likely to warrant outside referral. Between 75 and 95% of those with a diagnosed substance abuse disorder are regular smokers (Clemmey, Brooner, Chutuape, Kidorf, & Stitzer, 1997; Hurt et al., 1996). Additionally, while smoking cessation interventions do not negatively impact the effectiveness of substance abuse treatment, they do need appear to be effective at long-term follow-up (Prochaska, Delucchi, & Hall, 2004). For those with active substance abuse, a referral for specialty mental treatment is advised prior to engagement in tobacco cessation efforts.

While it may seem obvious that patients diagnosed with schizophrenia are not a good fit for brief integrated care treatments, it is important to note the high rates of smoking seen in this population. In a meta-analysis incorporating over 40 studies conducted across 20 nations, those diagnosed with schizophrenia were nearly six times more likely to be smokers (de Leon & Diaz, 2005). This relationship was still significant after accounting for severe mental illness more generally. There are several competing theories posited to account for this relationship which are outside the scope of this chapter (Gage & Munafo, 2015). What is important is that these patients are better suited for specialty mental healthcare, though BHPs may work with specialist providers to ensure they have evidence-based materials and resources available.

Finally, BHP should seek to refer to more intensive care any individuals who actively engage in provided cessation programs and are still unable to quit. This may be due to individual differences in coping with stress, high levels of anxiety sensitivity (Zvolensky, Farris, Schmidt, & Smits, 2014), or any number of variables specific to the patient. As always, PCPs should be kept apprised of any outside referrals made for their patients.

The Role of the Primary Care Provider/Medical Team in Treatment

Given the close working relationship with BHPs and surrounding medical staff in integrated care programs, it is unsurprising that the role of medical staff has been mentioned several times already. It is critical that PCPs engage patients in the first two As, Ask and Advise. They must also then make quick real-time handoffs to behavioral health staff to facilitate the Assess, Assist, and Arrange follow-up steps. As such, medical staff must be adequately trained prior to implementation of a smoking cessation program, and BHPs must ensure they have buy-in from their surrounding staff. Training health professionals in smoking cessation is associated with a 60% increase in cessation rates (Hartmann-Boyce et al., 2014). A cross-site analysis of a program which incorporated the 5As approach with systematic referrals to intervention in primary care settings found a 40% increase in cessation rate (Land et al., 2012). It is also recommended that

BHPs regularly check in with medical staff to ensure they are updated on shared patients and satisfied with the program.

How to Assess Impact on Care/Quality Improvement Processes

Concurrent with the national guidelines for treating tobacco use, the goal of any implemented program should be for 100% of smokers to receive at least Ask and Advise components (Fiore et al., 2008). This can most easily be accomplished by having the 5As documented inside EMRs. Quality improvement is likely to be primarily undertaken by increasing the rates at which the 5As are regularly completed. Secondarily, health impacts such as blood pressure can be tracked through EMR audits. Finally, medical staff satisfaction should be surveyed quarterly. Special attention should also be paid to improving programs such that they make medical staff more efficient, as opposed to slowing down their workflow.

References

Adams, C. E., Chen, M., Guo, L., Lam, C. Y., Stewart, D. W., Correa-Fernández, V., … Ahluwalia, J. S. (2014). Mindfulness predicts lower affective volatility among African Americans during smoking cessation. *Psychology of Addictive Behaviors, 28*(2), 580–585.

Alshaarawy, O., & Anthony, J. C. (2015). Month-wise estimates of tobacco smoking during pregnancy for the United States, 2002–2009. *Maternal and Child Health Journal, 19*(5), 1010–1015.

Banks, E., Joshy, G., Weber, M. F., Liu, B., Grenfell, R., Egger, S., … Beral, V. (2015). Tobacco smoking and all-cause mortality in a large Australian cohort study: Findings from a mature epidemic with current low smoking prevalence. *BMC Medicine, 13*(38), 1–10.

Bernstein, S. L., Yu, S., Post, L. A., Dziura, J., & Rigotti, N. A. (2013). Undertreatment of tobacco use relative to other chronic conditions. *American Journal of Public Health, 103*, e59–e65.

Brewer, J. A., Mallik, S., Babuscio, T. A., Nich, C., Johnson, H. E., Deleone, C. M., … Carroll, K. M. (2011). Mindfulness training for smoking cessation: Results from a randomized controlled trial. *Drug and Alcohol Dependence, 119*(1), 72–80.

Bricker, J., Wyszynski, C., Comstock, B., & Heffner, J. L. (2013). Pilot randomized controlled trial of web-based acceptance and commitment therapy for smoking cessation. *Nicotine & Tobacco Research, 15*(10), 1756–1764.

Bricker, J. B., Copeland, W., Mull, K. E., Zeng, E. Y., Watson, N. L., Akioka, K. J., & Heffner, J. L. (2017). Single-arm trial of the second version of an acceptance & commitment therapy smartphone application for smoking cessation. *Drug and Alcohol Dependence, 170*, 37–42.

Bricker, J. B., Leroux, B. G., Andersen, M. R., Rajan, K. B., & Peterson, A. V. (2005). Parental smoking cessation and children's smoking: Mediation by antismoking actions. *Nicotine & Tobacco Research, 7*(4), 501–509.

Bricker, J. B., Mann, S. L., Marek, P. M., Liu, J., & Peterson, A. V. (2010). Telephone-delivered acceptance and commitment therapy for adult smoking cessation: A feasibility study. *Nicotine & Tobacco Research, 12*, 454–458.

Bricker, J. B., Mull, K. E., Kientz, J. A., Vilardaga, R., Mercer, L. D., Akioka, K. J., & Heffner, J. L. (2014). Randomized, controlled pilot trial of a smartphone app for smoking cessation using acceptance and commitment therapy. *Drug and Alcohol Dependence, 143*, 87–94.

Bricker, J. B., Otten, R., Liu, J. L., & Peterson, A. V., Jr. (2009). Parents who quit smoking and their adult children's smoking cessation: A 20-year follow-up study. *Addiction, 104*(6), 1036–1042.

Brouwer, R. J. N., & Pomerleau, C. S. (2000). "Prequit attrition" among weight-concerned women smokers. *Eating Behaviors, 1*(2), 145–151.

Brown, D. W. (2010). Smoking prevalence among US veterans. *Journal of General Internal Medicine, 25*(2), 147–149.

Brown, R. A., Lejuez, C. W., Kahler, C. W., & Strong, D. R. (2002). Distress tolerance and duration of past smoking cessation attempts. *Journal of Abnormal Psychology, 111*(1), 180.

Brown, R. A., Palm, K. M., Strong, D. R., Lejuez, C. W., Kahler, C. W., Zvolensky, M. J., … Gifford, E. V. (2008). Distress tolerance treatment for early-lapse smokers rationale, program description, and preliminary findings. *Behavior Modification, 32*(3), 302–332.

Bull, E. R., Dombrowski, S. U., McCleary, N., & Johnston, M. (2014). Are interventions for low-income groups effective in changing healthy eating, physical activity and smoking behaviours? A systematic review and meta-analysis. *BMJ Open, 4*(11), e006046.

Cahill, K., Stevens, S., Perera, R., & Lancaster, T. (2013). Pharmacological interventions for smoking cessation: An overview and network meta-analysis. *Cochrane Database of Systematic Reviews, 5*, 1–44.

Carey, M. P., Kalra, D. L., Carey, K. B., Halperin, S., & Richards, C. S. (1993). Stress and unaided smoking cessation: A prospective investigation. *Journal of Consulting and Clinical Psychology, 61*(5), 831.

Carter, B. D., Abnet, C. C., Feskanich, D., Freedman, N. D., Hartge, P., Lewis, C. E., … Jacobs, E. J. (2015). Smoking and mortality—Beyond established causes. *New England Journal of Medicine, 372*(7), 631–640.

Casetta, B., Videla, A. J., Bardach, A., Morello, P., Soto, N., Lee, K., … Ciapponi, A. (2016). Association between cigarette smoking prevalence and income level: A systematic review and meta-analysis. *Nicotine & Tobacco Research, 19*(12), 1401–1407.

Catchpole, R. E., McLeod, S. L., Brownlie, E. B., Allison, C. J., & Grewal, A. (2016). Cigarette smoking in youths with mental health and substance use problems: Prevalence, patterns, and potential for intervention. *Journal of Child & Adolescent Substance Abuse, 26*, 41–55.

Centers for Disease Control and Prevention (CDC). (2002). Annual smoking-attributable mortality, years of potential life lost, and economic costs--United States, 1995-1999. *MMWR. Morbidity and Mortality Weekly Report, 51*(14), 300.

Chen, T. C., Hamlett-Berry, K. W., Watanabe, J. H., Bounthavong, M., Zillich, A. J., Christofferson, D. E., … Hudmon, K. S. (2015). Evaluation of multidisciplinary tobacco cessation training program in a large health care system. *American Journal of Health Education, 46*(3), 165–173.

Clair, C., Rigotti, N. A., Porneala, B., Fox, C. S., D'Agostino, R. B., Pencina, M. J., & Meigs, J. B. (2013). Association of smoking cessation and weight change with cardiovascular disease among adults with and without diabetes. *JAMA, 309*(10), 1014–1021.

Clemmey, P., Brooner, R., Chutuape, M. A., Kidorf, M., & Stitzer, M. (1997). Smoking habits and attitudes in a methadone maintenance treatment population. *Drug and Alcohol Dependence, 44*(2), 123–132.

Cnattingius, S. (2004). The epidemiology of smoking during pregnancy: Smoking prevalence, maternal characteristics, and pregnancy outcomes. *Nicotine & Tobacco Research, 6*(Suppl 2), S125–S140.

Cohen, S., & Lichtenstein, E. (1990). Perceived stress, quitting smoking, and smoking relapse. *Health Psychology, 9*(4), 466–478.

Davis, R. M. (1988). Uniting physicians against smoking: The need for a coordinated national strategy. *JAMA, 259*, 2900–2901.

de Leon, J., & Diaz, F. J. (2005). A meta-analysis of worldwide studies demonstrates an association between schizophrenia and tobacco smoking behaviors. *Schizophrenia Research, 76*(2), 135–157.

Dwyer-Lindgren, L., Mokdad, A. H., Srebotnjak, T., Flaxman, A. D., Hansen, G. M., & Murray, C. J. (2014). Cigarette smoking prevalence in US counties: 1996-2012. *Population Health Metrics, 12*(1), 1.

Eckert, T., & Junker, C. (2001). Motivation for smoking cessation: What role do doctors play? *Swiss Medical Weekly, 131*(35–36), 521–526.

Ekpu, V. U., & Brown, A. K. (2015). The economic impact of smoking and of reducing smoking prevalence: Review of evidence. *Tobacco Use Insights, 8*, 1–36.

Elwafi, H. M., Witkiewitz, K., Mallik, S., Thornhill, T. A., IV, & Brewer, J. A. (2013). Mindfulness training for smoking cessation: Moderation of the relationship between craving and cigarette use. *Drug and Alcohol Dependence, 130*(1), 222–229.

Farris, S. G., Zvolensky, M. J., Norton, P. J., Hogan, J., Smith, A. H., Talkovsky, A. M., … Schmidt, N. B. (2015). Smoking-specific experiential avoidance is indirectly associated with trait worry and smoking processes among treatment-seeking smokers. *Behavioral Medicine, 42*(4), 254–263.

Farris, S. G., Zvolensky, M. J., & Schmidt, N. B. (2015). Smoking-specific experiential avoidance cognition: Explanatory relevance to pre-and post-cessation nicotine withdrawal, craving, and negative affect. *Addictive Behaviors, 44*, 58–64.

Fiore, M. C., Jaen, C. R., Baker, T., Bailey, W. C., Benowitz, N. L., Curry, S. E. E. A., … Henderson, P. N. (2008). *Treating tobacco use and dependence: 2008 update*. Rockville, MD: US Department of Health and Human Services.

Fiore, M. C., Bailey, W. C., Cohen, S. J., Dorfman, S. F., Goldstein, M. G., Gritz, E. R., ... & Mecklenburg, R. E. (2000). Treating tobacco use and dependence: quick reference guide for clinicians. Rockville, MD: US Department of Health and Human Services. The Public Health Service.

Flegal, K. M. (2012). The conundrum of smoking cessation and weight gain. *Preventive Medicine, 54*(3), 193–194.

Gage, S. H., & Munafò, M. R. (2015). Rethinking the association between smoking and schizophrenia. *The lancet. Psychiatry, 2*(2), 118.

Garey, L., Farris, S. G., Schmidt, N. B., & Zvolensky, M. J. (2016). The role of smoking-specific experiential avoidance in the relation between perceived stress and tobacco dependence, perceived barriers to cessation, and problems during quit attempts among treatment-seeking smokers. *Journal of Contextual Behavioral Science, 5*(1), 58–63.

Gifford, E. V., Kohlenberg, B. S., Hayes, S. C., Antonuccio, D. O., Piasecki, M. M., Rasmussen-Hall, M. L., & Palm, K. M. (2004). Acceptance-based treatment for smoking cessation. *Behavior Therapy, 35*(4), 689–705.

Harrison, R., Preston, P., Bucur, C., & Fletcher, S. V. (2012). P205 smoking prevalence and smoking cessation amongst acute medical admissions. *Thorax, 67*(Suppl 2), A153–A154.

Hartmann-Boyce, J., Stead, L. F., Cahill, K., & Lancaster, T. (2014). Efficacy of interventions to combat tobacco addiction: Cochrane update of 2013 reviews. *Addiction, 109*(9), 1414–1425.

Hawkins, R. P., Kreuter, M., Resnicow, K., Fishbein, M., & Dijkstra, A. (2008). Understanding tailoring in communicating about health. *Health Education Research, 23*(3), 454–466.

Heckman, C. J., Egleston, B. L., & Hofmann, M. T. (2010). Efficacy of motivational interviewing for smoking cessation: A systematic review and meta-analysis. *Tobacco Control, 19*(5), 410–416.

Heffner, J. L., Vilardaga, R., Mercer, L. D., Kientz, J. A., & Bricker, J. B. (2015). Feature-level analysis of a novel smartphone application for smoking cessation. *The American Journal of Drug and Alcohol Abuse, 41*(1), 68–73.

Heppner, W. L., Spears, C. A., Correa-Fernández, V., Castro, Y., Li, Y., Guo, B., … Cinciripini, P. M. (2016). Dispositional mindfulness predicts enhanced smoking cessation and smoking lapse recovery. *Annals of Behavioral Medicine, 50*(3), 337–347.

Hettema, J. E., & Hendricks, P. S. (2010). Motivational interviewing for smoking cessation: A meta-analytic review. *Journal of Consulting and Clinical Psychology, 78*(6), 868–884.

Hitsman, B., Papandonatos, G. D., McChargue, D. E., DeMott, A., Herrera, M. J., Spring, B., … Niaura, R. (2013). Past major depression and smoking cessation outcome: A systematic review and meta-analysis update. *Addiction, 108*(2), 294–306.

Hoeppner, B. B., Hoeppner, S. S., Seaboyer, L., Schick, M. R., Wu, G. W., Bergman, B. G., & Kelly, J. F. (2015). How smart are smartphone apps for smoking cessation? A content analysis. *Nicotine & Tobacco Research, 118*(5), 1025–1031.

Hurt, R. D., Offord, K. P., Croghan, I. T., Gomez-Dahl, L., Kottke, T. E., Morse, R. M., & Melton, L. J. (1996). Mortality following inpatient addictions treatment: Role of tobacco use in a community-based cohort. *JAMA, 275*(14), 1097–1103.

Jamal, A., Dube, S. R., Malarcher, A. M., Shaw, L., Engstrom, M. C., & Centers for Disease Control and Prevention. (2012). Tobacco use screening and counseling during physician office visits among adults—National Ambulatory Medical Care Survey and National Health Interview Survey, United States, 2005–2009. *MMWR Morbidity and Mortality Weekly Report, 61*(Suppl), 38–45.

Jamal, A., Agaku, I. T., O'Connor, E., King, B. A., Kenemer, J. B., & Neff, L. (2014). Current cigarette smoking among adults—United States, 2005–2013. *MMWR Morb Mortal Wkly Rep, 63*(47), 1108–1112.

Jha, P., Ramasundarahettige, C., Landsman, V., Rostron, B., Thun, M., Anderson, R. N., … Peto, R. (2013). 21st-century hazards of smoking and benefits of cessation in the United States. *New England Journal of Medicine, 368*(4), 341–350.

Kabat-Zinn, J. (1994). *Wherever you go, there you are: Mindfulness meditation in everyday life*. New York, NY: Hyperion.

Kassel, J. D., Stroud, L. R., & Paronis, C. A. (2003). Smoking, stress, and negative affect: Correlation, causation, and context across stages of smoking. *Psychological Bulletin, 129*(2), 270.

King, B. A., Dube, S. R., Babb, S. D., & McAfee, T. A. (2013). Patient-reported recall of smoking cessation interventions from a health professional. *Preventive Medicine, 57*(5), 715–717.

Kreuter, M. W., Chheda, S. G., & Bull, F. C. (2000). How does physician advice influence patient behavior?: Evidence for a priming effect. *Archives of Family Medicine, 9*(5), 426–433.

Land, T. G., Rigotti, N. A., Levy, D. E., Schilling, T., Warner, D., & Li, W. (2012). The effect of systematic clinical interventions with cigarette smokers on quit status and the rates of smoking-related primary care office visits. *PLoS One, 7*(7), e41649.

Lawson, P. J., Flocke, S. A., & Casucci, B. (2009). Development of an instrument to document the 5A's for smoking cessation. *American Journal of Preventive Medicine, 37*(3), 248–254.

Lee, E. B., An, W., Levin, M. E., & Twohig, M. P. (2015). An initial meta-analysis of acceptance and commitment therapy for treating substance use disorders. *Drug and Alcohol Dependence, 155*, 1–7.

Lichtenstein, E., Zhu, S. H., & Tedeschi, G. J. (2010). Smoking cessation quitlines: An underrecognized intervention success story. *American Psychologist, 65*(4), 252–261.

Lindson-Hawley, N., Thompson, T. P., & Begh, R. (2015). Motivational interviewing for smoking cessation. *Cochrane Database of Systematic Reviews, 3*, 1–61.

Marlatt, G. A., & Kristeller, J. L. (1999). Mindfulness and meditation. In W. R. Miller (Ed.), *Integrating spirituality into treatment: Resources for practitioners* (pp. 67–84). Washington, DC: American Psychological Association.

Miller, W. R. (2012). MI and psychotherapy. *Motivational Interviewing: Training, Research, Implementation, Practice, 1*, 2–6.

Miller, W. R., & Rollnick, S. (2002). *Motivational interviewing: Preparing people for change* (2nd ed.). New York, NY: Guilford Press.

Mukhopadhyay, S., & Wendel, J. (2011). Is post-smoking-cessation weight-gain a significant trigger for relapse? *Applied Economics, 43*(24), 3449–3457.

Nagelhout, G. E., de Korte-de Boer, D., Kunst, A. E., van der Meer, R. M., de Vries, H., van Gelder, B. M., & Willemsen, M. C. (2012). Trends in socioeconomic inequalities in smoking prevalence, consumption, initiation, and cessation between 2001 and 2008 in the Netherlands: Findings from a national population survey. *BMC Public Health, 12*(303), 1–9.

Nelson, K. E., Hersh, A. L., Nkoy, F. L., Maselli, J. H., Srivastava, R., & Cabana, M. D. (2015). Primary care physician smoking screening and counseling for patients with chronic disease. *Preventive Medicine, 71*, 77–82.

Ng, M., Freeman, M. K., Fleming, T. D., Robinson, M., Dwyer-Lindgren, L., Thomson, B., … Murray, C. J. (2014). Smoking prevalence and cigarette consumption in 187 countries, 1980-2012. *JAMA, 311*(2), 183–192.

North American Quitline Consortium. (2009). *All Quitline facts: An overview of the NAQC 2009 annual survey of Quitlines*. Phoenix, AZ: North American Quitline Consortium.

Ossip-Klein, D. J., McIntosh, S., Utman, C., Burton, K., Spada, J., & Guido, J. (2000). Smokers ages 50+: Who gets physician advice to quit? *Preventive Medicine, 31*(4), 364–369.

Papadakis, S., McDonald, P., Mullen, K. A., Reid, R., Skulsky, K., & Pipe, A. (2010). Strategies to increase the delivery of smoking cessation treatments in primary care settings: A systematic review and meta-analysis. *Preventive Medicine*, *51*(3), 199–213.

Park, E. R., Gareen, I. F., Japuntich, S., Lennes, I., Hyland, K., DeMello, S., … Rigotti, N. A. (2015). Primary care provider-delivered smoking cessation interventions and smoking cessation among participants in the National Lung Screening Trial. *JAMA Internal Medicine*, *175*(9), 1509–1516.

Payne, T. J., Chen, C. I., Baker, C. L., Shah, S. N., Pashos, C. L., & Boulanger, L. (2012). National Ambulatory Medical Care Survey: Tobacco intervention practices in outpatient clinics. *Psychology of Addictive Behaviors*, *26*, 644–648.

Payne, T. J., Gaughf, N. W., Sutton, M. J., Sheffer, C. E., Elci, O. U., Cropsey, K. L., … Crews, K. M. (2014). The impact of brief tobacco treatment training on practice behaviours, self-efficacy and attitudes among healthcare providers. *International Journal of Clinical Practice*, *68*(7), 882–889.

Prochaska, J. J., Delucchi, K., & Hall, S. M. (2004). A meta-analysis of smoking cessation interventions with individuals in substance abuse treatment or recovery. *Journal of Consulting and Clinical Psychology*, *72*(6), 135–157.

Ridner, S. L., Ostapchuk, M., Cloud, R. N., Myers, J., Jorayeva, A., & Ling, J. (2014). Using motivational interviewing for smoking cessation in primary care. *Southern Medical Journal*, *107*(5), 314–319.

Rollnick, S., Miller, W. R., & Butler, C. C. (2007). *Motivational interviewing in health care*. New York, NY: The Guilford Press.

Rom, O., Reznick, A. Z., Keidar, Z., Karkabi, K., & Aizenbud, D. (2015). Smoking cessation-related weight gain—Beneficial effects on muscle mass, strength and bone health. *Addiction*, *110*(2), 326–335.

Rostron, B. L., Chang, C. M., & Pechacek, T. F. (2014). Estimation of cigarette smoking–attributable morbidity in the United States. *JAMA Internal Medicine*, *174*(12), 1922–1928.

Samet, J. M. (2013). Smoking cessation: Benefits versus risks of using pharmacotherapy to quit. *Circulation*, *129*, 8–10.

Sarna, L. P., Bialous, S. A., Kraliková, E., Kmetova, A., Felbrová, V., Kulovaná, S., … Brook, J. K. (2014). Impact of a smoking cessation educational program on nurses' interventions. *Journal of Nursing Scholarship*, *46*(5), 314–321.

Schuck, K., Otten, R., Kleinjan, M., Bricker, J. B., & Engels, R. C. (2014). Self-efficacy and acceptance of cravings to smoke underlie the effectiveness of quitline counseling for smoking cessation. *Drug and Alcohol Dependence*, *142*, 269–276.

Smith, A. (2015). *U.S. smartphone use in 2015*. Pew Research Center. Retrieved from http://www.pewinternet.org/2015/04/01/us-smartphone-use-in-2015/

Sobell, L. C., & Sobell, M. B. (2011). *Group therapy for substance use disorders: A motivational cognitive-behavioral approach*. New York, NY: The Guilford Press.

Stead, L. F., Perera, R., & Lancaster, T. (2007). A systematic review of interventions for smokers who contact quitlines. *Tobacco Control*, *16*(Suppl 1), i3–i8.

Steinberg, M. L., Williams, J. M., & Li, Y. (2015). Poor mental health and reduced decline in smoking prevalence. *American Journal of Preventive Medicine*, *49*(3), 362–369.

Suls, J. M., Luger, T. M., Curry, S. J., Mermelstein, R. J., Sporer, A. K., & An, L. C. (2012). Efficacy of smoking-cessation interventions for young adults: A meta-analysis. *American Journal of Preventive Medicine*, *42*(6), 655–662.

Thun, M. J., Carter, B. D., Feskanich, D., Freedman, N. D., Prentice, R., Lopez, A. D., … Gapstur, S. M. (2013). 50-year trends in smoking-related mortality in the United States. *New England Journal of Medicine*, *368*(4), 351–364.

Tran, B., Falster, M. O., Douglas, K., Blyth, F., & Jorm, L. R. (2015). Smoking and potentially preventable hospitalisation: The benefit of smoking cessation in older ages. *Drug and Alcohol Dependence*, *150*, 85–91.

Travier, N., Agudo, A., May, A. M., Gonzalez, C., Luan, J. A., Wareham, N. J., … Clavel-Chapelon, F. (2012). Longitudinal changes in weight in relation to smoking cessation in participants of the EPIC-PANACEA study. *Preventive Medicine*, *54*(3), 183–192.

Vidrine, J. I., Spears, C. A., Heppner, W. L., Reitzel, L. R., Marcus, M. T., Cinciripini, P. M., … Tindle, H. A. (2016). Efficacy of mindfulness-based addiction treatment (MBAT) for smoking cessation and lapse recovery: A randomized clinical trial. *Journal of Consulting and Clinical Psychology*, *84*(9), 824–838.

Vozoris, N. T., & Stanbrook, M. B. (2011). Smoking prevalence, behaviours, and cessation among individuals with COPD or asthma. *Respiratory Medicine*, *105*(3), 477–484.

Westbrook, C., Creswell, J. D., Tabibnia, G., Julson, E., Kober, H., & Tindle, H. A. (2013). Mindful attention reduces neural and self-reported cue-induced craving in smokers. *Social Cognitive and Affective Neuroscience*, *8*(1), 73–84.

Whitlock, E. P., Orleans, C. T., Pender, N., & Allan, J. (2002). Evaluating primary care behavioral counseling interventions: An evidence-based approach. *American Journal of Preventive Medicine*, *22*(4), 267–284.

Whittaker, R., McRobbie, H., Bullen, C., Rodgers, A., & Gu, Y. (2016). Mobile phone-based interventions for smoking cessation (review). *Cochrane Database of Systematic Reviews*, *4*, 1–46.

Zvolensky, M. J., Farris, S. G., Schmidt, N. B., & Smits, J. A. (2014). The role of smoking inflexibility/avoidance in the relation between anxiety sensitivity and tobacco use and beliefs among treatment-seeking smokers. *Experimental and Clinical Psychopharmacology*, *22*(3), 229–237.

Zwar, N. A., Zwar, N. A., Richmond, R. L., Zwar, N. A., & Richmond, R. L. (2006). Role of the general practitioner in smoking cessation. *Drug and Alcohol Review*, *25*(1), 21–26.

Specific Phobias

38

Ellen I. Koch and Michelle A. Fernando

Description of the Disorder

Diagnostic Criteria

Specific phobias are characterized by immediate, intense, and irrational fear when confronted with a particular object or situation [*Diagnostic and Statistical Manual-5* (*DSM-5*) American Psychiatric Association (APA), 2013]. When confronting the feared stimulus, the individual experiences an automatic physiological reaction that may include increased heart rate, sweating, and fainting in some cases (Fyer, 1998). As a result of this aversive reaction, an individual with specific phobia actively avoids situations that may involve the feared stimulus (*DSM-5*, APA, 2013). Avoidance behaviors can vary in severity and intrusiveness, ranging from taking a different work commute to refusing lifesaving medical treatment, e.g., claustrophobia leading to an inability to have a CT scan. Such behaviors are usually linked to escape from the stimulus, but if contact is unpreventable, avoidance behaviors such as diverting eye contact (Tolin, Lohr, Lee, & Sawchuk, 1999), distraction (Craske, Street, Jayaraman, & Barlow, 1991), or safety signals (Telch, 1994) may also serve to decrease fear. Generally, an individual with specific phobia experiences intense fear when confronting a specific object or situation and often exhibits avoidance behaviors to prevent or cope with this fear.

E.I. Koch (✉) • M.A. Fernando
Department of Psychology, Eastern Michigan University, Ypsilanti, MI, USA
e-mail: ellen.koch@emich.edu; mfernan3@emich.edu

Types

Individuals with specific phobias vary on the type of object or situation they fear. The *DSM-5* includes five different subtypes of specific phobia: animal, natural environment, situational, blood-injury-injection (BII), and other. Animal phobias involve fear of a living organism, such as dogs, spiders, or snakes. Individuals with natural environment phobias fear situations that commonly occur in the environment, such as inclement weather, heights, or water. Similarly, a situational phobia involves specific situations that evoke fear, such as flying, riding in elevators, or being in a large crowd. It is particularly important to differentiate situational phobias from agoraphobia. For example, if the fear is based on a concern regarding the plane crashing, that may suggest a specific phobia; whereas, if the fear is related to being trapped and not able to receive help, agoraphobia should be considered. The BII type involves aspects of medicine and bodily harm, including fear of seeing blood or open wounds, getting blood drawn, receiving an immunization, or going to the dentist. The "other"

A. Maragakis, W.T. O'Donohue (eds.), *Principle-Based Stepped Care and Brief Psychotherapy for Integrated Care Settings*, https://doi.org/10.1007/978-3-319-70539-2_38

subtype of specific phobias includes miscellaneous fears that do not fit into the categories described above, such as vomiting, loud noises, and costumed characters (*DSM-5*, APA, 2013). Under the diagnostic criteria, all potentially feared objects and situations fall under these five categories.

Onset

Specific phobias generally start in childhood and dissipate for some (Merckelbach, De Jong, Muris, & Van Den Hout, 1996). In general, the mean age of onset is 9.7 years old (Stinson et al., 2007), but this varies depending on the type of phobia. A study of adult females in Germany found an average age of onset of 6 years for animal and natural environment phobias (except for heights and water, which were 9 years), 7 years for BII, 9 years for physical phobias (i.e., doctors, vomiting, and infections), and 13 years for situational phobias (Becker et al., 2007). Another study found that BII phobias typically begin around 5.5 years old (Bienvenu & Eaton, 1998). Some phobias such as claustrophobia (Merckelbach et al., 1996) and driving have a later age of onset (Antony, Brown, & Barlow, 1997).

The manifestation of phobia symptoms differs among subtypes. Along with having a later onset, flying phobias can include panic attacks (Lipsitz, Barlow, Mannuzza, Hofmann, & Fyer, 2002). Heights and BII phobias involve more of an internal (i.e., bodily sensation) focus (Antony et al., 1997), while natural environment and situational phobias involve a focus on external danger (Lipsitz et al., 2002). Despite the differences in how phobias manifest, the cause is not different by phobia type (Lipsitz et al., 2002). Therefore, different types of specific phobias vary greatly in terms of symptomology, but not etiology.

Some evidence has suggested that specific phobias are somewhat heritable. Bolton et al. (2006) found that fears and phobias (both symptoms and full diagnosis) are more attributable to genetics than environment for younger children. Van Houtem et al. (2013) also indicated fears and specific phobia are moderately heritable with higher rates for animal and BII phobias. Therefore, individuals with family members diagnosed with specific phobia may be at a higher risk for developing specific phobia in the future.

Among adolescents in the United States, most individuals with specific phobia have more than one type, which in turn is associated with earlier onset and increased severity, impairment, and comorbidity (Burstein et al., 2012). Risk factors for developing specific phobia include being female, young, and having a low income; however, the risk is lower for Hispanic and Asian individuals (Stinson et al., 2007). The onset of specific phobia may lead to a range of other disorders, such as panic disorder, generalized anxiety disorder, and obsessive-compulsive disorder, as well as other anxiety, mood, pain, and eating disorders (Lieb et al., 2016). Therefore, it is important to assess for risk factors and comorbidities when diagnosing specific phobias.

Prevalence

There is a high prevalence of specific phobias from childhood to older adulthood. Paulus, Backes, Sander, Weber, and von Gontard (2014) found that 10% of preschoolers had specific phobia, including 7% of boys and 13% of girls. When based on parent interviews, 18% of children met diagnostic criteria for a phobia; when based on child interviews, this amount grew to 20% (Muris & Merckelbach, 2000). In adolescents, 20% of the sample experienced specific phobias, including 23% of females and 17% of males (Kessler, Petukhova, Sampson, Zaslavsky, & Wittchen, 2012). Among adults, approximately 12–18% of females and 6–10% of males meet diagnostic criteria for a specific phobia (Kessler et al., 2012; Stinson et al., 2007). Kessler et al. (2012) found a lifetime prevalence of 16% and a decreasing 12-month prevalence over time including 16% for adolescents, 10% for adults, and 5% for the elderly. Phobia rates may decrease steadily with age; in a 9-year follow-up study, specific phobia diagnoses decreased from 10% at age 70 to 4% at age 79 (Sigström, Skoog, Karlsson, Nilsson, &

Östling, 2016). Overall, the lifetime morbidity risk for specific phobia is 18.4%, which is the second most prevalent disorder (behind depression) and the most prevalent anxiety disorder (Kessler et al., 2012).

As reported, specific phobias are prevalent disorders; however, rates differ by location and country. In terms of international adult samples, rates range from 2 to 3% in China and Japan (Kawakami et al., 2005; Shen et al., 2005), 4–5% in South Korea (Cho et al., 2007; Park et al., 2013), 7–8% in New Zealand and Europe (Alonso et al., 2004; Wells et al., 2006), and 13% in Germany (Becker et al., 2007). In a sample of elderly individuals from Turkey, 11.5% had current and lifetime specific phobia, with the highest rates in the youngest elderly age group (Kirmizioglu, Dogan, Kugu, & Akyuz, 2009). In Spain, an adult primary care sample had 12-month and lifetime prevalence rates of 7% (8% for females and 5% for males; Serrano-Blanco et al., 2010).

The prevalence rates for types of specific phobias within international samples range from 2 to 8% for animal phobias, 0.4–13% for situational phobias, 0.5–4% for BII phobias, 1–2% for natural environment phobias (excluding heights), and 2–5% for height phobias (Becker et al., 2007; Bienvenu & Eaton, 1998; Depla, ten Have, van Balkom, & de Graaf, 2008; Fredrikson, Annas, Fischer, & Wik, 1996; Park et al., 2013; Stinson et al., 2007). Fredrikson et al. (1996) indicated that flying phobia increased and fear of injections decreased as a function of age in females only. Because specific phobia varies by location, it may be useful to look at area-specific base rates to guide diagnosis.

Specific phobias can last over 20 years, probably because few people (8–13%) seek treatment (Iza et al., 2013; Mackenzie, Reynolds, Cairney, Streiner, & Sareen, 2012; Stinson et al., 2007). Individuals take approximately 13 years to seek treatment, which represents the slowest and lowest percentage of treatment seeking among the anxiety disorders (Iza et al., 2013). For a Mexican adolescent population, only 6.5% of individuals with a phobia sought treatment (Benjet, Borges, Stein, Méndez, & Medina-Mora, 2012). Of those that do seek treatment, only 30% do so because of their fears (Zimmerman & Mattia, 2000). Individuals with more education, who are older, and sought treatment in the past are more likely to seek treatment for specific phobia (Iza et al., 2013). Despite specific phobias being extremely common, few people actually seek treatment for their fear.

Given the high prevalence and comorbidity rates of specific phobia, early identification and treatment is essential within a primary care setting. Appropriate screening is particularly important given that many individuals will not initiate treatment for specific phobias.

Screening Options in Integrated Care

A recent veteran study examining rates of anxiety diagnoses indicated that a significant number of specific phobia (45%) and anxiety not otherwise specified (NOS; 67%) diagnoses were made in a primary care setting compared to specialty mental health services. Additionally, individuals diagnosed in a primary care setting with anxiety NOS were less likely to receive treatment compared to those with a diagnosis in specialty mental health care (Barrera et al., 2014). Due to the high rates of disorders (particularly specific phobia) and the low level of treatment seeking, empirically validated assessments and interventions within primary care settings are essential (Chavira, Stein, Bailey, & Stein, 2004). Quality screening and brief interventions could potentially assist many patients presenting to primary care.

Although brief screening measures for multiple types of specific phobia are not currently available, clinicians are encouraged to ask patients if they have any items, objects, or situations that they fear or avoid, particularly if the fear is negatively impacting their lives. For example, if a patient is refusing medical tests or procedures, it will be important to determine if this is based on fear. A comprehensive list of possible fears is available with the Fear Survey Schedule-III (Wolpe & Lang, 1977) if screening for a wide range of fears is desired. If these broad screening approaches produce positive results, the clinician can conduct a more thorough assessment of the specific phobia(s).

Additional Assessment for Positive Screening

If a broad screening approach suggests the individual may have a specific phobia, a diagnostic interview can be completed, or the individual can be asked to complete a self-report questionnaire specifically designed for the type of phobia (see Table 38.1). One primary example is the widely used Spider Phobia Questionnaire (Klorman, Weerts, Hastings, Melamed, & Lang, 1974) and a more recently developed abbreviated version of the Spider Phobia Questionnaire with strong psychometric properties (Olatunji et al., 2009).

Table 38.1 Commonly used specific phobia measures

Measure	Phobia type	Number of items	Citation
Spider Phobia Questionnaire (SPQ)	Spiders	31	Klorman et al. (1974)
Fear of Spiders Questionnaire (FSQ)	Spiders	18	Szymanski and O'Donohue (1995)
Abbreviated Spider Questionnaire (SPQ-15)	Spiders	15	Olatunji et al. (2012)
Medical Fear Survey (MFS-short version)	BII	25	Olatunji et al. (2012)
Mutilation Questionnaire (MQ)	BII	30	Kleinknecht and Thorndike (1990)
Emetophobia Questionnaire (EmetQ-13)	Vomiting	13	Boschen, Veale, Ellison, and Reddell (2013)
Claustrophobia Questionnaire (CLQ)	Enclosed spaces	26	Radomsky, Rachman, Thordarson, McIsaac, and Teachman (2001)
Acrophobia Questionnaire (AQ)	Heights	40	Cohen (1977)
Driving Cognitions Questionnaire (DCQ)	Driving	20	Ehlers et al. (2007)

Typically, along with self-report scales, screening for specific phobia utilizes a behavioral approach test (BAT) if possible. A BAT involves the individual approaching the feared item or situation as much as they possibly can and providing a Subjective Units of Distress Scale (SUDS) rating for fear on a 0–100 scale where 0 is the *least anxiety ever experienced in the presence of the item/situation* and 100 is the *worst anxiety ever experienced with the item/situation*. The distance from the object and fear rating during approach are recorded along with any overt physiological responses from the individual.

Given that a specific phobia may not significantly interfere with functioning for a particular individual, it is important to assess both the negative impact the specific phobia is having for the person and the motivation and willingness to overcome the fear. If avoiding the feared item/situation is problematic (e.g., impacting ability to complete one's job, receiving medical care like an injection or MRI, etc.) or unavoidable confrontations are extremely distressing, the individual would be a good candidate for treatment. Treatment entails confronting the feared object/situation so it will be important to determine if the individual is motivated to overcome the fear even though it will be difficult and distressing. Additionally, given that some levels of stepped care will involve significant patient initiation, assessing treatment acceptability for the individual will be important to determine if any barriers exist.

Evidence-Based Care and Brief Psychotherapeutic Approaches

Specific phobias are highly treatable conditions that respond well to short-term and often exposure-based behavioral interventions (Choy, Fyer, & Lipsitz, 2007). In situations where it is difficult to conduct in vivo exposure (e.g., flying), virtual reality treatments are an effective alternative (Grös & Antony, 2006). Cognitive-based interventions are usually less effective for the treatment of specific phobias, although some evidence has been found for dental phobia and claustrophobia (Choy et al., 2007). A particularly good website reviewing treatment options for specific phobias is maintained by the Society of Clinical Psychology: http://www.div12.org/psychological-treatments/treatments/exposure-therapies-for-specific-phobias/. Because direct confrontation of the fear is difficult, the ability of the individual to do so on their own with guidance will help determine which level of stepped care is most appropriate.

Psychoeducation

Psychoeducation is important for any treatment program, not only to provide information for the patient and potentially correct misinformation but also to increase motivation for treatment. Psychoeducation for specific phobia should include discussing signs and symptoms of specific phobias, the protective function of fear and the fight-flight response, that this is a common and treatable condition, etiology, safety behaviors that may perpetuate or worsen fear, the negative reinforcement of escape behaviors and long-term impact of avoidance, treatment options, and the rationale for treatment.

Self-Help/e-Health/Bibliotherapy

A main resource for self-help/bibliotherapy is *The Anxiety and Phobia Workbook (6th edition)* by Bourne (2015). This book is designed to be utilized by the patient without the need for professional involvement (unless problems arise). Additional self-help books are available and could be reviewed for relevant content to recommend to patients.

One computer-assisted exposure (CAE) program, FearFighter (http://fearfighter.cbtprogram.com/), is available online with packages starting at approximately $125 addressing phobias and panic. The program has been empirically validated (Marks, Kenwright, McDonough, Whittaker, & Mataix-Cols, 2004). A novel CAE treatment option involves a video game and is currently being investigated in a randomized controlled trial for spiders (Miloff et al., 2016). These computer-based programs can be done independently without the clinician.

Although virtual reality equipment has historically been expensive, new equipment is now readily available for under $150 that utilizes a smartphone. However, the quality of the applications available for these systems has not been empirically validated. Therefore, the applications will require careful review by the clinician to determine if the program is appropriate for the patient and sufficiently generates anxiety facilitating effective exposure. In general, such programs and books should be carefully reviewed by the clinician before recommending any self-help treatment to a patient.

Guided Self-Help/Group

Animal

Since many integrated care sessions last from 20 to 30 min, treatment of animal phobias may need to be abbreviated or adapted to fit this time frame. In one study, researchers greatly reduced clinician time by switching to an Internet-aided treatment program. In this 4-week spider phobia program, patients used computer-based modules for psychoeducation and to watch a video modelling spider exposure. After watching the video, patients were instructed to safely conduct their own exposure therapy at home, paying special attention to avoidance and cognitions. Once the initial exposure was completed, the patient was then instructed on how to expand what was learned during exposure to other life situations. Because the majority of this program was self-administered from the patient's home, patients contacted the therapist for a total of 25 min over a 4-week span, not including initial and follow-up assessments. This therapy was shown to be comparably effective to one-session exposure treatment (OST), with no significant differences in the BAT posttreatment, and at 1-year follow-up

(Andersson et al., 2009). Similar results have been shown for an analogous snake phobia treatment (Andersson et al., 2013). In an integrated care setting, computer-aided exposure therapy can be supplemented with 20–30 min in-person therapy sessions to review progress or go over homework. When longer exposure sessions are not practical, computer-assisted and self-administered exposure therapy may be useful in time-limited, integrated care settings.

Situational

Although some situational phobias may be amenable to in vivo exposure in an integrated care setting, alternative methods may be used when this is not possible. For example, it is often not practical to purchase a plane ticket and ride through an entire flight with a patient, as is performed in in vivo flying exposure (Öst, Brandberg, & Alm, 1997). In these cases, the clinician may rely on virtual reality exposure (VRE) and CAE. In VRE, the patient wears an immersive head-mounted display that depicts takeoff, turbulence, and landing. VRE has been shown to decrease fear of flying both in multiple baseline studies (Botella-Arbona, Osma, Garcia-Palacios, Quero, & Banõs, 2004) and when compared to standard in vivo exposure (Rothbaum et al., 2006). It has also been effective for other types of situational phobias, such as claustrophobia (Malbos, Mestre, Note, & Gellato, 2008). CAE can also be used to treat flying phobia. In CAE, the patient uses a personal computer to view pictures of anxiety-provoking flying situations, such as packing for the flight, traveling to the airport, boarding the plane, flying, and hearing news about an airplane accident, and incorporates the use of sound similar to VRE (Tortella-Feliu et al., 2011). CAE has similar efficacy to VRE and cognitive therapy and can be used by the patient with minimal clinician interaction (Bornas, Tortella-Feliu, & Llabrés, 2006; Tortella-Feliu et al., 2011). When in vivo exposure is not available, the use of VRE or CAE may be a more practical exposure method.

Phobias in General

A particularly good treatment manual for phobias is *Mastering Your Fears and Phobias Workbook (2nd edition)* by Antony, Craske, and Barlow (2006). The workbook is designed to be completed by the patient with guidance from the clinician (an accompanying therapist guide is available). The clinician could be available for coaching by phone, email, face-to-face, chat, etc.; however, the patient would be primarily responsible for implementing the intervention.

Group treatment options would involve less clinician time; however, it may be difficult to gather a group of sufficient size to address one specific phobia. An option would be to have a general facing your fears group that can be attended by patients regardless of the content of their specific fear(s). The group should include homework assignments that allow the patient to engage in exposure for their fear between sessions and receive feedback on their progress during the group.

Brief Treatment

Blood-Injury-Injection (BII)

Given that individuals with BII phobia typically experience vasovagal syncope, a main component of treatment is teaching the individual to counteract the fainting response well before the process begins. Specifically, the clinician helps the patient identify the early warning signs that they are beginning to feel faint or identify the high-risk situations where fainting is most likely. The patient then engages in major muscle group contractions in order to stabilize their blood pressure and prevent fainting (see Öst & Sterner, 1987 for a complete description). It can be particularly helpful to measure blood pressure so that the patient can observe the change that applied tension produces during the initial training phase.

The applied tension technique can be effectively utilized in one session (Hellström, Fellenius, & Öst, 1996; Öst, Hellström, & Kåver, 1992).

A recent study found that rhythmic tension (brief 5 s of tension followed by 5 s of rest and repeating the process) was more effective at raising diastolic blood pressure than the constant tension approach (approximately 15 s followed by 20–30 s of release) as utilized in previous research (Bodycoat, Grauaug, Olson, & Page, 2017). However, because this study did not involve individuals with BII, it is difficult to confidently infer the effect remains for those with this type of specific phobia. Once the patient is reliably using the applied tension technique, the psychologist can implement the remaining treatment.

Situational

Cognitive therapy may also be a useful treatment, as individuals with situational phobia tend to misinterpret physical and cognitive symptoms (Craske & Sipsas, 1992). Although participants with claustrophobia showed slightly less reduction and fear after cognitive therapy, this therapy was comparably effective to OST and five session exposure techniques (Öst, Alm, Brandberg, & Breitholtz, 2001). Cognitive therapy for situational phobia should involve addressing irrational thoughts regarding the feared situation and teaching coping skills to cope with anxiety (Kraaij, Garnefski, & Van Gerwen, 2003). When exposure is not achievable, cognitive therapy may offer a good alternative for situational phobias.

Phobias in General

Other portions of interventions that could be completed by non-psychologists include problem-solving and relaxation to address general symptoms of anxiety. In terms of relaxation, *The Relaxation and Stress Reduction Workbook (6th edition)* by Davis, Eschelman, and McKay (2008) offers chapters on several relaxation strategies. This provides an opportunity to select relaxation procedures that may best fit the patient. Additionally, the relaxation chapter for *The Anxiety and Phobia Workbook (6th edition)* by Bourne (2015) is comprehensive and provides a variety of options for guided procedures.

Longer Treatment

Blood-Injury-Injection (BII)

Treatment for BII also involves exposure procedures to facilitate facing the fear. Once the patient is using the applied tension technique effectively, the clinician can begin to have the patient confront their fear hierarchy starting with items that produce moderate anxiety and eventually moving to tasks higher on the established hierarchy. The hierarchy is created by both the clinician and patient and ideally should have about 10–12 items that range from mildly, moderately, to severely anxiety producing. The clinician then systematically works with the patient to face hierarchy items both in session and outside of session. The additional work outside of session is important for generalization; however, it is expected that the patient will be able to confront items higher on the fear list with the clinician present than when working on their own. To increase generalization, the clinician should assign home confrontations that are realistic and not overwhelming for the patient, using tasks that are at least one step down on the fear hierarchy from what was achieved in session.

Given that a variety of stimuli (e.g., needles, blood draw stations, etc.) related to BII phobias are available in integrated care settings, this type of phobia can be successfully treated on site. Additionally, the integrated care setting would have access to blood pressure monitors that would allow the patient to have concrete evidence that they are utilizing the applied tension technique correctly (i.e., increase diastolic blood pressure to prevent fainting). Finally, as patients with BII phobias may also fear injury or illness, being present within the integrated care setting may allow for the patient to confront these fears simultaneously. Most integrated care settings already contain the equipment and setting needed for in vivo BII exposure therapy.

Animal

While there are a variety of treatment options available for animal phobia, the most effective includes an exposure component. Generally, exposure therapy is the treatment of choice for specific phobias, preferably in longer or more frequent sessions as opposed to abbreviated, infrequent sessions (Grös & Antony, 2006). For animal phobia, one-session exposure (OST) is a commonly used and well-established treatment method (Davis, Ollendick, & Öst, 2012; Öst, 1989). In this treatment, the patient gradually confronts the feared animal in vivo, beginning with approaching the animal and ending with directly handling the animal. Each step is first modeled by the clinician and then performed by the patient. The patient is encouraged to approach or stay with the animal until anxiety decreases, which prevents avoidance and promotes extinction of the feared response. Treatment is finished when the patient can complete the approach tasks with a greatly reduced anxiety level, usually about 50% of their original anxiety rating (Öst, 1989). The entire treatment is completed within one extended session, with a mean treatment time of 2.1 h (Davis et al., 2012). This therapy is most commonly clinician-administered on an individual basis, but it has also been shown to be effective in group settings (Öst, 1996; Öst, Ferebee, & Furmark, 1997) and to a lesser extent in self-administered manualized forms (Hellström & Öst, 1995). OST is the treatment of choice for animal phobias.

Although OST is a relatively short and successful treatment, it may not be practical in some integrated treatment settings. First, storage and care of live animals may not be possible in a healthcare setting that depends on cleanliness and sterility. Second, OST requires a prolonged session to achieve the desired behavior extinction; this time may not be practical in a clinic that usually sees patients in 20–30 min sessions. Therefore, OST may be difficult to implement in some integrated care settings.

It may be possible to adapt exposure treatment to better accommodate the unique features of integrated care. For example, virtual reality exposure (VRE) and augmented reality exposure (ARE) programs may be a good alternative option when the use of live animals is not possible. In VRE, exposure takes place within a completely computer-simulated setting in which the patient can interact with the feared animal. The patient accesses this virtual setting by viewing a computer monitor or wearing a virtual reality headset. To make interaction with the animal more realistic, tactile stimulation may be used when the patient is "handling" the virtual object (Carlin, Hoffman, & Weghorst, 1997; Hoffman, Garcia-Palacios, Carlin, Furness, & Botella-Arbona, 2003). Although VRE programs are still developing for a variety of specific phobia types, this treatment modality is an effective option when live exposure is not possible (Garcia-Palacios, Hoffman, Carlin, Furness, & Botella, 2002).

Similarly, ARE entails the use of virtual technology to project the feared stimulus onto the patient's immediate environment. When using ARE, the patient sees his or her actual environment (i.e., the office desk or floor) with the animal projected onto it. Because the patient maintains a sense of presence in the real world, ARE may seem more realistic and evoke an anxiety reaction more similar to in vivo exposure (Baus & Bouchard, 2014). Although this technology is still being developed, ARE is another potential treatment option (Botella et al., 2016).

Therefore, VRE and ARE may be good treatment options in settings that are not amenable to live exposure. For approximately $700, Virtually Better, Inc. (http://www.virtuallybetter.com/) offers empirically validated programs developed by psychologists and includes a package that covers the following fears: heights, elevators, spiders, storms, hurricanes, tornadoes, flying, and public speaking. Other companies include Virtual Reality Medical Center (fear of flying system that includes airplane seats and subwoofer: http://www.vrphobia.com/), VirtualRet (fears of flying, heights, blood-injury-injection, and public speaking along with agoraphobia: http://www.virtualret.com/en/), CleVR (fears of flying, heights, and social situations: http://clevr.net/en/), and Psious (online options for fears of flying, needles, heights, driving, animals, enclosed spaces, and public speaking as well as agoraphobia and generalized anxiety disorder: https://psious.com/). These virtual reality options provide greater flexibility for implementing exposure treatment.

Although OST is the most commonly used treatment for animal phobia, numerous technological advancements allow exposure to be adapted for use within an integrated care setting. In settings where one cannot access live animals for exposure, VRE or ARE may be helpful in navigating these obstacles. Similarly, in settings that rely on abbreviated treatment sessions, it may be helpful to use Internet-based treatment that encourages the patient to continue treatment at home. Regardless, there are a variety of exposure modalities that can be used to effectively treat animal phobia.

Situational

Similar to animal phobia, exposure therapy is most commonly used to treat situational phobia. OST has been shown to effectively decrease phobia of flying (Öst et al., 1997) and claustrophobia (Öst et al., 2001) at posttreatment and at 1-year follow-up. Unlike animal phobia, successive approach to the feared object is sometimes not possible; in these cases, the individual is either immersed fully in the situation or not. For claustrophobia, the clinician can successively increase the amount of time the patient stays in the enclosed space and alter whether the door is open, closed, or locked (Davis et al., 2012). For flying phobia, the clinician can have the patient successively confront the feared flying-related situations, such as going to the airport, checking into the flight, and ending with completing an entire flight (Öst et al., 1997). In either sense, the clinician and patient work together to create a hierarchy of situations related to the phobia and successively introduce feared situations starting from the least to most fearful-evoking.

For some situational phobias, in vivo OST can be performed conveniently within the integrated care setting. For claustrophobia exposure, the clinician can use a small windowless closet, elevator, or any confined space available within the clinic. However, it is important to note that, while OST can be completed within a single session, these sessions are quite long (typically 1–2 h) and require a large amount of clinician time (Davis et al., 2012). Although an integrated care setting may be amenable to situational phobia exposure, the time required for exposure may not fit into a brief therapy session.

When these exposure techniques are not practical in a fast-paced, integrated care setting, cognitive therapy can be used to target maladaptive thoughts and teach coping skills to help the patient cope with anxiety when they are in the feared situation. Such techniques may be especially useful for flying phobias, where the treatment goal may be just to "get through" an upcoming flight. In general, situational phobias offer some flexibility for treatment within the integrated care setting.

Natural

Natural environment phobias typically include fears of storms, heights, and water. In children, natural environment phobias are more difficult to treat than animal phobias (Ollendick, Raishevich, Davis, Sirbu, & Öst, 2010). Although case studies are available for natural environment phobias, only two studies have involved treating water phobia in children, and several studies have provided treatment for heights among adults. In relation to the fear of water, Menzies and Clarke (1993) found 20 min of in vivo exposure was superior to combining in vivo and vicarious exposure (modeling of non-fearful performance) in children aged 3–8. Additionally, Ultee, Griffioen, and Schellekens (1982) indicated eight sessions of in vivo treatment was superior to four sessions each of gradual imaginal desensitization and exposure in vivo for children 5–10 years old.

In terms of fear of heights with adults, one study found guided mastery to be more effective than desensitization alone (Williams, Turner, & Peer, 1985), and another study found 6-min trials involving exposure and opposite action to be significantly better at posttest and follow-up compared to exposure alone (Wolitzky & Telch, 2009). The remaining studies addressing height phobia for adults include the use of VRE as the primary exposure component (de Quervain et al., 2011; Glantz, Durlach, Barnett, & Aviles, 1996; Gregg & Tarrier, 2007; Huang, Himle, & Alessi, 2000; Krijn, Emmelkamp, Ólafsson, Schuemie,

& Van Der Mast, 2007; Ressler, Rothbaum, Tannenbaum, & Anderson, 2004; Smits et al., 2013).

Two VRE studies with height phobia found d-cycloserine added to two sessions produced significantly better results by enhancing extinction learning between session particularly when paired with successful fear reduction (Ressler et al., 2004; Smits et al., 2013). Additionally, one study found cortisol paired with three sessions of VRE was significantly better than VRE with placebo at both posttest and follow-up (de Quervain et al., 2011). One VRE study did not find any benefit to adding coping statements to the treatment (Krijn et al., 2007). Despite the fact that several studies have utilized VRE procedures, Gregg and Tarrier (2007) indicated that virtual reality exposure is not supported over traditional exposure treatment for height phobia.

In terms of addressing height phobia within an integrated care setting, a stairwell, elevator, or parking structure could be utilized to complete the BAT and facilitate the patient facing their fear. Similarly to approaches for other types of specific phobia, the clinician and the patient can work collaboratively to create an exposure hierarchy that includes situations that produce at least moderate anxiety with some feasible options for the integrated care setting. As it is not necessary to complete each item on the hierarchy within session, the patient should feel free to list some situations that cannot be completed within the integrated care setting. The clinician and patient begin to systematically confront the feared situations from moderately to severely anxiety provoking in session. Additionally, the clinician assigns homework for between session progress to promote generalization and additional fear reduction.

Other

Little empirical research is available for the "other" type of phobias; however, a recent study utilized cognitive behavioral treatment for fear of vomiting, and 58% of participants showed significant improvement (Riddle-Walker et al., 2016). Another researcher recently found a group intervention effective for fear of vomiting (Ahlen, Edberg, Di Schiena, & Bergstrom, 2015). Despite the lack of research focused on "other" phobias, the intervention should still utilize exposure-based procedures if possible. Similarly to how exposure-based procedures are utilized in integrated care settings described for the other phobia subtypes, these various phobias also respond to creating a hierarchy, accessing appropriate stimuli to facilitate fear confrontation, and systemic exposure to the feared stimulus until anxiety reduces both within and outside of the integrated care setting.

Other Treatment Options

In addition to the exposure-based treatment procedures described above, in situations where direct confrontation of feared stimuli is either very difficult or not possible, systematic desensitization or imaginal exposure procedures may be utilized. Cognitive therapy options can also be beneficial, and research supports the use of these interventions particularly with height phobia (Steinman & Teachman, 2014). However, the use of in vivo exposure procedures is still preferred for all specific phobias (Baldwin et al., 2014). Ideally these would be administered with direct confrontation in vivo, but in situations where that is not possible, VRE is a good alterative option for many specific phobias.

What Does Not Work

There is little published research on the treatment of specific phobias with non-psychotherapeutic methods, such as with pharmaceuticals. In one study, exposure therapy treatment had twice the effect size of benzodiazepine treatment alone, and combined treatment of exposure therapy and benzodiazepine did not increase treatment effects compared to exposure alone (Marks et al., 1993). There is some evidence to support the use of d-cycloserine to enhance the effects of exposure therapy, but this evidence is inconsistent (Guastella, Dadds, Lovibond, Mitchell, & Richardson, 2007; Smits et al., 2013). Therefore, there is little evidence to support the use of pharmacological treatment as the sole or primary treatment for specific phobia.

In both self-exposure and guided-exposure, it is necessary to remain in the situation until anxiety reduces (ideally at least by half), so it is important to have a sufficient block of time for this to occur. If the session is nearing the end, it is necessary to either finish the current step with reduced anxiety or move back a step or two on the hierarchy in order to "master" that step and finish at reduced anxiety. Additionally, it is unlikely that the patient will be able to conduct the same level of exposure at home as in the office. Therefore, homework assignments should entail something that will be challenging for the patient, but they are likely to experience success. Specifically, they will need to be able to tolerate the heightened anxiety and remain in the situation until their anxiety reduces. Leaving the exposure situation with heightened anxiety is likely to cause exacerbation of the fear or treatment dropout.

When to Refer to Specialty Mental Health

Although many clinicians could successfully treat specific phobias within an integrated care setting, given that many people do not seek treatment for specific phobia and the high prevalence rate of comorbidity for those with specific phobias may warrant referral to specialty mental health care. If a patient has high comorbidity, impairment, and distress, referral to specialty mental health care may be in the best interest of the patient. Patients with significant anxiety, mood, eating, or pain disorders in conjunction with specific phobia may benefit from a thorough mental health evaluation and course of treatment to fully address the various presenting issues and their severity.

Role of Primary Medical Provider in Treatment

Given the high prevalence but low rate of treatment seeking for specific phobia, the primary medical provider can assist the integrated care clinician by conducting effective screening of patients and routinely asking about specific phobias. Additionally, the medical provider can assist with evaluating the severity of comorbid conditions and determining if, in conjunction with the clinician, the patient may benefit from a combination of medication and psychological treatment to effectively address multiple presenting concerns. This may be particularly relevant if the patient is experiencing significant impairment or distress from their symptoms.

Assessing Impact on Care and Quality Improvement

Given the high prevalence rate of specific phobias, it will be important to monitor treatment and determine the extent that reducing the phobia and other comorbid conditions would successfully contribute to the patient's medical care. It is expected that successful treatment will result in less utilization of the medical system and significant cost savings. Additionally, determining the improvement in quality of life following treatment could indicate the overall impact of treatment for the individual. Clinicians working in integrated care settings can monitor the impact of psychological interventions on overall health particularly related to efficacy and efficiency. This process could facilitate improvements in our treatment techniques particularly within the integrated care setting to the benefit of patients and medical care providers.

References

Ahlen, J., Edberg, E., Di Schiena, M., & Bergstrom, J. (2015). Cognitive behavioural group therapy for emetophobia: An open study in a psychiatric setting. *Clinical Psychologist, 19*(2), 96–104. https://doi.org/10.1111/cp.12040

Alonso, J., Angermeyer, M. C., Bernert, S., Bruffaerts, R., Brugha, T. S., Bryson, H., … Vollebergh, W. A. (2004). Prevalence of mental disorders in Europe: Results from the European Study of the Epidemiology of Mental Disorders (ESEMeD) project. *Acta Psychiatrica Scandinavica Supplementum, 109*(420), 21–27. https://doi.org/10.1111/j.1600-0047.2004.00327.x

American Psychiatric Association. (2013). *Diagnostic and statistical manual of mental disorders* (5th ed.). Washington, DC: Author.

Andersson, G., Waara, J., Jonsson, U., Malmaeus, F., Carlbring, P., & Öst, L.-G. (2013). Internet-based exposure treatment versus one-session exposure treatment of snake phobia: A randomized controlled trial. *Cognitive Behaviour Therapy, 42*(4), 284–291. https://doi.org/10.1080/16506073.2013.844202

Andersson, G., Waara, J., Jonsson, U., Malmaeus, F., Carlbring, P., & Öst, L-G. (2009) Internet-based self-help versus one-session exposure in the treatment of spider phobia: A randomized controlled trial. *Cognitive Behaviour Therapy, 38*, 114–120. https://doi.org/10.1080/16506070902931326

Antony, M. M., Brown, T. A., & Barlow, D. H. (1997). Heterogeneity among specific phobia types in *DSM-IV*. *Behaviour Research and Therapy, 35*(12), 1089–1100. https://doi.org/10.1016/S0005-7967(97)00075-2

Antony, M. M., Craske, M. G., & Barlow, D. H. (2006). *Mastering your fears and phobias workbook* (2nd ed.). New York, NY: Oxford University Press.

Baldwin, D. S., Anderson, I. M., Nutt, D. J., Allgulander, C., Bandelow, B., den Boer, J. A., … Wittchen, H.-U. (2014). Evidence-based pharmacological treatment of anxiety disorders, post-traumatic stress disorder and obsessive-compulsive disorder: A revision of the 2005 guidelines from the British Association for Psychopharmacology. *Journal of Psychopharmacology, 28*, 403–439. https://doi.org/10.1177/0269881114525674

Barrera, T. L., Mott, J. M., Hundt, N. E., Mignogna, J., Yu, H. J., Stanley, M. A., & Cully, J. A. (2014). Diagnostic specificity and mental health service utilization among veterans with newly diagnosed anxiety disorders. *General Hospital Psychiatry, 36*(2), 192–198. https://doi.org/10.1016/j.genhosppsych.2013.10.013

Baus, O., & Bouchard, S. (2014, March). Moving from virtual reality exposure-based therapy to augmented reality exposure-based therapy: A review. *Frontiers in Human Neuroscience, 8*, 112. https://doi.org/10.3389/fnhum.2014.00112

Becker, E. S., Rinck, M., Türke, V., Kause, P., Goodwin, R., Neumer, S., & Margraf, J. (2007). Epidemiology of specific phobia subtypes: Findings from the Dresden Mental Health Study. *European Psychiatry, 22*(2), 69–74. https://doi.org/10.1016/j.eurpsy.2006.09.006

Benjet, C., Borges, G., Stein, D. J., Méndez, E., & Medina-Mora, M. E. (2012). Epidemiology of fears and specific phobia in adolescence: Results from the Mexican adolescent mental health survey. *Journal of Clinical Psychiatry, 73*(2), 152–158. https://doi.org/10.4088/JCP.11m07442

Bienvenu, O. J., & Eaton, W. W. (1998). The epidemiology of blood-injection-injury phobia. *Psychological Medicine, 28*(5), 1129–1136.

Bodycoat, N., Grauaug, L., Olson, A., & Page, A. C. (2017). Constant versus rhythmic muscle tension in applied tension. *Behaviour Change, 17*(2), 97–102.

Bolton, D., Eley, T. C., O'Connor, T. G., Perrin, S., Rabe-Hesketh, S., Rijsdijk, F., & Smith, P. (2006). Prevalence and genetic and environmental influences on anxiety disorders in 6-year-old twins. *Psychological Medicine, 36*(3), 335–344. https://doi.org/10.1017/S0033291705006537

Bornas, X., Tortella-Feliu, M., & Llabrés, J. (2006). Do all treatments work for flight phobia? Computer-assisted exposure versus a brief multicomponent nonexposure treatment. *Psychotherapy Research, 16*(1), 41–50. https://doi.org/10.1080/10503300500091058

Boschen, M. J., Veale, D., Ellison, N., & Reddell, T. (2013). The Emetophobia Questionnaire (EmetQ-13): Psychometric validation of a measure of specific phobia of vomiting (emetophobia). *Journal of Anxiety Disorders, 27*(7), 670–677. https://doi.org/10.1016/j.janxdis.2013.08.004

Botella, C., Pérez-Ara, M. Á., Bretón-López, J., Quero, S., García-Palacios, A., & Baños, R. M. (2016). *In vivo* versus augmented reality exposure in the treatment of small animal phobia: A randomized controlled trial. *PLoS One, 11*(2), 1–23. https://doi.org/10.1371/journal.pone.0148237

Botella-Arbona, C., Osma, J., Garcia-Palacios, A., Quero, S., & Banõs, R. M. (2004). Treatment of flying phobia using virtual reality: Data from a 1-year follow-up using a multiple baseline design. *Clinical Psychology and Psychotherapy, 11*(5), 311–323. https://doi.org/10.1002/cpp.404

Bourne, E. J. (2015). *The anxiety and phobia workbook* (6th ed.). Oakland, CA: New Harbinger Publications.

Burstein, M., Georgiades, K., He, J. P., Schmitz, A., Feig, E., Khazanov, G. K., & Merikangas, K. (2012). Specific phobia among U.S. adolescents: Phenomenology and typology. *Depression and Anxiety, 29*(12), 1072–1082. https://doi.org/10.1002/da.22008

Carlin, A. A., Hoffman, H. G., & Weghorst, S. (1997). Virtual reality and tactile augmentation in the treatment of spider phobia: A case report. *Behaviour Research and Therapy, 35*(2), 153–158.

Chavira, D. A., Stein, M. B., Bailey, K., & Stein, M. T. (2004). Child anxiety in primary care: Prevalent but untreated. *Depression and Anxiety, 20*(4), 155–164. https://doi.org/10.1002/da.20039

Cho, M. J., Kim, J.-K., Jeon, H. J., Suh, T., Chung, I.-W., Hong, J. P., … Hahm, B.-J. (2007). Lifetime and 12-month prevalence of *DSM-IV* psychiatric disorders among Korean adults. *Journal of Nervous and Mental Disease*, *195*, 203–210. https://doi.org/10.1097/01.nmd.0000243826.40732.45

Choy, Y., Fyer, A. J., & Lipsitz, J. D. (2007). Treatment of specific phobia in adults. *Clinical Psychology Review*, *27*, 266–286. https://doi.org/10.1016/j.cpr.2006.10.002

Cohen, D. C. (1977). Comparison of self-report and overt-behavioral procedures for assessing acrophobia. *Behavior Therapy*, *8*, 17–23.

Craske, M. G., & Sipsas, A. (1992). Animal phobias versus claustrophobias: Exteroceptive versus interoceptive cues. *Behaviour Research and Therapy*, *30*(6), 569–581. https://doi.org/10.1016/0005-7967(92)90002-X

Craske, M. G., Street, L. L., Jayaraman, J., & Barlow, D. H. (1991). Attention versus distraction during *in vivo* exposure: Snake and spider phobias. *Journal of Anxiety Disorders*, *5*(3), 199–211. https://doi.org/10.1016/0887-6185(91)90001-A

Davis, M., Eschelman, E. R., & McKay, M. (2008). *The relaxation and stress reduction workbook* (6th ed.). Oakland, CA: New Harbinger Publications.

Davis, T. E., Ollendick, T. H., & Öst, L.-G. (2012). *Intensive one-session treatment of specific phobias*. New York, NY: Springer. http://doi.org/. https://doi.org/10.1007/978-1-4614-3253-1

de Quervain, D. J.-F., Bentz, D., Michael, T., Bolt, O. C., Wiederhold, B. K., Margraf, J., & Wilhelm, F. H. (2011). Glucocorticoids enhance extinction-based psychotherapy. *PNAS*, *108*(16), 6621–6625. https://doi.org/10.1073/pnas.1018214108

Depla, M. F. I. A., ten Have, M. L., van Balkom, A. J. L. M., & de Graaf, R. (2008). Specific fears and phobias in the general population: Results from the Netherlands Mental Health Survey And Incidence Study (NEMESIS). *Social Psychiatry and Psychiatric Epidemiology*, *43*(3), 200–208. https://doi.org/10.1007/s00127-007-0291-z

Ehlers, A., Taylor, J. E., Ehring, T., Hofmann, S. G., Deane, F. P., Roth, W. T., & Podd, J. V. (2007). The driving cognitions questionnaire: Development and preliminary psychometric properties. *Journal of Anxiety Disorders*, *21*, 493–509. https://doi.org/10.1016/j.janxdis.2006.08.002

Fredrikson, M., Annas, P., Fischer, H., & Wik, G. (1996). Gender and age differences in the prevalence of specific fears and phobias. *Behaviour Research and Therapy*, *34*(1), 33–39.

Fyer, A. J. (1998). Current approaches to etiology and pathophysiology of specific phobia. *Biological Psychiatry*, *44*(12), 1295–1304. https://doi.org/10.1016/S0006-3223(98)00274-1

Garcia-Palacios, A., Hoffman, H., Carlin, A., Furness, T. A., & Botella, C. (2002). Virtual reality in the treatment of spider phobia: A controlled study. *Behaviour Research and Therapy*, *40*(9), 983–993. https://doi.org/10.1016/S0005-7967(01)00068-7

Glantz, K., Durlach, N. I., Barnett, R. C., & Aviles, W. A. (1996). Virtual reality for psychotherapy: From the physical to the social environment. *Psychotherapy*, *33*(3), 464–473.

Gregg, L., & Tarrier, N. (2007). Virtual reality in mental health. A review of the literature. *Social Psychiatry and Psychiatric Epidemiology*, *42*(5), 343–354. https://doi.org/10.1007/s00127-007-0173-4

Grös, D. F., & Antony, M. M. (2006). The assessment and treatment of specific phobias: A review. *Current Psychiatry Reports*, *8*(4), 298–303. https://doi.org/10.1007/s11920-006-0066-3

Guastella, A. J., Dadds, M. R., Lovibond, P. F., Mitchell, P., & Richardson, R. (2007). A randomized controlled trial of the effect of d-cycloserine on exposure therapy for spider fear. *Journal of Psychiatric Research*, *41*(6), 466–471. https://doi.org/10.1016/j.jpsychires.2006.05.006

Hellström, K., Fellenius, J., & Öst, L. G. (1996). One versus five sessions of applied tension in the treatment of blood phobia. *Behaviour Research and Therapy*, *34*(2), 101–112. https://doi.org/10.1016/0005-7967(95)00060-7

Hellström, K., & Öst, L. G. (1995). One-session therapist directed exposure vs two forms of manual directed self-exposure in the treatment of spider phobia. *Behaviour Research and Therapy*, *33*(8), 959–965. https://doi.org/10.1016/0005-7967(95)00028-V

Hoffman, H. G., Garcia-Palacios, A., Carlin, A., Furness, T. A., III, & Botella-Arbona, C. (2003). Interfaces that heal: Coupling real and virtual objects to treat spider phobia. *International Journal of Human Computer Interaction*, *16*(2), 283–300. https://doi.org/10.1207/S15327590IJHC1602

Huang, M. P., Himle, J., & Alessi, N. E. (2000). Vivid visualization in the experience of phobia in virtual environments: Preliminary results. *Cyberpsychology & Behavior*, *3*(3), 315–320. https://doi.org/10.1089/10949310050078742

Iza, M., Olfson, M., Vermes, D., Hoffer, M., Wang, S., & Blanco, C. (2013). Probability and predictors of first treatment contact for anxiety disorders in the United States: Analysis of data from the National Epidemiologic Survey on Alcohol And Related Conditions (NESARC). *The Journal of Clinical Psychiatry*, *74*(11), 1093–1100. https://doi.org/10.4088/JCP.13m08361

Kawakami, N., Takeshima, T., Ono, Y., Uda, H., Hata, Y., Nakane, Y., … Kikkawa, T. (2005). Twelve-month prevalence, severity, and treatment of common mental disorders in communities in Japan: Preliminary finding from the World Mental Health Japan Survey 2002-2003. *Psychiatry and Clinical Neurosciences*, *59*(4), 441–452. https://doi.org/10.1111/j.1440-1819.2005.01397.x

Kessler, R. C., Petukhova, M., Sampson, N. A., Zaslavsky, A. M., & Wittchen, H.-U. (2012). Twelve-month and lifetime prevalence and lifetime morbid risk of anxiety and mood disorders in the United States. *International Journal of Methods in Psychiatric Research*, *21*(3), 169–184. https://doi.org/10.1002/mpr

Kirmizioglu, Y., Dogan, O., Kugu, N., & Akyuz, G. (2009). Prevalence of anxiety disorders among elderly people. *International Journal of Geriatric Psychiatry*, *24*, 1026–1033. https://doi.org/10.1002/gps

Kleinknecht, R. A., & Thorndike, R. M. (1990). The mutilation questionnaire as a predictor of blood/injury fear and fainting. *Behaviour Research and Therapy*, *28*(5), 429–437.

Klorman, R., Weerts, T., Hastings, J., Melamed, B., & Lang, P. (1974). Psychometric description of questionnaires. *Behavior Therapy*, *5*, 401–409.

Kraaij, V., Garnefski, N., & Van Gerwen, L. (2003). Cognitive coping and anxiety symptoms among people who seek help for fear of flying. *Aviation Space and Environmental Medicine*, *74*(3), 273–277.

Krijn, M., Emmelkamp, P. M. G., Ólafsson, R. P., Schuemie, M. J., & Van Der Mast, C. A. P. G. (2007). Do self-statements enhance the effectiveness of virtual reality exposure therapy? A comparative evaluation in acrophobia. *Cyberpsychology & Behavior*, *10*(3), 362–370. https://doi.org/10.1089/cpb.2006.9943

Lieb, R., Miché, M., Gloster, A. T., Beesdo-Baum, K., Meyer, A. H., & Wittchen, H. U. (2016). Impact of specific phobia on the risk of onset of mental disorders: A 10-year prospective-longitudinal community study of adolescents and young adults. *Depression and Anxiety*, *33*(7), 667–675. https://doi.org/10.1002/da.22487

Lipsitz, J. D., Barlow, D. H., Mannuzza, S., Hofmann, S. G., & Fyer, A. J. (2002). Clinical features of four *DSM-IV*-specific phobia subtypes. *The Journal of Nervous and Mental Disease*, *190*(7), 471–478. https://doi.org/10.1097/01.NMD.0000022449.79274.48

Mackenzie, C. S., Reynolds, K., Cairney, J., Streiner, D. L., & Sareen, J. (2012). Disorder-specific mental health service use for mood and anxiety disorders: Associations with age, sex, and psychiatric comorbidity. *Depression and Anxiety*, *29*, 234–242. https://doi.org/10.1002/da.20911

Malbos, E., Mestre, D. R., Note, I. D., & Gellato, C. (2008). Virtual reality and claustrophobia: Multiple components therapy involving game editor virtual environments exposure. *Cyberpsychology & Behavior*, *11*(6), 695–697. https://doi.org/10.1089/cpb.2007.0246

Marks, I. M., Kenwright, M., McDonough, M., Whittaker, M., & Mataix-Cols, D. (2004). Saving clinicians' time by delegating routine aspects of therapy to a computer: A randomized controlled trial in phobia/panic disorder. *Psychological Medicine*, *34*(1), 9. https://doi.org/10.1017/S003329170300878X

Marks, I. M., Swinson, R. P., Basoglu, M., Kuch, K., Noshirvani, H., O'Sullivan, G., … Wickwire, K. (1993). Alprazolam and exposure alone and combined in panic disorder with agoraphobia: A controlled study in London and Toronto. *British Journal of Psychiatry*, *162*(1), 776–787.

Menzies, R. G., & Clarke, J. C. (1993). A comparison of *in vivo* and vicarious exposure in the treatment of childhood water phobia. *Behaviour Research and Therapy*, *31*(1), 9–15. https://doi.org/10.1016/0005-7967(93)90037-U

Merckelbach, H., De Jong, P. J., Muris, P., & Van Den Hout, M. A. (1996). The etiology of specific phobias: A review. *Clinical Psychology Review*, *16*(4), 337–361. https://doi.org/10.1016/0272-7358(96)00014-1

Miloff, A., Lindner, P., Hamilton, W., Reuterskiöld, L., Andersson, G., & Carlbring, P. (2016). Single-session gamified virtual reality exposure therapy for spider phobia vs. traditional exposure therapy: Study protocol for a randomized controlled non-inferiority trial. *Trials*, *17*(1), 60. https://doi.org/10.1186/s13063-016-1171-1

Muris, P., & Merckelbach, H. (2000). How serious are common childhood fears? II. The parent's point of view. *Behaviour Research and Therapy*, *38*(8), 813–818. https://doi.org/10.1016/S0005-7967(99)00119-9

Olatunji, B. O., Ebesutani, C., Sawchuk, C. N., Mckay, D., Lohr, J. M., & Kleinknecht, R. A. (2012). Development and initial validation of the medical fear survey – short version. *Assessment*, *19*(3), 318–336. https://doi.org/10.1177/1073191111415368

Olatunji, B. O., Woods, C. M., de Jong, P. J., Teachman, B. A., Sawchuk, C. N., & David, B. (2009). Development and initial validation of an Abbreviated Spider Phobia Questionnaire using item response theory. *Behavior Therapy*, *40*(2), 114–130. https://doi.org/10.1016/j.beth.2008.04.002

Ollendick, T. H., Raishevich, N., Davis, T. E., III, Sirbu, C., & Öst, L. G. (2010). Specific phobia in youth: Phenomenology and psychological characteristics. *Behavior Therapy*, *41*(1), 133–141. https://doi.org/10.1016/j.beth.2009.02.002

Öst, L. G. (1996). One-session group treatment of spider phobia. *Behaviour Research and Therapy*, *34*(9), 707–715. https://doi.org/10.1016/0005-7967(96)00022-8

Öst, L.-G. (1989). One-session treatment for specific phobais. *Behaviour Research and Therapy*, *27*, 1–7.

Öst, L. G., Alm, T., Brandberg, M., & Breitholtz, E. (2001). One vs five sessions of exposure and five sessions of cognitive therapy in the treatment of claustrophobia. *Behaviour Research and Therapy*, *39*(2), 167–183. https://doi.org/10.1016/S0005-7967(99)00176-X

Öst, L. G., Brandberg, M., & Alm, T. (1997). One versus five sessions of exposure in the treatment of flying phobia. *Behaviour Research and Therapy*, *35*(11), 987–996. https://doi.org/10.1016/S0005-7967(97)00077-6

Öst, L. G., Ferebee, I., & Furmark, T. (1997). One-session group therapy of spider phobia: Direct versus indirect treatments. *Behaviour Research and Therapy*, *35*(8), 721–732. https://doi.org/10.1016/S0005-7967(97)00028-4

Öst, L. G., Hellström, K., & Kåver, A. (1992). One versus five sessions of exposure in the treatment of injection phobia. *Behavior Therapy*, *23*, 263–282.

Öst, L. G., & Sterner, U. (1987). A specific behavioral method for treatment of blood phobia. *Behaviour Research and Therapy*, *25*(1), 25–29. https://doi.org/10.1016/0005-7967(87)90111-2

Park, S., Sohn, J. H., Hong, J. P., Chang, S. M., Lee, Y. M., Jeon, H. J., … Cho, M. J. (2013). Prevalence, correlates, and comorbidities of four *DSM-IV* specific phobia subtypes: Results from the Korean Epidemiological Catchment Area Study. *Psychiatry Research*, *209*(3), 596–603. https://doi.org/10.1016/j.psychres.2012.12.025

Paulus, F. W., Backes, A., Sander, C. S., Weber, M., & von Gontard, A. (2014). Anxiety disorders and behavioral inhibition in preschool children: A population-based study. *Child Psychiatry and Human Development*, 150–157. https://doi.org/10.1007/s10578-014-0460-8

Radomsky, A. S., Rachman, S., Thordarson, D. S., McIsaac, H. K., & Teachman, B. A. (2001). The claustrophobia questionnaire. *Journal of Anxiety Disorders*, *15*, 287–297.

Ressler, K. J., Rothbaum, B. O., Tannenbaum, L., & Anderson, P. (2004). Cognitive enhancers as adjuncts to psychotherapy. *Archives of General Psychiatry*, *61*, 1136–1144. https://doi.org/10.1001/archpsyc.61.11.1136

Riddle-Walker, L., Veale, D., Chapman, C., Ogle, F., Rosko, D., Najmi, S., … Hicks, T. (2016). Cognitive behaviour therapy for specific phobia of vomiting (Emetophobia): A pilot randomized controlled trial. *Journal of Anxiety Disorders*, *43*, 14–22. https://doi.org/10.1016/j.janxdis.2016.07.005

Rothbaum, B. O., Anderson, P., Zimand, E., Hodges, L., Lang, D., & Wilson, J. (2006). Virtual reality exposure therapy and standard (*in vivo*) exposure therapy in the treatment of fear of flying. *Behavior Therapy*, *37*(1), 80–90. https://doi.org/10.1016/j.beth.2005.04.004

Serrano-Blanco, A., Palao, D. J., Luciano, J. V., Pinto-Meza, A., Luján, L., Fernández, A., … Haro, J. M. (2010). Prevalence of mental disorders in primary care: Results from the diagnosis and treatment of mental disorders in primary care study (DASMAP). *Social Psychiatry and Psychiatric Epidemiology*, *45*(2), 201–210. https://doi.org/10.1007/s00127-009-0056-y

Shen, Y.-C., Zhang, M.-Y., Huang, Y.-Q., He, Y.-L., Liu, Z.-R., Cheng, H., … Kessler, R. C. (2005). Twelve-month prevalence, severity, and unmet need for treatment of mental disorders in metropolitan China. *Psychological Medicine*, *36*(2), 257. https://doi.org/10.1017/S0033291705006367

Sigström, R., Skoog, I., Karlsson, B., Nilsson, J., & Östling, S. (2016). Nine-year follow-up of specific phobia in a population sample of older people. *Depression and Anxiety*, *33*(4), 339–346. https://doi.org/10.1002/da.22459

Smits, J. A. J., Rosenfield, D., Otto, M. W., Powers, M. B., Hofmann, S. G., Telch, M. J., … Tart, C. D. (2013). D-cycloserine enhancement of fear extinction is specific to successful exposure sessions: Evidence from the treatment of height phobia. *Biological Psychiatry*, *73*(11), 1054–1058. https://doi.org/10.1016/j.biopsych.2012.12.009

Steinman, S. A., & Teachman, B. A. (2014). Reaching new heights: Comparing interpretation bias modification to exposure therapy for extreme height fear. *Journal of Consulting and Clinical Psychology*, *82*(3), 404–417. https://doi.org/10.1037/a0036023

Stinson, F. S., Dawson, D. A., Patricia Chou, S., Smith, S., Goldstein, R. B., June Ruan, W., & Grant, B. F. (2007, March). The epidemiology of *DSM-IV* specific phobia in the USA: Results from the National Epidemiologic Survey on alcohol and related conditions. *Psychological Medicine, 37*, 1047–1059. https://doi.org/10.1017/S0033291707000086

Szymanski, J., & O'Donohue, W. (1995). Fear of Spiders Questionnaire. *Journal of Behavior Therapy and Experimental Psychiatry*, *26*(I), 31–34.

Telch, J. (1994). Proximity to safety and its effects. *Behaviour*, *32*(7), 747–751.

Tolin, D. F., Lohr, J. M., Lee, T. C., & Sawchuk, C. N. (1999). Visual avoidance in specific phobia. *Behaviour Research and Therapy*, *37*(1), 63–70. https://doi.org/10.1016/S0005-7967(98)00111-9

Tortella-Feliu, M., Botella, C., Llabres, J., Breton-Lopez, J. M., del Amo, A. R., Banos, R. M., & Gelabert, J. M. (2011). Virtual reality versus computer-aided exposure treatments for fear of flying. *Behavior Modification*, *35*(1), 3–30. https://doi.org/10.1177/0145445510390801

Ultee, C. A., Griffioen, D., & Schellekens, J. (1982). The reduction of anxiety in children: A comparison of the effects of "systematic desensitization *in vitro*" and "systematic desensitization *in vivo*". *Behaviour Research and Therapy*, *20*, 61–67.

Van Houtem, C. M. H. H., Laine, M. L., Boomsma, D. I., Ligthart, L., van Wijk, A. J., & De Jongh, A. (2013). A review and meta-analysis of the heritability of specific phobia subtypes and corresponding fears. *Journal of Anxiety Disorders*, *27*(4), 379–388. https://doi.org/10.1016/j.janxdis.2013.04.007

Wells, J. E., Oakley Browne, M. A., Scott, K. M., McGee, M. A., Baxter, J., & Kokaua, J. (2006). Prevalence, interference with life and severity of 12 month *DSM-IV* disorders in Te Rau Hinengaro: The New Zealand Mental Health Survey. *Australian and New Zealand Journal of Psychiatry*, *40*(10), 845–854. https://doi.org/10.1111/j.1440-1614.2006.01903.x

Williams, S. L., Turner, S. M., & Peer, D. F. (1985). Guided mastery and performance desensitization treatments for severe acrophobia. *Journal of Consulting and Clinical Psychology*, *53*(2), 237–247. https://doi.org/10.1037/0022-006X.53.2.237

Wolitzky, K. B., & Telch, M. J. (2009). Augmenting *in vivo* exposure with fear antagonistic actions: A preliminary test. *Behavior Therapy*, *40*(1), 57–71. https://doi.org/10.1016/j.beth.2007.12.006

Wolpe, J., & Lang, P. J. (1977). *Manual for the fear survey schedule*. San Diego, CA: EdITS.

Zimmerman, M., & Mattia, J. I. (2000). Principal and additional *DSM-IV* disorders for which outpatients seek treatment. *Psychiatric Services*, *51*(10), 1299–1304. https://doi.org/10.1176/appi.ps.51.10.1299

Stress-Related Difficulties 39

Catalina Vechiu and William T. O'Donohue

An estimated one in three people in the United States report experiencing extreme stress, with approximately 75% of Americans endorsing physical and psychological symptoms related to stress (American Psychological Association, 2008). Excessive stress is associated with psychological distress and is often the precursor to many medical conditions. There is significant research identifying stress as an underlying factor in many health issues and illnesses. For instance, stress has been linked with many chronic diseases, such as hypertension, diabetes, allergies, and cardiovascular disorders (Segerstrom & Miller, 2004). Given the association between stress and a multitude of psychological and medical illnesses, behavioral healthcare providers are in an ideal position to evaluate and treat stress.

Given the ubiquitous nature of stress, there are a number of compelling reasons why early evaluation, prevention, and treatment of stress-related difficulties is important. First, there is a significant body of research that lends support to the cultural truism that stress has negative consequences and can lead to health issues. Second, stress-induced difficulties pose a significant cost to society in terms of lost work productivity (i.e., absenteeism), medical utilization, and outpatient treatment costs in addition to the escalated economic burden from physical and psychological comorbidities. Third, interventions aimed at reducing stress can provide valuable information regarding how stress causes disease. Therefore, preventing or ameliorating stress and stress-induced difficulties is beneficial both at the individual level, in the form of alleviating distress and suffering, as well as the societal level, in the form of reducing the costs of providing medical care. The aim of this chapter is to provide behavioral healthcare providers with the tools necessary to (1) screen and assess for stress, (2) provide stepped care psychotherapeutic interventions, and (3) streamline the referral process to specialty mental healthcare.

A Brief Description of the Problem

Stress is an omnipresent fact of modern day living, and it is used in a wide variety of contexts despite minimal conceptual clarity. Most individuals can identify the signs of stress, but the term has permeated both personal and professional language to a point of confusion. Stress is a popular buzzword used to describe social arrangements, work environments, and the increased pressure of urban living. For instance, the stereotype of the "stressed-out" student influences our understanding of what constitutes stress.

C. Vechiu, M.A. (✉) • W.T. O'Donohue, Ph.D.
Department of Clinical Psychology, University of Nevada, Reno, Reno, NV, USA
e-mail: cvechiu@gmail.com

A. Maragakis, W.T. O'Donohue (eds.), *Principle-Based Stepped Care and Brief Psychotherapy for Integrated Care Settings*, https://doi.org/10.1007/978-3-319-70539-2_39

Definitions of stress are multiple and varied, and reviewing each of these definitions is beyond the scope of this chapter (see Bartlett, 1998 for a description). One of the most popular conceptualizations of stress is Lazarus and Folkman's (1984) definition: "Stress is a particular relationship between the person and the environment that is appraised by the person as taxing or exceeding his or her resources and endangering his or her well being" (p. 19). In this model, stress is regarded as a process of appraisal and response; stressors (i.e., job loss) are appraised as either stressful or as non-threatening and insignificant. Stress-response mechanisms are triggered if external stimuli or conditions are perceived as stressful. An individual's stress-response includes psychological, behavioral, and physiological resources necessary to adapt to stressors.

Prevalence of Stress

In a survey of 2152 adults over the age of 18, more than half reported concerns with the amount of stress they experience in their lives (American Psychological Association, 2008). In a more recent survey of American adults, women and younger generations consistently reported higher levels of stress and that average stress levels have increased in the past year (American Psychological Association, 2016). Specific to primary care settings, 19% of patients in one study experienced a high degree of emotional distress in the month preceding a visit with their physician (Callahan et al., 1998). Additionally, 33% of Americans report experiencing extreme stress, and 48% feel that their stress levels have increased over the past 5 years (American Psychological Association, 2016). The top two sources of stress were money (67%) and work (65%). Other sources of stress include family responsibilities (54%), personal health concerns (51%), the economy (50%), and health problems affecting the respondent's family (50%) (American Psychological Association, 2016).

Individuals who experience stress are also more likely to report being diagnosed with depression, anxiety, obesity, hypertension, or a chronic illness. In fact, 67% of adults report receiving a diagnosis of a chronic illness (American Psychological Association, 2016). Although the true economic burden of stress is difficult to calculate, it is estimated that the United States spends $42 billion per year for stress-related disorders, more than half of which is due to healthcare utilization (Kalia, 2002). Additionally, work stress, in the form of absenteeism, lost productivity, stress-related psychological distress, substance use, and poor decision-making has led to an estimated loss of $150 billion in revenue (Kalia, 2002).

Although stress by itself many not necessarily cause poor health or increase vulnerability to particular diseases, it most likely interacts with various biopsychosocial factors (i.e., diet, genetics, trauma history) to produce a specific disease manifestation. Stress can affect the body's ability to resist disease and contributes directly to the progression of a disorder. Thus, there is high comorbidity between stress symptoms and illnesses such as heart disease and stress symptoms which are often indistinguishable from symptoms of anxiety and depression. Given the high prevalence rates of stress-related difficulties, it is important for providers to conduct systematic evaluation of stress during routine appointments.

Screening for Sexual Dysfunction in the Primary Care Setting

There is increased pressure on behavioral healthcare providers to deliver potent treatments that alleviate patients' stress-related concerns within a single visit, and "stress management" has become a catchall phrase that is often poorly defined. Without detailed assessment, most treatments will fail. Therefore, all patients should be screened and evaluated for high or extreme levels of stress. One option that may increase efficiency is the inclusion of one stress-related question to initiate conversations about stress.

1. On a scale of 0–10, where 0 indicates never and 10 indicates always, in the past month, how would you rate the amount of stress in your life (due to school, work, family, finances, etc.)?

Research suggests that single-item questionnaires are as valid and effective as longer questionnaires and can reduce patient burden and increase efficiency (Littman, White, Satia, Bowen, & Kristal, 2006). If the patient indicates a positive answer, the therapist can then conduct a detailed assessment for stress-related concerns by utilizing one of the following commonly utilized and empirically validated questionnaires:

- Perceived stress scale (PSS, Cohen & Williamson, 1988). The PSS is a ten-item questionnaire designed to measure the degree to which an individual appraises life events during the past month as stressful. A recommended cutoff score of ≥20 is indicative of high stress.
- The distress thermometer (DT, National Comprehensive Cancer Network (NCCN), 2010) assesses psychological distress during the previous week using a single-item visual analogue scale that ranges from 0 *no distress* to 10 *extreme distress*. The DT also includes a list of problems divided into five categories: (1) practical, (2) family, (3) emotional, (4) spiritual, and (5) physical. The NCCN recommends a cutoff score of ≥4 as indicative of stress.
- General health questionnaire (GHQ, Goldberg, 1978). The GHQ is a 12-item questionnaire designed to assess psychological distress across four domains: (1) social dysfunction, (2) anxiety/insomnia, (3) somatic symptoms, and (4) depression. It is generally accepted that a cutoff score of ≥15 indicates distress.

How to Further Assess If a Screen Returns Positive

If patients disclose experiencing difficulties with stress during the screening phase, assessment should focus on biopsychosocial factors that may interfere with health-promoting behaviors. Domains of health that have been found to impact stress include:

- *Psychological health*: Including self and familial history of psychological disorders (particularly depression and anxiety because of the high degree of symptom overlap)
- *Emotional functioning*: Including cultural beliefs and norms regarding appropriate emotional expression, modulation, and regulation
- *Environmental factors*: Including financial hardship, job status, academic pressure and performance, healthcare, and access to resources
- *Lifestyle factors*: Including diet, exercise, sleep patterns, medication and substance use, and past and current medical diagnoses
- *Cognitive factors*: Including history of intellectual disability, problem-solving skills, and coping strategies

Given the fast-paced nature of integrated care settings, behavioral healthcare providers may not have the time necessary to conduct a thorough assessment of the above domains. However, assessing functioning and difficulties within these areas does not necessarily have to be time-consuming. A useful framework for facilitating limited disclosure is the BATHE technique (Background, Affect, Troubling, Handling, Empathy; Stuart & Libermann, 1993). The BATHE technique was initially developed as a mode of time-limited psychotherapy delivery in primary care settings (Tesar, Austerman, Pozuelo, & Isaacson, 2010). The BATHE model provides standardization to the discussion of stress-related concerns and helps providers skillfully direct patients to

Table 39.1 The BATHE technique for initiating discussions of stress

Level	Scope	Examples
Background	Redirects patients from somatic focus to potential psychosocial stressors	"Tell me about what's been going on"
		"How have things been at work? With your family?"
		"What happened since your last visit?"
Affect	Gives permission to patients to comfortably discuss emotional functioning	"How do you feel about that?"
		"How have you been feeling about [condition/ stressor]?"
Troubling	Invites patients to discuss their perspective on their stress-related problems	"What about the [condition] bothers you the most?"
		"Can you tell me what you think is going on?"
		"Some of my patients who are under similar pressure/ stress describe having aches and pains. What has been your experience?"
		"From the difficulties you mentioned, which one is affecting you the most?"
Handling	Provides an assessment of self-management strategies and current level of dysfunction	"What do you do to cope?"
		"How have you been handling it?"
Empathy	Normalizes the patient's experience and reduces the emotional distance between patients and providers	"That must be very difficult for you"
		"I can understand why you would feel [emotion]"
		"This is a tough situation to be in"

disclose specific information regarding their environmental situations, behavior, emotional functioning, potential stressors, and current stressors. Refer to Table 39.1 for a description of each level.

Evidence-Based Stepped Care and Brief Psychotherapeutic Approaches

Once the BATHE technique is utilized to collect enough information regarding potential stressors and current functioning, a stepped care treatment plan can be developed for each patient that can reduce both cost and time. Integrated stepped care treatments are flexible approaches that provide cost-effective, efficient, and empirically supported care based on intensity, severity, and provider qualifications. The lowest levels of a stepped care model maintain cost and treatment effectiveness by providing low-intensity interventions to the largest number of patients. The other levels increase in cost, intensity, and provider time and qualification.

Successful implementation of a stepped care treatment program includes consistent monitoring and patient engagement and participation. Physicians and their treatment team can utilize the Client Satisfaction Questionnaire (CSQ; Larsen, Attkisson, Hargreaves, & Nguyen, 1979) to measure their patients' overall quality of experience and satisfaction with services. The CSQ is an eight-item questionnaire that is commonly used in mental health and medical settings and has been extensively studied. The following sections include a description of empirically based stepped care choices for the treatment of stress-related symptomatology.

Watchful Waiting

Watchful waiting is the least intensive tier in any stepped care intervention. It is a process of regular monitoring while delaying treatment to evaluate how stress progresses. At this level, patients and providers closely observe how stress levels change over time in order to better decide what type of treatment is necessary. Some patients may never need treatment, and others can delay more intensive treatments (i.e., medications). Watchful waiting may also be beneficial for patients who are reluctant to disclose psychosocial stressors during an initial visit. Watchful waiting does not ignore a patient's complaints or symptoms of stress but instead actively monitors the situation for any changes. The length of recommended time for watchful waiting varies from patient to patient and is affected by a number of issues, such as baseline level of stress and comorbid psychological and medical conditions. It may be prudent for the behavioral healthcare provider to schedule regular follow-up visits and administer one of the screening questionnaires to systematically monitor fluctuations in symptoms. If stress levels maintain or continue to rise, patients can then be "stepped up" to the next level.

Table 39.2 Changes for effectively managing stress

Lifestyle changes	Cognitive changes	Divert and distract
Decrease caffeine intake	Decrease dysfunctional beliefs	Take a short walk
Increase regular exercise	Positively reframe stressful situations	Listen to music
Decrease unhealthy food intake	Establish realistic expectations	Hang out with friends
Increase restful sleep	Keep a sense of humor	Take a hot bath
Incorporate relaxation exercises	Decrease indecisiveness	Balance work/leisure

Adapted from Posen (1995)

Psychoeducation

Psychoeducation integrates educational components with scientifically based psychotherapeutic techniques and is often used as a stress management tool. Successful psychoeducation interventions focus on well-being, improving health and coping skills, collaboration, and patient empowerment. Psychoeducation is a valuable tool, particularly during times of extreme stress because a patient's functioning and focus can be impaired when confronting major stressors or diseases. Psychoeducation can normalize stress-related difficulties by providing information about the stress-response cycle, internal and external sources of stress, the contribution of stress to the symptom development of disease, and education on managing and coping with chronic stress (see Appendix 1 for a list of the most commonly used stress management psychoeducational resources). Behavioral healthcare providers can continue to monitor stress levels and evaluate the practical, psychological, patient, and medical considerations mentioned in the next section to determine if patients should receive more intensive treatments.

Self-Help and Bibliotherapy

Patients who do not show a decrease in stress levels after receiving psychoeducation may require further treatment. Self-help and bibliotherapy is cost-effective and convenient and is well suited for patients who are highly motivated. An essential component of self-help and bibliotherapy is teaching patients various physiological approaches to stress management. For instance, various relaxation skills such as progressive muscle relaxation, abdominal breathing techniques, and visualization reverse the physiological stress reaction by slowing the breath and pulse, lowering blood pressure, and they produce a calming effect. In addition to relaxation techniques, self-help and bibliotherapy should also include problem-solving skills. An example is teaching patients to identify the contributing factors to stress (i.e., lifestyle, cognitive) and take steps toward changing them (see Appendix 2 for a list of the most commonly utilized self-help resources) (see Table 39.2).

Group Therapy

One of the most challenging aspects of stress management is that stress is implicated in the pathogenesis of numerous diseases. Part of this challenge is teaching patients stress management techniques that can be applied to different situations and stressors to avoid exceeding the optimum level of stress, which varies for each patient. A potential solution for this challenge is stress management in a group format. Group therapy can also reach a larger number of patients, create a sense of shared purpose, and provide a support system for individuals who experience stress-related symptoms. The duration of a group therapy session is typically approximately 90 min, and the associated cost is usually half of an individual session. Additionally, group stress management has been found to be effective in settings such as primary care, general medical practice, and hospital settings (Kabat-Zinn et al., 1992). The availability of stress management group programs will vary by geographical location; however, the most effective groups include the following components:

1. An individualized assessment of each patient's particular stressful difficulty
2. Stress management training
3. Relaxation skills
4. Homework assignments
5. An individual and specific action plan for each patient (Coffman & Katz, 2007)

Another option is Mindfulness-Based Stress Reduction (MBSR) which was developed for the treatment of stress for medical patients, and it has demonstrated good efficacy for various psychological and physiological disorders. MBSR is an intensive 8-week training comprised of three techniques: mindfulness meditation (cultivation of nonjudgmental awareness and mindful attention to the breath), body scanning (gradual attention to the body from the feet to the head), and Hatha yoga (simple postures and breathing exercises designed to strengthen and relax the body) (Chiesa & Serretti, 2009). MBSR may be beneficial for patients with stress-related difficulties and can be a cost-effective option particularly because it was developed for use in a group format.

What Does Not Work

Medical Interventions

Pharmacological management of stress-related symptoms is an essential component of a patient's treatment plan. For patients with complex disease presentations and medication regimen, psychopharmacological interventions may seem like a solution. However, it is critical that physicians consider lower-level interventions prior to medical interventions. A comprehensive review of the patient's medication history, potential drug interaction, safety and risk associated with adding specific medications, proper use and monitoring, and treatment adherence should be conducted prior to the implementation of medical interventions. Additionally, although antibiotics, antacids, steroids, and cardiovascular treatments are often utilized in treating physiological symptoms, they may not alleviate the causes of stress-related difficulties. Research indicates that environmental, lifestyle, psychosocial factors, and psychological distress contribute to the development of stress. These difficulties are better treated by psychological interventions and are less time-consuming, more cost-effective, and flexible.

When to Refer to External Specialty Mental Health

One of the key components of any stepped care intervention is a plan for referral to specialty mental healthcare services that are more time intensive. The following factors should be considered simultaneously to develop a decision tree that triages patients to the most appropriate level in the stepped care plan and helps providers decide when to refer to external services:

- *Practical considerations*: Including scheduling, payment, staff availability, patient insurance, patient flow and retention, and provider resources
- *Patient considerations*: Including skills, preferences, motivation, willingness, level of psychological distress, and patient adherence
- *Psychological considerations*: Including stress level, comorbidity with other psychological disorders, psychosocial and lifestyle factors, and functional impairment
- *Medical considerations*: Including medical diagnoses, cause, course and progression, adherent to treatment regimen, and medication use

Beyond these considerations, behavioral healthcare providers should also evaluate the patient's preferences, comorbidities, his or her own limitations in knowledge and experience, and cultural background. Often, symptoms of stress are culturally specific manifestations, and it may behoove providers to refer patients to external specialty mental health services that may better assist them. Options for treatment include:

Individual Therapy

Stress management techniques are well suited for individual therapy, particularly because a mental health professional can perform a thorough evaluation and assessment of each patient's idiosyncratic problems and can identify the causes of stress and subsequently devise an individualized stress management plan. Individual therapy is also beneficial for patients who (1) exhibit complex problems that are beyond the scope of the physician and the medical team; (2) patients who may lack the motivation, willingness, or skills necessary to engage with self-directed treatment; (3) patients who display high psychological distress; and (4) patients who prefer to circumvent the lower steps. Empirically support techniques utilized in individual therapy include:

- Relaxation and mindfulness techniques for patients who may experience depression, anxiety, or chronic pain
- Cognitive behavioral therapy (CBT) for patients who struggle with changing maladaptive beliefs
- Emotion regulation skills for patients who may have difficulty processing emotions
- Behavior therapy for patients who may struggle with changing health-related behaviors
- Problem-solving skills for patients who lack the repertoire necessary to self-manage their illness
- Stress prevention and resilience for patients who may require the skills necessary to cope with future stressors

Finally, although individual therapy has been shown to be effective in the treatment of a host of psychological disorders, there are practical drawbacks that may prevent patients from following through with a referral. The most common are time and expense constraints. Therefore, it is often beneficial for patients to enter treatment at a lower level before considering individual therapy.

The Role of the Primary Care Provider/Medical Team in Treatment

Because a patient's first point of contact with a healthcare practitioner is typically with a primary care physician, the starting point for stress management often occurs within this setting. Therefore, the role of the physician is to routinely screen and assess for stress and stress-related difficulties. The greatest barrier to addressing mental health concerns is the time-limited nature of the patient-doctor relationship. This concern is not unfounded; the average medical visit in the United States is 10–20 min, although due to economic issues of the managed care model, the standard is closer to 10–12 min per patient (Camasso & Camasso, 1994; du Pré, 2002). However, within an integrated care setting, physicians can start the screening and assessment process and engage in a "warm handoff" with the behavioral healthcare provider who can conduct a more thorough assessment. With effective communication between the patient, the physician, and the behavioral health providers, helping patients cope with stress can be successfully initiated during routine medical visits and continued during behavioral health visits. This increases collaboration between the various members of the medical team and normalizes any psychological distress patients may experience.

Quality Improvement (QI) and Impact on Care

Systematic QI is necessary for improving physician knowledge and satisfaction, enhancing patient outcomes, improving the health of the target population, and reducing the costs of care. Given the complexity of healthcare and stress-related difficulties, QI efforts and the methods used are likely to vary based on the primary care setting, their goals and priorities, and resources. Specific areas that could be evaluated might be the identification, evaluation, monitoring, and follow-up of patients in the stepped care model of treatment for stress, improving the delivery of stepped care treatments for stress-related difficulties, or improving the referral process for patients with complex stress-related problems.

Although there has been a recent surge in QI development and implementation across the United States, the complexity of healthcare delivery poses a challenge to the systematic measurement of QI. However, there are various organizations that have developed standardized and validated measures for use in healthcare, chief among them, the Agency for Healthcare Research and Quality (AHRQ) and the Joint Commission. Many of these scientifically evaluated measures can be found at AHRQ's website (www.qualitymeasures.ahrq.gov). Although process-improvement techniques may be initially difficult, physicians have the opportunity to begin QI in the first visit and at every step in the evaluation, treatment planning, and stepped care model of treatment for stress.

Some strategies for initiating QI include (1) provider reminder systems (computerized reminders), (2) facilitated communication between providers (transmission of clinical data between various providers via systems other than medical chart), (3) patient and medical team education (workshops, classes, brochures), (4) organizational change (multidisciplinary teams, systematic QI initiatives), and (5) continuous assessment and monitoring (QI is a dynamic process of change and quality indicators should be identified and communicated) (Shojania, McDonald, Wachter, & Owens, 2004). By adopting QI initiatives and implementing a standardized QI questionnaire into a patient's regular or follow-up visits, providers have the opportunity to improve efficiency, manage or reduce the costs of healthcare utilization, and increase provider knowledge and satisfaction.

Conclusion

Stress has become a notorious concept with the lay public and the idea that everyone experiences stress to one degree or another, or that stress is at the root of many diseases, or that stress affects academic performance and can impair social relationships has been widely accepted as fact. The psychological and medical literature has extensively studied stress although it remains an "imprecise construct" with multiple theoretical explications. Stress is a complex and highly prevalent condition associated with a myriad of negative physiological and psychological sequelae. This chapter has provided suggestions and guidelines for the effective evaluation and treatment of stress-related difficulties that could aid providers in providing high-quality healthcare to all of their patients. The key to an efficient visit is effective time management and increasing communication between physicians and behavioral health provider communication skills. The BATHE model (Stuart & Libermann, 1993) provides a framework for the timely discussion of stress-related concerns and provides standardization that can help providers expertly uncover behavioral, situational, emotional, and medical stressors in order to initiate treatment planning for stress-related difficulties. This chapter also provides suggestions for a stepped care model of treatment that is cost-effective and has the potential to reduce costs associated with healthcare utilization. How effectively stepped care for stress is implemented in any particular practice is dependent on continuous quality improvement initiatives, and providers are encouraged to employ standardized measures for monitoring patient outcomes and satisfaction.

Appendix 1: Psychoeducational Resources for Stress Management

- *University of Massachusetts Medical School*: Provides free handouts for mindfulness, managing stress, guided meditation, and information regarding the stress cycle.

http://www.umassmed.edu/psychiatry/resources/wellness/stress_management/stress_handouts/

- *University of Texas, Austin:* Provides psychoeducation regarding stress and stress management.
https://www.cmhc.utexas.edu/stress.html
- *Wellness Proposals:* Provides free handouts for stress management aimed at different populations (i.e., middle/late life) and for different stressors (i.e., marriage, divorce).
http://wellnessproposals.com/wellness-library/stress-management/stress-management-handouts-vol-1/
- *Regent University:* Provides a brochure for managing stress and anxiety.
https://www.regent.edu/acad/schcou/psc/images/brochures/print_brochures/managing_stress_and_anxiety.pdf
- *In-House Physicians:* Provides free psychoeducational materials and suggestions for further resources for stress management, nutrition, and fitness.
http://www.inhousephysicians.com/patient-handouts/

Appendix 2: Self-Help and Bibliotherapy Resources for Stress Management

- *US Department of Veterans Affairs*: Provides a free workbook for managing stress.
http://www.prevention.va.gov/mpt/2013/docs/managestressworkbook_dec2013.pdf
- *Northwest Territories Literacy Council:* Provides a free stress management workbook.
http://www.nwtliteracy.ca/resources/adultlit/career_life_work/dealing_with_stress_workbook.pdf
- Davis, M., Eshelman, E., McKay, M., & McKay, M. (1993). *The Relaxation & Stress Reduction Workbook*. Oakland, CA: New Harbinger Publications.
- Kabat-Zinn, J. (2005). *Full Catastrophe Living, Using the Wisdom of Your Body and Mind to Face Stress, Pain, and Illness.* New York: Bantam Dell.
- LaRoche, L. (1998). *Relax—You May have Only a Few Minutes Left: Using the Power of Humor to Overcome Stress in Your life and Work*. New York: Villard.
- Rechtschaffen, S. (1996). *Time Shifting: Creating More Time to Enjoy Your Life.* New York: Doubleday.

References

American Psychological Association. (2008). *Stress in America. Stress in America Survey.*

American Psychological Association. (2016). *Stress in America: The impact of discrimination. Stress in America Survey.*

Bartlett, D. (1998). Stress perspectives and processes. Buckingham. Philadelphia: Open University Press.

Callahan, E. J., Jaen, C. R., Crabtree, B. F., Zyzanski, S. J., Goodwin, M. A., & Stange, K. C. (1998). The impact of recent emotional distress and diagnosis of depression or anxiety on the physician-patient encounter in family practice. *The Journal of Family Practice, 46*, 410–418.

Camasso, M. J., & Camasso, A. E. (1994). Practitioner productivity and the product content of medical care in publicly supported health centers. *Social Science & Medicine, 38*, 733–748.

Chiesa, A., & Serretti, A. (2009). Mindfulness-based stress reduction for stress management in healthy people: A review and meta-analysis. *The Journal of Alternative and Complementary Medicine, 15*(5), 593–600.

Coffman, D., & Katz, C. (2007). *Stress management. The Clearinghouse for Thematic Groups*, 1–64.

Cohen, S., & Williamson, G. (1988). Perceived stress in a probability sample of the United States. In S. Spacapan & S. Oskamp (Eds.), *The social psychology of health: Claremont Symposium on applied social psychology*. Newbury Park, CA: Sage.

du Pré, A. (2002). Accomplishing the impossible: Talking about body and soul and mind during a medical visit. *Health Communication, 14*(1), 1–21. https://doi.org/10.1207/S15327027HC1401_1

Goldberg, D. P. (1978). *Manual of the general health questionnaire*. Windsor, England: NFER Publishing.

Kabat-Zinn, J., Massion, A. O., Kristeller, J., Peterson, L. G., Fletcher, K. E., Pbert, L., … Santorelli, S. F. (1992). Effectiveness of a meditation-based stress reduction program in the treatment of anxiety disorders. *American Journal of Psychiatry, 149*, 936–943.

Kalia, M. (2002). Assessing the economic impact of stress—The modern day hidden epidemic. *Metabolism, 51*(6), 49–53.

Larsen, D. L., Attkisson, C. C., Hargreaves, W. A., & Nguyen, T. D. (1979). Assessment of client/patient satisfaction: Development of a general scale. *Evaluation and Program Planning, 2*, 197–207.

Lazarus, R. S., & Folkman, S. (1984). *Stress, appraisal and coping*. New York: Springer.

Littman, A. J., White, E., Satia, J. A., Bowen, D. J., & Kristal, A. R. (2006). Reliability and validity of 2 single-item measures of psychosocial stress. *Epidemiology, 17*, 398–403.

National Comprehensive Cancer Network (NCCN). (2010). *NCCN clinical practice guidelines in oncology. Distress Management*. National Comprehensive Cancer Network. Retrieved from www.nccn.org

Posen, D. B. (1995). Stress management for patient and physician. *The Canadian Journal of Continuing Medical Education*. Retrieved from http://www.mentalhealth.com/mag1/p51-str.html

Segerstrom, S. C., & Miller, G. E. (2004). Psychological stress and the human immune system: A meta-analytic study of 30 years of inquiry. *Psychological Bulletin, 130*(4), 601–630. https://doi.org/10.1037/0033-2909.130.4.601

Shojania, K. G., McDonald, K. M., Wachter, R. M., & Owens, D. K. (2004). Closing the quality gap: A critical analysis of quality improvement strategies. *Technical Reviews, 9*(1).

Stuart, M. R., & Libermann, J. A. (1993). *The fifteen minute hour: Applied psychotherapy for the primary care physician*. Westport, CT: Praeger.

Tesar, G. E., Austerman, J., Pozuelo, L., & Isaacson, J. H. (2010). *Behavioral assessment of the general medical patient*.

40 Treatment Engagement and Multicultural Considerations

Mana K. Ali and Melody Mickens

Culture is generally defined as a set of attitudes, values, behaviors, and symbols shared by a large group of people and usually communicated from one generation to the next (Hays, 2001). People are multicultural, often identifying with various cultural categories (e.g., sex, age, disability, religion, national origin, race) that are layered and intersect in every possible way. It is insufficient to understand a person's worldview without appreciating the social positions of their cultural memberships (Crenshaw, 1989; Hays, 2001). An individual's social position can be best understood by examining how their cultural identities influence their role in Hofstede's power distance relationship paradigm (Hofstede & Bond, 2016). Belonging to various cultural groups that have historically faced oppression, discrimination, stigmatization, or exclusion may exacerbate barriers in biological, psychological, and social areas of the human experience. Belonging to lower-power groups does not determine poor life experiences, and belonging to a higher-power group does not guarantee positive life experiences (see Table 40.1). The factors that contribute to life inequities are multifactorial, interrelated, and complex. This holds true for health inequities, which are rooted in an amalgamation of individual, provider, health system, societal, and environmental factors. Health inequities have been noted across a number of lower-power cultural groups including disability, minority race/ethnicity, homo- or bi-sexual orientation, female or transgender, and lower socioeconomic status (Farber, Ali, Van Sickle, & Kaslow, 2017).

Table 40.1 Broad power differentials in the United States

Cultural group	More power	Less power
Age	Adults	Children, adolescents, elders
Mental/physical disability	Able-bodied	Persons with disability
Race	White	People of color
Religion	Christian	Jews, Muslims, other non-Christian
Social class	Upper and middle class	Poor and working class
National origin	Born in United States	Immigrants, refugees
Gender	Male	Female, transgendered
Sexual orientation	Heterosexual	Gay men, lesbians, bisexual

Adapted from Hays (2001). ADDRESSING: a model of cultural influences and their relationship to the social construct of power

M.K. Ali, Ph.D. (✉)
Department of Physical Medicine and Rehabilitation, Johns Hopkins University, Baltimore, MD, USA
e-mail: ms.manaali@gmail.com

M. Mickens, Ph.D.
Hunter Holmes McGuire Veterans Affairs Medical Center, Richmond, VA, USA
e-mail: mnmick@gmail.com

A. Maragakis, W.T. O'Donohue (eds.), *Principle-Based Stepped Care and Brief Psychotherapy for Integrated Care Settings*, https://doi.org/10.1007/978-3-319-70539-2_40

Culture and Power in Primary Care

Within a primary care setting, each member of the patient-provider dyad brings aspects of their own culture to primary care interactions intentionally or unintentionally. Power positions in the United States (US) permeate primary care and both members are largely shaped by the nexus of their cultural identities, stereotypes, biases, and personal life experiences. Cultural differences between health provider and patient may reinforce objective or assumed power differences. Moreover, there are inherent power differentials between the patient and health provider that can exist in immutable (e.g., age and race), tangible (e.g., white coats), and intangible (e.g., style of communication, education differences) forms.

Professional boundaries coupled with the brief nature of primary care appointments create a challenge to openly explore differences in culture between the provider and patient. Nonetheless, the health provider is still tasked with identifying power differentials that may contribute or impede understanding of how the patient negotiates health affairs such as provider-patient alliance, as well as health behaviors and decisions. The major aims of this chapter are to (1) identify patient and provider-level factors that interfere with cross-cultural collaboration in the primary care setting, (2) review indicators of power dynamics that may impede rapport building and treatment engagement, and (3) introduce specific interventions designed to help providers understand cultural differences.

The Patient

The environmental and societal level barriers that disproportionately affect lower-power groups' health trajectories, such as poverty, institutional-level discrimination, and systemic racism (Clark, Anderson, Clark, & Williams, 1999; Fiscella, Franks, Gold, & Clancy, 2000) may have low visibility and mutability during a primary care appointment. Nevertheless, it is necessary to recognize that such larger-scale variables may prevent access to, utilization of, and adherence to engagement with health care. Patients with access to primary care appointments may be armored with values, attitudes, and beliefs that are significantly influenced by their social position. Unique patient-level barriers to health-care engagement include but are not limited to medical and cultural mistrust, provider preference, acculturation status, and health literacy. These barriers could be interrelated with cumulative effects on health care.

Medical Mistrust

Medical mistrust, which has been defined as the patient's belief that the medical community, health-care providers and systems, seeks to exploit the needs of individuals from cultural communities of lower power, has been associated with decreased health-care utilization across various groups. Arguably, this is an adaptive response to numerous examples of historic mistreatment of oppressed cultural groups by medical providers and research scientists (Ashby, 1986; Suite, La Bril, Primm, & Harrison-Ross, 2007). In one study where older Black patients reported less trust in their physicians compared to White patients, Black patients had decreased utilization of routine checkups and preventative services (Musa, Schulz, Harris, Silverman, & Thomas, 2009). Compared to the general population of the US, Native American consumers demonstrate more medical mistrust and less satisfaction with health care (Guadagnolo et al., 2009). In other research, men who have sex with men and report higher medical mistrust had longer time periods between medical appointments (Eaton et al., 2015).

Provider Preference

Racial and ethnic minorities are more likely to report less satisfaction, patient-centered care, and continuity of care, as well as poorer quality of care from health providers (Institute of Medicine, 2002). Lower ratings of trust, lower positive affect, shorter appointments, and more verbally dominant communication by the medical provider may contribute to difficulty with establishing rapport and a patient-provider alliance (Cooper & Powe, 2004; Johnson, Roter, Power, & Cooper, 2004). Poor quality working alliance variables have been linked to decreased delivery of preventive care services and proper referrals by the provider and disparities in patient follow-up care for racial/ethnic minorities (Jackson, 2005; Little et al., 2001; O'Malley, Sheppard, Schwartz, & Mandelblatt, 2004).

Concordance, or similar demographic characteristics such as age, sex, and race between patient and provider, has been associated with greater trust and satisfaction with provider (Street, O'Malley, Cooper, & Haidet, 2008). Particularly among racial and ethnic minorities, perceived shared identity with provider has been associated with increased utilization of medical services and involvement in medical decision-making (Peek et al., 2010). Despite racial and ethnic minority groups representing about 25% of the US population, they are represented in less than 6% of doctors (Cooper & Powe, 2004). There is evidence that language, shared values, education, age, and sex concordance between patient and provider are also associated with positive health outcomes (Johnson Thornton, Powe, Roter, & Cooper, 2011). It is possible that patient-provider concordance has positive effects on rapport and health outcomes via several mechanisms. The provider may share cultural values and life experiences, which in turn may increase empathy and sensitivity to patients (Cooper & Powe, 2004). Furthermore, increasing similarities within this dyad reduces perceived power differences. Shrinking power differences increases sense of control for the vulnerable partner and may encourage their participation and agency during health-care appointments.

Acculturation

Research has consistently demonstrated that immigrants have better health and lower mortality rates than US natives, but this advantage disappears with longer residence in the United States (Ali, Mwendwa, Sims, Ricks, & Sumner, 2016; Koya & Egede, 2007; Singh & Siahpush, 2002). Growing research has at least in part attributed this trend to acculturation, or a shift from native cultural values and orientation toward the Western, mainstream society (Oh, Koeske, & Sales, 2002; Singh & Siahpush, 2002). There are several pathways that may link mainstream orientation to poor health. Acclimating to one's host community has been linked to poor health through behavioral pathways such as changes in lifestyle patterns, unhealthy diets, cigarette smoking, and alcohol use (Morales, Lara, Kington, Valdez, & Escarce, 2002). For example, in one study Hispanic immigrants in a lower socioeconomic position were more likely to smoke cigarettes and have sedentary lifestyles (i.e., health habits) (Morales et al., 2002). Lower socioeconomic status was also associated with overweight conditions (i.e., precursor to biological outcomes) in Hispanic immigrants (Morales et al., 2002).

Furthermore, a pathophysiological pathway may also link the immigrant experience to disease susceptibility, quite possibly due to the considerable amount of stress associated with migration and acculturation, which may overactivate the hypothalamic-pituitary-adrenal axis and autonomic nervous systems and result in serious life-threatening health conditions (Davidson, Jonas, Dixon, & Markovitz, 2000; Suarez, 2003). Immigrants report higher levels of stress compared to their native counterparts (Breslau & Chang, 2006; Lashley, 2000).

As a lower-power group in the US, immigrants often experience a myriad of intersecting barriers to health care that include (1) reduced access to health care and providers in local communities and limited means of transportation to primary care appointments; (2) financial barriers such as lower incomes and lack of health insurance; (3) cultural barriers to health care such as linguistic factors that may prevent successful patient-provider communication, as well as cultural beliefs (e.g., trust in providers); and (4) psychological processes of acculturation, which in its negative form can be linked to stress, depression, anxiety, insecurity, anger/hostility, and loneliness/isolation (Lashley, 2000; Marmot & Wilkinson, 2001). These barriers and the psychological stressors associated with acculturation may independently or in tandem negatively affect patient attendance and engagement in primary care appointments. As such, immigrants may have increased risk for and susceptibility to chronic diseases due to chronic stressors and may have decreased opportunities for disease prevention, detection, and intervention due to barriers that interfere with health-care access, utilization, and adherence.

Cultural Beliefs Regarding Medicine and Physical Health

Across different cultures, individuals have conceptualized medicine, particularly non-Western medicine, as a source of healing often tied to religious and spiritual beliefs. For example, traditional Eastern models of medicine incorporate natural elements, integrative practices such as acupuncture, and dietary changes and characterize illness as a state of imbalance between the self, the social climate, and the natural environment (Carteret, 2011; Micozzi, 2015). Similarly, in Native American and indigenous cultures, individuals and providers ascribe to traditional healing practices that include a bio-psycho-social-spiritual model that focuses on integration of spiritual legends, individual responsibility, use of community healers, respect for laws of nature, and ceremonial interventions (Koithan & Farrell, 2010) for treatment and to achieve overall wellness.

In Latino and Hispanic cultures, medicine and health interventions may include consultation with traditional and folk healers such as curanderos, brujos and brujas, yerberas, or parteras as well as an emphasis on treating "hot" and "cold" illnesses (Juckett, 2013). These community-based approaches not only incorporate natural elements but are often used in place of or in conjunction with traditional Western practices. Although they are revered by many who use them, traditional Western providers often dismiss or discount their effectiveness or may be unaware of the prevalence of their use. In Latino/Hispanic communities, communication with providers often includes family members, particularly males, and a need for interventions that focus on addressing the needs of the entire family while respecting the role of elders in the family. While many of these cultures may be hesitant to engage with traditional Western medicine, incorporating aspects of their cultural health beliefs and practices or inquiring about non-Western traditional health practices may enhance their engagement with care and assist with communication.

Health Literacy

Health literacy is the "degree to which individuals have the capacity to obtain, process, and understand basic health information and services needed to make appropriate health decisions" (Institute of Medicine, 2004). By contrast, low health literacy can decrease a patient's confidence and ability to manage their health as well as interfere with efforts to share information with providers, understand and adhere to recommended treatment guidelines, and navigate health systems (e.g., filling out forms and finding services and providers). Vulnerable or low-power groups in the US are at greater risk for limited health literacy. Older adults or individuals over 65 years old are disproportionately affected by chronic illness and are the largest group in the US with limited health literacy (Kutner, Greenberg, & Baer, 2005). Health literacy was found to mediate racial/ethnic disparities and contribute to education disparities in health status and flu vaccinations (Bennett, Chen, Soroui, & White, 2009).

The Provider

Health-care providers, driven by their compassion to help patients achieve maximum health and recovery as well as institutional demands on their time, may find themselves conveying a position of power by falling into "traps" identified by Miller and Rollnick (2013). These traps are often the effect of educational practices that endow health-care providers with medical expertise and organizational beliefs and norms that expect the provider to lead and guide the health-care interaction. These traps are associated with patient disengagement in care and can undermine the patient's expertise on their own values, attitudes, beliefs, and goals. Moreover, frequent use of these traps often diminishes a collaborative alliance between patient and provider and decreases the likelihood of building rapport.

Expert Trap

Health providers have many years of formalized coursework, supervised clinical training, degrees, certifications, and/or independent practice, which create a high likelihood of being more knowledgeable about illness, disease, risks and benefits of treatment options, and evidence base than the patient. In fact, the patient is likely pursuing a primary care appointment for help from someone they hope and expect to be more informed about a particular problem. However, it is erroneous to assume that providers have the best solution to a patient's problem without considering the patient's unique experiences. Miller and Rollnick (2013) suggest that relying on a myopic view dictated solely by the provider's experience constitutes the expert trap, and they caution against being directive with knowledge and directions without involving the patient's expertise, as this perspective promotes patient passivity and disengagement. This unbalanced contribution to the provider-patient alliance is mutually exclusive with patient-centered care and shared decision-making. Shared decision-making model emphasizes active patient involvement in identifying areas of concern and treatment goals. Racial/ethnic consumers have reported a greater preference for this model compared to White consumers (Peek et al., 2009).

Assessment and Premature Focus Traps

Asking too many questions, assuming the problem, and determining the focus of encounters may lead to the assessment and premature focus traps (Miller & Rollnick, 2013). Focusing and assessing before a collaborative relationship and common goals are established with a patient can decrease opportunities for active listening by the provider. The assessment role also minimizes the patient's role as an expert by putting them in the passive position of answering questions. Research has demonstrated possible effects of the assessment in trap (i.e., less participation) in lower-power groups including racial/ethnic minorities, patients with poorer health, older patients, and patients with less than high school education (Cooper & Roter, 2003). Moreover, patients with psychiatric disability were found to actively repeat and ask questions and express concerns important to them that appeared to be disregarded by the provider (McCabe, Heath, Burns, & Priebe, 2002).

Blaming and Labeling Traps

Health providers are problem solvers, seeking understanding of the etiology of a problem to guide interventions and solutions. At times, a genuine effort to understand a patient's health concerns may lead to the error of blaming or faultfinding, rather than emphasis on change. This is known as the blaming trap and can be off-putting to the patient and lead to defensiveness (Miller & Rollnick, 2013). Holding patients accountable, without assigning fault, is key for health behavior change or treatment plan adherence. Holding patients accountable entails emphasis on their control to change rather than what led to the problem at hand, as well as expressing empathy without promoting the problematic behavior to foster a nonjudgmental environment.

The labeling trap may be partly attributed to providers' persistence and appreciation of a patient's presentation and health profile. Health providers are diagnosticians by training, and their wealth of knowledge and expertise in diagnostic procedures allows characterization of signs and symptoms. Medical intervention hinges on proper medical diagnoses and serves the purpose of helping patients achieve optimal health. The good intention of determining medical diagnoses may lead to the error of engaging in power struggles or unproductive dialogues to convince patients to accept their label or diagnosis. When forcing patients to accept a label or diagnosis without understanding the patient's perspective or ambivalence, providers risk disregarding the patient and their concerns.

Implicit Bias

Power differences, whether objective or assumed, are exacerbated by bias, prejudice, and stereotypes. All human beings are predisposed to development of bias, prejudice, and stereotypes. On one hand this predisposition is useful; heuristics and categorizing the environment facilitates quick and efficient cognitive processing. On the other hand, mental shortcuts may lead to unequal and unfair treatment, particularly in the health arena. A seminal report from the Institution of Medicine, *Unequal Treatment*, elucidates racial inequities in quality of health services despite the presence of confounding variables such as insurance, socioeconomic status, stage of health presentation, and comorbidities. The report notes this is partly contributed to stereotyping. Social groups with lower power/privilege, who have historically been disenfranchised, are at risk for being recipients of implicitly biased stereotypes and discrimination. Perceived differential negative treatment based on class and racial group memberships was associated with lower positive affect and lower ease of communication between patient and provider (Hausmann et al., 2011).

Power Struggle Indicators

Power struggles within patient-provider relationships may lead miscommunication between patients and providers that can result in frustration for both. Residual effects of power struggles may manifest as patient refusals to engage in discussion or try recommended treatments, avoidance of health-care providers via missed primary care appointments, nonadherence to medication regimens or interventions, disengagement, indecision, and passive engagement styles. The following section delineates many, but not all, indicators of power struggles in primary care visits.

Ambivalence

Ambivalence, or simultaneous conflicting thoughts, feelings, or behaviors, may indicate oversight of the patient's expert role in their health care (Miller & Rollnick, 2013). One example is the patient that attends doctor's appointments regularly, but is noncompliant with treatment recommendations or demonstrating poor medication adherence. Another example is the patient who agrees with information and advice provided, then offers reasons to disagree. The conjunction "but" is a sign of guarded optimism rooted in ambivalence.

Doctor: Smoking increases your risk of having another stroke. You should consider quitting.

Patient: I know it is horrible for my health, ***but*** *it helps me relax.*

Using smoking cessation as an example, patients typically can identify risks of tobacco use. Ambivalence is not an issue of ignorance or intentional strive to be unhealthy. It is better understood as difficulties with confidence or lack of importance or a combination of both (Miller & Rollnick, 2013). The provider must accept their inability to change the patient. Relinquishing control increases the presence of acceptance and compassion for the patient.

Disengagement

Engagement in health care is differentiated from participation or appointment attendance because it includes emotional involvement, commitment, and deliberate effort toward goals (Lequerica & Kortte, 2010). Consistent with patients' motivation for responsibility and an active role and control in their health care, patients express a desire to share power with health-care providers. Feelings of powerlessness have been linked to poor engagement in health care among socially vulnerable groups including ethnic minorities, older aged persons, persons of low socioeconomic status, and those with multiple chronic health conditions (Sheridan et al., 2015). Neglect to acknowledge emotional, spiritual, and sociocultural factors that contribute to lived experience of a chronic condition can increase risk of patient disengagement. Sensitivity to these areas of a patient's life during health-care visits facilitates engagement and retention for high-need minority groups such as transgender women living with human immunodeficiency virus and those with serious mental illness (Farber et al., 2017; Sevelius, Patouhas, Keatley, & Johnson, 2014).

Passive and Too Agreeable

It is rare that health providers complain about the patient who was too agreeable. Yet, this can be an indicator of poor understanding, lack of satisfaction, or feeling powerless in the patient-provider dyad. Patients that are passive or too agreeable rarely ask questions or offer suggestions and information or express excessive reverence of their health providers. Patients from socioeconomically disadvantaged groups and the elder are more likely to demonstrate submissiveness and unassertiveness (Bismark et al., 2006).

Fear

Fear in the presence of medical professionals or procedures may be rooted in feelings of vulnerability and lack of control, both tenets of decreased sense of power. Fear in medical environments has been most closely linked to research on white-coat hypertension. This phenomenon is a pattern of elevated blood pressure in medical setting, but normal levels across other settings (Franklin, Thijs, Hansen, O'Brien, & Staessen, 2013). The clinical setting activates the body's stress response, also known to aid "fighting or flighting" in the presence of perceived danger. Relatedly, fear may manifest as anger and defensiveness (fight) or disengagement and withdrawal (flight). The flight or fight response is associated with temporary increase in blood pressure explaining white-coat hypertension. Women and older adults have demonstrated greater frequency of this white-coat hypertension (Franklin et al., 2013). Increasing patients' sense of control, through inviting collaboration, ensuring patient understanding, and building patient confidence, can alleviate fear.

Reducing Power Distance

In order to facilitate a working alliance and build rapport, health-care providers and patients can benefit from a collaboration that allows an open exchange of culturally relevant information. Using cultural humility and aspects of motivational interviewing, engaging patients in shared medical decision-making, and modifying delivery of medical information, health-care providers can create an environment that transcends cultural barriers, empowers patients, and reduces barriers to medical adherence and consistent use of medical services (Fig. 40.1).

Cultural Humility

At times, patients' refusals, disengagement, ambivalence, and fear during primary care appointments are fueled by mismatched goals between the patient and provider. Values, attitudes, and beliefs drive

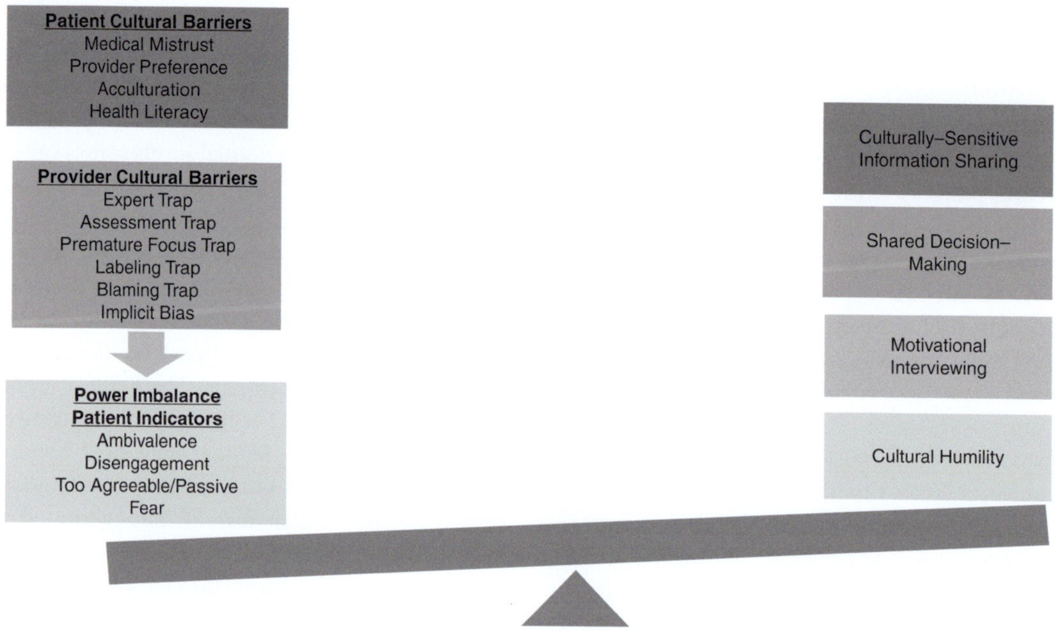

Fig. 40.1 Reducing power imbalance in primary care settings

goals. Providers' awareness and acceptance of possibility for mismatched goals is fundamental in creating positive collaboration with patients. Given the complexity of multiculturalism, providers should continue to strive for cultural humility. This is a lifelong process marked by self-awareness and self-critique of one's own culture and its influence on understanding and interacting with patients. Cultural humility also recognizes an intention to close power distances, advocate for patients, create partnerships, and interact with diverse people (Tervalon & Murray-Garcia, 1998).

Motivational Interviewing

Motivational interviewing is an empathic interviewing strategy used by clinicians working in a variety of medical settings. The major principles of motivational interviewing can be summarized in the following way (Miller & Rollnick, 2013): express empathy, roll with resistance, develop discrepancy, and support self-efficacy. Providers can express empathy in several ways. First, providers can use their behaviors and nonverbal actions to communicate empathically to their patients.

- Maintaining eye contact with the patient throughout the visit
- Shaking the patient's hand upon entering and exiting the exam room
- Sitting across from or next to the patient instead of standing and talking to the patient while maintaining open posture (e.g., arms unfolded)
- Listening silently and attentively as patient's disclose concerns

Providers can also verbally express empathy by using four skills from motivational interviewing.

1. Open-ended questions
   (a) Open-ended questions allow patients to speak about their concerns and to explain these concerns to their health-care providers.
   (b) They engage the patient and help the provider understand how the patient comprehends the medical problem and cultural aspects to address when recommending treatments.
   (c) Examples: What are your concerns right now? How did the medication help? When are you eating? Who can help you remember to track blood glucose readings?

2. Affirmations
   (a) Are statements of praise that demonstrate the provider's interest in patient's successful behaviors.
   (b) Help to point out changes that the patient has made, thus potentially building their confidence to adopt additional behavioral changes.
   (c) Build rapport and help patient and provider create a working alliance.
   (d) Examples: It sounds like you've been working hard on eating more vegetables! It is impressive that you were able to remain tobacco-free for the past 30 days; you are clearly dedicated to your health and I want to support your efforts.
3. Reflections
   (a) Are a statement of observed feeling, emotion, or affect.
   (b) Encourage a patient to explore or elaborate on a topic.
   (c) Examples: You seem angry about hearing that you've lost your insurance. I hear a lot of frustration in what you're saying right now.
4. Summaries
   (a) Let the client know that you have been listening attentively.
   (b) Allow client to clarify information you may have misunderstood.
   (c) Example: Let me see if I understand the problem; you're having trouble tracking your blood glucose readings because you take them at different times during the week and you've been forgetting to write them down?

Shared Decision-Making

Shared decision-making (SDM) emphasizes both the patient and provider as experts who work collaboratively to determine health goals. The provider is an expert in the field of medicine, and the patient is the expert on their values, treatment preferences, and health goals (Makoul & Clayman, 2006). Research has found that patients may speak uninterrupted for an average 12 seconds, are interrupted twice, and speak for about one-third of the appointment time during primary care visits (Rhoades, McFarland, Finch, & Johnson, 2001). Such data suggests unequal contribution between health providers and patients in health discussion and decision-making. For shared decision-making to be effective, both the patient and provider should have all necessary information to make a decision. Important pieces of information include an agreed upon decision and timeline in which the decision should be made, clarity of health conditions, diagnoses, and courses of disease, all available prevention and intervention options (with risks and benefits), and which of the identified risks and benefits are most important to the patient (Agency for Healthcare Research and Quality (AHRQ) SHARE approach). Shared decision-making has been linked to better health outcomes, increased patient engagement and compliance with treatment regimens, increased sense of control, and greater patient satisfaction ratings (Agency for Healthcare Research and Quality, 2016). Clarify collaborative roles at the outset of appointments and identify both the patient's and provider's expertise.

- Ask patients about their concerns as related to health-care recommendations.
- Demonstrate active listening.
- Include the patient in evaluating the decision.
- Help patient problem solve identified barriers and challenges.
- Maintain eye contact with the patient.
- Provide patient with decision aids such as brochures, fact sheets, lists of complications, or videos and diagrams to explain complex biological processes or procedures.

Culturally Sensitive Information Delivery

If patients are unable to understand information received, they are less likely to find it important or valuable leading to poor health-care engagement. The following recommendations may facilitate understanding in the presence of cultural patient barriers:

- Do not assume level of understanding based on formal educational level.
- Ask for permission to give information ("Are you interested in additional information on risks of cigarette use?").
- Vet health information so patients are responsible for only learning three pieces of information (Partnership for Clear Health Communication "Ask Me 3"). Encourage and help patients with answering the following three questions:
  - What is my main problem?
  - What do I need to do about the problem?
  - Why is doing this important for me?
- Avoid asking "Do you understand?" Instead, have patients teach you what they understand about their condition.
- Use bullet points vs. paragraph form when providing written information.
- Avoid graphs and tables. Consider visual illustrations of conditions and procedures.
- Normalize asking questions to create a safe and shame-free environment.
- Use plain language instead of medical jargon and slow down.

Conclusions

Societal and environmental factors that disproportionately affect low-power groups and perpetuate health inequities, such as poverty and systemic racism, have low mutability during primary care appointments. Health providers may have greatest access and impact on patient- and provider-level health barriers in vulnerable cultural groups. These barriers can be rooted in perceived lack of concordance or unbalanced power between patient and provider. Particularly in the presence of barriers that may be rooted in power dynamics, providers should use techniques to reduce power distance and promote collaborative care.

References

Agency for Healthcare Research and Quality. (2016). Shared decision-making. Rockville, MD.

Ali, M., Mwendwa, D. T., Sims, R., Ricks, M., & Sumner, A. (2016). Age at immigration and kidney function among self-identified healthy Africans in the United States. *Journal of Immigrant and Minority Health, 18*, 194.

Ashby, H. U. (1986). Mislabeling the Black client: A reply to Ridley. *American Psychologist, 41*, 224–225.

Bennett, I. M., Chen, J., Soroui, J. S., & White, S. (2009). The contribution of health literacy to disparities in self-rated health status and preventive health behaviors in older adults. *Annals of Family Medicine, 7*(3), 204–211.

Breslau, J., & Chang, D. (2006). Psychiatric disorders among foreign-born and US-born Asian Americans in a US national survey. *Social Psychiatry and Psychiatric Epidemiology, 41*, 943–950.

Bismark, M. M., Brennan, T. A., Paterson, R. J., Davis, P. B., & Studdert, D. M. (2006). Relationship between complaints and quality of care in New Zealand: a descriptive analysis of complainants and non-complainants following adverse events. *Quality & Safety in Health Care, 15*(1), 17–22.

Carteret, M. (2011). Traditional Asian health beliefs & healing practices. Retrieved March 27, 2017, from http://www.dimensionsofculture.com/2010/10/traditional-asian-health-beliefs-healing-practices/

Clark, R., Anderson, N. B., Clark, V. R., & Williams, D. R. (1999). Racism as a stressor for African Americans: A biopsychosocial model. *American Psychologist, 54*, 805–816.

Cooper, L. A., & Roter, D. L. (2003). Patient-Provider communication: the effect of race and ethnicity on process and outcomes. In Institute of Medicine (US) Committee on Understanding and Eliminating Racial and Ethnic Disparities in Health Care; Smedley BD, Stith AY, Nelson AR, editors. Unequal Treatment: Confronting Racial and Ethnic Disparities in Health Care. Washington (DC): National Academies Press (US).

Cooper, L. A., & Powe, N. R. (2004). *Disparities in patient experiences, health care processes, and outcomes: The role of patient-provider racial, ethnic, and language concordance*. Commonwealth Fund.

Crenshaw, K. (1989) Demarginalizing the intersection of race and sex: A black feminist critique of antidiscrimination doctrine, feminist theory, and antiracist politics, University of Chicago Legal Forum, 139.

Davidson, K., Jonas, B., Dixon, K., & Markovitz, J. (2000). Do depression symptoms predict early hypertension incidence in young adults in the CARDIA study? Coronary Artery Risk Development in Young Adults. *Archives of Internal Medicine, 160*, 1495–1500.

Eaton, L. A., Driffin, D. D., Kegler, C., Smith, H., Conway-Washington, C., White, D., & Chauncey, C. (2015). The role of stigma and medical mistrust in the routine health care engagement of black men who have sex with men. *American Journal of Public Health, 105*(2), e75–e82.

Farber, E., Ali, M. K., Van Sickle, K. S., & Kaslow, N. J. (2017). Psychology in patient-centered medical homes: Reducing health disparities and promoting health equity. *American Psychologist, 72*(1), 28–41.

Fiscella, K., Franks, P., Gold, M. R., & Clancy, C. M. (2000). Inequality in quality: Addressing socioeconomic, racial, and ethnic disparities in health care. *Journal of the American Medical Association, 283*, 2579–2584.

Franklin, S. S., Thijs, L., Hansen, T. W., O'Brien, E., & Staessen, J. A. (2013). White-coat hypertension: New insights from recent studies. *Hypertension, 62*, 982–987.

Guadagnolo, A. B., Cina, K., Helbig, P., Molloy, K., Reiner, M., Cook, E. F., & Petereit, D. G. (2009). Medical mistrust and less satisfaction with health care among Native Americans presenting for cancer treatment. *Journal of Health Care for the Poor and Underserved, 20*(1), 210–225.

Hausmann, L. R. M., Hannon, M. J., Kresevic, D. M., Hanusa, B. H., Kwoh, K., & Ibrahim, S. A. (2011). Impact of perceived discrimination in health care on patient-provider communication. *Medical Care, 49*(7), 626–633.

Hays, P. A. (2001). *Addressing cultural complexities in practice: Assessment, diagnosis, and therapy*. Washington, DC: American Psychological Association.

Hofstede, G., & Bond, M. H. (2016). Hofstede's culture dimensions. *Journal of Cross-Cultural Psychology, 15*(4), 417–433.

Institute of Medicine. (2002). In B. D. Smedley, A. Y. Stith, & A. R. Nelson (Eds.), *Unequal treatment: Confronting racial and ethnic disparities in health care*. Washington, DC: Institute of Medicine.

Institute of Medicine. (2004). *Health literacy: A prescription to end confusion*. Washington, DC: National Academies Press.

Jackson, J. L. (2005). Communication about symptoms in primary care: Impact on patient outcomes. *Journal of Alternative and Complementary Medicine, 11*(Suppl 1), S51–S56.

Johnson, R. L., Roter, D., Power, N. A., & Cooper, L. A. (2004). Patient race/ethnicity and quality of patient-physician communication during medical visits. *American Journal of Public Health, 94*(12), 2084–2090.

Johnson Thornton, R. L., Powe, N., Roter, D., & Cooper, L. A. (2011). Patient-physician social concordance, medical visit communication and patients' perceptions of health care quality. *Patient Education and Counseling, 85*(3), e201–e208.

Juckett, G. (2013). Caring for Latino patients. *American Family Physician, 87*(1), 48–54.

Koithan, M., & Farrell, C. (2010). Indigenous Native American healing traditions. *Journal of Nursing Practices, 6*(6), 477–478.

Koya, D., & Egede, L. (2007). Association between length of residence and cardiovascular disease risk factors among an ethnically diverse group of United States immigrants. *Journal of General Internal Medicine, 22*, 841–846.

Kutner, M., Greenberg, E., & Baer, J. (2005). *Adult literacy in America: A first look at the findings of the National Adult Literacy Survey*. Washington, DC: National Center for Educational Statistics.

Lashley, M. (2000). The unrecognized social stressors of migration and reunification of Caribbean families. *Transcultural Psychiatry, 37*, 201–215.

Lequerica, A. H., & Kortte, K. (2010). Therapeutic engagement: A proposed model of engagement in medical rehabilitation. *American Journal of Physical Medicine & Rehabilitation, 89*, 415–422.

Little, P., Everitt, H., Williamson, I., Warner, G., Moore, M., Gould, C., … Payne, S. (2001). Observational study of effect of patient centredness and positive approach on outcomes of general practice consultations. *British Medical Journal, 323*(7318), 908–911.

Makoul, G., & Clayman, M. L. (2006). An integrative model of shared decision making in medical encounters. *Patient Education and Counseling, 60*, 301–312.

Marmot M., & Wilkinson R.G. (2001). Psychosocial and material pathways in the relation between income and health: a response to Lynch et al. *British Medical Journal, 322*(7296):1233–6.

McCabe, R., Heath, C., Burns, T., & Priebe, S. (2002). Engagement of patients with psychosis in consultation: Conversation analytic study. *British Medical Journal, 325*, 1148–1151.

Micozzi, M. S. (2015). Characteristics of complementary and alternative medicine. In M. S. Micozzi (Ed.), *Fundamentals of complementary and alternative medicine* (pp. 3–12). St. Louis, MO: Elsevier Saunders.

Miller, W. R., & Rollnick, S. (2013). *Motivational interviewing: Helping people change*. New York, NY: Guilford Press.

Morales, L. S., Lara, M., Kington, R. S., Valdez, R. O., & Escarce, J. J. (2002). Socioeconomic, cultural, and behavioral factors affecting Hispanic health outcomes. *Journal of Health Care for the Poor and Underserved, 13*, 477–503.

Musa, D., Schulz, R., Harris, R., Silverman, M., & Thomas, S. B. (2009). Trust in the health care system and the use of preventive health services by older black and white adults. *American Journal of Public Health, 99*, 1293–1299.

Oh, Y., Koeske, G. F., & Sales, E. (2002). Acculturation, stress, and depressive symptoms among Korean immigrants in the United States. *Journal of Social Psychology, 142*(4), 511–526.

O'Malley, A. S., Sheppard, V. B., Schwartz, M., & Mandelblatt, J. (2004). The role of trust in use of preventive services among low-income African-American women. *Preventative Medicine, 38*(6), 777–785.

Peek, M. E., Odoms-Young, A., Quinn, M., Gorawara-Bhat, R., Willson, S. C., & Chin, M. H. (2010). Race and shared decision making: Perspectives of African Americans with diabetes. *Social Science & Medicine, 71*(1), 1–9.

Peek, M. E., Wilson, S. C., Gorawara-Bhat, R., Odoms-Young, A., Quinn, M. T., & Chin, M. H. (2009). Barriers and facilitators to shared decision-making among African-Americans with diabetes. *Journal of General Internal Medicine, 24*(10), 1135–1139.

Rhoades, D. R., McFarland, K. F., Finch, W. H., & Johnson, A. O. (2001). Speaking and interruptions during primary care office visits. *Family Medicine, 33*(7), 528–532.

Sevelius, J. M., Patouhas, E., Keatley, J. G., & Johnson, M. O. (2014). Barriers and facilitators to engagement and retention in care among transgender women living with human immunodeficiency virus. *Annals of Behavioral Medicine*, *47*(1), 5–16.

Sheridan, N.F., Kenealy, T.W., Kidd, J.D., Scmidt-Busby, J., Hand, J.E., Raphael, D.B., McKillop, A.M. & Rea, H.H. (2015). Patients' engagement in primary care: powerlessness and compounding jeopardy. A qualitative study. *Health Expectations*, *18*, 32–43.

Singh, G. P., & Siahpush, M. (2002). Ethnic-immigrant differentials in health behaviors, morbidity, and cause-specific mortality in the US: An analysis of two national databases. *Human Biology*, *74*, 83–109.

Street, R. L., O'Malley, K. J., Cooper, L. A., & Haidet, P. (2008). Understanding concordance in patient-physician relationships: Personal and ethnic dimensions of shared identity. *Annals of Family Medicine*, *6*(3), 198–205.

Suarez, E. C. (2003). Joint effect of hostility and severity of depressive symptoms on plasma interleukin-6 concentration. *Psychosomatic Medicine*, *65*, 523–527.

Suite, D. H., La Bril, R., Primm, A., & Harrison-Ross, P. (2007). Beyond misdiagnosis, misunderstanding and mistrust: Relevance of the historical perspective in the medical and mental health treatment of people of color. *Journal of National Medical Association*, *99*(8), 879–895.

Tervalon, M., & Murray-Garcia, J. (1998). Cultural humility versus cultural competence: A critical distinction in defining physician training outcomes in multicultural education. *Journal of Health Care for the Poor and Undeserved*, *9*, 117–125.

Trichotillomania and Excoriation Disorder

41

E.B. Lee, C.W. Ong, and M.P. Twohig

A Brief Description of the Disorders

Trichotillomania, or hair-pulling disorder, is characterized by the recurrent pulling out of one's hair, leading to hair loss. The *Diagnostic and Statistical Manual of Mental Disorders, Fifth Edition* (DSM-5; American Psychiatric Association, 2013), specifies additional diagnostic criteria for trichotillomania: (a) repeated attempts to reduce or stop hair pulling, (b) the hair pulling causes clinically significant distress or functional impairment, and (c) the hair pulling or hair loss is not due to a medical or other mental condition. Hair pulling can be observed in any region of the body, including the scalp, eyebrows, and axillary region.

Excoriation disorder is functionally very similar to trichotillomania. It involves skin picking that leads to damage or lesions. The DSM-5 includes additional criteria:

(a) Repeated attempts to stop picking.
(b) Clinically significant distress.
(c) It is not caused by a substance such as cocaine or methamphetamine or another medical condition such as scabies.
(d) It is not explained by another psychological condition such as psychosis.

E.B. Lee (✉) • C.W. Ong • M.P. Twohig
Utah State University, Logan, UT, USA
e-mail: eric.lee@usu.edu; clarissa.ong@usu.edu

An important functional and descriptive feature of hair pulling and skin picking is that there are generally two styles of pulling: *focused* and *automatic*. Focused pulling/picking occurs consciously and is often accompanied by thoughts about the process (e.g., "this hair feels thicker," or "once I get this piece of skin I'll stop"), whereas automatic pulling/picking occurs outside of awareness such as while driving, reading, working at a computer, or watching television. Some individuals predominantly use one type of pulling, but most engage in both.

Screening for Trichotillomania and Excoriation Disorder in the Primary Care Setting

Depending on the pulling/picking location, signs of trichotillomania and excoriation can be quite conspicuous. Simply being aware of the disorders and looking for signs of hair pulling and skin picking can help the professional recognize problems before even speaking with patients. Individuals with trichotillomania and excoriation disorder frequently pull/pick from visible areas (i.e., scalp, eyebrows, eyelashes, face, arms), often leaving bald patches or sores that may be difficult to cover up and are easily discernable if one is looking for them. Similarly, attempts to cover the damage with scarfs, wigs, or pinning of hair occur for trichotillomania, and attempting to

A. Maragakis, W.T. O'Donohue (eds.), *Principle-Based Stepped Care and Brief Psychotherapy for Integrated Care Settings*, https://doi.org/10.1007/978-3-319-70539-2_41

cover or hide skin occurs for excoriation. Because patients might not volunteer this information, simply asking patients who might be more likely to pull/pick whether they engage in these behaviors can be an effective way to screen for these disorders. Many patients are unaware that medical professionals can address hair pulling and skin picking and may not bring it up without a prompt.

There are multiple psychometrically sound measures of trichotillomania and excoriation disorder that may be used for screening purposes. While not exhaustive, the following lists of assessment are recommended and provide quick, effective methods of screening for these disorders. At the time of this writing, we were able to find freely available copies of each of these measures at www.bfrb.org/clinicalscales.

Screening Measures for Trichotillomania

National Institute of Mental Health Trichotillomania Questionnaire (NIMH-TQ; Swedo et al., 1989). The NIMH-TQ consists of two semi-structured, clinician-rated scales: The Trichotillomania Severity Scale (NIMH-TSS) and the Trichotillomania Impairment Scale (NIMH-TIS). The NIMH-TSS is a short, six-item scale that broadly examines trichotillomania symptom severity, function of pulling behavior, attempts to resist pulling, and levels of distress and impairment caused by hair pulling. The NIMH-TIS is a global impairment scale with scores ranging from 0 to 10 within four broad categories: no impairment (0), minimal impairment (1–3), mild impairment (4–6), and moderate/severe impairment (7–10). Scores are dependent upon factors such as degree of distress, shame, interference with daily life, and hair loss.

Massachusetts General Hospital Hair Pulling Symptom Severity Scale (MGH-HPS; Keuthen, O'Sullivan, Ricciardi, & Shera, 1995). The MGH-HPS is a commonly used, self-report measure of trichotillomania severity. It assesses frequency and control over urges to pull and pulling behavior as well as the level of associated distress. The measure consists of seven items, rated on a 5-point scale, with higher scores indicating greater trichotillomania severity.

Trichotillomania Scale for Children (TSC; Tolin et al., 2008). The TSC is a self-report measure of trichotillomania derived from the MGH-HPS that is tailored for children and adolescents. There is a child and parent version of the measure that both share similar items and the same scoring structure. Assessment can consist of the child or the parent alone; however, gathering both the child and parent report is recommended for a thorough assessment, especially for younger children. The TSC consists of 12 items, rated from 0 to 2, with higher scores indicating greater severity, distress, and impairment.

Screening Measures for Excoriation Disorder

Yale-Brown Obsessive Compulsive Scale (YBOCS) Modified for Neurotic Excoriation (NE-YBOCS; Arnold et al., 1999). The NE-YBOCS is a ten-item, semi-structured, clinician-rated measure of excoriation disorder severity. The scale is a modified version of the original YBOCS that simply replaces the words "obsessive" and "compulsive" with "skin picking." The scale includes five items assessing urges to pick and five questions assessing picking behavior, with higher scores indicating greater excoriation severity.

Skin Picking Scale-Revised (SPS-R; Keuthen et al., 2001). The SPS-R is a six-item, self-report measure of excoriation disorder severity, with higher scores indicating greater excoriation severity. It is essentially a self-report version of the NE-YBOCS, assessing urges to pick and picking behavior.

How to Further Assess If a Screen Returns Positive?

The previous screening measures provide a quick, simple overview of the severity of these disorders. If, following the screening, the patient would benefit from further assessment and treatment, we recommend a thorough functional analysis of the pulling/picking. Utilizing one of the following measures is a simple first step of this analysis. The measures quickly examine whether the pulling/picking behavior is predominantly automatic or focused in nature. Following this, we recommend further assessment and analysis of the behavior. Session one of the treatment outline below explains what should be included in a functional analysis for these disorders.

Milwaukee Inventory of Subtypes of Trichotillomania: Adult and Child Versions (MIST-A and MIST-C). The MIST-A and MIST-C are short, self-report measures developed to help patients and clinicians identify patterns of hair-pulling behavior, specifically, whether it is automatic or focused in nature. While most individuals with trichotillomania utilize both types of pulling, understanding whether one type is more predominant can inform treatment. Both the MIST-A and MIST-C will provide automatic and focused total scores that will help identify how much someone is engaging in these types of pulling.

The Milwaukee Inventory for the Dimensions of Adult Skin Picking (MIDAS; Walther, Flessner, Conelea, & Woods, 2009**)**. The MIDAS is a 12-item, self-report measure similar to the MIST-A, but developed for populations with skin picking behavior. Like the MIST-A, the MIDAS was developed to identify patterns of picking behavior. It provides a total score for both automatic and focused picking behavior.

Evidence-Based Stepped Care and Brief Psychotherapeutic Approaches

The methods for treating trichotillomania and excoriation disorder are essentially identical, as both involve a behavior (hair pulling or skin picking) that functions as way to regulate urges and internal thoughts and emotions. Evidence-based treatment for trichotillomania and excoriation disorder consists of basic behavioral skills in the form of habit reversal training, which is the process of increasing patients' awareness of their urges and behavior, teaching behavioral skills to decrease pulling/picking, and facilitating social support for the patient, and some form of modern cognitive behavior therapy that generally correspond to the automatic and focused types of pulling behavior. This manual will focus on acceptance and commitment therapy (Woods & Twohig, 2008a), as it is the most well-researched treatment for these disorders; however, dialectical behavior therapy (Keuthen et al., 2012; Keuthen & Sprich, 2012) and traditional cognitive behavior therapy (Ninan, Rothbaum, Marsteller, Knight, & Eccard, 2000) may also be utilized in its place if you are more familiar with those modalities. The following walks through five sessions that can be completed in 20–30 min each.

Session 1. This session will largely consist of a functional assessment of the patient's problematic behavior and psychoeducation. The functional assessment will include a history of pulling/picking, current symptoms, pre- and post-pulling/picking behaviors, settings in which pulling/picking occurs, and emotional states and cognitions that are present before, during, and after pulling/picking. Assess the following issues: When and where does it usually occur (e.g., driving, studying, watching TV, in front of mirror, in bed, etc.)? What emotions are present (e.g., stress, anxiety, lonely, frustration, etc.)? What types of cognitions are present (e.g., thinking they are out of control, unattractive, or shameful or thoughts about needing to "just get one more hair" or "fix this uneven part of my skin," etc.)? What is done with the hair/skin after pulling/picking (e.g., discard it, rub it between fingers or on face or lips, bite the bulb of the hair, ingest it)? For all patients with trichotillomania, be sure to ask whether they ingest their hair as it can be a significant health concern (see Role of Primary Care Provider section for more details).

As patients provide these details, it is useful to begin getting an idea of how much the pulling/picking are automatic or focused, as this will inform the treatment plan. Most people experience both automatic and focused types of pulling/picking to some degree, and it is recommended to include all portions of the treatment plan. However, if the patient predominantly engages in automatic pulling/picking, emphasize the interventions found in sessions 2 and 3. Likewise, if the patient predominantly engages in focused pulling/picking, emphasize the methods provided in sessions 4 and 5.

Once the role of pulling/picking is understood, it is important to provide psychoeducation about the disorder. The TLC Foundation's website offers free, quality psychoeducational information for trichotillomania and excoriation disorder (bfrb.org/learn-about-bfrbs/tools-a-info-for/for-clinicians). Many with trichotillomania or excoriation disorder unfortunately feel as though they are the only one who pulls their hair or picks their skin. Providing basic information about the prevalence of the disorder can reduce shame and feelings of isolation. It may also be helpful to give information about online resources such as the TLC Foundation for Body-Focused Repetitive Behaviors website (www.bfrb.org) that can provide further education, support, and resources.

Leave the patient with homework to record the behavior. For hair pulling, the patient can record how many hairs are pulled and how many urges to pull are experienced each day. For skin picking, the minutes spent picking and how many urges to pick are experienced each day can be recorded. Additionally, at least one time per day, the patient should write down an urge to pull/pick. This should include what the urge felt like, what emotions and thoughts were noticed, and what was done to reduce the urge (e.g., pull/pick, distract themselves, seek help, etc.). We recommend providing the patient with a premade self-monitoring form such as the one found at this website: www.oxfordclinicalpsych.com/view/10.1093/med:psych/9780195336054.001.0001/med-9780195336054-appendix-10.

Session 2. This session will involve teaching the first of two basic behavioral skills borrowed from habit reversal training that largely target automatic pulling/picking. Before introducing this skill, check in with the patient about the assigned, self-monitoring homework. While discussing urges, compile a list of pulling/picking "warnings." These warnings are used to inform the patient that pulling is likely or has already begun. The warnings can be behaviors (e.g., hand moving to head, rubbing hair/skin, looking in a mirror, etc.) or sensations (e.g., pressure under skin, itching, burning, tingling, etc.). Once a list has been created, introduce the first skill: competing responses. Competing responses, referred to as "exercises," are behaviors that can be easily and discretely performed in nearly any situation that are incompatible with pulling/picking. A commonly used competing response is to place one's hands by their side while making gentle fists. Help the patient to commit to perform the agreed upon competing response for one full minute whenever a warning sign is noticed. If another warning occurs following the minute, begin the exercise again for another minute.

Instruct your patient to practice using the competing response each time a warning sign occurs between this and the next session. Take a moment to ask what might be difficult about the task, and offer solutions or reasons to engage in the exercises, even when it is difficult. It is common for people to feel that they are having to do the exercises nearly constantly, especially in the beginning. The need to do the competing response will drop quickly as the warning signs decrease.

Finally, using the self-monitoring data provided, help the patient set an achievable goal to reduce the amount of hairs pulled or time spent picking between this and the next session. Agree upon a specific number of hairs or minutes each day. Ask for a commitment to work toward this goal and to use the exercises each time a pulling/picking warning occurs.

Session 3. This session utilizes stimulus control procedures, the second behavioral skill that targets automatic pulling/picking. The purpose of stimulus control procedures are to essentially find ways to make pulling/picking more difficult or effortful to do, therefore, making these behaviors less likely to occur. Begin by helping identifying common settings where pulling/picking occurs and any tools that are used such as tweezers, mirrors, needles, etc. Once this information has been gathered, work with the patient to come up with ways to modify the environment. Some common examples are removing or covering mirrors or bright lights that assist in pulling/picking; using a timer to limit the amount of time spent in a setting (like the bathroom); holding an object in free hand when reading, studying, or driving; and relocating tools, such as tweezers, to a location that requires effort to obtain (e.g., a distant room, the possession of a supportive person). Additionally, if social support exists, informing friends or family of high-risk settings or times and recruiting them to check in can be helpful. At the end of the session help the patient set meaningful and specific goals to reduce the amount of pulling/picking between this and the next session.

Session 4. People generally think that they can control urges to pull or make them go away if they work hard enough or if they could simply find a magic trick, perfect exercise, or way of thinking about their problem. This thought process often leads to people who place great energy in attempting to control, change, or distract themselves from their urges. Help the patient understand that urges are not something to fight or control, instead, understanding that urges come and go and that pulling and picking actually increase the urge. Thus, practicing emotional acceptance may be the most useful way to deal with urges to pull or pick. Essentially, the patient can control actions such as using competing responses, stimulus control, not pulling/picking, and engaging in meaningful actions, but controlling internal experiences such as urges is likely to backfire. The term "willingness" is often used to describe this approach to the urge to pull or pick.

Before introducing willingness, it is important to help the patient understand why it might be worth trying a new strategy. Therefore, the first step to the introduction of willingness is helping the patient recognize that attempts to control internal events, like urges, are not only ineffective but actually the heart of the problem. It is helpful to create a list of strategies that one uses to control, change, or distract from urges and to examine the effectiveness of each one. Some examples of control strategies include trying to think of something else, playing with a toy, placing tape on her fingers, and avoiding certain locations or activities. The most notable control strategy is pulling/picking, but the professional may have to bring this up, as patients often do not think of it as such. Make four columns on a sheet of paper. The list of control strategies goes on the left-most column. In the next column place an "X" if the strategy works in the short-term (it usually does). Similarly, in the next column place an "X" if the strategy works in the long-term (it usually does not, as urges return). Finally, ask the patient, "what are the costs of using these strategies?" and list them in the right-most column. Once filled out, use open-ended questions to allow the patient to contemplate the ultimate futility of these control strategies.

Leave the patient with homework to monitor the picking/pulling. Additionally, instruct the patient to add to the list as different attempts to control the urge show. Finally, set a specific goal with the patient to reduce the amount of picking/pulling each day.

Session 5. Before moving forward, the patient should recognize that control strategies are not effective at reducing urges. It might be helpful to review the list of control strategies made in the previous session and added to as homework. Additionally, it might be useful to do a short exercise to illustrate how ineffective control strategies are at regulating internal events. For example, the patient can place a hand on any area where picking occurs and not find an interest in picking. Next, instruct the patient to do everything in her power to not think about pulling/picking for the next 60 s. Point out how even when the patient tries really hard at it, urges or thoughts are very hard to control. Finally, point to an object in the room and instruct her to see if she can go for a full minute without touching the object. Obviously, the patient will be capable of this task. Illustrate the difference between controlling a thought or a feeling and an action (like picking or pulling). Explain that the strategies used to control the outside world (e.g., don't touch the object, don't pull/pick) do not work to control our internal world (e.g., don't have urges, don't think that).

Once the patient sees that control is part of the problem, propose an alternative strategy: willingness. A simple and concrete way to practice willingness is to create the urge to pick or pull and practice sitting there with it. This is easily accomplished by touching the area where one picks or pulls from. The patient should vocalize the thoughts that are occurring. The health professional can direct the patient to focus on the particular stimuli (e.g., thicker hairs or bits of skin hanging off) and allow urge to remove them to occur. The patient should practice allowing those urges to occur and build the skill of allowing those feelings to be present. Reminding the patient that these urges have been there for many years and that they will continue to be there in the future, thus, they should not choose the patients actions. For more detail on these exercises, there is a therapist guide and client workbook (Woods & Twohig, 2008a, 2008b).

Instruct the patient to continue monitoring behaviors each day and to continue to set daily and weekly goals. Additionally, review the importance of employing competing responses and stimulus control procedures. Finally, instruct the patient to practice experiencing the urge every day for at least 10 min.

What Does Not Work

The main roadblock we run into in our work is with children and adolescents who are not interested in receiving treatment for their trichotillomania or excoriation disorder, but the parents are motivated to get help for the issue. Assessing motivation for treatment and willingness to participate is important. Usually, when the child/adolescent has little motivation, no gains occur and the parent gets frustrated with the child/adolescent. If treatment ends up being aversive to the patient, then it is possible that when motivation is high at a later date, the patient may not seek services. Basically, we suggest starting treatment when there is some interest in receiving treatment. Assessing interest from children and adolescents can be difficult, but it is important to ask. We recommend inquiring about treatment interest when away from parents or caregivers when possible to reduce the likelihood of the patient simply complying because they feel that they should.

Similarly, the caregivers of the child may experience frustration from slow behavior change. This is reasonable. The caregiver needs to focus on reinforcing the behaviors they want to see and not punishing what they do not want to see. Specifically, do not punish picking and pulling. Praise the use of competing responses or times when the child/adolescent is seen not picking or puling in situations where it would usually occur.

When to Refer to External Specialty Mental Health

Trichotillomania and excoriation are difficult disorders. Availability of specialized treatment is rare, so medical professionals may be the best option even when experience is low. Guidance based on step-by-step manuals such as material described here (Woods & Twohig, 2008a) is available, and the session length is pretty reasonable (ten sessions). Web-based treatment is also available (www.stoppicking.com; www.stoppulling.com). If help with guided aides or the use of the website does not reduce pulling, it may be time to seek a professional who has experience working with trichotillomania or skin picking. The TLC Foundation for Body-Focused Repetitive Behaviors (www.bfrb.org) maintains a list of treatment providers. Change can be slow, so even if pulling/picking has not ceased, as long as a general reduction is occurring, continuing course is prudent.

The Role of the Primary Care Provider/Medical Team in Treatment

First and foremost, the role of the primary care provider is to ensure the safety of patients through thorough examination and screening. An estimated 5–18% of individuals with trichotillomania ingest their hair after pulling. This puts them at risk of developing masses of hair in the stomach or intestines called trichobezoars. These growths can cause considerable problems including abdominal pain, weight loss, nausea, gastrointestinal bleeding, and even death (Bouwer &

Stein, 1998). All patients who report hair pulling should be asked about hair ingestion and receive education regarding the risks of this behavior. Those who do ingest their hair should be examined for potential trichobezoars. This might include physical examination and x-rays or computed tomography scans of the abdomen for masses. Individuals with excoriation disorder are at risk of infection, tissue damage, and blood loss. We recommend that primary care providers examine all picking sites and refer to appropriate medical professionals as necessary.

In addition to the patient's physical well-being, the medical team should be aware of the shame, stigma, and alienation that those with trichotillomania and excoriation disorder often experience (Singh, Wetterneck, Williams, & Knott, 2016). The team should work to normalize and destigmatize the patient's urges and behavior whenever possible. This is largely done by the manner in which the team communicates with the patient. Efforts should be made to not make patient's feel weird or different because of their behavior. Additionally, patients should be made aware of just how common these disorders are and informed that quality, evidence-based treatments are available.

How to Assess Impact on Care/Quality Improvement Processes

Assessment tools described earlier in this chapter can be similarly used to evaluate impact of interventions by examining changes in scores before and after treatment. Various operationalizations of treatment response have been proposed, including (a) complete abstinence from hair pulling/skin picking, (b) at least a 25% reduction in symptom scores, (c) functioning within normal range based on measure cutoffs, and (d) clinical significance, defined as both functioning within normal range and reliable change, which takes score variability into account when calculating change in score over time (Nelson et al., 2014).

Less formal ways of assessing improvement include visual inspection of areas affected by pulling/picking, as well as behavior tracking measures (e.g., daily frequency of hair pulling). These methods should be used both at the start and end of treatment to allow for appropriate comparisons. In addition, if treatment goals and personal values are established at the start of treatment (e.g., nurturing family relationships), progress may be evaluated based on how closely the individual is living according to those goals and values. For example, an individual who has significantly reduced her hair-pulling behavior, but who still struggles with maintaining close family ties may benefit from further intervention. Ultimately, both the clinician and patient need to collaboratively determine the extent of the latter's progress.

References

American Psychiatric Association. (2013). *Diagnostic and statistical manual of mental disorders: DSM-5™* (5th ed.). Arlington, VA: American Psychiatric Publishing.

Arnold, L. M., Mutasim, D. F., Dwight, M. M., Lamerson, C. L., Morris, E. M., & McElroy, S. L. (1999). An open clinical trial of fluvoxamine treatment of psychogenic excoriation. *Journal of Clinical Psychopharmacology, 19*(1), 15–18.

Bouwer, C., & Stein, D. J. (1998). Trichobezoars in trichotillomania: Case report and literature overview. *Psychosomatic Medicine, 60*(5), 658–660.

Keuthen, N. J., O'Sullivan, R. L., Ricciardi, J. N., & Shera, D. (1995). The Massachusetts General Hospital (MGH) hairpulling scale: I. Development and factor analyses. *Psychotherapy and Psychosomatics, 64*(3–4), 141–145.

Keuthen, N. J., Rothbaum, B. O., Fama, J., Altenburger, E., Falkenstein, M. J., Sprich, S. E., … Welch, S. S. (2012). DBT-enhanced cognitive-behavioral treatment for trichotillomania: A randomized controlled trial. *Journal of Behavioral Addictions, 1*(3), 106–114.

Keuthen, N. J., & Sprich, S. E. (2012). Utilizing DBT skills to augment traditional CBT for trichotillomania: An adult case study. *Cognitive and Behavioral Practice, 19*(2), 372–380.

Keuthen, N. J., Wilhelm, S., Deckersbach, T., Engelhard, I. M., Forker, A. E., Baer, L., & Jenike, M. A. (2001). The skin picking scale: Scale construction and psychometric analyses. *Journal of Psychosomatic Research, 50*(6), 337–341.

Nelson, S. O., Rogers, K., Rusch, N., McDonough, L., Malloy, E. J., Falkenstein, M. J., … Haaga, D. A. (2014). Validating indicators of treatment response: Application to trichotillomania. *Psychological Assessment, 26*(3), 857.

Ninan, P. T., Rothbaum, B. O., Marsteller, F. A., Knight, B. T., & Eccard, M. B. (2000). A placebo-controlled trial of cognitive-behavioral therapy and clomipramine in trichotillomania. *The Journal of Clinical Psychiatry*, *61*(1), 47–50.

Singh, S., Wetterneck, C. T., Williams, M. T., & Knott, L. E. (2016). The role of shame and symptom severity on quality of life in obsessive-compulsive and related disorders. *Journal of Obsessive-Compulsive and Related Disorders*, *11*, 49–55. https://doi.org/10.1016/j.jocrd.2016.08.004

Swedo, S. E., Leonard, H. L., Rapoport, J. L., Lenane, M. C., Goldberger, E. L., & Cheslow, D. L. (1989). A double-blind comparison of clomipramine and desipramine in the treatment of trichotillomania (hair pulling). *New England Journal of Medicine*, *321*(8), 497–501.

Tolin, D. F., Diefenbach, G. J., Flessner, C. A., Franklin, M. E., Keuthen, N. J., Moore, P., … Trichotillomania Learning Center Scientific Advisory Board. (2008). The trichotillomania scale for children: Development and validation. *Child Psychiatry and Human Development*, *39*(3), 331–349. https://doi.org/10.1007/s10578-007-0092-3

Walther, M. R., Flessner, C. A., Conelea, C. A., & Woods, D. W. (2009). The Milwaukee Inventory for the Dimensions of Adult Skin Picking (MIDAS): Initial development and psychometric properties. *Journal of Behavior Therapy and Experimental Psychiatry*, *40*(1), 127–135. https://doi.org/10.1016/j.jbtep.2008.07.002

Woods, D. W., & Twohig, M. P. (2008a). *Trichotillomania an ACT-enhanced behavior therapy approach: Therapist guide*. Oxford; New York: Oxford University Press.

Woods, D. W., & Twohig, M. P. (2008b). *Trichotillomania: An ACT-enhanced behavior therapy approach: Workbook*. New York: Oxford University Press.

Index

A. Maragakis, W. T. O'Donohue (eds.), *Principle-Based Stepped Care and Brief Psychotherapy for Integrated Care Settings*, https://doi.org/10.1007/978-3-319-70539-2

P

Q

R

T

MIX
Papier aus verantwortungsvollen Quellen
Paper from responsible sources
FSC® C105338

If you have any concerns about our products,
you can contact us on
ProductSafety@springernature.com

In case Publisher is established outside the EU,
the EU authorized representative is:
Springer Nature Customer Service Center GmbH
Europaplatz 3, 69115 Heidelberg, Germany

Printed by Libri Plureos GmbH
in Hamburg, Germany